A Practical Guide to Decontamination in Healthcare

A Practical Guide to Decontamination in Healthcare

Gerald McDonnell BSc, PhD
Vice President of Research & Technical Affairs
STERIS Limited
Basingstoke, UK

Denise Sheard RGN, RMW, CHN, OTN, ON,
Diploma Nursing Ed, MSc Nursing
Sterile Services Training Consultant
Cape Town, South Africa

WILEY-BLACKWELL

A John Wiley & Sons, Ltd., Publication

Library of Congress Cataloging-in-Publication Data

McDonnell, Gerald E.
    A practical guide to decontamination in healthcare / Gerald McDonnell, Denise Sheard.
       p.   cm.
    Includes bibliographical references and index.
    ISBN 978-1-4443-3013-7 (hardcover : alk. paper)
1. Infection–Prevention.   2. Hospital buildings–Disinfection.   3. Disinfection and disinfectants.   4. Sterilization.   I. Sheard, Denise.   II. Title.
    QR69.S75M35 2012
    614.4′8–dc23

                                        2012010293

A catalogue record for this book is available from the British Library.

Contents

Foreword

Having spent a lifetime's career in healthcare and in particular developing a great interest in the decontamination of medical devices and other patient associated equipment, I am greatly honoured and privileged to be invited to write this foreword.

This text book is intended for worldwide use as a reliable reference book for those interested in the science, technology and practice of decontaminating devices. As such, the book provides great detail, translated into easy reading and understanding.

In the opening chapter we see the scene set through a look at past notable events relating to decontamination practices. A basic introduction is then given to the associated areas of anatomy and physiology, microbiology, chemistry and the various types of medical/surgical devices the reader is likely to be confronted with in practice. This is followed by a detailed description of each step in the decontamination process, including cleaning, disinfection, inspection, sterilization and storage, with a final consideration being given to the key aspects of safety and management.

Bear in mind that although the principles of decontamination remain the same internationally, their interpretation is necessarily different according to where you are practicing. This is brought about by varying cultures, national economics, and availability of resources, both human and material, and the perception of safe healthcare in differing situations. Within this book, therefore, you will find a variety of solutions to similar problems aimed at giving the most appropriate advice to suit local circumstances.

The book provides a comprehensive approach and guide to all aspects of device decontamination and is essential reading for all involved in the reprocessing of re-usable devices either in healthcare or similar situations.

Gillian A. Sills
Consultant and Director of Education
IDSc (Institute for Decontamination Sciences)
UK
2012

Glossary of terms

For the purpose of discussion, many general terms are used throughout the book. These include words such as "cleaning", "disinfection", "sterilization", "decontamination", etc. These are specifically defined here. They can have very specific meanings and are often misused. These definitions can vary from country to country or depending on their particular use in certain applications. In many cases there is currently no universal acceptance of some definitions, but wherever possible internationally accepted definitions have been used. Further definitions related to specific discussions in the book, for example in the chapters on anatomy, physiology and biochemistry (Chapter 2), microbiology and infection control/prevention (Chapter 5), and chemistry (Chapter 6) are provided in these respective chapters.

Anatomy　The study of the structure of living things.

Anion　Negatively charged atom or molecule, with examples being Cl^- (the chloride ion) and OH^- (the hydroxide ion).

Antibiotics　Drugs that kill or inhibit the growth of bacteria and some fungi by interfering with their normal functions. They are used to prevent ("prophylactic") or treat bacterial and some fungal infections.

Anti-infectives　Drugs that can kill or inhibit the growth of infectious agents. These drugs are usually specific in the way they work; they are therefore classified as antibacterials, antifungals, antivirals and antiprotozoal agents.

Antimicrobial　The ability of a process or product to be effective against microorganisms by either killing them or inhibiting their growth. Antimicrobials include drugs that are particularly used therapeutically within patients to control infections. These are often referred to as anti-infectives or "drugs" and include antibiotics, antifungals and antiviral agents. These are generally specific in their activity, being active against a very limited range of microorganisms. For example, antibiotics only work against some kinds of bacteria (and sometimes some

fungi) and most antiviral agents only target certain classes of viruses. These are not discussed in any detail in this book. The antimicrobial chemicals that are used in disinfection and sterilization applications are often referred to as "biocides" or "microbiocides".

Antisepsis　Destruction or inhibition of microorganisms on the skin, mucous membranes or wounds. An antiseptic is a product used for this purpose. Hand hygiene is an example of antisepsis, including the use of hand washes (soap-based products, water-based applications) and hand rubs (alcohol-based products, waterless applications).

Antiseptic　An antimicrobial product or process used on the skin or other living tissues. In some countries antiseptics are labelled as disinfectants or antiseptic disinfectants. They are often further classified based on their particular use, to include hand washes, hand rubs and hygienic hand disinfectants, pre-operative preparations ("pre-op preps") and surgical scrubs (or "surgical hand disinfectants").

Archaea　A group of unicellular, prokaryotic microorganisms that are distinct from bacteria. In general these microorganisms are not described as being pathogenic to man, plants or animals, but are found to survive in extreme environmental conditions (such as hot springs).

Aseptic　Free of microorganisms. An aseptic process uses means to keep something free of microbial contamination.

Bacteria　Also known as *eubacteria*. A class of microorganisms that are prokaryotic (no defined nucleus) and unicellular (one-celled, in comparison to multicellular organisms). Examples include *Bacillus, Staphylococcus* and *Pseudomonas*.

Bioburden　The "microbial load" or number and type of microorganisms on a surface or object. Note: the bioburden from patient-derived materials such as body fluids (or "soil") may include non-viable (abiotic) substances such as proteins and lipids.

Biochemistry   The study of the chemical processes in living organisms and the structure and function of cells and their components.

Biocide   A general term referring to any chemical or physical antimicrobial agent that inhibits or inactivates life. Chemical biocides include chlorine, iodine, alcohols and hydrogen peroxide. Physical biocides include heat and radiation. "Microbiocides" or "microbicides" are those biocides that are effective against microorganisms. Sub-categories of microbicides include bactericides, bacteriostatic and viricidal or virucidal.

Biofilm   Communities of microorganisms (either single or multiple types) that have developed on or with surfaces.

Carbohydrate   An essential structural component of cells/microorganisms and a source of food/energy. They include sugars (such as sucrose, glucose) and starch. Also known as "saccharides".

Cation   Positively charged atom or molecule, with examples including Na^+ (the sodium ion) and Ag^+ (the silver ion).

Cell   From the Latin "small room", a cell is the basic structural and functional component of living organisms. Humans, for example, are multicellular organisms consisting of many billions of cells and cell types (such as muscle cells and skin cells), while bacteria are single-celled. They can be further sub-classified into two groups based on their basic, microscopic structure: prokaryotic cells (prokaryotes) and eukaryotic cells (eukaryotes). Prokaryotes are considered smaller and simpler in structure, while eukaryotes are larger and more compartmentalized.

Chelating agent   A compound which attaches to a component (e.g. metal ion) and forms a stable complex. It therefore removes metal ions from water or another solution.

Chemical indicators (CI)   Test systems that reveal a change in one or more pre-defined process variables based on a chemical or physical change resulting from exposure to a process (e.g. a color change).

Chemistry   The study of chemicals and chemical reactions.

–cidal   A suffix (the ending of a word) that means the ability to kill a group of microorganisms. As an example, sporicidal designates the ability to kill bacterial spores. Others include bactericidal (kills bacteria), fungicidal (kills fungi) and viricidal (kills viruses). In certain countries these terms are defined by the demonstration of being able to pass certain standardized tests (e.g. a known level of kill in a defined test against certain types of microorganisms). Compare *–cidal*, to *–static*.

Cleaner   A formulation designed for cleaning purposes. Also referred to as a "detergent", because it contains chemicals known as detergents (or surfactants).

Cleaning   The removal of contamination (often referred to as "soil") from a surface to the extent necessary for further processing (e.g. disinfection, sterilization) or for intended use.

Cleaning chemistry   A formulation (or mixture of chemicals) designed for cleaning purposes. Cleaning chemistries are often referred to as "detergents", but detergents are usually only one part of these mixtures that can include biocides, enzymes, buffers, chelating agents and other components.

Conductivity   Measure of the concentration of ions and therefore various metals and molecules in solution.

Contamination   The presence of dirt or "soil" that can include various materials, chemistries and bioburden (such as microorganisms). Depending on the situation, contamination may be visible (e.g. a blood spill) or invisible (e.g. the presence of microorganisms). Contamination of a device (e.g. an endoscope) following patient use is generally referred to as "soil".

Cyst (or oocyst)   In microbiology, a cyst or oocyst is the dormant form of a microorganism, particularly protozoa.

Decontamination   Physical and/or chemical means to render a surface or item safe for handling, use or disposal. In many cases decontamination is at least a two or even three-step process, to include cleaning and disinfection and/or sterilization; however, cleaning alone or a multi-step process of cleaning, disinfection and sterilization may also be required for decontamination, depending on the final use of the surface/item. In this book, the terms "decontamination" and "reprocessing" are used interchangeably.

Detergent   A compound, or a mixture of compounds, intended to assist cleaning. Detergents are a sub-class of surface active agents ("surfactants"). Also commonly referred to as cleaners or cleaning chemistries, but detergents are only one part of these mixtures.

Device   Any instrument, apparatus, appliance, material or other article which is intended to be used for the purpose of diagnosis, prevention, monitoring, treatment or alleviation of disease or other medical/surgical use. A re-usable device is designed to be used many times on different patients, being provided with detailed instructions on how it can be safely reprocessed between each patient. A single-use device (SUD) has been designed by a manufacturer to be used on a single patient only and then discarded. The terms device and instrument are used interchangeably throughout the book.

Diagnosis   A variety of observations and/or tests that can be performed in order to identify ("diagnose") the cause of a particular disease or medical problem, and providing the supporting evidence of such as the cause.

Disinfectant   A physical or chemical product for disinfection.

Disinfection   The antimicrobial reduction of the number of viable microorganisms on a product or surface to a level previously specified as appropriate for its intended further handling or use. Different levels of disinfection are traditionally defined, such as high, medium or low, which refers to the spectrum of microbicidal activity of a given product or process; the exact meaning and usage of these terms may vary from country to country. Other terms, such as pasteurization and antisepsis are forms of disinfection.

Endospores   Types of spores that are produced within a cell, such as bacterial spores.

Endotoxin   Components of certain types of microorganisms (e.g. lipopolysaccharides of Gram negative bacteria) that are released only upon the death and disintegration of their cells. Endotoxins can cause fever (pyrogenic) when injected.

Enzyme   A protein molecule that speeds up a chemical reaction, but is not changed during the process. They are widely used in formulation with chemicals for cleaning applications (e.g. enzymatic cleaners) because of their ability to break down (or "digest") various types of molecules found in soils (such as proteins, lipids and carbohydrates). Enzymes are classified based on mechanism of action, to include *proteases* (enzymes that break down proteins) and *lipases* (enzymes that break down lipids).

Epidemiology   A branch of science dealing with the transmission and control of disease; an "epidemiologist" is a specialist in this area.

Eukaryotic   Defines a type of cell that is much larger than that of bacteria and contains a well-defined nucleus and other organelles; examples of eukaryotic cells include those of fungi, protozoa, plants and humans (see the section on human cells).

Exotoxin   A class of toxins produced and secreted by certain types of microorganisms (e.g. the tetanus toxin from *Clostridium tetani*) while they are fully functional.

Formulation   A combination of ingredients, including active and inert ingredients, into a product for its intended use. Examples include liquid chemical cleaning and disinfection formulations. Although products used for antisepsis, disinfection and cleaning have common names such as "enzymatics", "alkalines", "peracetic acid" and "glutaraldehyde", these only refer to the active ingredients and their individual activities can vary dramatically. The benefit of formulation is to optimize the activity of these ingredients while minimizing any negative effects (such as poor water quality and surface damage).

Fumigation   The delivery of a disinfectant to an area by aerial dispersion, usually in the form of a gas, vapor or aerosol.

Fungi   A group of cell wall-containing eukaryotic microorganisms, that can be further sub-divided into molds (or filamentous fungi, as they can form long filaments or lines of cells) and yeast (unicellular, single-celled forms).

Germ and germicide   A germ is a general term referring to any microorganism, but is often used to refer to bacteria in particular (e.g. in the USA). Therefore, germicidal refers to a product or process which kills microorganisms, but sometimes only refers to bactericidal activity (as in US EPA disinfectant registrations). "Germ" is a colloquial term and its use is discouraged.

Guideline   Document used to communicate recommended procedures, processes or usage of particular practices.

Hardness   Concentration of calcium and magnesium ions in water, expressed as parts per million (ppm) or milligrams per liter (mg/L) of calcium carbonate ($CaCO_3$) equivalents.

Helminths   A large group of multicellular eukaryotic microorganisms that include worms (such as tapeworms and roundworms) and flukes. Examples include *Ascaris* and *Taenia*.

Hydrophilic (polar)   Refers to "water-loving", being a substance that attracts and can absorb water; similar to lipophilic, meaning "loves lipid".

Hydrophobic (non-polar)   A substance that repels and does not absorb water ("water-hating"); similar to lipophobic, meaning "lipid-hating".

Inactivation   Loss of ability of microorganisms to grow and/or multiply.

Infection   The detrimental introduction and colonization of a host (human/animal) by a microorganism.

Infection prevention/control   Discipline concerned with preventing the spread of microorganisms and infection; it is therefore part of the branch of the science known as epidemiology. Often used interchangeably, "prevention" is more correctly used to describe practices to prevent infection, while "control" may also include practices to control the infection after it has taken place (e.g. isolation precautions, antibiotic or other drug-based therapy, etc.).

Prevention strategies including antisepsis, disinfection and vaccination; control strategies may include the use of anti-infectives (drugs) to treat or even prevent infections, investigating outbreaks and managing outbreaks of infection. Experts in this area may be known as infection control practitioners, infection preventionists or epidemiologists.

Inorganic   Non-carbon based molecules. Inorganic chemistry is the study of non-carbon based molecules such as table salt (NaCl) or water (H_2O). The exception to this rule is a group of chemicals like the carbonates (such as calcium carbonate, $CaCO_3$, and sodium carbonate, Na_2CO_3) that are known as "inorganic carbon".

ISO   International Standards Organization.

Label   An identification indication on a product or other article. This can include the manufacturer, their address, product/item identification (e.g. serial or part number), instructions for use, etc. A product label can include what is physically written on the product (the attached label), but also any other accessory information such as additional instructions for use, the material safety data sheets (MSDS) and technical literature.

Lipid   An essential structural component of cells/microorganisms and a source of food/energy. They are generally described as being insoluble in water (hydrophobic) and include fats, oils and cholesterol.

Material safety data sheets (MSDS)   A document provided with a chemical product by the manufacturer/supplier that describes any chemicals that are present, and pertinent safety information including safe handling and emergency procedures.

Matter   Any living or non-living thing that takes up space.

Medicine   The science of and ability to heal. "Medical" refers to the study and practice of medicine.

Microbiology   The study of microorganisms.

Microorganism   Entity of microscopic size, including bacteria, fungi, protozoa and viruses.

Nucleic acid   A class of macromolecules that make up the genetic material of cells and viruses. There are two main classes, DNA and RNA.

Oocyst   See cyst.

Organic   Carbon-based: organic chemistry is the study of carbon-based molecules, which are a diverse group including proteins, lipids and plastics like polyurethane and polypropylene. The exception to this rule is a group of chemicals, like the carbonates (such as calcium carbonate, $CaCO_3$, and sodium carbonate, Na_2CO_3) that are known as "inorganic carbon". Strictly speaking, "organic" refers to chemicals with carbon (C) and hydrogen (H).

Packaging system   Combination of the sterile barrier system and protective packaging.

Parasite   A microorganism that can live in or on a host (animal, plant or other organism), without benefiting or killing the host, but may cause damage/sickness.

Pasteurization   A form of heat-based disinfection used to reduce the number of harmful microorganisms on a surface or in a liquid.

Pathogen   Disease-causing microorganism.

pH   A measure of the activity of hydrogen ions (H^+) in a solution and, therefore, its acidity or alkalinity. The pH value is a number without units, between 0 and 14 that indicates whether a solution is acidic (<7), neutral (~7, generally 6–8) or basic/alkaline (>7).

Physiology   The study of how living structures function.

PPE   Personal protective equipment.

Preservation   The prevention of the multiplication of microorganisms in products.

Pressure   The effect that occurs when a force is applied on a surface or the force applied per unit area. For example, atmospheric pressure is the pressure exerted by the earth's atmosphere and at sea level is known to be ~101.3 kPa (= 14.7 lb in^{-2}, 1 bar, 760 mmHg or 760 Torr).

Prion   Unusual transmissible agents considered to be composed only of protein.

Process   A designed sequence of operations or events, possibly taking up time, space, expertise or other resources, which produces some outcome.

Prokaryote   Defines a type of cell that is considered less organized in structure than eukaryotic cells; bacteria are the most common examples of prokaryotic cells.

Protein   An essential structural component of cells/microorganisms and a source of food/energy. They are made up of nitrogen-containing molecules known as amino acids, and protein examples include enzymes, collagen and keratin.

Protozoa   A diverse group of cell-wall free, unicellular, eukaryotic microorganisms. Examples include *Cryptosporidium* and *Plasmodium*.

Pyrogen   A fever-producing substance. Many microorganisms produce pyrogens (known as toxins), which can be an important cause of disease or other patient complications. Examples include bacterial endotoxins and exotoxins.

Qualification   Process of obtaining and documenting evidence. With decontamination equipment, this can include installation (IQ), operational (OQ) and performance qualification (PQ). Installation qualification refers to evidence that equipment has been provided and installed in accordance with its specification; OQ indicates that the installed equipment operates within predetermined limits when used in accordance with its operational procedures; and PQ refers to evidence that the equipment consistently performs in accordance with predetermined criteria and meets its specification.

Qualitative The quality of something, usually referring to the various types of chemicals present in a sample.

Quality A measure of meeting an expectation or a standard. In device decontamination, this will be to provide a device that is safe for patient use and to meet the requirements of those needing to use the device (medical/surgical staff). Quality control (QC) is a procedure or set of procedures to ensure that a manufactured product or performed service adheres to a defined set of criteria or meets the requirements of a customer. Quality assurance (QA) is similar, being a procedure or set of procedures intended to ensure that a product or service under development (before work is complete, as opposed to afterwards) meets specified requirements. QC and QA are often expressed together as quality assurance and control (QA/QC). A quality management system (QMS) describes the organizational structure, procedures, processes and resources needed to implement quality management in any facility.

Quantitative The amount of something (from "quantity"), for example the various amounts of a chemical type in a given sample.

Regulation A rule or order issued by a country, community or administrative agency, generally under authority granted by statute, that enforces or amplifies laws enacted by the legislature and has the force of law.

Reprocessing See decontamination.

Resistance The ability (natural or acquired) of a microorganism to survive treatment with an anti-infective or biocide.

Resistivity The ability of water (or any liquid) to resist the flow of electricity; a measure of the resistance of water and the inverse of conductivity (being the ability to transmit electricity).

Safety The condition of being protected from danger, harm or injury.

Soil Contamination on a surface following a patient procedure (also see contamination and bioburden).

Spore A stage in the reproductive cycle of certain types of bacteria and fungi where the cell becomes condensed in a thick coat. It is a dormant, reproductive structure of a microorganism that is adapted for dispersal and surviving for extended periods of time in unfavorable conditions. They form part of the life cycles of various types of fungi and bacteria. Bacterial spores are also known as *endospores*. Sporulated organisms can survive much longer in the environment and are also more resistant to inactivation by physical and chemical agents. Many spores are known to be highly resistant to disinfection and even sterilization methods.

Standard A document that specifies the minimum acceptable characteristics of a product or material, issued by an organization that develops such documents. Note: publication of standards can include international and/or local standards. Standard organizations include ISO (International Standards Organization).

–static A suffix (the ending of a word) that refers to the ability to inhibit the growth of a group of microorganisms, but not to kill. Examples include bacteriostatic (inhibits vegetative bacteria), fungistatic (inhibits the growth of fungi) and sporistatic (inhibits the growth of spores, generally bacterial and fungal spores).

Sterilant (or sterilizing agent) is a chemical or physical (e.g. heat) agent that can be used for sterilization, but is only effective for sterilization when provided as part of a defined process.

Sterile Free from viable organisms.

Sterile barrier system A package that provides a barrier to microorganisms and allows aseptic presentation of a product at the point of use.

Sterility assurance level (SAL) The probability of a single viable microorganism occurring on a product after sterilization. This is generally expressed as 10^{-n}. For example, it is common in healthcare applications to use an SAL of 10^{-6}, implying a <1 in a million chance that an item may be contaminated when a starting population of 10^6 of the test organism is present on the test surface.

Sterilization A defined and validated process to render an item free from viable microorganisms, including bacterial spores.

Surfactant Surface active agent: an agent that can emulsify oils and hold dirt in suspension. They are widely used in cleaning chemistries. Detergents are a sub-class of surfactants.

Surgery A specialty in medicine that investigates or treats disease or injury by an operative procedure. Surgical procedures (or "operations", "surgery") involves entering the body or body cavities by incision (breaking through the skin or other area of the body).

Total dissolved solids (TDS) Sum of all ions in a solution, often approximated by means of electrical conductivity or resistivity measurements.

Total organic carbon (TOC) Measure of organic (or carbon-based) substances that are present in a solution or on a surface. Strictly speaking, this excludes "inorganic carbon" such as carbonates. In water analysis it is usually residual carbon material from natural microbial, plant and animal decomposition.

Toxin   A poisonous ("toxic") substance produced by microorganisms and other life forms. Toxins produced by many types of pathogens are the primary cause of the signs and symptoms of infection, such as an increase in temperature and tissue damage. They can be further described in many ways, such as how they are produced by a microorganism (endotoxins or exotoxins) and by what type of microorganism they are produced by (e.g. mycotoxins are produced by certain types of fungi). Many toxins, such as endotoxins, are also "pyrogens", referring to their ability to cause a dramatic rise in body temperature.

Validation   Documented procedure for obtaining, recording and interpreting the results required to establish that a process will consistently yield a product complying with predetermined specifications.

Vegetative   In microbiology, refers to an actively growing and multiplying form of a microorganism. The opposite of a vegetative microorganism would be a dormant form (e.g. bacterial and fungal spores or protozoan cysts).

Viable   Indicates that something is alive and capable of reproducing.

Virus   A class of microorganisms that cannot replicate without a living, susceptible host cell (human, plant or bacterial). They are, therefore, called "obligate parasites". They have no cell structure typical of other microorganisms (see eukaryote and prokaryote).

Washer-disinfector   A machine that cleans and disinfects medical devices and other articles used in the context of medical, dental, pharmaceutical and veterinary practice.

Acknowledgements

The authors would sincerely like to thank all those who critically reviewed various sections and chapters of the book. Their feedback was invaluable. They include:

Georgia Alevizopoulou, Greece
Richard Bancroft, UK
Peter Burke, USA
Jackie Daly, USA
Anthony Fiorello, USA
John Harrison, UK
Xana Jardine, South Africa
Marietta Jungblut, Netherlands
Herbert Kaiser, USA
Terry McAuley, Australia
Susan Meredith, UK

Val O'Brien, UK
Birte Oskarsson, Sweden
Yaffa Raz, Israel
Wim Renders, Belgium
Syed Sattar, Canada
Richard Schule, USA
Gillian Sills, UK
Wayne Spencer, UK
Susan Springthorpe, Canada
Bengt Ternström, Sweden
Rene Viss, Netherlands

1 Introduction

What is decontamination?

First "to do no harm"
Of the Epidemics, Hippocrates (~400 BC)

Health is an important subject to all. It affects us as individuals, our families and the communities in which we live. Our health is improved by promoting well-being and preventing disease or other negative health impacts. A disease may be defined as any effect that impairs/harms the body's normal function and therefore has an impact on our health (mild, moderate or even severe). Diseases can be infectious or non-infectious (such as cancer, effects of drug abuse, stress, chemicals, etc.). Infectious diseases are a leading cause of sickness and death worldwide. They are caused by living creatures that cannot be seen by the naked eye, known as "microorganisms", such as viruses and bacteria. It is estimated that infectious diseases affected our breathing, digestive and immune systems are responsible for ~17% of human death worldwide (the next highest cause of death is coronary heart disease at ~12%). These rates are estimated across the whole world, but are even higher in lower income regions. Examples of health efforts to reduce these risks in the general public include improving drinking water quality (chemical and microbiological), immunization (vaccination), and safe handling/disposal of waste. Many of these efforts influence our daily lives, but the risk of infectious disease significantly increases when we are sick or when our bodies are otherwise compromised (e.g. when undergoing a surgical procedure). For these reasons, healthcare institutions (such as hospitals and clinics) have many procedures and practices in place to control the spread of infectious disease within these facilities, and to protect patients, staff and the general public. It is an important philosophy in medical practice: First "to do no harm" or in Latin "*primum non nocere*". These are collectively referred to as "safe" or "infection control/prevention" practices that prevent the spread of disease or other negative effects from one patient to another (or to/from staff or visitors within these facilities). These practices include:

- Immunization
- Isolation of patients with specific diseases
- Decontamination of equipment and various surfaces

As "contamination" refers to something being "dirty" or "soiled", "decontamination" is the means to render it safe for handling, use or disposal. Dirt or soil may include things like dust, patient materials (such as blood, feces, various tissues from surgical procedures, etc.) and associated microorganisms that can cause disease. In this book, the terms "decontamination" and "reprocessing" are used interchangeably. In healthcare facilities a variety of physical and/or chemical products or processes are used for decontamination. These include:

- Cleaning, the removal of soil to make something "clean"
- Disinfection, the antimicrobial reduction of microorganisms; other widely used terms that refer to disinfection can include antisepsis, pasteurization, sanitization and fumigation
- Sterilization, the complete eradication of all microorganisms

These are all methods of decontamination and are explained further in this book. Examples of specific decontamination practices will include:

- Hand and skin hygiene, including routine hand disinfection and preparation of the skin for a surgical procedure
- Taking surgical or medical instruments that have been used on one patient and decontaminating them in preparation for use on another

A Practical Guide to Decontamination in Healthcare, First Edition. Gerald McDonnell and Denise Sheard.
© 2012 Gerald McDonnell and Denise Sheard. Published 2012 by Blackwell Publishing Ltd.

• Cleaning and disinfection of linens or other materials (including patient bed sheets, sterile towels and cottons fabrics)
• Disinfection of water for drinking or sterilization of water for injection use
• Cleaning and disinfecting environmental surfaces such as floors and beds
• Sterilization of contaminated waste materials for safe disposal (including incineration)

In some cases decontamination is a one-step process, for example sterilization of contaminated waste materials, but is most often a two-step process to include cleaning (the physical removal of soil) and disinfection or sterilization (as the antimicrobial process to inactivate the various types of microorganisms that we cannot see). For re-usable medical and surgical instruments this will normally include at least cleaning and disinfection, but will often include sterilization, this being the highest level of safety. Decontamination is therefore an integral part of infection prevention and should not be underestimated.

A brief history of decontamination

It is clear from many ancient documents that decontamination practices have been considered to have health benefits. Examples include:
• In approximately 1400–1200 BC (estimated to be at the time of Moses), a sanitary code was outlined in the Leviticus, Numbers and Deuteronomy chapters of the Bible. It was noted even at this time that when dealing with disease that hands should be washed under running water and that there was a value in boiling water to make it safe for drinking or other purposes.
• The Eber's Papyrus, a medical document from about 1500 BC, describes a method of combining animal and vegetable oils with alkaline salts to form a soap-like material used for treating skin diseases, as well as for washing hands.
• The world's oldest known medical text outlines the procedures for wound management practiced by the Sumerians (~2000 BC). The wound was cleansed with beer (which contained alcohol) and then bandaged with a cloth soaked in wine and turpentine. The practice of using alcoholic beverages and turpentine would remain the treatment of choice until the modern era.
• Similar examples of wound, water or air treatments have been described by the ancient Greek and Roman cultures. Aristotle (384–322 BC), a Greek philosopher, even described boiling to treat water. Homer (~850 BC),

in his epic poem the *Odyssey*, described the use of sulfur as an area disinfectant.
• Ancient methods of preserving foods from rotting during storage (which we now know is caused by microorganisms) included drying, heating and use of sugar or vinegar.

From these ancient times to the 19th century, infection was a major cause of mortality and morbidity in humans. It would take many thousands of years for the microbiological origin and transmissibility of infection to be discovered. A recurring theme in history was the belief that epidemic diseases were spread by something in the air. Hippocrates (460–370 BC) was an ancient Greek doctor and is often referred to as the father of medicine, being still referred to today by new doctors taking the Hippocratic oath. He put this belief into practice when attempting to drive the plague (now know to be a bacterial disease) from Athens by lighting fires of aromatic wood in the streets. This belief that diseases were spread by something in the air continued throughout history.

Many ancient physicians well understood that when the skin was broken in any way (by a wound or during attempts at surgery) the risks of "bad" things happening was significantly increased. It was unknown at the time that wound infections were caused by various types of microorganisms, particularly bacteria, with dramatic consequences, including destruction of limbs and death. Infections in such cases of skin damage were the major contributor to death and suffering, which is why surgical procedures were attempted only as a last resort. Through the ages operations were performed with little regard for a "clean" environment. Surgeons' hands, rarely washed, were placed directly into the patient's wounds. Frequently, onlookers were encouraged to "take a feel" for educational purposes. Surgical instruments used in such procedures were crudely wiped, placed back into their velvet carriers, and re-used, some having been sharpened on the sole of the surgeon's boot. The floors of the surgical wards were covered with whatever came from the patient, which could include feces, urine, blood and pus, and hygiene practices in other areas of such facilities (if indeed dedicated facilities where used) at the time were also unknown. Not surprisingly, surgical site infection was the major contributor to morbidity and mortality rates, occurring after practically all operations and taking the lives of almost half of all surgical patients.

Hippocrates was one of the first recorded to hold an opinion on the cause of such problems, stating that the formation of pus (suppuration) was not a natural part of the healing process and should be avoided. His recommendations for managing wounds were: cleansing with wine, applying a bandage, and then pouring wine on the bandage. Another Greek physician Claudius Galen (~AD 130–200) recommended soap for both medicinal and cleansing purposes. He, however, disagreed with Hippocrates, that the formation of pus was not a normal occurrence; he believed that pus was essential for wound healing. It is often considered that this was originally an Arabic idea. Suppuration was actively encouraged by surgeons in traumatic and painful procedures. This disagreement would continue to be debated for centuries.

One thousand years later, the Italian Theodoric Borgognoni (1205–1298) challenged Galen's view of suppuration. He dedicated his career to finding the ideal conditions for wound healing and became one of the most famous surgeons during the Middle Ages. He argued that a wound should be maintained clean and closed (sutured) to control infection (and preserve life). Because his views were contrary to the established teachings, he was denounced by his colleagues and even by the church. Indeed, the surgeon would often welcome the signs of suppuration, depending on how it looked. Wounds were classified into two categories: those with suppuration and those without. Wounds with "laudable pus" (a creamy yellow ooze) tended to run a chronic course, taking months to heal, but the patients were generally free of other negative signs and did not die! Wounds with a thin, watery discharge were associated with a fatal outcome, with the patient dying of sepsis within days. It is not, therefore, surprising that even the most conscientious surgeons preferred and even encouraged the formation of pus. Galen's doctrine of suppuration would remain the rule for wound management until the late 19th century.

In addition to wound infection, general standards of public hygiene and their impacts on public health were not widely appreciated. As an example in Europe, following the eventual fall of Rome in AD 467 many simple hygiene practices were neglected. Examples included a decline in bathing habits, lack of personal cleanliness and unsanitary living conditions (lack of waste disposal, etc.). It is well appreciated that such conditions contributed heavily to the great plagues of the Middle Ages, and especially to the Black Death of the 14th century. At the same time, it was understood that contact with sick individuals could rapidly spread a disease, as highlighted by the fear associated with bacterial diseases such as leprosy and bubonic plague; in fact, infected bodies have been used over the ages as effective weapons in battles and sieges! Equally, infected bodies and materials were often dealt with by burning (incineration).

Hieronymus Fracastorius (1478–1553) suggested that the cause of infectious disease was from invisible living "seeds" (*seminaria contagionum*). He even at this period described three modes of disease spread: direct contact with infected persons, indirect contact with fomites and airborne transmission. Ambroïse Paré (1510–1590), considered one of the fathers of modern surgery, believed that infection was introduced from the environment. In 1625 Francis Bacon described some methods to prevent or control wound infections, such as by the use of salt or excluding air. In the 1670s Anton van Leeuwenhoek was the first microbiologist to observe individual, live microorganisms, by using a simple microscope. He called these animalcules or "little animals". He also described the first direct evidence of disinfection in observing the death of animalcules treated with pepper (in water) or vinegar. Similar disinfection studies were described shortly after by Edmund King and John Pringle. It could be argued that this was the start of the modern era of understanding infectious diseases and their control, but even then the "microbial theory" remained debated for the next few centuries.

In the meantime, the benefits of disinfection practices continued to be better understood. Ancient disinfection methods had been previously recognized, such as the benefits of storing water and other liquids in copper or silver vessels (as a preservative method from the release of copper or silver into the water), burning with fire (as a method of incineration) and boiling water. In the modern era further advances where made such as:

• In 1680 Dennis Papin developed the first recognizable steam generating machine.

• In 1774 Scheele discovered chlorine and its antimicrobial effects.

• In the 1830s William Henry published studies on the "disinfection power of increased temperatures".

• In the mid-1800s copper sulphate, zinc chloride and sodium permanganate, acids, alkalis, sulfurs and alcohols were recognized as disinfectants.

In the late 1840s, Dr Ignaz Semmelweis, whilst working in the maternity wards of a Vienna hospital, observed that the mortality rate in a delivery room staffed by medical students was up to three times higher than in a second delivery room staffed by midwives. Expectant mothers were terrified of the room staffed by the medical students! Semmelweis observed that the students were coming straight from their lessons in the autopsy room to the delivery room. He believed that they were carrying infectious agents from the lab to their patients. When he implemented a hand washing protocol at the hospital the mortality rate dropped to less than 1%. Today, he is recognized as the father of hand hygiene, one of the most important measures to be taken by healthcare practitioners to reduce cross-contamination. Due to the lack of indoor plumbing at the time, it was difficult to get water to wash hands, making this an unpopular idea. In order to make the water comfortably warm, it would have to be heated over a fire. Besides, contact with water was associated with diseases such as malaria and typhoid fever. Unknown to him, similar results had been described a few years previously by the American scientist Oliver Wendell Holmes. Both suggestions fell on deaf ears. Semmelweis, for his efforts, was committed to an asylum and died of a blood infection.

Despite the earlier work by others such as van Leeuwenhoek, the prevailing theory at the time was known as "spontaneous generation". This is often originally attributed to the Greek philosopher Aristotle (384–322 BC) and simply regards the origins of life as being from inanimate matter or non-living substances. Many famous names in the modern history of infection control, such as Pouchet, Nightingale and Virchow subscribed. Louis Pasteur was born in 1822 in France and in 1857 he proposed the "germ theory of disease", which is regarded as one of the most important discoveries in decontamination history. The theory proposed that most infectious diseases are caused by germs; he also specifically described the existence of bacteria. In the 1860s Pasteur commenced his anti-spontaneous generation experiments and demonstrated that "microorganisms are present in air but not created by air", thereby disproving the concept of spontaneous generation. This was vigorously debated for many years after, with many leading scientists refusing to accept this idea, but the modern era of microbiology had begun. Pasteur proved that protection from air, by sealing or providing a tortuous path, prevented contamination; if growth media was exposed to air it resulted in contamination by microorganisms. With the development of the germ theory by Pasteur and its subsequent application to surgical practices, surgeons were able to operate with a substantially reduced risk of infection. Pasteur was also able to show that bacteria could be killed by various processes. "Pasteurization" is a heat-based process to control microorganisms that still bears his name and he also designed some simple steam cabinet sterilizers (with Charles Chamberland in 1880).

During the 1700–1800s, various scientists described the phenomenon that by injecting healthy people with fluids (such as blood) from patients suffering from certain diseases, particularly with milder or similar types of disease, they could be protected from disease. This became known as vaccination and was previously described by the Chinese, Indians and Turks. Worthly-Montague and Jenner used such methods to prevent smallpox, a prevalent infectious disease at the time and now eradicated. Pasteur also developed vaccination methods (e.g. against rabies). Vaccination is now an important part of public health, including the prevention of common diseases such as measles, mumps and seasonal flu. Polio has all but been eradicated due to immunization.

Pasteur's work accelerated other investigations in microbiology and infection control/prevention. As an example, Agostino Bassi (1773–1856) described the use of a variety of disinfectants in the control of different diseases such as cholera; these included alcohol, acids and chlorine. Joseph Lister (1827–1912), a professor of surgery in Glasgow, Scotland, quickly noticed the connection between Pasteur's work and the suppuration of wounds. He concluded that microbes in the air were most likely causing the infection and had to be destroyed before they entered the wound. Lister began to clean wounds and dress them using a solution of carbolic acid (phenol). Little did he know that at the same time other European surgeons were already practicing similar methods with other chemicals. In 1867 he published a paper on antisepsis, stating that "all the local inflammatory mischief and general febrile disturbance which follow severe injuries are due to the irritating and poisoning influence of decomposing blood or sloughs". Lister began applying phenol to compound fracture wounds; wounds healed without infection. The application of germ theory to wound healing changed the practice of surgery. Lister also campaigned for heat or chemical sterilization (and for surgeons to use something other than sawdust swept up from the floors of the mills for surgical dressings!).

During the Franco-Prussian war (1870–1871) antiseptic practices were shown to have an impact on saving soldiers' lives. German surgeons were beginning to practice antiseptic surgery, using sterilized instruments and materials. In 1876, Lister presented his ideas at the International Medical Congress in Philadelphia. William W. Keen (1837–1932) attended the presentation and became one of the first American surgeons to implement Lister's ideas. During the American Civil War, Keen was one of the first physicians in the world to adopt aseptic surgical technique. During the American Civil War, 90% of the deaths on both sides were due to infectious disease rather than direct death from military trauma. While bayoneting killed less outright, minor scratches from other injuries often festered into mortal wounds. Keen recommended and practiced the following surgical set-up in hospitals at the time:

• All carpets and unnecessary furniture were removed from the patient's room.

• Walls and ceilings were carefully cleaned the day before the operation, and the woodwork, floors, and remaining furniture were scrubbed with carbolic solution. This solution was also sprayed in the room on the morning preceding but not during the operation.

• The day before the operation, the patient was shaved, scrubbed with soap and water, and ether, and covered with wet corrosive sublimate dressing until operated on, and then ether and mercuric chloride washings were repeated.

• The surgical instruments were boiled in water for two hours, and sponges for use during the procedures were treated with carbolic acid before use.

• The surgeon's hands were cleaned and disinfected with soap, water and alcohol.

It is interesting to note that many of these practices are still in use today (such as washing or the use of alcohol on the hands), while others are not (such as the use of mercury). As the knowledge on the use of various chemicals improved, it was realized that while many of these practices could kill or prevent the growth of microorganisms, many could also do harm to human health (or were "toxic" either in the short or long term).

As scientific knowledge expanded during the late 19th century so did the advancement of infection prevention. Another important milestone was when Robert Koch (1843–1910), a German physician, was able to demonstrate the cause-and-effect relationship between a specific bacterium (*Bacillus anthracis*) and the disease anthrax. He used a sequence of experimental steps to directly relate a specific microbe to a specific disease; these steps of disease association, isolation, inoculation, and re-isolation became known as Koch's Postulates. These still form the basis of defining an infectious agent today. In 1882 Koch also discovered the causative agent of tuberculosis, the bacteria *Mycobacterium tuberculosis*. Tuberculosis was the cause of one in seven deaths in the mid-19th century; interestingly, in the 21st century tuberculosis is once again a major problem due to the development of drug (antibiotic) resistant forms of the bacterium. Koch also published a book (*On Disinfection*) that described various types of disinfectants and the differences in their abilities to kill various types of microorganisms (with *Mycobacterium tuberculosis* and

Bacillus anthracis being particularly difficult to inactivate, the latter due to its ability to form heat/chemical resistant spores). Other advances before the end of the 19th century included:

• In 1883, Gustav Neuber introduced the use of sterile gowns and caps during surgery.

• In 1890, William Stewart Halsted introduced surgical gloves after he commissioned the Goodyear rubber company to fashion gloves for his nurse to protect her hands from the mercuric chloride solutions used to disinfect the instruments. Rubber gloves were routinely used after 1890.

• In 1891 Ernst von Bergmann introduced routine heat sterilization of instruments, which proved superior to chemical methods used at the time.

• In 1897, Mikulicz introduced the use of surgical masks. During the early part of the 20th century a variety of other chemicals began to be used for infection prevention purposes, including hydrogen peroxide, various types of phenols, dyes and quaternary ammonium compounds. During the 1920s, Sir Alexander Fleming (1881–1955), working in London, made the accidental discovery of penicillin, one of the first and most widely used antibiotics. Antibiotics are drugs used to treat or prevent bacterial infections. It was not until the Second World War (in the 1940s) that penicillin was widely introduced, as an extract from the fungus (another type of microorganism) known as *Penicillium*. This led to a revolution in the development and manufacturing of various types of antibiotics (such as tetracycline and methicillin). It seemed that bacterial infections might be something of the past, but quickly it was shown that bacteria could develop resistance to antibiotics and in the present day there are less antibiotics available to treat a greater variety of antibiotic-resistant bacteria (such as methicillin-resistant *Staphylococcus aureus*, MRSA and multi-drug resistant *Mycobacterium tuberculosis*, MDR-TB). Despite this, antibiotics became and still remain widely used for treating bacterial infections and also in preventing them (known as prophylaxis, such as when given prior to surgery). With increasing rates of antibiotic-resistant bacteria today, there is a re-focus on efforts to prevent infection by isolating and eliminating any variable that could pose a risk, including decontamination.

Up until the 1940s, medical/surgical supplies were mainly decontaminated (or "reprocessed") and maintained in the surgery or patient care area in which they were to be used. Under this system, there was duplication of both time and equipment at various locations within larger healthcare facilities, and it was difficult to maintain consistently high standards. As the number and variety of surgical procedures grew and the types of medical/surgical devices, equipment and supplies increased, it became apparent that centralized reprocessing areas were needed for efficiency, economy and patient safety. The work of scientists such as W.B. Underwood and J.J. Perkins was instrumental in encouraging healthcare facilities to establish separate and distinct areas/departments with specialized expertise and direct responsibility for providing clean and sterile medical/surgical supplies and equipment to patient care areas. These areas are often referred to by a variety of names, such as decontamination service (DS), central sterile services department (CSSD), sterile services department (SSD), sterile processing centre (SPD) and theatre sterile services unit (TSSU) to mention but a few. It was also in the 1940s that various organizations (such as the British Medical Research Council) advocated that in order to reduce surgical sepsis and other associated infections in healthcare facilities, "fulltime special officers" should be appointed to supervise the control of infection. These officers became experts in infection control and prevention practices within facilities, such as infection control nurses (ICN) and doctors. Further recommendations included the establishment of an infection control committee with multidisciplinary representatives, including doctors, nurses and administrators. It is now normal practice worldwide to employ ICNs and to have established infection control committees with a mandate to monitor and prevent hospital or healthcare-acquired infections (HAIs).

Advances in various sterilization methods including those based on steam, dry heat and even low temperature chemical methods, such as those based on ethylene oxide, became standard practices in the preparation of surgical devices. Focus was also placed on the variety of devices and instruments that where being developed and used on patients, both medically and surgically. Examples included flexible endoscopes that allowed internal structures of the body to be examined by entering through natural openings (such as through the mouth). During the 1950s a classification system was proposed by Dr E. Spaulding that suggested devices could be considered as critical (entering the "sterile" areas of the body, including blood contact), semi-critical (contacting non-intact skin or mucous membranes) and non-critical (intact skin contact). While sterilization was recommended for critical devices, various levels of disinfection (ranging from low to high level) could be safely used for the other device classification. New types of high-level disinfectants (sometimes even referred to as "sterilants"), such as those based on glutaraldehyde, became widely

used as effective and more rapid alternatives to heat and chemical sterilization methods. Medical/surgical devices continue to show new innovations, including replacement parts of the body (e.g. hips and knees), as well as allowing for robotic surgery. In parallel, newer and even safer disinfectants and sterilization processes have been developed to meet the decontamination demands for traditional and advanced instrumentation.

Our knowledge of the various different types of microorganisms that cause infections has continued to develop. Examples include the ever increasing types of bacteria, fungi and protozoa that are implicated as causing various diseases. At the end of the 19th century, a further group of infectious agents were first described that appeared to be much more basic in nature than previously considered: viruses. It was not until the 1930s, with the invention of powerful electron microscopes that their nature was truly understood. Viruses are now well known as the causative agents in many diseases such as measles (the measles virus), AIDs (HIV), flu (influenza), hepatitis (e.g. Hep A and B) and some forms of cancer (e.g. papillomavirus). During the 1970–1980s further groups known as "prions", were identified as causative agents in diseases such as "mad cow disease" in animals and humans. Indeed, the range of microorganisms that are implicated in disease continues to grow.

In the modern era, with increasing microbial resistance to drugs (not only in bacteria but in other microorganisms) and greater risks of infections (e.g. more invasive surgical procedures, etc.) there is a much greater emphasis than ever before on the prevention of infection. Decontamination practices play a central role in infection prevention strategies and ensuring patient safety.

Goals of decontamination and the Spaulding classification

Decontamination practices are designed to render devices, instruments and materials "safe" for handling, use and/or disposal. It has already been highlighted that the primary goal is to reduce or even completely remove microbial contamination, but in fact it is more than that. Overall, it is to ensure safety: safety for the patient, staff, the devices and even the environment. The goals of decontamination are:

• To reduce or completely remove microbial contamination to a level that is safe for use by medical staff and with/in a patient.

• To ensure that no toxic substances remain on the surface that could cause other negative patient reactions. This can include patient soil (even in some cases at low concentrations), water or decontamination chemistry (e.g. cleaning and disinfection chemicals) residues and even parts of microorganisms that have been killed.

• To ensure that the decontamination process does not damage the device and that the process is therefore "compatible" with the device. Negative effects can include visual and undetected damage that may lead to device failure or breakage during use. Even cosmetic changes in the device can sometimes impact its use (e.g. loss of color-coding marks).

• A growing concern is the impact of decontamination on the environment. On the positive side, decontamination reduces the risks of general public exposure to contamination. But equally it requires the use of energy (e.g. generation of steam or use of an automated washing-disinfection process), water and many different types of chemicals. The negative effects of these chemicals need to be minimized, particularly in the use and disposal of chemicals that have a minimum impact on the environment. There are other issues that may need to be considered, such as costs, but these are secondary to the primary aim of patient and staff safety.

Given the range of potential decontamination issues in healthcare facilities, various methods may be considered acceptable to ensure safety. First, inanimate objects are treated separately to animate (or living). Consider, for example, the various types of physical and chemical antimicrobial methods that can be used on medical and surgical devices; these will include various heat and/or chemical methods, but many of these could not be safely used on the skin. Disinfection of skin ("antisepsis") can include the washing of hands and the preparation of the skin for an injection or surgical incision. Only a limited number of antimicrobial methods may be used, due to the sensitive nature of the skin. Therefore, the decontamination of the skin (and mucous membranes) is considered separate to various "hard" surfaces such as tables, benches and surgical devices. Second, different classification systems can be used that define the level of decontamination that is applicable depending on the use of the surface, device or instrument. The most widely used classification for medical/surgical devices is known as the Spaulding classification (as introduced briefly in the previous section). During the 1950s, Dr Earl Spaulding defined the minimum levels of disinfection/sterilization to be employed according to the infection risk associated with a device/surface when used with a patient. It was assumed that the first step was to ensure that the surface was visually clean; this was to ensure the effectiveness of any antimicrobial process/product in reducing the level of soil or dirt that could interfere with their activity. The required use of the device then dictates the recommended antimicrobial process:

• Non-critical devices or surfaces are considered to have the lowest risk to patients, being any surface that only contacts intact skin. Examples could include table tops, bedrails and chairs, as well as some medical devices such as stethoscopes and blood-pressure monitoring cuffs. For such non-critical devices, cleaning alone may be sufficient (to physically remove microorganisms and visual signs of soiling). In other cases, disinfection (to a low level) may be recommended, encompassing certain types of viruses (especially enveloped viruses such as influenza and HIV), most bacteria and some fungi. Cleaning and disinfection may sometimes be achieved in a one-step process, but is most often achieved using a two-step process of cleaning followed by disinfection. Remember, disinfection only reduces the level of microorganisms present and is not expected to completely remove all microorganisms.

• Semi-critical devices pose a higher risk as they may come into contact with mucous membranes or non-intact (broken) skin. These devices may include a variety of endoscopes, probes or even re-usable thermometers. In these cases disinfection is recommended as a minimum, but to a higher level to ensure the inactivation of a wider range of microorganisms. This would include certain types of microorganisms that are considered much more difficult to inactivate. To ensure efficacy, cleaning is a necessary first step, followed by disinfection.

• Critical devices pose the highest risk as they enter or have contact with a normally "sterile" (or microorganism-free) area of the body, such as the blood or tissue. Sterilization is recommended for these devices. Sterilization is a process used to render a surface or product free from viable microorganisms, including bacterial spores. Sterilization therefore includes disinfection, but provides a great level of safety.

Note that in this system a device can change its classification depending on how it is used with a patient. For example, the same device may be critical when used for a surgical procedure or semi-critical if used for a non-invasive diagnostic purposes. Although other classification systems may be used (e.g. class 1, 2a, 2b and 3), the Spaulding classification is a practical and widely used system worldwide. Examples of other systems include the classification of antiseptics as being used with water (e.g.

soap-based hand washes) or without water ("waterless", such as alcohol hand rubs) or for use for routine hand hygiene, higher risk applications (such as in preparation for surgery by surgeons, using surgical scrubs or on patients using a pre-operative skin preparation antiseptic) and even therapeutic applications (such as treatment of skin acne or fungal infections).

These exact requirements ensure the safety and effectiveness of cleaning, disinfection (including antisepsis) and sterilization products/processes, which vary from country to country and region to region. Various different guidelines, standards and regulations can be consulted or are even required to be followed to ensure such products/processes are effective. These will include compliance to international standards (section 1.6), standardized test methods (for antimicrobial efficacy and toxicity), routine or periodic tests and compliance to local registration requirements. As these can vary considerably, particular care should be taken by those purchasing or using decontamination products to ensure that they do provide the required level of safety.

The decontamination process

A summary of the decontamination process for patient-used devices, instruments and materials is given in Figure 1.1.

Healthcare devices can be classified in a variety of ways, such as purpose of use, materials of construction and the risk of contamination/infection transmission to a patient (as defined by the Spaulding classification, in the previous section). A further classification is if the device is for single use (on a single patient) or re-use (with many patient). A single-use device can be simply defined as a device that has been designed and provided by a manufacturer to be used on a single patient. These are usually discarded following use on that patient, although in some cases this may be used once or a limited number of times but with the same patient. A re-usable device has been designed to be used on a patient, decontaminated and then used again.

This can be repeated many times with the use of the device until it is no longer needed, damaged, unsafe to use or otherwise replaced. The emphasis is therefore placed on ensuring that the device is safely handled and decontaminated between patients. The decontamination cycle describes this process as used in healthcare facilities today. Devices enter the cycle as either new devices

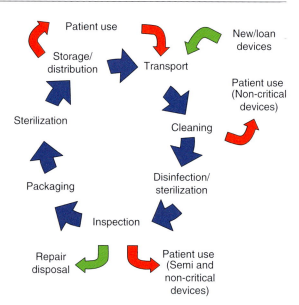

Figure 1.1 The decontamination cycle.

provided by a manufacturer (that need to be prepared for use for the first time) or following clinical use. The various steps in the process are briefly discussed here and in more detail in the subsequent chapters of this book. They include:

• Post-procedure handling and transport (Chapter 7). Medical or surgical procedures using devices and materials can be performed in various locations within a healthcare facility. Post-procedure it is important that these are handled correctly to ensure that they are not damaged or lost and do not pose any safety risks to staff, visitors and subsequent patients. They should be sorted (e.g. disposable from non-disposable items) and then safely contained and transported to an area designated for decontamination. This can be within the same room, a separate room/area or even at another facility.

• Cleaning (Chapter 8) is the removal of contamination (or "soil") from an item to the extent necessary for its further processing and its intended subsequent use. This may include the removal of various materials such as patient materials (blood, tissues, etc.), microorganisms and even different chemicals used during a procedure (e.g. cements, gels, etc.). Cleaning may be the only decontamination step required (e.g. for some non-critical devices/surfaces), but is always a required step before any further decontamination steps in the cycle (such as disinfection and/or sterilization).

• Disinfection (Chapter 9) is the antimicrobial reduction of microorganisms from a surface to a level determined to be appropriate for its intended further handling or use. Various different levels of disinfection may be required, depending on the risk associated with the device/surface. In some cases, sterilization may be directly applied at this stage as an alternative to disinfection and for immediate use with/or a patient. Again, many devices may leave the decontamination cycle at this stage, for patient use (following some inspection to ensure they are safe for use). Disinfection may also be conducted at this stage to allow for staff to safely handle devices in preparation for sterilization.

- Inspection and packaging (Chapter 10). Prior to direct patient use or further decontamination, instruments or materials are checked for cleanliness and functionality. Devices may be identified at this point for repair or even disposal (although this may occur at any stage during the decontamination cycle). They may then be safely transported to a site of patient use or for further assembly/packaging in preparation for sterilization. Packaging is designed to protect a single device or set of assembled devices during sterilization, storage and transport, for future use with or on a patient. Surgical devices are generally assembled into dedicated trays designed for specific types of surgical procedures (Chapter 3).
- Sterilization (Chapter 11) is a process used to render a surface or product free from viable organisms, including bacterial spores. Following sterilization, devices may be transported for direct patient use or stored until required for a specific procedure.
- Storage and distribution (Chapter 12). The correct storage (if applicable) and distribution of re-usable devices is an essential step to complete the decontamination cycle.

Other considerations in this cycle will include the acquisition of devices and raw materials, and the handling of wastes. In addition to these specific decontamination steps and sections, further consideration is given in this book to various background subjects that are important, such as:

- Human anatomy and physiology (Chapter 2)
- Various different types of medical and surgical procedures (Chapter 3)
- The variety of medical and surgical devices used (Chapter 4)
- Principles of microbiology and infection prevention/ control (Chapter 5)
- Basic understanding of chemistry and physics (Chapter 6)
- Safety considerations (Chapter 13)
- Management principles (Chapter 14)

The design of a decontamination area

Decontamination (or reprocessing) areas may be at or adjacent to the procedure area (e.g. a theatre sterile services unit, TSSU, or decontamination room/area), at a remote location within the hospital (e.g. a central sterile services department, CSSD, or decontamination service departments) or even at a completely different facility (e.g. a "super-center" or contract sterilization facility). Despite the location, the primary purpose of the area, department or facility is to ensure the safe reprocessing of devices. It should be dedicated and appropriate for that purpose. The area should be designed to:

- Allow for the safe reprocessing of devices and/or materials, should they require cleaning alone; cleaning and disinfection; or cleaning, disinfection and sterilization, as examples. Safety considerations should include patient as well as staff and visitor risks.
- Ensure it can meet the workload demands to maintain a supply of re-usable devices. This will include budget, available space, equipment and staffing requirements.
- Reduce the risk of accidental mixing of "dirty", "clean" or disinfected/sterilized devices or cross-contamination. This can be achieved by workflow design.

An important factor in running an effective decontamination service is good area design and workflow. Workflow must always be from dirty to clean to disinfected/sterile. Such workflow systems are designed to prevent the accidental mixing of dirty and decontaminated devices/ materials. They may be part of a room, a dedicated room or a whole, purposely build decontamination department. Examples of area layouts that highlight such workflows are shown in Figure 1.2.

To maintain good workflow implies proper functioning and coordination between the various distinct decontamination areas. These include:

- "Dirty" area: here devices/materials are received, disassembled and washed. For washing the area will include at least a manual cleaning area, but consideration should also be given to include automated washer or washer-disinfectors. For manual cleaning, a double (two) sink arrangement is optimal, one for cleaning and one for rinsing. Automated washers or washer-disinfectors are often preferred and can be provided as single or double-door designs (the latter to allow for physical separation of the dirty and clean areas of the decontamination area).
- "Clean" area: cleaned, and often disinfected, devices/ materials are inspected and reassembled for use and

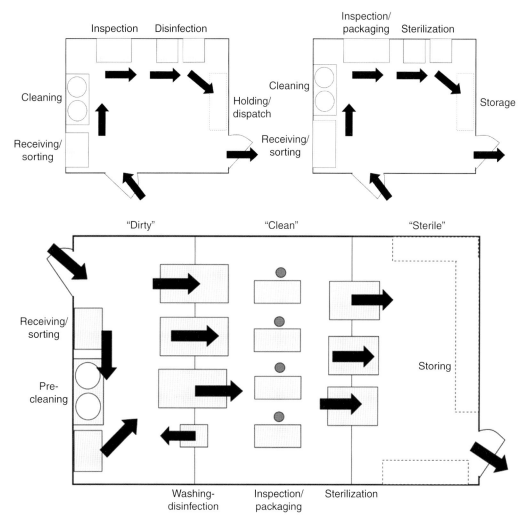

Figure 1.2 Examples of decontamination area/facility workflow plans. On the upper panel are examples of single rooms for cleaning-disinfection (left) and cleaning-sterilization (right). In the disinfection example, devices are received in one area, passed through the process and held in a separate area waiting for release for the new patient procedure. The sterilization example is identical, but in this case the devices/sets are packaged, sterilized and stored ready for patient use. The lower panel shows a typical physically separated area design, designated areas for receiving/pre-cleaning, cleaning-disinfection, inspection-packaging, sterilization and storage. Physical separation in this case is enabled by using two-door designs of washer-disinfector machines and sterilizers (that open on one end for loading and on the other for unloading); note that an additional pass-through hatch is shown between the clean and dirty area, to allow for devices that have not been adequately cleaned to pass back to the dirty area for additional cleaning.

subsequently packaged for sterilization (if applicable). There may be provisions made for specific transfer methods (e.g. transfer hatches) between physically separated department designs (Figure 1.2).

• Sterilization area (if applicable), where devices/materials are subjected to a sterilization process.

• Processed goods storage and distribution: this may be at the same area or in a separate, designated area of the facility (e.g. with other sterile stores).

Serious consideration should always be given to the correct layout of a decontamination area/facility. Too often decontamination areas are found to be inadequate.

Figure 1.3 The layout of a modern decontamination facility, designed to have physical separation between dirty, clean and sterile storage/dispatch areas.

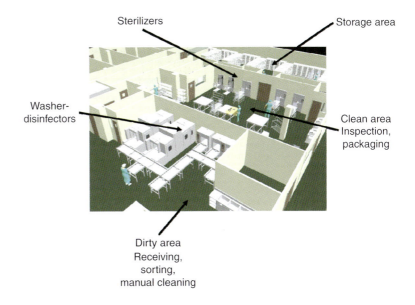

Sterilizers

Storage area

Washer-disinfectors

Clean area
Inspection,
packaging

Dirty area
Receiving,
sorting,
manual cleaning

The area should be designated for decontamination purposes only (e.g. not mixed with food or drink preparation areas) and of ample size for the required procedures/workload. These can include single or multiple room/area designs (Figure 1.2). In single room set-ups, correct layout and staff training is essential to prevent cross-contamination. These risks are minimized in larger, physically separated area designs (Figure 1.3). It is important to remember that in addition to the receiving, decontaminating and storage/dispatch of re-usable devices/materials, provision should also be made for the handling of supplies or raw materials for the decontamination process. This will include chemicals, packaging materials (single use or re-usable), labels, indicators, etc. Equally, the area can have many items (contaminated or non-contaminated) that will be designated for waste disposal and will need to be considered. Finally, any equipment within the area (and their associated utilities such as electricity, water/steam supply, drainage, etc.) will require periodic maintenance and testing; therefore access to such equipment should be considered and with minimum disruption to the decontamination needs of the facility.

There are many other environmental concerns to be considered in the design of a decontamination area. These include:

• Access to the area should be limited and controlled. This should prevent any unauthorized person from entering the area without permission.

• Comfort of staff: temperature and humidity control (air conditioning), in particular in areas where heat-associated equipment (such as steam sterilizers and thermal washer-disinfectors are used), is preferred. Consideration may also be given to ensure there is adequate lighting (preferably natural) and noise control.

• Ventilation: the cleaning area, in particular with manual cleaning, can pose a safety risk to staff and visitors (from microorganisms, patient tissues and various chemicals used in the cleaning process). These areas should be adequately ventilated, so as to provide ~20 air changes/hour. It is also recommended that these areas should have dedicated air handling systems and be maintained at ambient pressure or even at a slight negative pressure (e.g. −5 to −10 Pa) that acts to keep contamination within the area. Equally, the clean or sterile packaging area should also be similarly ventilated (~20 air changes/hour), reducing any risks of airborne contamination and under a slightly positive pressure (e.g. +10 Pa) to keep contamination out.

• The area should be designed to allow for periodic ease of routine cleaning or, particularly in dirty areas, for handling of accidental spillages.

• Sterile or otherwise decontaminated items should be stored in a suitable area designed to reduce any potential for cross-contamination such as from the air, water, damage, etc.

• Staff/visitors should have access to hand washing facilities, separate to those used for cleaning devices, before entering or leaving the areas.

• For larger facilities/departments, provisions may need to be made for management offices, general staff areas (for eating and drinking) and storage that are separated from the decontamination area.

An effective management system should be in place to control the entire decontamination system, from patient use to the next patient use. This may require a coordinated effort from all staff involved, particularly in larger facilities that will include operating room, transport, decontamination and inventory control staff, as examples. For the decontamination process, written procedures should be in place and staff trained on these procedures to ensure that the various decontamination steps are conducted correctly. Once in place, deviations to established procedures should not be tolerated. If deviations are demanded by medical/surgical staff due to patient needs it is recommended that written authorization is obtained from management that accepts any associated patient risk.

For an effective decontamination, other considerations to be considered will include:
• Adequate water supply: this will include cold and hot tap (potable) water, and may also include the provision of a higher water quality for rinsing and other purposes (e.g. for generation of steam). Water, and the various types of chemicals and other materials that can be present in it, can play an important role in the decontamination of devices and patient safety.
• Sufficient draining, with consideration of any local or regional requirements regarding disposal of chemicals or other materials into drains.
• Automated decontamination processes (for cleaning, disinfection and sterilization) are preferred over manual methods. Any equipment provided should be installed correctly and verified to be fit for purpose; for example any equipment that requires temperature control should be routinely checked to ensure it is working at the correct, set temperatures, and only authorized staff should be able to change cycle parameters. Equipment will require periodic maintenance and testing.
• Staff and visitor safety is important: safety equipment (personal protective equipment (PPE)), such as safety glass and proper gloves (e.g. heavy duty for cleaning) should be provided and used. Specific safety equipment will depend on the various procedures or equipment being used within the area.
• International, regional and local guidelines regarding decontamination should be considered.
A correctly designed decontamination area is the first step to ensuring patient safety, but is closely followed by staff training. Designated staff should be trained on the correct procedures (including equipment used) for decontamination within the area and have sufficient allocated time to ensure a quality process. It is important that

training should be conducted when any changes in these procedures are made, such as the introduction of new equipment, chemicals, devices, etc. Periodic re-training should also be considered to ensure that standards are maintained.

Where to start

This book provides a practical guide to decontamination principles and practices from an international perspective. As introduced in the previous section, this includes many background concepts to the subject, such as an introduction to anatomy, chemistry and microbiology, as well as detailed consideration of the various steps of the decontamination process. This book should be used in conjunction with available international, regional and local regulations, standards and guidelines. These will include various aspects of decontamination, including quality control, the design of decontamination facilities, minimal steps for device/materials reprocessing, waste disposal, use of chemicals, selection of equipment and their use, etc.

Regulations are rules or orders issued by a region, country, community or administrative agency, under legal authority, and have the force of law. Depending on the region or country you live in, there may be various laws or directives concerning the safe use of medical/surgical equipment, as well as various products and processes used for their decontamination. Examples, at the time of writing, include:
• European Union (note that C€ mark stands for Conformité Européenne or "European conformity", which when attached to a device is a manufacturer's claim that it meets all the requirements of applicable European legislation). This can vary depending on the type of product, with examples including:
  ○ Medical Device Directive (the most recent version being 2007/47/EC). This directive covers the essential requirements for any medical device, defined as any instrument or other article (used alone or in combination) intended to be used for human beings for the purpose of diagnosis, prevention, monitoring, treatment or alleviation of disease. Medical devices are further sub-classified based on their risk to patients, ranging from class 1 (low risk, such as beds and wheelchairs), class 2a (low-medium risk, such as hearing aids), class 2b (medium-high risk, such as many surgical devices and equipment used to reprocess them like sterilizers and washer-disinfectors) and class 3

(e.g. implants like heart valves). Equipment and products used in the reprocessing of devices (disinfectants, sterilizers, etc.) are also considered "medical devices" under this directive. The manufacturer, with reference to the "essential" requirements of the directive as well as other standards (international and/or European) that are specific to the types of device/equipment, ensures compliance and should provide a certificate (or "declaration") of conformance. In most cases this is reviewed and approved by an independent organization known as a Notified Body. Note that a separate directive may be in place for specific types of medical devices, such as the Active Implantable Medical Devices (including pacemakers) under Directive 90/385/EEC.

○ Machinery Directive (2006/42/EC), defining essential health and safety requirements for machinery. "Machinery" is any assembly using moving parts and therefore would apply to equipment like washers and sterilizers. Compliance is similar to that described for the medical devices directive.

○ Biocidal Products Directive (98/8/EC). "Biocides" are defined active substances/preparations supplied to destroy, deter, render harmless, prevent the action of or otherwise exert a controlling effect on any harmful organism. Interestingly, this includes the use of chemical disinfectants/sterilants using on general surfaces, but excludes their specific use on medical devices (as when used as such they are required to meet the requirements of the medical devices directive). In addition to these essential requirements, at the time of writing a series of specific test methods are under development in Europe that should be used to confirm any efficacy claims (e.g. kills bacteria or viruses) used with disinfectants (these are discussed in further detail in Chapter 9.

○ REACH (Registration, Evaluation and Authorization of Chemicals; Regulation (EC) 1907/2006). Regulation on the production and use of any chemical, with an emphasis on human and environmental health. This would include a wide range of chemicals used, for example in cleaning chemistries or chemical disinfectants. Other directives/regulations apply to specific types of chemicals such as biocides (98/8/EC, as discussed above) and detergents (regulation (EC) 648/2004).

These directives are applicable for all EU countries and compliance allows for the devices to be legally sold in all countries; however, in some cases additional requirements can be put in place in individual countries.

- United States of America (USA):
  ○ The Federal Drug Administration's (FDA) Center for Devices and Radiological Health (CDRH) is responsible for regulating those who manufacture, repackage, re-label, and/or import medical devices sold in the United States. Medical devices are classified based on their risk, to include class 1, 2 and 3 (from low to high risk). These include surgical devices and decontamination processes such as washer-disinfectors, sterilizers and device disinfection chemistries. Class 2 (such as sterilizers and device disinfectants) and class 3 devices, specifically, require a formal approval by the FDA known as a Premarket Notification 510(k) or Premarket Approval (PMA). In either case, the safety and efficacy of a product/process is reviewed and formally approved prior to selling in the USA. The FDA also provides guidance documents to manufacturers regarding device/process specific requirements, such as for sterilizers, high-level disinfectants/sterilants and reprocessing instructions.
  ○ The Environmental Protection Agency (EPA) regulates the use of general/environmental surface disinfectants under Federal Insecticide, Fungicide and Rodenticide Act (FIFRA). Note: any disinfectants used on medical devices are registered for use in the USA by the FDA, while those for environmental surface disinfection should be registered by the EPA. They refer to biocides or antimicrobial chemistries as "antimicrobial pesticides". The EPA requires that special tests (such as those described by AOAC International) are used to ensure disinfectant efficacy, as well as or any human and ecological risks from exposure. The EPA also provides guidance documents on various aspects of disinfectant registration, such as testing for specific antimicrobial claims and dental issues.

- Australia:
  ○ The Therapeutic Goods Administration (TGA), a division of the Department of Health and Ageing, is the regulatory authority for therapeutic goods, including medical devices and their reprocessing methods. Medical devices are registered under the Therapeutic Goods (Medical Devices) Regulations (2002). All products are required to be listed in the Australian Register of Therapeutic Goods (ARTG) before they can be supplied in Australia. The Office of Devices Authorization (ODA) is responsible for initial registration of medical devices, while the Office of Product Review (OPR) is responsible for any post-registration issues. Devices are also classified based on risk ranging from low (class 1) to high (class 3 or active implantable devices

separately). Device disinfectants, for example, are considered class 2b devices. Liquid chemical disinfectants and sterilants, for example, are regulated under Therapeutic Goods Order No. 54 (1996), but this excludes antiseptics (disinfectants used on the skin) and water treatment. The TGA also provide various guidance documents such as infection control guidelines for the prevention of transmission of infectious diseases and reducing public health risks associated with re-usable medical devices.

- Canada:
  ○ Medical Devices Regulations are under the authority of the Food and Drugs Act. Health Canada reviews all medical devices to assess their safety, effectiveness and quality before being authorized for sale in Canada. Medical devices are classified based on risk, ranging from class 1 to class 4. For example, equipment/products used for disinfecting or sterilizing a medical device are classified as class 2. Health Canada also provides guidelines such as for reporting problems with medical devices.

As can be seen from this brief but not exhaustive review, the specific requirements can be complicated and are regularly updated or changed. These laws/directives generally control the legal marketing and use of medical/surgical devices, as well as requirements for decontamination, within those specific areas. It is the responsibility of the healthcare facility to understand these requirements and ensure that they are correctly applied. Many of these regulations are general and include specific requirements in further standards and guidelines. Examples of various standard/guideline organizations are shown in Table 1.1.

Standards are documents that specify the minimum acceptable characteristics of a product or material, issued by a standards organization (e.g. ISO, International Organization for Standardization and CEN, European Commission for Standardization). Most countries will have some legal requirements, directly or indirectly, regarding decontamination of re-usable devices/materials; these may or may not include such standards within a given country/region. International standards (such as those developed by ISO) are continually under development for various different aspects of decontamination procedures and practices. A summary of some of these standards is provided in Table 1.2. Other regional (e.g. CEN within Europe) and local standards and best practice guideline documents are also important to consider, and are often mandated in certain countries (Chapter 14). Guidelines are documents used to communicate regional recommended procedures, processes or usage of particular practices; they are often considered best practice at the time of writing. During the course of this book, various different standards and guidelines are referenced for each phase of the decontamination cycle.

A particularly important standard that should be considered in decontamination is ISO 17664 (2004) *Sterilization of medical devices – information to be provided by the manufacturer for the processing of resterilizable medical devices*. Although it is the responsibility of a healthcare facility to safely decontaminate re-usable items, it is the responsibility of the suppliers of these items to provide detailed instructions on how they should be safely reprocessed. These instructions should be verified as being effective by the manufacturer. The title of this standard does specifically apply to "resterilizable medical devices", but it is a useful and practical reference for all re-usable devices/materials (e.g. for cleaning alone or cleaning/disinfection). Instructions provided should include:

- The device manufacturer and their contact information.
- Device(s), by model number and device description or generic type.
- Any appropriate warnings or limitations, such as care on handling (e.g. sharp edges), restrictions on reprocessing conditions (e.g. "cannot be immersed in water" or "electrical hazard".
- Instructions on handling the device at its point of use and for transport to a decontamination area. Examples include inspections, pre-cleaning, care in handling, etc.
- Instructions on preparation for decontamination, including disassembly. The use of specific tools and procedures may need to be described, depending on the device design.
- Cleaning instructions, manual and automated. This will include the cleaning chemistries and procedures to be used. At a minimum, a manual cleaning method should be described in detail. A further automated cleaning should be described, although this is sometimes not possible due to the device design.
- Disinfection (if applicable). Manual and automated procedures should be described, unless automated processes cannot be employed. This should include applicable thermal and/or chemical disinfection methods, equipment required and requirements for rinsing (in particular with chemical disinfection to ensure the device is safe for patient use or further reprocessing).
- Drying (if applicable). Instructions for the drying of the device should be provided.

Table 1.1 Examples of various standard and guideline publishing organizations internationally. This list is by no means exhaustive.

Title	Notes
International Standards Organization (ISO)	A non-governmental, international body based in Geneva, Switzerland. Develops draft standards through technical committees (e.g. ISO/TC 198 *Sterilization of healthcare products*) that are then approved by a majority of country (national) member bodies[1]. ISO collaborates closely with the International Electrotechnical Commission (IEC) on all matters of electrotechnical standardization and with CEN on harmonized international standards[2].
Comité Européen De Normalisation (CEN). European Committee for Standardization	A not-for-profit European organization based in Brussels, Belgium. Develops draft standards through technical committees (e.g. CEN/TC 204 *Sterilization of medical devices* and CEN/TC 216 *Disinfectants and antiseptics*) that are then approved by European country (national) member bodies[3]. CEN collaborates closely with CENELEC (Comité Européen de Normalisation Électrotechnique; European Committee for Electrotechnical Standardization) on matters of electrotechnical standardization and with ISO on the development of harmonized international standards[2].
British Standards Institute (BSI)	National standards body in the UK. BSI also use the "kite mark" to indicate that a product has been independently tested to conform with a relevant British Standard.
(DIN)	National standards body in Germany.
Association Française de Normalisation (AFNOR)	National standards body in France.
American National Standards Institute (ANSI) Association for the Advancement of Medical Instrumentation (AAMI)	National standard and guideline bodies in the USA. AAMI develop standards and recommended practices, with many being approved by (ANSI) as American National Standards. For example, a TIR (Technical Information Report) provides guidance on a particular aspect (e.g. use of disinfectants/sterilants or water quality).
ASTM International (previously known as the American Society for Testing and Materials, ASTM)	Standards body in the USA, particularly in the development of test method (e.g. chemical and microbiological) standards.
AOAC International (previously known as the Association of Analytical Communities (AOAC))	Standards body in the USA, particularly in the development of test method (chemical and microbiological) standards.
Standardization Administration of China (SAC)	Standards body in China. Mandatory standards are prefixed with "GB", while recommended standards are prefixed "GB/T"
Standards Australia	Standard bodies in Australia and New Zealand. Joint Australian (AS) and New Zealand (NZS) Standards and Guidelines are often developed (known as AS/NZS). An example is AS/NZS 4187 (2003) on cleaning, disinfection and sterilization of re-usable devices in healthcare facilities.

[1] Examples of national standard bodies include BSI (UK), AFNOR (France), DIN (Germany) and AAMI (United States), see above.
[2] The Vienna Agreement (1991) is an agreement on technical cooperation between ISO and CEN in the development of standards. As an example, ISO/TC 198 *Sterilization of healthcare products* and CEN/TC 204 *Sterilization of medical devices* cooperate to develop harmonized standards in the reprocessing or sterilization of devices. An example of a harmonized standard is EN ISO 14937 *Sterilization of healthcare products – general requirements for characterization of a sterilizing agent and the development, validation and routine control of a sterilization process for medical devices*. Despite these efforts, sometimes the standard is not adopted in all countries or modifications of the standard are made/published by the national standard body.
[3] CEN members are the national standards bodies of different European countries. Members should comply with the CEN/CENELEC regulations that stipulate a European Standard should be given the status of a national standard without any alteration.

Table 1.2 Examples of international standards that consider various decontamination aspects. These may or may not apply to a given region or country.

Standard Number[1]	Title	Description
ISO 13485 (2003)	*Medical devices – quality management systems – requirements for regulatory purposes.*	The requirements for the development, implementation and monitoring of a quality management system for the manufacturer of medical devices. Generally for device manufacturers, but can also apply to healthcare facilities decontaminating devices.
ISO 17664 (2004)	*Sterilization of medical devices. Information to be provided by the manufacturer for the processing of resterilizable medical devices.*	Instructions to be provided by the device manufacturer to ensure safe reprocessing/decontamination of the device of re-use.
ISO 15883-1 (2005)	*Washer-disinfectors. General requirements, definitions and tests.*	Design, performance and testing of washer-disinfectors, including cleaning and disinfection requirements. Provided in a series, part 1 describes the requirements for all washer-disinfectors and subsequent parts provide more details on specific types of machines (e.g. surgical instruments and flexible endoscopes).
ISO TS 15883-5 (2005)	*Washer-disinfectors. Part 5: test soils and methods for demonstrating cleaning efficacy of washer-disinfectors.*	Technical specification that provides information about various methods used around the world to test cleaning efficacy.
ISO 9398 series	*Specifications for industrial laundry machines.*	Series of standards on laundry machines, including definitions, testing of capacity and consumption characteristics.
ISO 14937 (2009)	*Sterilization of healthcare products – general requirements for characterization of a sterilizing agent and the development, validation and routine control of a sterilization process for medical devices.*	Development, validation and routine control of any sterilization process used for healthcare devices and other materials.
ISO 17665-1 (2006)	*Sterilization of healthcare products – moist heat. Part 1: requirements for the development, validation and routine control of a sterilization process for medical devices*	Development, validation and routine control of moist heat (steam) sterilization processes for devices.
ISO 20857 (2010)	*Sterilization of healthcare products – dry heat – requirements for the development, validation and routine control of a sterilization process for medical devices*	Development, validation and routine control of a dry heat sterilization process for devices.
ISO 11135-1 (2007)	*Sterilization of healthcare products. Ethylene oxide. Part 1: requirements for development, validation and routine control of a sterilization process for medical devices.*	Development, validation and routine control of an ethylene oxide sterilization process for medical devices.

[1] International standards, as published by ISO, are designated by a specific number, but also the date or issue (as they are periodically updated). When (and if) the standard is accepted regionally or within a specific country it may be designated, for example BS EN ISO xxxx (designated a harmonized standard for the United Kingdom, European Union and International) or AMMI ISO xxxx (designates a USA-AAMI version of an international standard); note, in such cases modifications, specific to that region or country, may be included before publication in these areas. All attempts are made internationally to harmonize such standards, but at the time of writing this is not always possible.

• Maintenance, inspection and testing. This will include instructions for periodic testing, lubrication, inspections, etc., to ensure that the device can be safely used on the next patient.

• Packaging (if applicable), in preparation for storage and/or terminal sterilization.

• Sterilization (if applicable). At least one method of sterilization should be provided, but the instructions may also include restrictions on what should or should not be applied, such as "should not be immersed", not subjected to low pressure levels or should not exceed certain temperatures.

• Storage. Any recommendations for the time or conditions of storage prior to use, if required.

Reprocessing instructions are essential in order to ensure patient safety. They require close cooperation between medical/surgical device manufacturers, those using the devices and the suppliers of cleaning, disinfection and sterilization products/processes. Although it is often difficult for manufacturers to provide detailed instruc-tions to meet individual requirements for each country, it is important that they consider local decontamination standards and guidelines. In the absence of adequate instructions, it will not be possible to ensure patient safety and the healthcare facility may decide not to use such devices/materials.

In conclusion, this book has been written for a wide interdisciplinary, international audience, and whilst it dis-cusses the basic principles of decontamination and related guidelines, it should not be used as a replacement for local legislative or guidance documents issued in respective countries or regions. However, regardless of your loca-tion, the same basic principles should be applied to decontamination practices throughout the world, using a combination of processes which include as a basic mini-mum adequate cleaning and disinfection or sterilization in order to render a re-usable item safe for further use on patients and for handling by staff. Decontamination of re-usable devices and materials is essential in minimizing the risk of transmission of infectious agents.

2

Basic anatomy, physiology and biochemistry

Introduction

Anatomy is the study of the structure of living things and physiology is the study of how these structures function. This chapter gives a brief introduction into human anatomy and physiology, and in particular aims to give a basic understanding of the many terms that are used during surgical or interventional procedures. Similar language is used for the anatomy and physiology of animals, which may be a helpful introduction to some readers. Microbiology and microorganisms are specifically discussed in Chapter 5.

Let us consider the structure of the human body, from what we can see, down to the very basis of life itself. A useful analogy is to consider the human body as an encyclopaedia, with various parts (i.e. organ systems) all the way down to the individual words and even letters (i.e. molecules and atoms) that make up the complete work (see Table 2.1). The human body is a complex, organized structure of various systems. There are eleven systems to consider and each one has a unique function. Examples include the nervous, respiratory, digestive and cardiovascular systems, which will be discussed later in further detail. As an example, the digestive system consists of various parts that allow us to eat and drink, breaking down food into various components, allowing nutrients to be absorbed into the body and ridding the body of any remaining wastes. Each system can be subdivided into individual organs. In the digestive system organs include the mouth, stomach and intestines (small and large). It is important to note that many organs have shared functions; examples include the mouth being used for breathing (as part of the respiratory system) and eating/drinking (the digestive system).

Each individual organ is made up of various tissues that work together to perform a specific function. There

Table 2.1 The various human body structures and examples.

Structures	Examples
Systems	Nervous, respiratory, digestive and cardiovascular systems
Organs	Stomach, heart, kidney, liver, brain
Tissues	Epithelial, muscular, nervous, connective tissues
Cells	Nerve, muscle, skin, blood cells
Molecules	Water (H_2O), proteins, carbohydrates, lipids, nucleic acids
Atoms	Carbon (C), hydrogen (H), oxygen (O), nitrogen (N)

are only four basic types of tissues in the adult body: epithelial, muscular, nervous and connective:

• Epithelial tissues provide coverings or linings to organs, in addition to forming various types of glands that can produce substances (or secretions). Examples of epithelial tissues include the epithelium (or outermost) layer of the skin (where specific glands excrete sweat) and, in the case of the stomach, the inner mucous membrane (containing mucus producing glands) and outer serous membrane. Others examples are glandular tissues which produce hormone chemicals that secrete into the bloodstream and function to direct other cells in the body to act or respond.

• Nervous tissue allows for communication within the body directly.

• Muscular tissue allows for movement (i.e. in the beating of the heart). There are three types of muscular tissue: cardiac, smooth and skeletal. Cardiac and smooth muscle are controlled by involuntary commands, whereas skeletal muscle can move by way of voluntary commands.

A Practical Guide to Decontamination in Healthcare, First Edition. Gerald McDonnell and Denise Sheard.
© 2012 Gerald McDonnell and Denise Sheard. Published 2012 by Blackwell Publishing Ltd.

Figure 2.1 Human cell structure. Examples are given (top) of the various different shapes of cells that can be observed, but they practically all have the same essential structure (shown below).

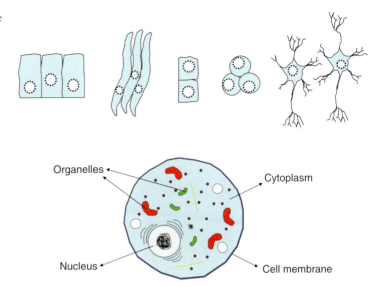

Organelles

Cytoplasm

Nucleus

Cell membrane

• Connective tissue provides support and connections (i.e. bones, blood).

It should be noted that the four basic tissue types can be further sub-divided into specific kinds based on their structures and functions, such as the many kinds of muscle and connective tissues.

When the structural and functional integrity of tissues is compromised, the result can lead to disease of the organ of which it is comprised. Pathology is the study and diagnosis of disease through examination of the whole body, including the various organs, tissues and cells. To explore further the structure of the various types of tissues, microscopic examination is now required. Specifically, histology is the science that studies the microscopic structure of organs and tissues. Each type of tissue is made up of specialized cells that are similar in function and structure. A single cell is the basic unit structure and function of life. Human cells are found to be in different shapes and sizes, depending on their function and structure, and organized together to give the various types of tissues. Despite these differences, cells are all essentially of the same basic design (Figure 2.1).

As we begin to look into the structure of these cells, we now consider the science of biochemistry. This is the study of the chemical processes in living organisms, focusing on the structure and function of cells and their components. Human cells consist of an outer cell membrane, enclosing a liquid-like cytoplasm (Figure 2.1). The cytoplasm holds various different structures (known as "organelles") that provide the various functions to the

cell. Organelles are comprised of macromolecules such as proteins, lipids and carbohydrates, with each type of cell having a unique mix of organelles based on the primary function of the cell. Key organelles include mitochrondria (that make energy in the cell), microfilaments (allowing for movement and support), lysosomes (which contain enzymes for food digestion and destruction for invading microorganisms) and the nucleus. The nucleus is particularly prominent and is separated from the rest of the cell by a further membrane. This is the heart of the cell, containing the genetic material DNA (deoxyribonucleic acid). In human cells the DNA is organized into specialized structures called chromosomes and most cells in the body contain 46 (23 pairs, one of each pair inherited from the mother and the other from the father). These are important structures, as the DNA is like a blueprint for the cell and is made up of individual genes. It is the expression (whether they are turned off or on) of these genes that allow the cell to produce all the necessary molecules (biomolecules) that are required for cell structure and function (described in the following section). It is therefore the same gene expression that allows the cell to survive or die, divide, communicate with other cells, change structure or function, and essentially dictates during the development of the human body whether that cell becomes any of the various types of cells that make up the tissues and organs. It is quite a remarkable structure.

All cells are made up of four basic structures, referred to as biomolecules: proteins, lipids, carbohydrates and nucleic acids. Their structures can vary from simple to

Table 2.2 Examples of the four biomolecules that make up cellular structure and function.

Biomolecule	Examples	Basic unit
Nucleic acids (polynucleotides)	DNA[1], RNA[2]	Nucleotides
Proteins (peptides, polypeptides)	Enzymes, keratin, albumin	Amino acids
Carbohydrates (saccharides)	"Sugars", starch, cellulose, polysaccharides	Monosaccharides
Lipids	Fat, oil, glycolipids, sterols	Structurally diverse but many based on fatty acids

[1]DNA: Deoxyribonucleic acid.
[2]RNA: Ribonucleic acid.

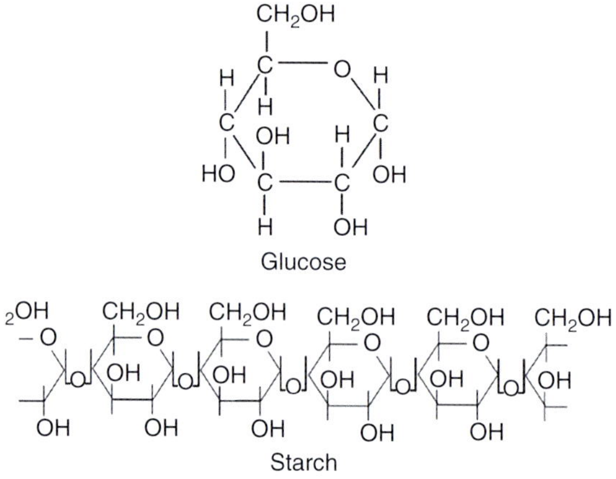

Figure 2.2 The chemical structure of glucose and starch, types of sugars or carbohydrates. Glucose is made up of atoms from three types of chemical elements: carbon (C), hydrogen (H) and oxygen (O). The chemical way of describing glucose is $C_6H_{12}O_6$, with the numbers of each type of element identified. Note that starch is essentially a polymer of glucose, consisting of long lines of glucose bound together.

very complex, but they combine together to perform all the functions and provide all the structures of the cell. Each chromosome, for example, that was described as being present in the nucleus of the cell contains one long thread of DNA (a nucleic acid) which is wrapped around various types of proteins. The cell membrane is made up of a double layer of lipid-based molecules (one to the outside and one to the inside), but includes various types of proteins integrated into the lipid structure such as "glycoproteins" (proteins that have attached carbohydrates). Examples of each type of biomolecule are given in Table 2.2.

If we look at one of the structures of these biomolecules (for example, starch), we find that it is made up of a basic unit of structure (glucose) that is itself constructed from various different types of chemical elements (Figure 2.2).

Chemistry is the study of chemicals and chemical reactions. Chemical elements are the essential building blocks of chemistry, including all living and non-living things. Examples include oxygen (also known as its chemical symbol O), nitrogen (N), calcium (Ca), silver (Ag) and gold (Au). Elements can exist on their own (e.g. gold, silver) or combine together to form molecules (e.g. H_2O, the chemical symbol of water, made up of two hydrogens and one oxygen). A molecule is therefore made up of two or more elements. There are over one hundred types of elements that have been identified, but only six are actually used in the various different types of biomolecules that make up the various cells, tissues, organs and systems

of the body: carbon, hydrogen, nitrogen, oxygen, sulfur and phosphorus. As shown in Figure 2.2, glucose and starch (which are types of carbohydrates) are made up of only three elements (hydrogen, oxygen and carbon). One unit (or molecule) of glucose is actually composed of six carbon (C), twelve hydrogen (H) and six oxygen (O) atoms and can be written in chemical terms as $C_6H_{12}O_6$. Starch is a polymer of glucose, being a rather large molecule consisting of repeated units of glucose linked together. In another example, DNA is a polymer of nucleotides. In the structure of DNA there are only four types of nucleotides (as defined by their bases: adenine, thymine, cytosine and guanine); it is remarkable to think that all the genes in human DNA are made up of only these four types and it is the sequence of these that dictates all the structure and functions that make us human and all different.

Anatomy terminology

In work with surgical or diagnostic practice, there are a number of key definitions that will help you in understanding the terminology that can be frequently used. The human body can be examined in an upright position, with the palms of the hands turned out (Figure 2.3). This

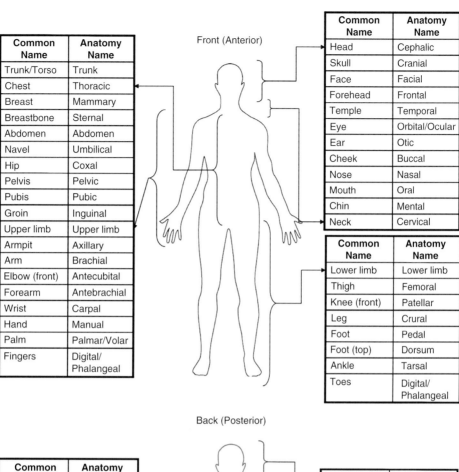

Front (Anterior)

Common Name	Anatomy Name
Trunk/Torso	Trunk
Chest	Thoracic
Breast	Mammary
Breastbone	Sternal
Abdomen	Abdomen
Navel	Umbilical
Hip	Coxal
Pelvis	Pelvic
Pubis	Pubic
Groin	Inguinal
Upper limb	Upper limb
Armpit	Axillary
Arm	Brachial
Elbow (front)	Antecubital
Forearm	Antebrachial
Wrist	Carpal
Hand	Manual
Palm	Palmar/Volar
Fingers	Digital/ Phalangeal

Common Name	Anatomy Name
Head	Cephalic
Skull	Cranial
Face	Facial
Forehead	Frontal
Temple	Temporal
Eye	Orbital/Ocular
Ear	Otic
Cheek	Buccal
Nose	Nasal
Mouth	Oral
Chin	Mental
Neck	Cervical

Common Name	Anatomy Name
Lower limb	Lower limb
Thigh	Femoral
Knee (front)	Patellar
Leg	Crural
Foot	Pedal
Foot (top)	Dorsum
Ankle	Tarsal
Toes	Digital/ Phalangeal

Back (Posterior)

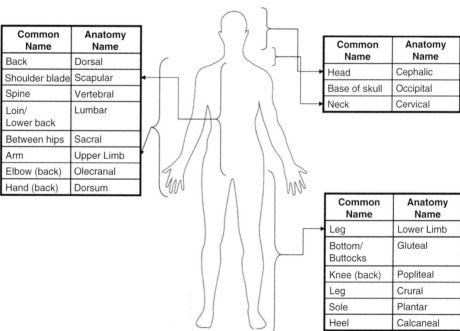

Common Name	Anatomy Name
Back	Dorsal
Shoulder blade	Scapular
Spine	Vertebral
Loin/ Lower back	Lumbar
Between hips	Sacral
Arm	Upper Limb
Elbow (back)	Olecranal
Hand (back)	Dorsum

Common Name	Anatomy Name
Head	Cephalic
Base of skull	Occipital
Neck	Cervical

Common Name	Anatomy Name
Leg	Lower Limb
Bottom/ Buttocks	Gluteal
Knee (back)	Popliteal
Leg	Crural
Sole	Plantar
Heel	Calcaneal

Figure 2.3 Common and anatomical names for various parts of the human body.

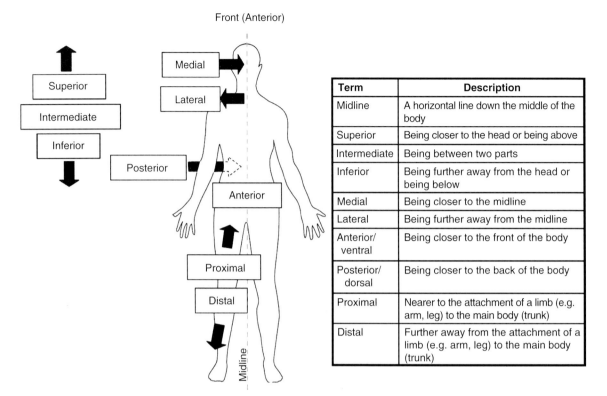

Term	Description
Midline	A horizontal line down the middle of the body
Superior	Being closer to the head or being above
Intermediate	Being between two parts
Inferior	Being further away from the head or being below
Medial	Being closer to the midline
Lateral	Being further away from the midline
Anterior/ ventral	Being closer to the front of the body
Posterior/ dorsal	Being closer to the back of the body
Proximal	Nearer to the attachment of a limb (e.g. arm, leg) to the main body (trunk)
Distal	Further away from the attachment of a limb (e.g. arm, leg) to the main body (trunk)

Figure 2.4 The most common directional anatomical terms used in anatomy.

is referred to as the anatomical position. In this position, the body can be considered as five major sections: the head, neck, trunk/back, upper limb and lower limb. The front of the body is considered as the 'anterior' and the back as the 'posterior'. A summary of the various different regions of the body, with both their common and anatomical names, is given in Figure 2.3. Many of these terms may already be familiar to you. These regions can be further sub-divided. For example the trunk (or torso) can be sub-divided into various regions from the top of the chest to just above the pubic area, such as the epigastric (just below the nipples), umbilical (the area of the belly button) and hypogastric (upper pubic) regions.

Another position of the human body under examination when the body is face up on a surgical table is referred to being in a "supine" position, the most commonly perceived position for surgical procedures, and in contrast to being face down (in the "prone" position). In fact, the surgical procedure may take place in a variety of positions, depending on many factors such as the type of surgery, the surgeon and available surgical equipment.

Next, let us consider some of the most common terms that are used to describe the position of one part of the body to another part, which are also referred to as "directional" terms. For the purpose of this description, the same anatomical position is considered with a single line drawn through the centre of the body from the top to the bottom, referred to as the "midline". The most widely used directional terms are summarized in Figure 2.4. These terms can be used to refer to various organs and structures both on the outside of (external) and inside (internal) the body.

As we now begin to move into the body, before we describe the various anatomical systems, there are a number of defined body spaces (known as "cavities") that should be mentioned. A cavity may be defined as a space within the body that contains supports, protects and separates the various internal organs. In the human body, a cavity can be either open or closed from the external environment. For example, open cavities consist of the oral, nasal, alimentary (or digestive) cavities. There are two major closed cavities within the body: the ventral and

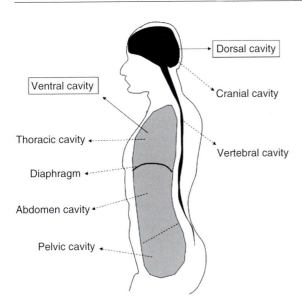

Figure 2.5 Major human body cavities. Note that the abdominal and pelvic cavities are not physically separated and are continuous. This cavity is also referred to as the abdominopelvic (a dotted line shows the approximate area of separation). The diaphragm physically separates the ventral cavity into the thoracic and abdomen-pelvic cavities.

the dorsal that can be further sub-divided as follows (Figure 2.5). The dorsal cavity is made up of the cranial (containing the brain) and vertebral (containing the spinal cord) areas. The ventral cavity, the largest body cavity is divided into two parts: the thoracic and the abdominal-pelvic area, which are separated by the diaphragm. The thoracic cavity contains the lungs (referred to as the "pleural cavity") and the other organs in the area (such as the heart, esophagus and trachea within the mediastinal cavity); the heart may be considered in a separate area in its own right known as "pericardial cavity". The abdominal-pelvic cavity is sub-divided into two sections: the abdominal (including the stomach, liver, pancreas and most of the intestines) and the pelvic (including the bladder and reproductive organs).

The anatomical systems of the human body

All in all, the human body is a complex organization of systems. There are eleven major systems of the human body and these are summarized in Table 2.3. A very brief

description of each system, their functions and major organs are described in the following sections.

Cardiovascular

Introduction

The cardiovascular system consists of the heart, various blood vessels and the blood itself that circulates around the body (Figure 2.6). Blood is itself a type of connective tissue consisting of two parts: the plasma (a watery-type liquid) and various types of cells/cell fragments (often called the "formed elements"). Plasma is similar to the "interstitial" fluid that surrounds the various cells in the body and to the lymph that circulates through the lymphatic system (see section on lymphatic system). The blood moves around the body through the various types of blood vessels and is pumped by the heart.

Structure

Blood consists of two major components; the plasma and the cell/cell fragment component. The plasma is a pale, yellow liquid that consists of ~92% water, the remaining being various types of plasma proteins and other components (such as nutrients, waste products and dissolved gases). The cell/cell fragment part consists of red blood cells (RBCs), white blood cells (WBCs) and platelets. They are all produced in a process known as hemopoesis, primarily from the red bone marrow of the skeletal system (see section on skeletal system). The platelets are not cells but cell fragments, produced from specialized cells known as megakaryocytes; they are primarily involved in the generation of blood clots to prevent the loss of blood from the cardiovascular system (e.g. due to blood vessel rupture or skin cuts). Red blood cells and WBCs are living cells. Red blood cells (also known as erythrocytes) give blood its characteristic red color due to the presence of a unique protein (or pigment) called hemoglobin. Hemoglobin plays an important role in the transport of oxygen through the blood (and in a certain part carbon dioxide). White blood cells (also known as leukocytes) consist of many different types of cells such as neutrophils, eosinophils, lymphocytes and monocytes; they are all involved in the body's immune system, protecting the body from the invasion of various types of microorganisms (e.g. bacteria and viruses).

The blood is carried through the body through a series of blood vessels (the vascular system). They are referred to as arteries, arterioles, capillaries, venules and veins. Blood vessels are similar but vary in their individual structures. For example, arteries have thicker muscle

Table 2.3 A summary of the anatomical systems of the human body.

System	Common names	Organ and component examples	Function
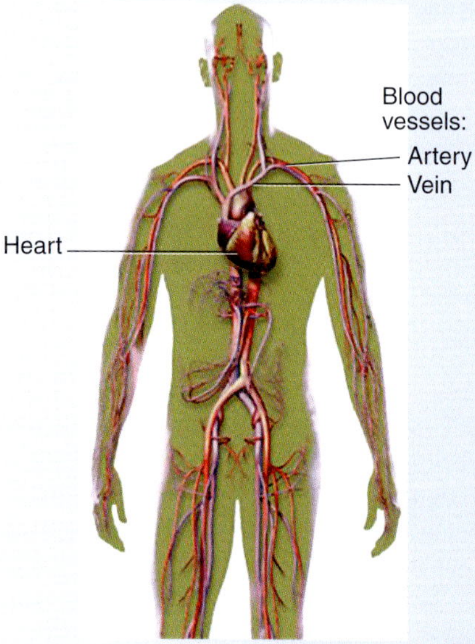 Cardiovascular	Circulatory system, blood	Heart, veins, arteries	Circulation of blood around the body. Carries oxygen, nutrients and wastes to and from cells. Regulates temperature and water levels. Defends against disease and repairs damaged tissues.

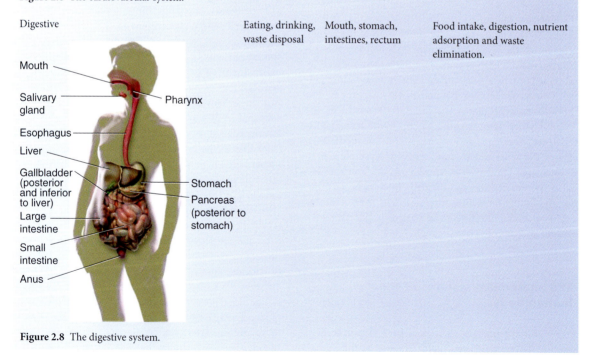

Figure 2.6 The cardiovascular system.

Digestive	Eating, drinking, waste disposal	Mouth, stomach, intestines, rectum	Food intake, digestion, nutrient adsorption and waste elimination.

Figure 2.8 The digestive system.

Table 2.3 (*cont'd*).

System	Common names	Organ and component examples	Function
Endocrine	Hormones	Adrenal glands, pituitary glands, ovaries, testes, thyroid	Controls various functions in the body by releasing special chemicals known as hormones (e.g. insulin, oestrogen and testosterone).
Integumentary	Skin	Skin, hair, nails	Senses (touch, taste, pain, etc.), protection, temperature regulation.

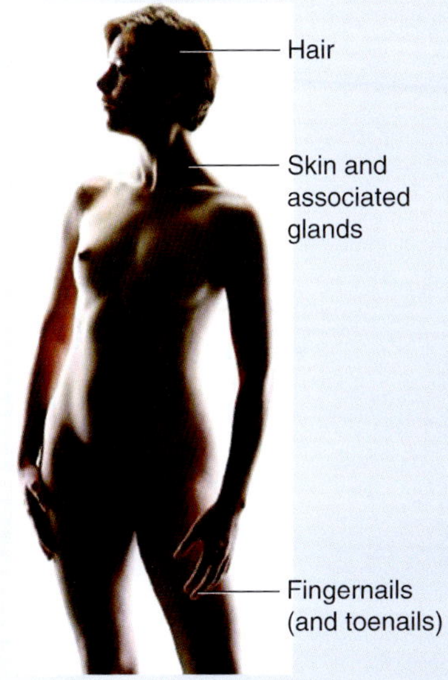

Figure 2.10 The integumentary (or "skin") system.

Lymphatic	Immune system	Spleen, tonsils, lymphatic vessels	Water and nutrient circulation, defence against microorganisms.

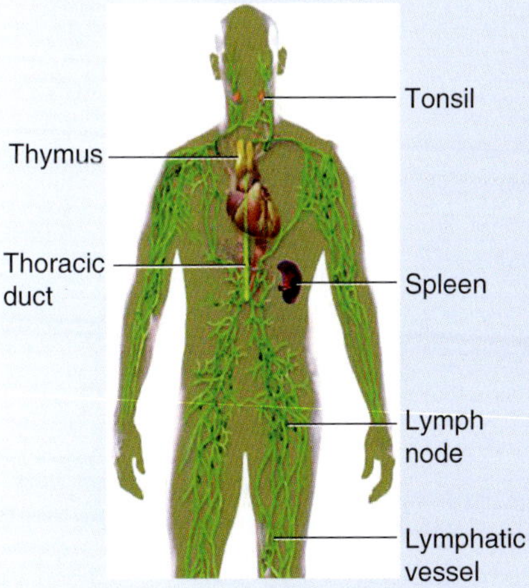

Figure 2.12 The major components of the lymphatic system, a parallel transport system to the venous part of the circulatory (blood) system.

(*continued*)

Table 2.3 (*cont'd*).

System	Common names	Organ and component examples	Function
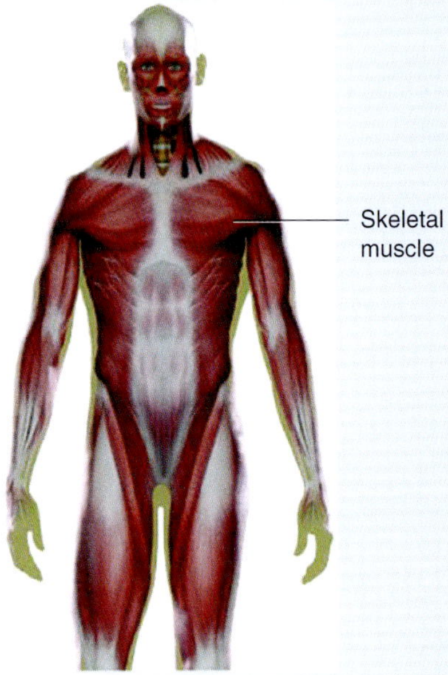 Muscular	Muscle, movement	Biceps, triceps, hamstrings	Movement, heat generation.

Figure 2.13 The muscular system.

System	Common names	Organ and component examples	Function
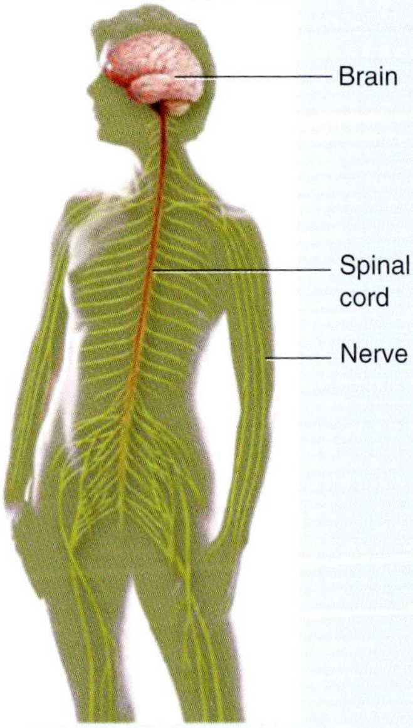 Nervous	Nerves, brain	Brain, spinal cord, optic nerve	Regulates the body activities.

Figure 2.14 The nervous system.

Table 2.3 (*cont'd*).

System	Common names	Organ and component examples	Function
Reproductive	Sex	Testes, ovaries, uterus	Reproduction.

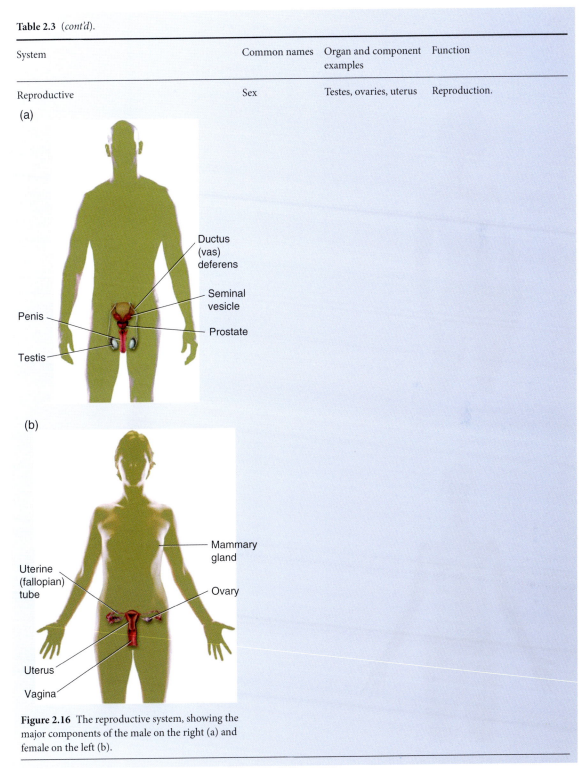

(a)

Ductus (vas) deferens

Seminal vesicle

Penis

Prostate

Testis

(b)

Mammary gland

Uterine (fallopian) tube

Ovary

Uterus

Vagina

Figure 2.16 The reproductive system, showing the major components of the male on the right (a) and female on the left (b).

(*continued*)

Table 2.3 (*cont'd*).

System	Common names	Organ and component examples	Function
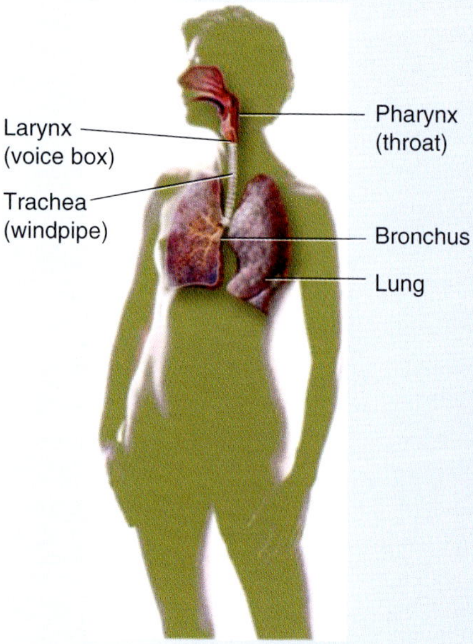 Respiratory	Breathing	Lungs, larynx, bronchus	Bring in oxygen and remove wastes such as carbon dioxide. Speaking.

Larynx (voice box)
Pharynx (throat)
Trachea (windpipe)
Bronchus
Lung

Figure 2.17 The respiratory system, consisting of the upper and lower tracts/systems.

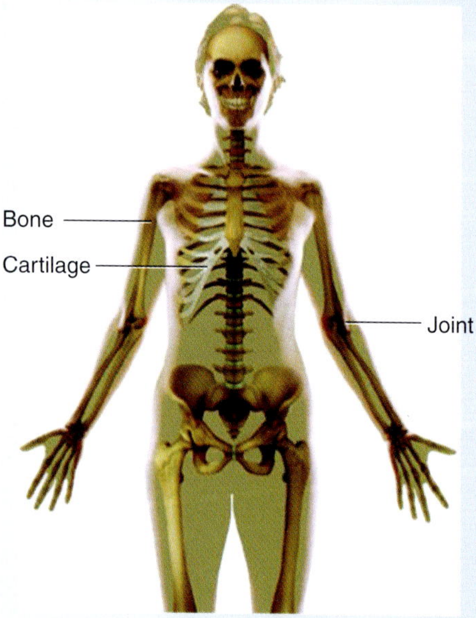 Skeletal (including dental)	Bones, teeth, skeleton	Skull, femur, pelvis, molars	Body support and protection.

Bone
Cartilage
Joint

Figure 2.18 The skeletal system.

Table 2.3 (*cont'd*).

System	Common names	Organ and component examples	Function
Urinary	Urine, excretion	Kidneys, bladder	Urine generation and excretion, maintain mineral balance.

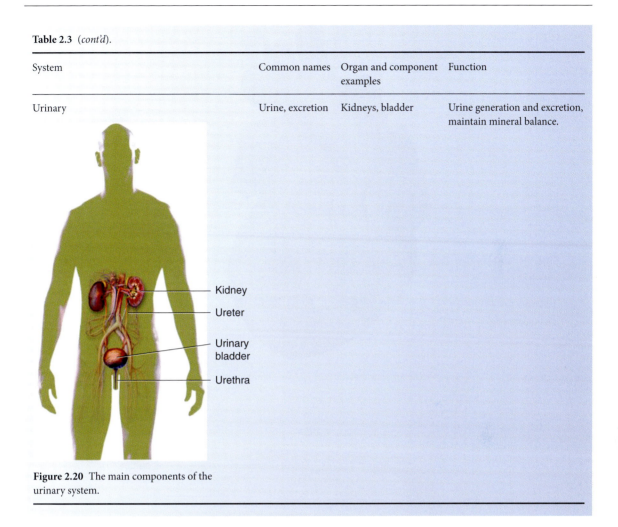

Kidney

Ureter

Urinary bladder

Urethra

Figure 2.20 The main components of the urinary system.

layers in their structure than most veins. The arteries are larger vessels that take blood from the heart to the various organs and parts of the body. Arteries sub-divide into arterioles and then into capillaries that supply the various cells of the body. In converse, venules and then the larger veins take blood back to the heart. The blood vessels have various names depending on the areas of the body they provide blood to. Examples include

Coronary: to and from the heart muscle tissue

Pulmonary: to and from the lungs

Others have specific names, such as the aorta (the largest artery in the body providing blood to the body) and the vena cava (superior and inferior veins being two of the main veins from the upper and lower parts of the body, respectively).

The heart lies slightly to the left side of the thoracic cavity, just above the diaphragm in an area known as the mediastinum (Figure 2.7). It does vary in size depending on the individual, but is approximately the size of a clenched fist in the same person. From the outside in, the heart consists of an external membrane (the pericardium) and a three-layered wall (consisting of an epicardium, myocardium and endocardium layer, from the outside in). The myocardium contains the muscle cells of the heart that are responsible for its pumping action. The endocardium is the innermost layer that lines the cavities of the heart and forms part of the heart valves. The heart is divided into four inner chambers (Figure 2.7). They make up two distinct pumping systems (a "right" and "left" system). Each pumping

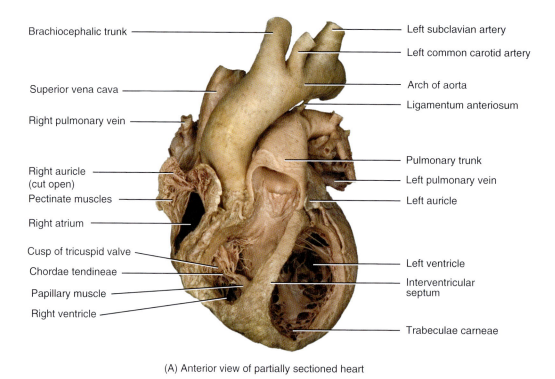

(A) Anterior view of partially sectioned heart

(B) Inferior view of transverse section of thoracic cavity
showing the heart in the mediastinum

Figure 2.7 The position and structure of the heart. (*Principles of Human Anatomy*, Gerard J. Tortora and Mark T. Nielsen, and John Wiley & Sons, 2011. This material is reproduced with permission of John Wiley & Sons, Inc.)

system consists of an upper chamber (called an atrium) and a lower chamber (the ventricle; Figure 2.7). In each system, the blood enters the atrium from the supplying veins, passes into the lower ventricles and is pumped out into the various arteries. The right system is called the pulmonary system, which takes blood being returned from the body and pumps it to the lungs to take up oxygen. The left system receives the oxygenated blood returning from the lungs and pumps it to the rest of body through the aorta. In both cases, the blood flowing through the heart is controlled by the muscles and four major valves (two in each system) to ensure a one-way flow of blood.

Function

The cardiovascular system has three major functions: transportation, protection and regulation:
- Transportation: blood carries various substances to and from the various cells of the body. Nutrients absorbed from the digestive system (see the section on the digestive system) and oxygen from the lungs (see section on respiration) are transferred to cells through the interstitial fluid surrounding them. Similarly, various wastes (including carbon dioxide) are taken up by the blood and transferred to various organs for elimination from the body (such as the skin, lungs, digestive system and kidneys).
- Protection from disease/damage: blood (in particular the platelets) can form clots that stop the loss of blood from the cardiovascular system (e.g. due to a cut on the skin) and allow for a platform from which the body can repair the damage. The blood also contains various types of cells (the white blood cells) and proteins (such as antibodies) that are actively involved in the body's immune system to protect it against the invasion of various microorganisms and associated diseases.
- Regulation: the blood system is involved in regulating the various body fluids, temperature and pH balance (how acidic or alkaline the blood is; see Chapter 6) to ensure proper functioning of the various organs and body parts.

Additional comments

Hematology is the study of blood, the tissues that form blood and the various types of blood diseases and disorders. The various different types of blood types are defined in hematology. For example, the ABO-type system of defined blood type is based on the presence of different types of proteins (in this case referred to as antigens) that are present on the surface of red blood cells;

individuals with only type A or B antigens are called types A or B respectively; those with both A and B are called type AB and those with neither are called type O. Similar antigens are used to define an individual as being type Rhesus$^+$ or Rhesus$^-$ (being the presence or absence of another type of antigen). These are important where the blood is being taken from one person and placed into another in a process known as transfusion, to ensure that the recipient does not have an adverse reaction to the transfused blood.

Other commonly used terms in the study of blood are "septicemia" (commonly known as blood poisoning), describing where microorganisms (particularly bacteria and their associated toxins) have entered the blood during an infection (Chapter 5), and "hemorrhage" describing the loss of a large amount of blood from the system either internally (inside the body) or externally (outside the body).

Cardiology is the study of the heart and associated diseases. An important example is coronary artery disease or disease of the arteries supplying the heart muscles. This is a leading cause of death in humans due to the development of restrictions in these blood vessels, which can in its most severe case lead to heart attacks. These conditions can be treated surgically in a procedure known as coronary artery by-pass grafting (CABG or by-pass surgery), where a blood vessel from another part of the body is taken out and attached to the affected artery to by-pass the blockage. Alternatively, this can be treated non-surgically by percutaneous transluminal coronary angioplasty (PTCA or balloon angioplasty), where a special type of device (known as a balloon catheter) is entered into the affected area, inflated to squash the blockage and then withdrawn.

Digestive

Introduction

The digestive system is responsible for the breakdown ("digestion") and absorption of the various foods and nutrients required for the structure and function of the body. The system consists of two parts: the gastrointestinal (GI) tract (or alimentary canal) and its associated organs (such as the liver and pancreas; Figure 2.8). The alimentary canal part is a continuous tube or tract that starts at the mouth, through the esophagus, stomach, small and large intestines, rectum and exits at the anus. It is extremely long (being ~6.5 m in length in a typical adult), but is folded in a way to fit into a smaller area. The basic structure in humans is described further in this section, but it is essentially similar in other mammals, although distinct in other ways (e.g. some mammals have a multi-chambered stomach, as opposed to a single chambered human stomach).

Structure

The GI tract, being one long continuous tubular structure, is made up of the same basic structure along its length, although there are distinct differences that reflect the various functions of the different areas of the tract (e.g. the stomach being primarily for mixing and initial digestion in contrast to the optimal structure in the small intestine for absorption of the various nutrients). The structure consists of four layers, from the outside into the body, being the outer serosa layer, the muscularis externa (containing various types and thicknesses of muscle tissue depending on the particular part of the GI tract), the submucosa (being rich in blood vessels and nerves) and finally the inner mucosa layer (including the innermost lining of epithelial cells that secrete fluids such as mucus and are also responsible for the absorption of nutrients to be taken up by the blood system). The GI tract consists of various organs; starting at the entry point these are the mouth, pharynx, esophagus, stomach, small intestine, large intestine, rectum and anus. The first part of the tract is referred to as the upper GI, extending from the mouth to the stomach, with the lower GI referring to the intestines and rectum/anus.

In addition, the accessory organs to the digestive system include the salivary glands, the liver, pancreas and gall bladder. These are briefly described in the following section.

The entry of the digestive system is the mouth (the oral or "buccal" cavity), which includes three types of accessory organs, namely the salivary glands, the tongue and the teeth (for further discussion on the teeth, refer to skeletal section). This area provides initial mechanical digestion of food (by mastication or chewing), as well as providing taste (or "gestation") due to the location of special sensory organs mainly on the surface of the tongue known as taste-buds). The accessory salivary organs (three types known as the parotid, submandibular and sublingual glands) produce a watery type secretion (known as saliva) into the mouth, which aids in lubrication and chemical digestion. Saliva consists mainly of water (~99%), but contains various types of enzymes (amylase and lipase) and salts. Enzymes are protein molecules that speed up a chemical reaction (but are not themselves changed in doing so); their primary role in digestion is in the breakdown of various types of food molecules. In this case, amylase breaks down starch

(a type of carbohydrate) and lipase breaks down fats (types of lipids) into smaller parts to allow their absorption further down the GI tract. Further discussion on enzymes and their use in cleaning chemistry applications is given in Chapter 6.

The food next moves into an area after the mouth known as the pharynx (or the throat), which acts in swallowing and passing food/liquids into the esophagus. The esophagus is a tube that runs from the pharynx to the stomach. Swallowing, or deglutition, is controlled by voluntary muscle contraction in the upper esophagus, to force food into the lower esophagus, where a process known as peristalsis ensures that the food is pushed along to the stomach. Both the pharynx and esophagus produce mucus, which aids in this process by lubrication. The stomach is an enlarged, J-shaped organ that acts as a mixing and digesting area before the intestine. As part of the digestive process it produces gastric juice (produced by gastric glands) and provides a more acidic environment for digestion. Gastric juice contains a low concentration of hydrochloric acid (HCl) and enzymes, such as pepsin (a protease) and gastric lipase that work optimally under acidic conditions; it is the combination of enzymatic and acidic processes that digest the various foods.

The stomach also controls thet rate of entry of food into the first part of the small intestine called the duodenum. Further digestion in this area is dependent on various accessories of the GI tract: the liver, gall bladder and pancreas, all adjacent to the duodenum. The liver is the largest organ in the body and is divided into lobes. Its structure is primarily made up of specialized cells known as hepatocytes; these cells perform many key roles in body metabolism including, as part of the digestive process, secretion of a substance known as bile (that is involved in the digestion and absorption of lipids). Other important functions include controlling carbohydrate (glucose) levels in the blood, controlling lipid and protein metabolism, detoxification of various substances harmful to the body, and nutrient storage (including carbohydrate, vitamins and minerals). Bile is stored in the gall bladder, located just outside the liver (Figure 2.8). The pancreas is also located adjacent to the duodenum and has two key functions: the majority of the cells that make up the pancreas are involved in the digestion process and produce pancreatic juice (its so-called exocrine function) and a smaller proportion of cells (known as the "islets of Langerhans") specifically produce hormones as part of the endocrine system (see section on the endocrine system and are therefore referred to as the endocrine function; the hormones include glucagon and insulin, both involved in the maintenance of glucose levels in the blood). Pancreatic juice contains multiple enzymes involved in the digestion of carbohydrates (e.g. amylase and trypsin), a lipase and others, in combination with water and salts.

The small intestine is made up of three regions (from the stomach to the large intestine): the duodenum, the jejunum and the longer part known as the ileum. It is in the small intestine that digestion continues and particularly absorption of nutrients into the body takes place, primarily due to its length and increased surface area due to the presence of many folds and finger-like projections known as villi on its internal surface. Specific types of cells produce mucus (known as goblet cells) and absorb nutrients ("absorptive cells"). Digestion is performed over time by a combination of the presence of bile, pancreatic juice and the production of intestinal juice. Intestinal juice is at a slightly neutral pH (pH 7.6) and is made up of primarily water, mucus and further enzymes (including those breaking down protein and carbohydrate). In all, about 90% of nutrients and water are absorbed in the small intestine. The remaining material next moves into the larger intestine, which is sub-divided into four regions known as the cecum, colon, rectum and the anal canal. It is in this area that any final absorption takes place, but particularly water, various vitamins and minerals, with any remaining material considered as feces and passed out of the body. The inner wall of the large intestine also contains specific absorptive and goblet (mucus-secreting, but in this case not enzyme secreting) cells, but does not have the same convoluted structure as the small intestine structure. Large amounts of bacteria are also present in the large intestine, which play an important role in the digestive and adsorption processes.

Functions

The major role of the digestive system is the acquisition of nutrients for the body and can be sub-divided into four functions:

• Ingestion, including the eating of food and drinking of liquids. This is performed in the mouth in combination with various accessory organs such as the tongue and teeth, to provide mixing.
• Digestion, which is performed both mechanically (e.g. in the mouth with the aid of teeth and in the stomach) and chemically. Chemical digestion includes the use of both acid and alkaline pH conditions, as well as the various enzymes produced during passage through the GI tract. During this process the various proteins, carbohydrates and lipids are broken down into smaller, absorbable molecules that are taken up by the body.
• Absorption, or the uptake of nutrients into the body (blood system; see the section on the cardiovascular system) is performed by specialized epithelial cells lining the inner surfaces of the system, and particularly in the small and large intestines.
• Defecation or waste removal, with the ridding of feces from the system.

In addition to their digestive functions the pancreas and liver, as accessory organs of the system, have other key roles. The pancreas is a major part of the body endocrine system (see the section on the endocrine system) and the liver is involved in toxic substance detoxification, nutrient metabolism and storage.

Additional comments

Gastroenterology is the study of the structure, function and diseases of the stomach and intestines, while proctology specifically relates to lower part of the GI tract (the rectum and anus).

Flexible endoscopes are instruments (or devices) that are used for minimal invasive diagnostic and surgical procedures (Chapters 4 and 15). Although they were initially designed for diagnostic purposes, for the direct visualization of various internal parts of the body and in particular the digestive system, they are being increasingly used for surgical procedures penetrating the internal surface of the various parts of the system. There are many types of endoscopes designed for use in different areas of the GI tract. these include:

• Colonoscopes: for "lower endoscopy" viewing, particularly the large intestine, by entering the anus
• Gastroscopes: for "upper endoscopy" viewing of the stomach by insertion through the mouth
• Duodenoscopes: for observing the duodenum and associated ducts (e.g. to the liver, gall bladder and pancreas) by insertion through the mouth and stomach

Endocrine
Introduction

The endocrine and nervous systems (see section on nervous systems) work together to control the various functions of the body. In the nervous system this is controlled by a connecting system of specialized cells (called neurons) that rapidly communicate with each other and various organs. In the endocrine system this is due to the production of specialized chemical substances, known as hormones. The system is made up of a diverse number of

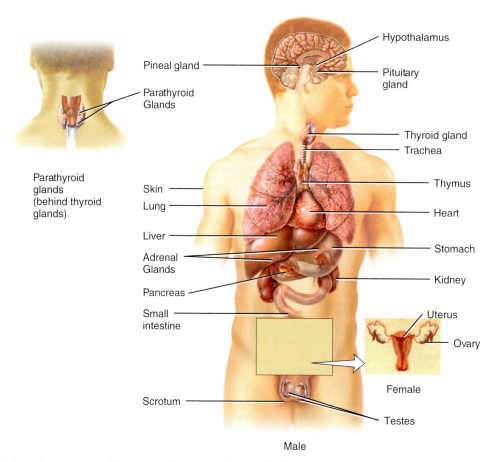

Parathyroid glands (behind thyroid glands)

Figure 2.9 The endocrine system. The location of the major endocrine glands is shown, in addition to various other parts of the body that contain endocrine tissue. (*Principles of Human Anatomy*, Gerard J. Tortora and Mark T. Nielsen, and John Wiley & Sons, 2011. This material is reproduced with permission of John Wiley & Sons, Inc.)

organs known as the endocrine glands and parts of other organs that contain endocrine tissue (Figure 2.9).

Structure

Endocrine tissue, either as part of a whole organ (specifically known as a "gland") or as part of another organ with other functions, is composed of specialized cells that produce the various different types of hormones. Glands are defined as specialized groups of cells within the body that secrete various substances and are sub-divided in anatomy into two types: the endocrine and exocrine glands. The endocrine glands secrete hormones into the body (being taken up into the blood that then transfers them to the various cells of the body) and exocrine glands secrete substances into specialized ducts for transfer to and even outside the body (e.g. the sweat glands in the skin, see the

section on the integumentary system, and the various digestive glands, see section on the digestive system). A summary of the major endocrine glands, the hormones they produce and their specific effects are given in Table 2.4. Many glands are primarily involved with hormone production (such as the adrenal and thyroid glands, they are known as the primary endocrine glands), while other organs are involved in many other functions for other systems. In addition to the organs listed in Table 2.4, these secondary organs include:

• The kidneys (urinary section) produce many hormones such as erythropoietin that controls red blood cell production.

• The heart (cardiovascular section) produces a hormone known as atrial natriuretic peptide (ANP) that is involved in controlling blood pressure.

Table 2.4 A summary of the major primary endocrine glands and secondary organs that contain endocrine tissue, with examples of the associated hormones they produce and their functions.

Endocrine gland/organ	Hormones produced	Function(s)
Major glands		
Hypothalamus	Hypothalamic releasing and inhibitory hormones	Control the release of various hormones from the pituitary gland

Pituitary gland	• Major hormone-producing gland of the body, including:
	  ○ Human growth hormone (somatotropin)
	  ○ Thyroid-stimulating hormone (thyrotropin) prolactin
	  ○ "Gonadotropins"
	  ○ Antidiuretic hormone (vasopressin)
		• Produces many hormones that control the functions of other endocrine glands:
		  ○ Stimulates production of a range of hormones that regulate growth and metabolism
		  ○ Control of the thyroid gland
		  ○ Milk production from the mammary glands
		  ○ A number of hormones involved in controlling the ovaries/testes
		  ○ Controls water loss from the body

Pineal gland	• Melatonin	• Involved in regulating the body's "biological clock" or rhythms. Other hormones and functions are proposed but are not fully defined.
Thyroid gland	• Thyroid hormones (thyroxine, triiodothyronine)	• Multiple functions including growth and cell metabolism.
Parathyroid gland	• Parathyroid hormone (parathormone)	• Bone breakdown ("reabsorption"; see section on skeletal system).
Thymus	• Thymosin • Thymic factor	• Control the production of cells involved in immunity (e.g. T-cells, section on lymphatic system).
Adrenal glands	• Produces a variety of hormones including: aldosterone, cortisol, epinephrine ("adrenaline")	• Water/salt blood level control. • Stress response (affecting glucose metabolism). • Stress response ("flight or fight").
Secondary organs (examples)		
Pancreas	Variety of hormones, but particularly glucagon and insulin	Blood sugar (glucose) level control. Glucagon raises and insulin decreases the levels in the blood.
Ovaries (in females)	Female sex hormones (e.g. estrogens and progesterone)	Regulates female productive cycle and the female body characteristics.
Testes (in males)	Male sex hormones (e.g. testosterone)	Regulates production of sperm and the male body characteristics.

• Various parts of the gastrointestinal tract (see digestive section) produce hormones that regulate digestion, such as gastrin (produced in the stomach and stimulate the local production of acid) and secretin (produced in the duodenum that stimulates secretion from the pancreas, e.g. the pancreas in the section on the endocrine system, the kidneys in the section on the urinary system and the testes/ovaries in the section on the reproductive system).

Hormones are released at very low concentrations, but have powerful effects on the cells they contact; but not all cells are capable of reacting with the various hormones when they are released, it will depend on the types of cells and the specific hormone. They are often classified into three types based on structures:

• Amino acid-derived, specifically from the amino acids tyrosine and tryptophan (e.g. thyroxine, adrenalin)
• Peptide or protein based (e.g. insulin)
• Lipid-based (e.g. testosterone)

Functions

The endocrine system, along with the nervous system (see the section on nervous system), are the informational and signalling systems of the body, essentially controlling the various body functions. The major roles of the endocrine system are:

- Controlling body growth and metabolism
- Controlling the expression of the male or female characteristics and reproduction (the process of generating offspring)
- Control of body rhythms and stress responses
- Regulation of body fluids, metabolism, various secretions and some immune (protection) functions

The specific functions of some of the major hormones produced from the endocrine system and that have been described in some detail are given in Table 2.4.

Additional comments

Endocrinology is the study of the endocrine system, including associated diseases. Hormone balance is importance to the various functions of the body, so much so that even slight imbalances can have significant physiological and emotional effects. For example, the various forms of diabetes are due to the inability of the body (specifically the pancreas) to produce or to use insulin effectively. Insulin is involved in stimulating (and therefore controlling) the lowering of glucose levels in the blood. Diabetes remains a major cause of death in humans. Other examples of endocrine-based diseases include polycystic ovary syndrome, hypothyroidism, osteoporosis and Addison's disease.

"Growth factors" are substances (or chemicals) that stimulate cell production, growth, differentiation (into the various types of cells) and even cell death. They include various types of hormones and cytokines. Cytokines are in many ways similar to hormones; they are protein based substances, with examples including the interleukins. They all essentially allow communication between cells/organs. In addition to their natural functions in the body, various growth factors are also used artificially in the treatment of certain blood and cancer diseases.

Integumentary

Introduction

The integumentary system includes the skin and its associated structures, taking its origin from Latin, meaning "to cover the body" (Figure 2.10).

The skin is actually the largest system in the body. It includes the skin itself, but also the various external structures attached to the skin that we can see, such as the hair and nails, and those within the skin structure that we do not see (such as sweat glands and sensory receptors).

Dermatology is the study of the structure and treatment of the integumentary system and its associated diseases.

Structure

If we section ("cut through") and examine the structure of the skin microscopically we find that it consists of three layers: the outer epidermis, the inner dermis and the lower hypodermis (or subcutaneous) layer (Figure 2.11). The epidermis is a thin, external layer of cells (a type of epithelial tissue; see introductory section); it is a tough structure, being composed of high concentrations of a certain type of protein called keratin that protects the more sensitive internal layers from damage. It is also this area that gives the skin color due to the production of a specific pigment known as melanin. The epidermis is continually growing from the inside out, accumulating more keratin as they grow out, to eventually become released from the surface as skin flakes or, in obvious excessive conditions such as "peeling" following sunburn or with dandruff. Beneath

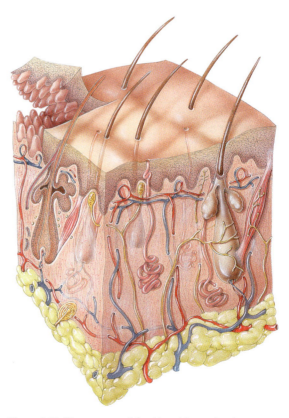

Figure 2.11 The structure of the skin, with associated components. (*Principles of Human Anatomy*, Gerard J. Tortora and Mark T. Nielsen, and John Wiley & Sons, 2011. This material is reproduced with permission of John Wiley & Sons, Inc.)

the epidermis is the dermis layer which is primarily composed of different types of tissues (connective tissues containing proteins such as collagen and elastin). The dermis gives the skin flexibility, but also strength. It is within this layer that we see many of the associated structures of the integumentary system, like the various glands, receptors and the basis for hair attachment, but in addition this layer includes blood vessels and nerves that provide nutrients/remove wastes (blood vessels) and allow for various sensing reactions (nerves). Glands include those that produce sweat ("sudoriferous") and oil ("sebaceous") glands. Finally, the subcutaneous (or "below the skin") layer is the innermost and is strictly not considered part of the true skin structure. This area also includes larger blood vessels and nerves supplying the dermis, but particularly is where fat (technically included in a further type of tissue known as "adipose tissue") is stored.

The main accessory structures of the skin are the hair, nails and glands. The hair is based in the dermis and grows out through the outer layers. The outer portion of the hair that we see is made up of dead cells containing keratin and other proteins. Nails are the same, but are more packed or dense to give them a harder, clear structure; the lower part of the nail is actively growing (alive), but then becomes inactive and dead as the structure grows out of the tips or fingers/toes. The final structures are glands; these are defined as groups of specialized cells or even organs (as in the case of the pancreas; see the section on digestive system) that produce various types of substances. These include hormones (referred to as the endocrine glands and discussed in the section on the endocrine system) and the exocrine glands that secrete salt, enzymes, water and other liquids. Examples of exocrine glands in the skin are the sebaceous and sudoriferous (sweat) glands. The sebaceous glands are generally associated with the base of hairs in the dermis (Figure 2.11) and secrete an oily liquid known as sebum (a mixture of proteins, lipids and salts); acne in teenagers, although a complicated condition, is often associated with over-production of sebum, but sebum has an important role in the various functions of skin (such as preventing drying). The sweat glands of various types (e.g. eccrine and apocrine) are also found in the dermis, but extend up to and at the surface of the epidermis (as in the case of the sweat pores on the skin surface). They produce mainly a mixture of water and salts, but may also include various types of proteins, lipids and other chemicals; it is interesting to note that in their excreted form they have little to no odor, but their presence on the skin can also allow for the growth of various types of bacteria/

fungi that naturally live on or in the skin (see below) and it is these that give rise of the various smells associated with sweat. They aid in regulating body temperature, protection from microorganisms (such as bacteria) and disposal of wastes. A further example of a modified sweat gland is the mammary gland (or breast); this actually gives the name to "mammals" or a group of animals that have these types of glands and produce milk as food for their young.

Overall, the skin is a remarkable, active and resilient structure.

Functions

The skin has many functions, many of which are not obvious. The most important and well-described of these are:

• Outer covering for and protection of the internal organs of the body. The skin essentially keeps us together. In addition to the obvious protection mechanism to prevent physical damage, including active repair of this damage as observed due wound healing, it also provides chemical inhibition to various types of microorganisms (such as bacteria and viruses) that may otherwise infect, damage and even penetrate the skin. A further mechanism is the production of melanin, which in addition to giving the color to the skin also offers some limited protection against damaging ultraviolet rays from the sun.

• Detection of various environmental conditions and sensory functions, such as cold, heat, chemical or microbial irritation (e.g. itching) and pain, which in itself is a protective mechanism for the body to prevent more serious damage.

• Temperature control, by sweat production and heat insulation (afforded by adipose tissue in the subcutaneous layer).

• Waste disposal, via sweat for example, which can include ammonia and urea as breakdown products within the body.

• Adsorption (the accumulation or taking-up) of some substances can occur at the skin surface, including some vitamins (A and D) and gases (oxygen, but to a limited extent). Medicine has often made use of this fact by the application of drug-impregnated patches onto the skin.

• Vitamin D-synthesis. Vitamin D is essential to human life and the skin is involved in its production.

• Blood reservoir. Up to 10% of the total blood in the body can be contained within blood vessel in the skin (particularly the dermis), which allows the body to control the need for blood (oxygen) at various times and control the body temperature.

Additional comments

As the outermost external structure of the body, the skin not only contains the various types of human cells, but actually co-exists with an even greater number of other microorganisms (Chapter 5). The actual numbers and types of microorganisms will depend on many factors, such as lifestyle and wet/dry areas of the skin. In general, the microbial flora or ecosystem of the skin is considered as being "resident" and "transient". The resident types are found on the skin of most people and are considered permanently present, including a variety of bacteria (e.g. *Staphylococcus* such as *S. epidermidis*, *Micrococcus*, *Propionbacterium*, and *Corynebacterium* species) and fungi (*Candida* and the dermatophytes such as *Microsporum*). Transient microorganisms can include any that are temporarily picked up by the skin and can include viruses (e.g., noroviruses), a variety of fungi and bacteria such as *Staphylococcus aureus* (including MRSA strains), *Clostridium difficile* (in vegetative and spore forms) and *Escherichia coli*.

Hand washing and skin cleaning therefore plays an essential role in preventing the transmissions of microorganisms from a patient or contaminated surface (such as medical or dental instrument) to another person (including yourself). This topic is further considered as an important strategy for infection prevention and control (Chapter 5).

Lymphatic

Introduction

In parallel to the circulatory (or blood) system, which transfers various nutrients, chemicals and gases around the body (see section on cardiovascular system), this is another transport system known as the lymphatic system. This system is closely linked to the structure and functions of the circulatory system. The system consists of various lymphatic tissues/organs, a series of lymph vessels and a watery substance that flows through the system known a lymph.

Structure

The lymphatic system is composed of the lymph, lymph vessels (conducting system for the lymph) and various lymphatic tissues and organs (Figure 2.12).

The lymph is essentially the same as the interstitial fluid that surrounds the various cells of the body. As a clear fluid, it is mostly composed to water (~92%) and various types of proteins, lipids/fats, minerals, hormones and white blood cells (WBCs; see the section on structure

under cardiovascular system). The WBCs are involved in protecting the body against the attack of various microorganisms, as part of the immune system (discussed later in this section). The blood system provides various components to this fluid, which exchanges nutrients (in) and wastes (out) of the various cells of the body. Part of this fluid exchanges back into the blood veins and through the circulatory system; the other part drains into the lymph system, where it is then referred to as lymph. The lymph is filtered into a network of lymph capillaries that form together to form larger lymph vessels. Lymph capillaries and vessels are similar in this sense to the structure of the veins (see the section on cardiovascular system). The vessels further drain into larger lymph trunks and finally into two major ducts (the thoracic and right lymphatic ducts), which are located just below the neck and feed directly into specific veins in this area.

The lymphatic system tissues and organs are distributed around the body, being associated with the lymph vessels. Lymphoid tissue itself consists of connective tissues, with associated types of WBCs (in particular, the lymphocytes). They consist of two major types:
• Primary tissues/organs, being the thymus and bone marrow. It is in these that the lymphocytes (known as T and B-lymphocytes) are made.
• Secondary tissues/organs, including the lymph nodes and lymphatic follicles present in various organs such as the tonsils, skin and spleen.

The lymph nodes vary in size and are present along the various lymph vessels through which the lymph passes on its return to the blood system. This allows for a close interaction with the various types of immune cells present, and they act as natural filters for the body to remove unwanted agents. The spleen is the largest organ consisting of lymphoid tissue in the body; in addition to its role in the lymphoid system, it is also responsible for the removal of aged red blood cells from the blood. Overall, there is a close connection between the circulatory and lymphatic systems of the body.

Functions

The lymphatic system has essentially three major functions in the body:
• Provides defence against the various microorganisms, or other foreign substances found in the body, playing a vital role in the immune system.
• Links to the functions of the digestive system; various lipids and lipid-soluble materials (such as vitamins A, D, E and K) are taken up by the lymph and transported to the blood through the lymphatic system.

• Controlling the levels of fluids around the various cells of the body, by draining into the lymphatic circulatory system and transferring lymph back to the blood system.

Additional comments

Immunity (or the body's resistance) is the ability of the body to protect itself against disease or damage. The human immune system consists of two main parts:

• Innate, non-specific immunity: this consists of the various organs, tissues, cells and substances that we are born with and defend the body from microorganisms in a non-specific manner. It can be further sub-divided into the front line of defence (such as the skin and mucous membranes providing a physical barrier to attack from these agents) and the second line defence. The second line includes types of cells known phagocytes, the body's inflammation and fever reactions, and the production of various antimicrobial chemicals (such as cytokines, further discussed in section on the endocrine system under additional comments). The innate system also interacts and actually activates adaptive immunity.

• Adaptive, specific immunity: this is composed of various types of cells (known as T and B-lymphocytes) that recognizes and attacks the presence of various microorganisms when it encounters them in a specific way. Therefore, this type of immunity is constantly developed through life, based on what we are exposed to. In addition to the specific reactions to the invading microorganism, this type of immunity provides a memory to the immune system, acting quickly against the microorganism if it is experienced in the future.

The adaptive response is the basis of immunization (or vaccination), where the body is exposed to a part of or an injured microorganism, allowing for the development of the response in the absence of disease. Examples include the BCG vaccine against tuberculosis (a disease caused by bacteria known as *Mycobacterium tuberculosis*) and the MMR vaccine (a combined vaccination against three viral diseases: measles, mumps and rubella).

When immunity is lowered (in patients this is described as being "immunocompromised"), the body can become very susceptible to infection from the various types of disease-causing microorganisms (that are known as pathogens; Chapter 5). A common example is observed during the progression of a disease known as AIDS (acquired immunodeficiency syndrome). This is caused by a virus known as HIV (human immunodeficiency disease), which actively attacks the human immune system. The virus specifically attacks certain types of T-lymphocytes, which over time are no longer available as part of the adaptive immune response. This leads to the patient becoming immunocompromised and open to infection by a variety of bacteria, viruses and fungi. It is the combination of infections with these microorganisms that eventually leads to death in these patients.

Muscular

Introduction

The muscular system (Figure 2.13), consisting of the various sizes and shapes of muscles, makes up about 45% of the body mass and is distributed around the body. It is the action of these various muscles that provide movement, internally and externally, in coordination with various other systems such as the nervous, circulatory and skeletal systems.

Structure

Muscle cells (also known as myocytes or muscles fibers) are arranged into bundles ("fascicles"), which are combined to give individual muscles. In the body there are three principal types of muscle tissue: skeletal, cardiac and smooth tissues. This classification is based on their structures, locations and functions. Skeletal muscles are primarily associated with the bones, being attached through specific connective tissues known a tendons (also see the section on the skeletal system); they are often referred to as "voluntary" muscles as they work when we decide to use them (e.g. for lifting and walking). Muscle tissues allow for movement by contracting and relaxing, primarily under control of the nervous system and expending energy. Cardiac tissues, as the name would suggest, are found in the walls of the heart; their control is considered "involuntary" in that we do not decide if they work or not and they play an important role in the pumping of blood (by the heart) around the circulatory system. Smooth muscles are also considered involuntary and are located within the structures of various other systems, such as blood vessels, the stomach and intestines, the skin, uterus and eye.

Functions

The primary functions of the muscular system are:
• Allowing for movement, including walking and lifting, as well as providing support and posture.
• It is the action of various tissues that allow for the passage of various substances through the body, including the intestines, airways and blood/lymph vessels.
• Heat generation: the heat generated by movement is used by the body to regulate the body temperature, being necessary for normal metabolism.

Additional comments

Myology is the study of muscles. All muscles of the body have specific names, such as the orbicularis oris (surrounding the mouth), rectus abdominus (in the belly), deltoid (shoulder) and soleus (lower leg).

Muscle cells consume a lot of energy during movement, which is generated by the production and expenditure of a chemical known as ATP (adenosine triphosphate); ATP is also used by other cell systems such as in bacteria. Note that ATP detection methods are sometimes used to evaluate bacterial contamination and/or presence of residual, patient soil on instrument surfaces (Chapter 8).

Some common medical problems associated with muscles include strains and tendonitis. A strain (also known as tear or pulled muscle) is due to the muscle becoming torn or broken, generally due to some kind of physical exertion (e.g. in sports). Tendonitis may also be caused by similar exertion, injury or disease, leading to inflammation of the tendons.

Nervous

Introduction

The nervous system, together with the endocrine system (see the section on the endocrine system), are responsible for communication and control in the body. The nervous system senses various stimuli (both outside and within the body) and can cause a reaction to senses, as well as providing the control of walking, talking, exercising, etc., and higher order effects such as memory. The major components are the brain, spinal cord and various nerves around the body (Figure 2.14).

Structure

Nervous tissue is made up of two unique types of cells: nerve cells (known as neurons) and glia cells ("neuroglia" or "glia"). Neurons are specialized cells that conduct signals (nerve impulses) along the nervous system; they can respond to various types of stimuli (e.g. heat sensors in the skin), cause an effect to happen (e.g. movement away from a source of heat) and even lead to the development of memory (e.g. hot may not be good). The glia cells support, maintain and protect the neurons.

The nervous system can be considered in two ways: functionally and anatomically. Functionally, the system can be considered in three parts: sensory (those parts that detect various stimuli, both external to and within the body), motor (that cause an effect, such as stimulating a muscle to move in connection with the skeletal system) and integrative (connecting between the sensory and motor functions, including the storing of information). Anatomically the nervous system can be sub-divided into two parts: the central nervous system (CNS) consisting of the brain (in the skull) and the spinal cord (that runs from the brain through the vertebral column of the back), and the peripheral nervous system (PNS), consisting of all the nerves extending from the spinal cord and through the rest of the body. The peripheral system includes various nerves (consisting of neurons, glia, connective tissue and blood vessels), ganglia (groups of neurons) and sensory receptors (e.g. in the skin, responding to various stimuli).

Think of the brain as a central computer that controls the body by sending and receiving messages, between the brain and various parts of the body through the spinal cord and a network of peripheral nerves. When the brain receives a message it sends a reply instructing the body in how to act. For example, if you touch a hot surface the nerves in the skin automatically send a message to the brain that registers as pain and sends a message back telling the muscles in the hand to pull away.

The brain is one of the larger and more complex organs of the body. Different areas have been identified as dealing with different functions, such as speech, hearing, smell, sight, movements, salivating, etc. Some of these centres are concerned with the information coming into the brain (sensory areas) and others are concerned with sending messages from the brain and making things happen (motor centres). The brain can be further sub-divided into three main sections (Figure 2.15):

• The forebrain (or "cerebrum") is the main part of the brain and further sub-divided into various sections known as lobes (e.g. the frontal lobe). In addition, various parts of the forebrain have been mapped to the control of various body functions, such as vision to the back of the cerebrum and speech/hearing more centrally.

• The midbrain is located underneath the middle of the forebrain, and is considered the master coordinator for all the messages going in and out of the brain.

• The hindbrain, sits underneath the back end of the forebrain, and consists of the cerebellum, pons and medulla. The cerebellum is responsible for balance, movement and coordination. The pons and the medulla, along with the midbrain, are often referred to as the "brainstem". The brainstem takes in, sends out and coordinates all of the brain's messages. It also controls many of the body's automatic functions, like breathing, heart rate, blood pressure, swallowing, digestion and

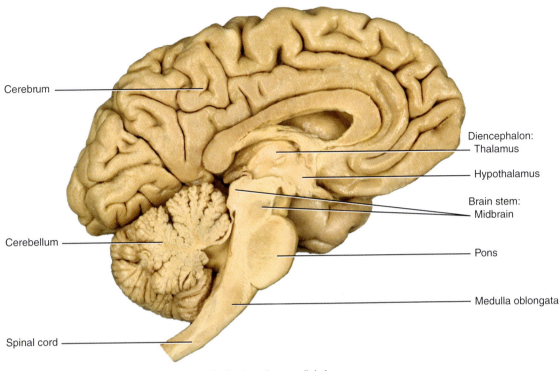

Cerebrum

Diencephalon:
Thalamus

Hypothalamus

Brain stem:
Midbrain

Cerebellum

Pons

Medulla oblongata

Spinal cord

Sagittal section, medial view

Figure 2.15 The basic structure of the brain, with main sections indicated. (Courtesy of Mark Nielsen, The University of Utah, Salt Lake City, UT, USA.)

blinking. If an individual has an injury to the brainstem they generally cannot survive without significant medical assistance.

The spinal cord extends from the hindbrain and through the vertebrae of the back (approximately to the lumbar area of the back); various nerves extend from the cord at various intervals along its length into various parts of the body.

The CNS (brain and spinal cord) is surrounded by three layers of protective membrane known as the meninges. These layers are called, from the outside in, the dura mater, arachnoid and pia mater. Between the inner two layers of the meninges is a water-like substance known as cerebrospinal fluid (CSF); it is a colorless fluid that is composed mostly of water, as well as various chemicals and nutrients. It is the combination of bones (the skull or vertebrae), the meninges and the CSF that protect the CNS from movement and damage.

Functions

The nervous system is overall responsible for communication and control in the body, by reacting to various

stimuli and causing reactions around the body. These include:

• Sensing, such as the five senses (sight, taste, touch, hearing and smell). This includes both external and internal environment sensing, as well as other functions such as movement and balance.

• Motor effects, causing movement or other responses to occur around the body (e.g. movement of muscles and release of hormones).

• Control and coordination of the various functions of the organs and systems of the body, including collaboration with the endocrine system and its associated hormones.

• Memory and intelligence.

Other comments

Neurology is the study of the nervous system (including its functions and associated diseases) and therefore a neurologist is a specialist in this area. Encephalopathy is any disorder of the brain.

Neurons are unique cells in the body as they do not have the ability to divide or reproduce; therefore they survive for the whole of our lives unless they are lost due to injury or disease. Therefore, loss or degeneration of neurons can lead to severe disease in patients, such as Parkinson's disease, Alzheimer's disease and Creutzfeldt-Jakob disease. Damage to the brain or spinal cord can lead to a variety of effects, including coma (a state of unconsciousness), encephalitis (inflammation of the brain, for example due to a virus infection), meningitis (inflammation of the meninges due to infection), dementia (loss of intelligence ability, often associated with the progression of age), and paralysis (loss of function/control of one or many limbs).

Reproductive
Introduction
Reproduction is the process of generating offspring. In humans and animals this is achieved by "sexual" reproduction, where the goal is the union of specialized cells (known as "gametes") in a process known as fertilization. The introductory section explained that most cells of the body contain the nucleic acid DNA in organized structures known as chromosomes; there are 46 chromosomes (23 pairs) in each cell, with the exception of the gametes that only contain one set (only 23 chromosomes). The males gametes are called sperm (or spermatozoa), which are produced in the testes (or testicles) and the female gametes are called oocysts that are produced from the ovaries. The testes and ovaries are organs known as "gonads". During fertilization (in the female), the gametes join together to form a new cell known as a zygote that contains 46 chromosomes (half from the mother and half from the father) and develops by cell division into an embryo. Over time, referred to as gestation or pregnancy, the embryo develops into a fetus and when fully developed is born (during parturition or labor) as an infant.

The human reproductive systems in males and females consists of the gonads (that not only produce the gametes but also the sex hormones as part of the endocrine system; see the section on the endocrine system), a system of ducts (to store and/or transfer the gametes), accessory glands and supportive structures (such as the penis in males and the vagina in females).

Structure
The male reproductive system (Figure 2.16a) consists of the testes (or testicles, held in the scrotum), various ducts (such as the epididymis that is attached to each testicle, storing the sperm, and vas (or ductus) deferens that transports the sperm from the epididymis to the urethra and out of the penis during ejaculation), accessory glands (such as the seminal vesicle and prostate gland) and supportive structures (in this case the penis and scrotum). The sperm are developed in the testes and the different associated glands add various substances to this (for transportation and protection purposes) to produce semen for ejaculation from the system into the female system. The testes also contain specific cells that produce the male sex hormone testosterone as part of the endocrine system (see section on the endocrine system).

The female reproductive system (Figure 2.16b) consists of the ovaries (on either side of the uterus), the uterine (or Fallopian) tubes (that transfer the oocysts released from the ovaries into the uterus), the uterus (where fertilization usually occurs, as well as the development of the fetus), the vagina (for receiving the penis during sexual intercourse and for passage of the fetus out of the system during birth) and also the mammary glands (or "breasts", for the production of milk and feeding of the newborn). The ovaries produce, develop and release the female gametes (oocysts) during a process known as ovulation during the female reproductive cycle. The cycle ends in menstruation ("period") or in fertilization and fetus development. Similar to the testes, the ovaries also produce various female sex hormones, such as progesterone and the estrogens, as part of the endocrine system (see the section on the endocrine system).

Functions
The primary function of the reproductive system is to produce offspring and the survival of the species. For this purpose the specific functions include:
- The generation of gametes (sperm in the testes and oocysts in the ovaries).
- Sexual intercourse.
- Fertilization and development of the fetus (in the female, specifically the uterus).
- Nourishment during development of the fetus, delivery and initial feeding (with milk) of the newborn infant.
- Production of the various sex hormones that determine the principle male or female traits (see section on endocrine system).

Additional comments
Gynecology is the branch of medicine that specializes in the study of the health associated diseases and disorders of the female reproductive system. Similarly, andrology is the branch of medicine associated with the male system. Both branches are closely related to urology, or the study of the urinary tract or "urogenital" systems (see the section on the urinary system).

In medical literature, a female is often designated by the symbol ♀ and males by the symbol ♂.

Respiratory

Introduction

Cellular respiration is the process used in human cells to produce energy (in the form of a molecule called ATP) from the various nutrients acquired through the digestive system (see the section on the digestive system). In addition to nutrients, cells also require oxygen (O_2) for respiration and the respiratory system provides a mechanism of acquiring oxygen for the body by breathing in air (that contains ~21% oxygen). In addition, the system expels a further gas (carbon dioxide, CO_2) that is a by-product of respiration; at high levels this can be toxic to cells, and it therefore is continually removed and expelled from the body. The respiratory system works closely with the cardiovascular (blood) system (see the section on the cardiovascular system) to take in oxygen (inspiration) and expel CO_2 (expiration). The system consists of various airways that passage air into the system and the lungs that allow gas (O_2 and CO_2) exchange. As examples of accessory functions, the respiratory system allows for speech and the sense of smell.

Structure

The respiratory system (Figure 2.17) is generally divided into two parts: the upper tract and the lower tract. The upper tract consists of the nose/mouth and pharynx (in the head/neck region) and the lower tract including the larynx (voice box), trachea (windpipe), bronchi and lungs (in the neck/thoracic cavity region).

The upper respiratory system channels air into the lower system and is mostly shared with the digestive system (mouth and pharynx; see the section on the digestive system). The nose and mouth provide the entry/exit points for air. The nose structure is part of the skull (being bone) but also a more flexible tissue known as cartilage (at the outer part of the nose; see the section on the skeletal system). Internally it contains the nasal cavities that extend back and deep into the head, below the brain and above the oral cavity (mouth); the nasal and oral cavities join at the back of the throat. The nasal passages are covered by mucous membranes that secrete mucus and also contain specialized sensing cells that are responsible for "olfaction" (the sense of smell). The area extending from the back of the nasal passages and the mouth, down towards the lower tract is known as the pharynx (or throat). Muscles in the pharynx play a role in digestion (swallowing) and contain the tonsils (part of the lymphatic system; see the section on the lymphatic system). For device and surgical reference, the pharynx is subdivided into three sections, from the back of the nose down: the nasopharynx, oropharynx and laryngopharynx. The pharynx channels air through the system and at the base of the laryngopharynx is the point at which the respiratory and digestive systems separate, at the larynx (voice box). The larynx connects to the trachea (windpipe); it contains cartilage in its structure that gives it strength but also contains the inner vocal cords (made of mucous membrane folds). Vibrations of the cords on the passage of air across them give sound. The trachea also has an internal mucous membrane layer and a rigid, external cartilage ring structure. The trachea separate into two bronchi just as they enter into either lung. The lungs are found in the thoracic cavity, in the rib cage and on either side of the sternum (see Figure 2.18 and the skeletal system). Each lung is maintained in a separate subcavity and protected by a pleural membrane. The lung itself is divided up into various lobes and contains the various extensions of the bronchi and other supportive tissues (such as connective tissues, blood vessels and lymph vessels). As the bronchi enter the lungs they further sub-divide to give a continuous airway deep in the lung structure; bronchi sub-divide into smaller diameter bronchi and even smaller bronchioles, similar to the roots of a tree and changing structure (e.g. losing cartilage) as they get smaller in size. At the ends of each bronchiole are alveolar ducts and various grape-like sub-divisions called alveoli. The alveoli are lined with specialized types of cells that allow for the diffusion (or passage) of gases in and out of the various capillary blood vessels of the lungs.

Functions

The primary functions of the respiratory system include:
- Intake of oxygen and removal of carbon dioxide as part of cellular respiration (the generation of energy in the body).
- Regulation of water and heat content in the body, along with other systems, as both are also expelled during expiration (breathing out).
- Regulation of the acidity/alkalinity (pH) levels in the blood, due to gas and water exchange.
- Providing the ability to speak/make sounds and smell, through associated organs and receptors.

Additional comments

The medical specialty dedicated to the lungs and associated parts of the respiratory system is known as pulmonary medicine (or pulmonology); therefore, the term "pulmonary" is linked in some way to this system. Specifically, the ENT ("ear, nose, and throat") specialty is known as oto-rhino-laryngology.

Anesthesia is defined as the ability to block or take away the sensation of pain. It is an important procedure during surgical and other procedures. Anesthetics can include processes and, more commonly, various types of drugs. It can be include local or regional anesthesia that has an effect at a certain region or even smaller area of the body; in these cases the drugs work outside the brain and are applied directly to the region/area in preparation for surgery/procedure. In contrast, as in the case of "general" anesthesia, the drugs work on the brain and can cause the patient to partially or fully lose consciousness ("sleep") and cannot be woken even when in pain. A variety of drugs are used for anesthesia and, in the case of general anesthesia this is usually administered to a patient intravenously (through a vein) or more commonly by inhalation (breathing) through the lungs. In this latter case the drugs are mixed with a carrier gas and are absorbed into the body through the respiratory system. This can be a complex process, in preparing, administering, monitoring and reviving the patient; those specializing in anesthesiology are called anesthesiologists or anesthetists.

Asthma, where a patient is diagnosed with repeated difficulty in breathing, is due to reoccurring inflammation of the lungs and associated airways (particularly the bronchi, which become narrower and restrict the passage of air); the condition can range from mild to severe, even leading to respiratory failure and death. Its exact cause is often unclear, but it is known to be affected by the genetics of the patients and his/her environment. Other diseases/conditions of the respiratory tract include:
- Laryngitis: inflammation of the inner membranes of the larynx, often associated with a loss of voice and commonly due to microbial infections.
- Bronchitis: inflammation of the bronchi (mucous membranes), often associated with viral infections such as influenza (common cold) but also some bacteria.
- Pneumonia: inflammation of the lungs, also commonly due to a wide range of microorganisms including bacteria (such as *Steptococcus pneumoniae* and *Mycobacterium tuberculosis*), viruses and fungi.

Upper respiratory tract (ear, nose and throat (ENT)) endoscopy and bronchoscopy are types of procedures using special types of devices known as endoscopes (see Chapters 4 and 15) for direct visualization of the upper and lower respiratory tracts, respectively.

Skeletal (including dental)
Introduction
The human skeletal (or bone) system consists of 206 bones that are organized in a structure known as the skeleton (Figure 2.18). It is the skeleton structure that gives the body its characteristic shape and support. In the study of anatomy, the skeleton is sub-divided into two parts: the axial and appendicular. The axial skeleton consists of the central part of the structure, including the cranium (skull), vertebral column (running down the back), the sternum (long flat bone in the centre of the chest), hyoid bone (in the neck), and the associated ribs (in the chest). The appendicular skeleton consists of the pectoral (or shoulder) girdle (consisting of two clavicles (collar bones) and two scapula (shoulder blades) bones), the pelvic (or hip) girdle (consisting of two coxal or hip bones) and their associated limbs (the arms and legs respectively, also known as the upper and lower limbs).

In addition to the skeleton, the dental system is considered briefly in this section. These are made up of the teeth (or "dentes") in the mouth and are specific organs associated both the skeletal and the digestive system (see the section on the digestive system).

Structure
Due to their strength and structure, it is a common misconception that bones are dead; bones are actually active, continually regenerating structures consisting of unique types of cells and tissues. Bone (or osseous) tissue is made of four types of bone cells: osteogenic cells, osteoblasts, osteocytes and osteoclasts. Osteogenic cells are actively dividing cells in the inner bone structure, which subsequently stop dividing and develop into osteoblasts and then osteocytes. The osteoblasts produce an external matrix that surrounds the cells, which gives bone its unique, hardened structure. This matrix consists of 25% water, 25% collagen (a type of protein) and 50% salt crystals. The crystals are made up primarily of hydroxyapatite (a combination of two salts: calcium phosphate $[Ca_3(PO_4)_2]$ and calcium hydroxide $[Ca(OH)_2]$) mixed with other salts (e.g. calcium carbonate) and ions (e.g. fluoride). It is the combination of collagen and salt crystal production and deposition that give bone strength, in a process known as calcification. As the osteoblasts become entrapped in the calcification process, they develop into osteocytes; osteocytes are not dormant but are actively involved in maintaining bone structure in the exchange of nutrients and waste materials with blood supply. As bone is generated, it is also continuously broken down by

Table 2.5 The various types of bones in the skeletal system.

Skeleton structure	Common name	Description
Axial		
Cranium	Skull, head	The skull is composed of various cranial and facial bones. The cranial bones surround and protect the brain. The facial bones give the face structure and support, while also supporting the dental system (teeth) and, along with the cranial bones, other organs such as the eyes, nose and ears. Example of facial bones include the mandible or lower jaw bone that is the only movable bone in the skull, carrying the lower teeth and the maxillae, supporting the upper teeth.
Vertebral column	Spine or backbone	Consists of 33 bones known as vertebrae arranged in a column. They protect the spinal cord and give upright support. They are further sub-divided into the cervical (neck), thoracic (chest or upper back), lumbar (loin or lower back), sacral (consisting of four fused bones) and the coccyx (four fused bones) vertebrae.
Sternum	Breastbone	Large flat bone in the centre of the chest
Ribs	Ribs	24 bones arranged in 12 pairs. They all are attached to the vertebrae and some are also attached to the sternum. The ribs and sternum provide protection to the main organs in the chest, such as the heart and lungs.
Appendicular		
Pectoral girdle	Shoulder	Consists of two clavicles (collar bones, along the front) and two scapula (shoulder blades, to the back). Can be considered part of, and are attached to, the upper limbs.
Upper limbs	Arms	Consists of 30 bones and divided into three areas (from the girdle end down): the humerus (upper arm), the ulna and radius (forearm), and the hands. The hands are divided into eight carpal bones (carpus or wrist), five metacarpals (the palm of the hand) and 14 phalanges (making up the fingers and thumb; each bone is a *phalanx*).
Pelvic girdle	Hips	Two hip bones (coxal or pelvic bones). They are joined together at the front (anterior) of the body and interact with the vertebral column (the sacrum). Can be considered part of, and are attached to, the lower limbs. There is a distinct difference between the structures of male and female pelves.
Lower limbs	Legs	Consists of 30 bones, similar to the upper limbs, and divided into four areas (from the girdle end down): the femur (upper leg), the patella (kneecap), the tibia and fibula (lower leg) and the feet. The feet are divided into seven tarsal bone (tarsus or ankle), five metatarsals (in the centre of the foot) and 14 phalanges (making up the toes).

the final type of bone cells, the osteoclasts. These specialized cells are found in the inner bone structure and break down the bone tissue by the production of acids and enzymes (this process is referred to as readsorption).

There are two main types of bone tissue, compact (or "dense") and spongy (or "cancellous") bone, which differ in overall structure; in general, compact bone tissue is found on the surface of bones and spongy tissue in the interior. Finally, as an active structure, the various bones are supplied by nerves (nervous system), muscles and a blood supply (as part of the cardiovascular system). A brief summary of the major parts and bones of the skeletal system is given in Table 2.5.

A joint (or "articulation") is where two bones meet, being designed to allow for movement between bones and for mechanical support. There are many types of joints that vary in structure, including fibrous, cartilaginous and synovial joints. In all of these cases, muscles are attached to bones by specialized structures known as tendons (or sinews). Ligaments join bones together and fascias connect muscles to each other. All of these are similar in structure, composed of collagen fibers.

Special consideration should also be given to the dental system or teeth. They are associated (in the mouth) with the mandible (lower jaw) and maxillae (upper jaw) bones of the cranium (Table 2.5). Humans have 20 deciduous (or primary) and 32 permanent (or secondary) sets of teeth. The first set develop early in life, consisting of (from the back of the mouth forward and on each side of the mouth) two molars, one canine and two incisor teeth in each jaw. These are lost typically between the ages of 6 and 12 and replaced by the permanent teeth consisting of (from the back of the mouth forward and on each side of the mouth) three molars, two premolars, one canine and two incisor teeth in each jaw (Figure 2.19); the innermost molars (known as the third molars or "wisdom" teeth) are often not formed or displayed in the mouth.

A single tooth consists of three sections: the outer and visible crown, the neck (at the gum line) and the root (Figure 2.19). From the outside in, a tooth has an external covering of white enamel composed of hydroxyapatite (composed of calcium phosphate and calcium carbonate, being stronger than even bone structures). Within the enamel is the dentin layer, also an extremely strong structure consisting of calcified connective tissue (produced by cells known as odontoblasts) and a central space known as the pulp cavity, consisting of connective tissue, nerves, blood and lymph vessels. Teeth are embedded and supported in the mouth by the periodontium. This consists of four parts: the cementium (being part of the tooth, surrounding the dentin in the root of the tooth; Figure 2.19), periodontal ligaments, alveolar bone and gingiva (or "gum"). The ligaments attached the tooth (specifically the cementium) to the alveolar bone, which is covered externally by the gingiva (consisting of mucosal tissue).

Functions

There are five main functions of the skeletal system:
- Providing support to the body and its structures, such as various types of attached tissues and associated organs.
- Protection for various essential organs, including the lungs, brain and heart.
- Allowing for movement, with the interaction of the muscular system.
- Blood cell production: some bones contain a specific type of tissue known as red bone marrow (or myloid tissue). These include the hip bone, ribs, femur and humerus. This tissue produces various types of blood cells, such as red blood cells (RBCs), white blood cells (WBCs) and platelets (see the section on the cardiovascular system). These cells are produced in the marrow and broken down in the liver.
- Storage: the bone provides storage of various types of essential minerals (such as calcium and phosphate) and lipids (triglycerides). The triglycerides are stored in "yellow bone marrow", which is primarily made up of adipose (or "fat") tissue. Triglycerides are an important source of energy and yellow marrow is most commonly found in the inner parts of bones such as the femur, tibia and humerus. The dental system is used for biting and grinding food, as part of the digestive system (see the section on the digestive system).

Additional comments

Cartilage is a similar structure to bone, but is more flexible in structure. It is a type of connective tissue made up of specific cells known as chondrocytes, that also produce an extracellular matrix including protein (collagen or elastin) fibers and a gel-like substance (chondroitin sulphate). Cartilage is primarily found at the end (or joints) of bones as well as in specific structures such as the nose, ears and bronchial tubes (see the section on the respiratory system).

"Osteo-" is a prefix associated with bone. Examples include the various types of bone cells (e.g. osteoblasts) and associated diseases. Osteoathritis is a joint-based disease, where the cartilage around the bone ends in joints degenerates (or breaks down) over time due to wear and tear. Similarly, rheumatoid arthritis (RA) is also associated with degeneration of cartilage, but in this case due to the body's reaction against itself. In these cases the body's immune system (see section on lymphatic system) reacts against the joint structure, leading to damage and breakdown. A further commonly used suffix is "arthro-", which is in reference to a joint; examples include arthroplasty (a surgical procedure relating to the reconstruction or replacement of a joint) and arthroscopy (the surgical examination and repair of the interior of a joint by minimal invasive surgery (MIS) using specific type of endoscope known as an arthroscope).

Rheumatism refers to any naturally (not due to infection or injury) occurring pain associated with the skeletal system (including the bones, tendons, ligaments and associated muscles).

A "fracture" is a break in any bone. Examples include open, closed, simple, multi-fragmentary and stress fractures. An open (or compound) fracture is where the bone breaks and penetrates through the skin so that it can be seen; a closed fracture is therefore where the bone does not break through the skin. A simple fracture is when the bone breaks along one line, while multi-fragmentary (or *comminuted*) are more serious in that the bone is broken at multiple sites. A stress fracture is composed of smaller or minor fractures in the bone but not necessarily showing any obvious break in the bone.

Dentistry is the science of diagnosing, preventing and treating diseases of the teeth, gums, and related structures of the mouth. Specifically, endodontics is concerned with the more inner structures of the teeth (the pulp, root and alveolar bone) and periodontics relating to those tissues around the teeth (such as the gums). Orthodontics is concerned with the prevention and correction of teeth alignment within the mouth.

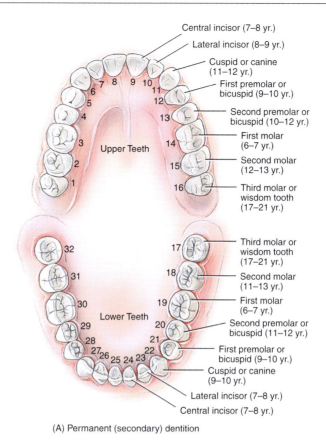

Central incisor (7–8 yr.)
Lateral incisor (8–9 yr.)
Cuspid or canine (11–12 yr.)
First premolar or bicuspid (9–10 yr.)
Second premolar or bicuspid (10–12 yr.)
First molar (6–7 yr.)
Second molar (12–13 yr.)
Third molar or wisdom tooth (17–21 yr.)

Upper Teeth

Third molar or wisdom tooth (17–21 yr.)
Second molar (11–13 yr.)
First molar (6–7 yr.)
Second premolar or bicuspid (11–12 yr.)
First premolar or bicuspid (9–10 yr.)
Cuspid or canine (9–10 yr.)
Lateral incisor (7–8 yr.)
Central incisor (7–8 yr.)

Lower Teeth

(A) Permanent (secondary) dentition

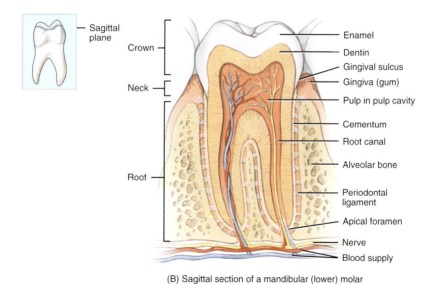

Sagittal plane

Crown
Neck
Root

Enamel
Dentin
Gingival sulcus
Gingiva (gum)
Pulp in pulp cavity
Cementum
Root canal
Alveolar bone
Periodontal ligament
Apical foramen
Nerve
Blood supply

(B) Sagittal section of a mandibular (lower) molar

Figure 2.19 The dental system. (A) The permanent teeth of an adult human (third molars shown) and (B) The structure of a tooth. (*Principles of Human Anatomy*, Gerard J. Tortora and Mark T. Nielsen, and John Wiley & Sons, 2011. This material is reproduced with permission of John Wiley & Sons, Inc.)

Urinary

Introduction

The urinary (or excretory) system works closely with the cardiovascular system (see the section on the cardiovascular system) for waste disposal and maintenance. It consists of the kidneys (two) and a series of transport tubes and storage vessels. The kidneys are constantly filtering the blood to remove various wastes (such as urea and ammonia that can be toxic at high concentrations in the body), but also in reabsorbing back into the blood various components (such as water and salts) necessary for fluid/electrolyte balance; the end result is a concentrated liquid waste known as urine. The urine is initially stored in the body and then discharged from by the body during urination.

Structure

The urinary system includes the kidneys, ureters, the bladder and urethra (Figure 2.20).

The kidneys are the main organs of the system, being responsible for most of its primary functions. Internally they are divided into two distinct areas: the external cortex and the internal medulla. Blood enters the kidneys and is transferred via the blood vessels to specialized structures known as nephrons, which start in the cortex and extend into the medulla. At the cortex level, the blood vessels make contact with the entry to the nephrons and, under pressure, cause various components of the blood to filter into nephrons. The resulting fluid (which is notably some hundred times the volume of the final urine) then passes through the rest of the nephron structure where various components are reabsorbed back into the surrounding blood supply (such as water and minerals) and further exchange of wastes from the blood vessels to the nephrons can occur. The resulting urine is collected by various tubules in the medulla region that combine to exit the kidney structure and into a ureter tube that extends from each kidney to collect into the bladder for storage. The bladder acts as a hollow reservoir. When the bladder fills, this creates a pressure that triggers the requirement and eventually necessary release of urine through the urethra and out of the body. The release of urine from the body is referred to as urination or micturition.

Functions

The urinary system functions include:
• The removal of various wastes and foreign chemicals (such as drugs and/or their by-products) from the blood and release from the body.
• Regulation of blood composition and volume. In addition to the removal or water, salts and wastes, essential chemicals (such as water, sodium and calcium) can be reabsorbed, pH levels are regulated (by uptake of ions) and blood pressure can be controlled.
• The kidneys produce some hormones, as part of the endocrine system (see the section on the endocrine system), including erythropoietin that is involved in the control of red blood cell production.

Additional comments

Urology is the branch or medicine that deals with the urinary system, while nephrology particularly relates to the study of the kidneys. The term "renal" also pertains to the kidneys. There is a physically close relationship between the urinary and reproductive systems (see the section on the reproductive systems), which are often medically referred to together as the genito-urinary (or urogenital) system.

Urinalysis is the analysis of the urine for the purpose of medical diagnosis or monitoring. A urine sample is taken from a patient and can be subjected to various chemical and (if required) microbiological analysis as an indication of health or disorder. Urine is normally ~95% water, with the remaining 5% containing various chemicals such as urea, uric acid, ammonia and minerals/salts (such as sodium and potassium). In various conditions, the composition of urine can change dramatically and can indicate different internal disorders, diseases, diets, etc. Urine, for example, is generally free of bacteria and the presence of certain types of bacteria can be indicative of a urinary tract infection (called a UTI). Chemically, the presence of blood (and therefore bleeding) may indicate damage to the various tissues/components of the system.

The system can be very robust, but when it is not working effectively it can be life threatening. Dialysis is a medical intervention that can act as an alternative, artificial system and is used in patients with damaged or diseased kidneys. "Hemodialysis" uses a machine to take blood from a patient, remove the wastes in the machine and then return it to the patient. "Peritoneal" dialysis is performed within the patient, where a sterile fluid is added into the abdominal cavity and the surrounding peritoneal membrane that encloses the cavity acts as a substitute membrane for the exchange process with the blood; the fluid is maintained for a given time and then removed/discarded.

Like many other natural orifices of the body, endoscopes can be used for the direct visualization, investigation and treatment of various parts of the urinary system. Procedures include cystoscopy (investigating the bladder by entry through the urethra) and ureteroscopy (entry through the urethra and bladder to access the ureters).

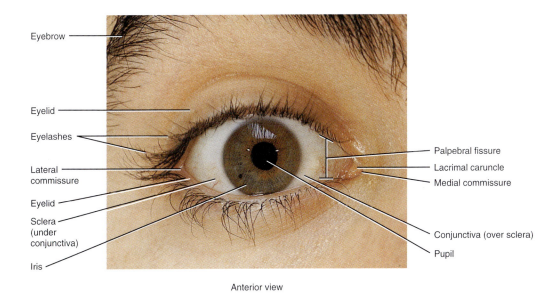

Anterior view

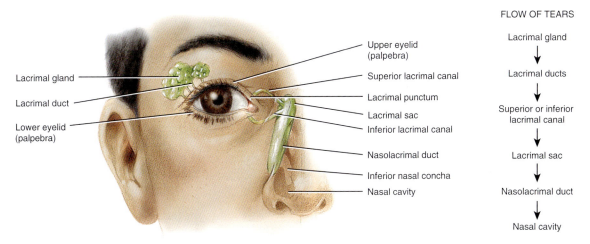

Anterior view of the lacrimal apparatus

Figure 2.21 The external and internal structure of the eye. (*Principles of Human Anatomy*, Gerard J. Tortora and Mark T. Nielsen, and John Wiley & Sons, 2011. This material is reproduced with permission of John Wiley & Sons, Inc.)

Additional structures

There are two additional structures of the body that are briefly introduced and described in this section. They are the eyes and the ears, both of which work closely with the nervous system for the full scope of their functions.

Eyes

The eyes (Figure 2.21) are responsible for the sense of sight (the detection of light). They are ball-shaped and associated with the skull (see the section on the skeletal system). From the outside we can see some of the internal structures at the front of the eye, including the sclera (the white surface that surrounds most of the eye), the iris (which is colored) and the central pupil (central black circle). The front of the eye contains various structures such as the cornea, pupil, iris and lens; they are all involved with allowing light to enter and be focused into the eye. Most of the eye's innermost wall is a specialized surface known as the retina. The retina contain the photoreceptors that respond to the presence of light; there are two types of receptors known as the rods (that react to dimmer

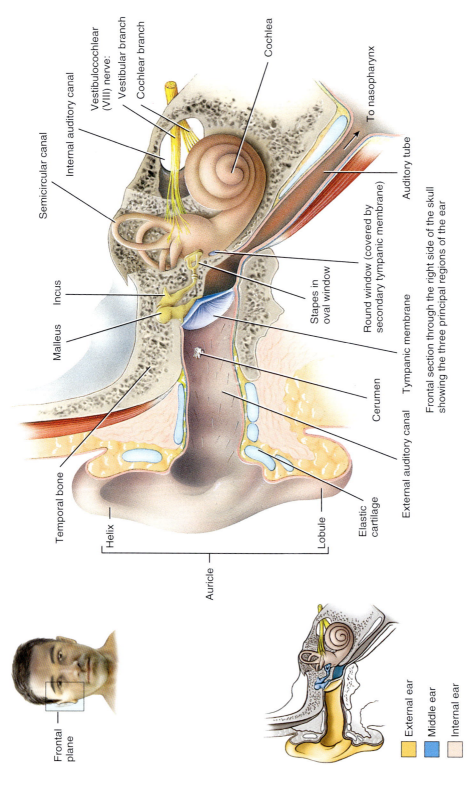

Figure 2.22 The external and internal structures of the ear. (*Principles of Human Anatomy*, Gerard J. Tortora and Mark T. Nielsen, and John Wiley & Sons, 2011. This material is reproduced with permission of John Wiley & Sons, Inc.)

Frontal plane

Semicircular canal

Internal auditory canal

Vestibulocochlear (VIII) nerve:

Vestibular branch

Cochlear branch

Cochlea

Temporal bone

Incus

Malleus

Helix

Lobule

Auricle

Stapes in oval window

Round window (covered by secondary tympanic membrane)

Tympanic membrane

Cerumen

External auditory canal

Elastic cartilage

To nasopharynx

Auditory tube

Frontal section through the right side of the skull showing the three principal regions of the ear

External ear

Middle ear

Internal ear

light, showing blacks, whites and grays) and the cones (that react to show various other colors). These receptors convert light to nerve pulses along nerve fibers that collect at the back of the eye to form the optic nerve. The eyeball is filled with a jelly-like substance known as vitreous humor that helps maintain the eyeball shape and protects the retina.

Ophthalmology (or optometry) is a medical speciality dealing with the eye and associated structures. The terms "ocular" and "optic" pertain to the eye and/or to light (e.g. fiberoptic or ocular diseases).

Ears

The ears (Figure 2.22) are responsible for the sense of sound (detection of vibrations). They are located on either side of the head and project into the skull. The ear structure consists of three areas: the outer, middle and inner ear. The main, external part of the ear is called an "auricle" and functions in funnelling sound waves into the ear. The auricle leads to the entry into the ear, along the auditory canal and to the eardrum (known as the tympanic membrane); the outer ear consists of the region from the auricle to the eardrum. The middle ear, on the other side of the eardrum, is a small cavity containing some of the smallest bones in the body known as the ossicles: malleus (hammer), incus (anvil) and stapes (stirrip). In that order the joint

formed by these three ossicles provides a link from the eardrum to the oval window, a membrane that separates the middle and inner ear. The middle ear is also linked, by the auditory (or Eustachian) tube, to the upper pharynx (see the sections on digestive system and respiratory system). The inner ear (or "labyrinth") consists of a series of fluid filled channels, such as the semicircular canals and the cochlea. Sound is detected by directing sound waves into the outer ear leading to vibrations on the eardrum; these vibrations are amplified through the bones of the middle ear and the interaction of the stapes along the oval window causes pressure changes in the inner ear structures. These pressure changes are converted into nerve pulses along a network of nerves in the inner ear that combine and leave the ear structure as the vestibulocochlear nerve. Although the ear detects sound, it is the transmission and interpretation of the signals that are transmitted to the brain that also form differentiation of language, music, etc. In addition to hearing, the ear plays an important role in maintaining body balance.

Otology is the study of the ear and accessory structures, including various diseases and disorders. The ear, nose and throat are all connected through the pharynx (see the sections on digestive system and respiratory system) and are often considered under the same medical speciality (ENT and by ENT specialists).

3 Medical and surgical procedures and facilities

Introduction

The word "medical" refers to the study and practice of medicine, which is the science of and ability to heal. Generally, it refers to the specialty concerned with the diagnosis, management and particularly, non-surgical treatment of diseases, either of one particular organ system or of the body as a whole. Examples of medical procedures include observation (visually inspecting the patient's skin color, weight, teeth, temperature, blood pressure and pulse rate) and specific therapeutic treatment (prescribing drugs, dialysis, chemotherapy, wound therapy, etc.). An important medical term that is worth defining is "diagnostic", which refers to a variety of observations and/or tests that can be performed in order to identify (diagnose the cause of) a particular disease or medical problem, and providing the supporting evidence such as the cause. Examples of diagnostic procedures include various types of endoscopy, cardiac stress tests, blood tests, X-rays, etc. The term "surgical" refers to a specialty in medicine that investigates or treats disease or injury by an operative procedure. Surgical procedures (or "operations", "surgery") involve entering the body or body cavities by incision (breaking through the skin or other area of the body). Surgical specialties focus on the various operative and instrumental techniques to treat disease/injury, generally classified according to the organ, organ system or tissue involved (Chapter 2). It should also be pointed out that many surgical procedures are not specifically for the treatment of disease or injury, with examples being to enhance body appearance or function (such as in many cases of cosmetic surgery), and for various physical, cultural and even religious reasons (such as circumcision and tatoos). In medical, diagnostic and surgical procedures, a variety of instruments and devices can be used with, on or in patients. When these are re-used from patient to patient, decontamination plays an essential role in reducing any health risks.

Medicine can be further sub-divided into three areas of care: primary, secondary and tertiary:
• Primary care is care provided by health professionals who have first contact with a patient seeking treatment. This contact most often occurs in a doctor's office, clinic, nursing home, school, etc.
• Secondary care is provided to patients who are generally referred to hospitals, specialists and specialized clinics by primary care providers, either for diagnosis or further specialist treatment.
• Tertiary care is specialized, highly technical care that includes diagnosis and treatment of disease and disability. The patient is usually referred by primary or secondary medical care personnel for specialized care, for example intensive care, advanced diagnostics, long-term care, etc. Various types of diagnostic, surgical and medical procedures can be performed in any of the above areas depending on the nature of the procedure, risks of patient complications and available facilities. Minor procedures can be considered routine and performed in a physician's office, dental office or opticians, whereas more complicated procedures require a full medical team and are usually restricted to dedicated hospital or clinic settings. These facilities can range from a procedure room to a specially designed area equipped with modern imaging, lighting, equipment and self-contained air handling systems (Figure 3.1).

Despite the design of these facilities, and regardless of the economic status of different geographic regions of the world, the same essential policies and procedures can be enforced to ensure the safe reprocessing of re-usable instrumentation and devices used for these procedures. The various different types of instruments are described further in Chapter 5. As outlined in Chapter 1, in the section on goals of decontamination and the Spaulding

A Practical Guide to Decontamination in Healthcare, First Edition. Gerald McDonnell and Denise Sheard.
© 2012 Gerald McDonnell and Denise Sheard. Published 2012 by Blackwell Publishing Ltd.

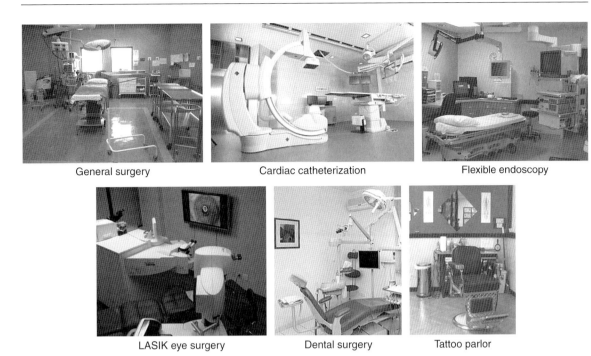

General surgery   Cardiac catheterization   Flexible endoscopy

LASIK eye surgery   Dental surgery   Tattoo parlor

Figure 3.1 Examples of the various types of facilities in which medical and surgical techniques are in use worldwide. Although the design and investment in such facilities can range dramatically depending on the patient procedure and country-specific economic situation, the essential practices of decontamination of instrumentation should remain the same.

classification a variety of medical and surgical instrumentation is used across the world; a standard system is recommended for the reprocessing of instrumentation and devices based on the risk to an individual or patient. This system, known as the Spaulding classification, is based on the use of the instrument or device on a patient, recommending a higher standard of reprocessing (e.g. disinfection or sterilization) as the risks of the introduction of microbial contamination to that patient are considered greater (Chapter 1, in the section Goals of Decontamination and the Spauldings Classification). For example, if an instrument is introduced into or comes in contact with a patient's blood supply or sterile space it carries a higher risk to that patient than a procedure that would only touch the intact skin. This classification system is not always as simple to apply as it appears, given the design of a facility or area in which a medical or surgical procedure is being conducted. It is expected that the highest levels of reprocessing standards should be applied to the higher risk surgical instruments and devices that enter essentially sterile areas of the body, such as those used in neurosurgery (into the brain or spinal cord), orthopedic surgery (e.g. knee and hip implants) and cardiothoracic (e.g. heart) surgery. Most, if not all, of

these types of procedures should be conducted with sterile instruments and devices and in dedicated surgical rooms (surgical theatres/suites). However, procedures that may also be considered as requiring sterile instrumentation and techniques are often performed in other facilities such as dental practices, cosmetic surgery clinics, procedure rooms and tattoo parlors, where the patient blood system may be entered. Although the design of such facilities may be dramatically different, the reprocessing standards should remain the same as the risk to the patient is just as high.

Historical methods of surgical intervention often were associated with exposing internal body organs and tissues to the air for long periods of time, therefore exposing the patient to a greater risk of infection. Newer methods and techniques of medical and surgical interventions (e.g. using various types of endoscopic instrumentation for "keyhole" or minimally invasive surgery) are less invasive than historical methods, shortening the surgery time and reducing trauma to the patient. The complex equipment used today for these procedures can present a challenge for any reprocessing area as it is often more difficult to perform safe and effective decontamination and can therefore result in an increased risk of infection.

An infection is a type of disease caused by microorganisms (Chapter 6, see the introductory section). Surgical site infections (SSIs) are defined as infections that occur in or around surgical sites (usually incisions), typically when microorganisms are introduced at the time of surgery (e.g. when a contaminated device is introduced into a patient). Surgical site infections can be, but are not always, acquired during an operation either from the operating room environment, medical equipment or staff ("exogenous"), or from microorganisms on the patient's skin ("endogenous"). The risk of infection is also dependent on the patient's general health, length of the procedure, wound classification, etc. Other predisposing factors include the surgical technique used, the presence of foreign bodies, such as implants, drains, pre-operative shaving (if used), and the experience and skill of the surgical team. A clean operating room environment with sterile (or correctly decontaminated) equipment, with restricted access and appropriately attired staff can go a long way to reducing the risks of surgical site infections.

Procedures and techniques

When a cure is unlikely naturally over time or through medication alone, various medical, diagnostic and surgical procedures can be performed to identify causes and alleviate disease and suffering. A variety of devices and instrumentation can be used to perform these procedures. The terms "device" and "instrument" are used interchangeably throughout the book as generally meaning any inanimate object that is used for medical, diagnostic or surgical procedures. In some countries these terms are used specifically from a legal point of view, such as the term "medical device". For example, a common classification of devices (which can include surgical, medical or diagnostic instruments) that is used internationally is based on how the device is used and the risks associated with them (not unlike the Spaulding classification system; in the section on goals of decontamination and the Spaulding classification). These include:

Class 1: considered low risk and include most types of non-invasive devices, meaning that they do not penetrate through or into the body. Examples can include: surgical lights, surgical tables, examination gloves, packaging materials and stethoscopes.

Class 2: considered medium risk, which can include various types of most invasive devices (or even products that are used with such devices) that penetrate into or through the body, but also the length of time used. Note: in some countries this is even sub-divided further into sub-classes such as Class 2a and 2b).

Class 3: considered the highest risk, which can include various types of implantable devices (those that can remain in the body long term or even permanently).

This is a general example, as the exact classification of a device can be different, depending on various rules or regulations in individual countries or regions, and such classification may change over time.

Medical and surgical procedures are generally categorized according to their urgency, body system involved, department they are conducted in (e.g. dedicated operating rooms for specialized procedures such as orthopedics, cardiac, neurosurgery, as different equipment is used), type of procedure, degree of invasiveness, and any special instrumentation that may be used (e.g. an endoscopic suite or catheterization laboratory). Based on the diagnosis and need for surgical intervention, patient admission is generally classified according to the organ, organ system or tissue involved (Chapter 2). Dentistry, while a separate discipline from medicine, is also considered a part of the medical field.

There may also be various options on how the procedure will be performed, for example:

• Elective procedures – these may not be essential but may improve the quality of life. The patient can choose if and when to have the procedure.

• Required procedures – these need to be done to prevent future complications, but do not necessarily have to be done immediately.

• Emergency procedures – often a matter of life or death and are required due to an urgent medical or traumatic event.

Medical disciplines and common procedures

Medical procedures are generally performed and/or supported by a medical team in hospitals, doctor's offices, clinics, dental offices, etc. The medical team consists of experts in various disciplines of medicine.

The medical team
The hospital medical team consists of a consultant, registrars, head nurse, senior nurse, bedside nurse, pharmacist, dietician and physiotherapists, with possible support from microbiologists, or surgeons. Depending on the medical discipline, a multidisciplinary team cares for the patient throughout the patient's stay. In many cases,

a smaller team or even an individual may be responsible for immediate care, such as in the case of emergency treatment, local surgery and dental procedures.

Types of medical disciplines

Examples of the most common types of medical disciplines are given in Table 3.1.

Table 3.1 Types and descriptions of medical disciplines.

Discipline	Explanation
Alternative medicine	Acupuncture, chiropractic, homeopathy, naturopathy, osteopathy.
Cardiology	Disease of the cardiovascular system dealing with congenital heart defects, coronary artery disease, heart failure, valvular heart disease and cardiac emergencies.
Dermatology	Skin and its appendages (hair, nails, sweat glands, etc.).
Emergency medicine	The primary management of medical emergencies, often in hospital emergency departments or at point of injury.
Endocrinology	The endocrine system (i.e. endocrine glands and hormones Chapter 2, section on endocrine system) and its diseases, including diabetes and thyroid diseases.
Gastroenterology	The alimentary tract and associated organs (see Chapter 2, section on digestive system).
Geriatrics	Care of elderly patients.
Obstetrics/gynecology	Deals with childbirth, reproductive and fertility medicine, the female reproductive system and associated organs (see Chapter 2, section on reproductive system).
Hematology	Deals with the blood, the blood-forming organs, and blood diseases.
Hepatology	Liver and biliary tract, usually a part of gastroenterology.
Immunology	Deals with the immune system.
Infectious disease	Diseases caused by biological agents.
Critical care medicine	Deals with life support and management of critically ill patients, often in an ICU.
Nephrology	Diseases involving the kidneys.
Neurology	Diseases involving the central, peripheral, and autonomic nervous systems (Chapter 2, section on nervous system).
Oncology	Cancer and other malignant diseases (due to uncontrolled growth of tissues).
Ophthalmology	Diseases of the visual pathways, including the eyes, brain, etc.
Palliative care	Pain and symptom relief and emotional support in patients with long-term or terminal illnesses.
Paediatrics	The medical care of infants, children and adolescents (newborn to 16–21, depending on the country).
Pathology	The study and diagnosis of disease, including studying tissues, organs and the whole body (e.g. an autopsy) and by other laboratory analysis (e.g. analyzing blood and urine samples).
Psychiatry	The diagnosis, treatment and prevention of cognitive, perceptual, emotional and behavioural disorders.
Pulmonology/respirology	The lungs and respiratory system (Chapter 2, section on respiratory system).
Rheumatology	Autoimmune and inflammatory diseases of the joints and other organ systems (e.g. arthritis and other rheumatic diseases).
Urology	The urinary tract system of males and females, and the male reproductive system (see Chapter 2, section on urinary system).
Medical genetics	Diagnosis and management of hereditary disorders.
Radiology	Imaging of the human body, for example by X-rays, computed tomography, ultrasonography and nuclear magnetic resonance tomography.
Nuclear medicine	The study of various systems of the body, for diagnostic and therapeutic reasons, using radioisotopes or radioactive methods. An example is using a PET (positron emission tomography) scanner and radioactivity sources such as Technetium-99m.
Neurophysiology	Physiology or function of the central and peripheral nervous system.

Medical and diagnostic equipment

Medical and diagnostic equipment is designed to aid in the diagnosis, monitoring or treatment of medical conditions. They can include a variety of devices and it is not within the scope of this book to describe all of these in detail. A number of the more common examples in a modern hospital or clinic are described further.

Some of the most obvious examples of simple and widely used medical devices include:
- A stethoscope used to listen to breathing, lung and heart sounds
- A Baumanometer/blood pressure machine used to check a patient's blood pressure (BP)

More complicated examples can include:
- Therapeutic equipment used to assist with patient treatment, including infusion pumps and dialysis equipment.
- Life support equipment is used to maintain a patient's basic bodily functions (breathing, kidney function) and includes medical ventilators, anesthetic machines, heart-lung machines, extracorporeal membraneous oxygenation (ECMO), and dialysis machines.
- Diagnostic equipment, such as electrocardiography (ECG), a non-invasive trans-thoracic recording of the electrical activity of the heart captured and externally recorded by skin electrodes and direct imaging devices.

The range of diagnostic imaging equipment that is available, giving the ability to look into the body without the need for surgery, is an example of some of the greatest advances in medicine in recent years. Traditionally, X-rays were used for this purpose, in particular to view damaged (broken or fractured) bone. But technological advances now include:
- Magnetic resonance imaging (MRI) is an imaging technique used in radiology to visualize detailed internal structures. The imaging makes it possible to differentiate between healthy and unhealthy/abnormal tissue, it is especially useful in brain, muscles, heart and cancer diagnosis.
- Computed tomography (CT) is a medical imaging X-ray procedure which uses ionizing electromagnetic radiation (tomography) for processing the X-rays.
- Positron emission tomography (PET) is a nuclear medicine imaging technique which produces a three-dimensional image or picture of functional processes in the body.
- Cardiac catheterization is now considered a common and routine medical procedure in many parts of the world. It uses a number of device types in order to diagnose or treat cardiac disease. A catheter is a flexible or rigid tube that is inserted into the body for the purpose of introducing or withdrawing a fluid, creating an opening (e.g. for another device) or to keep any passageway open; examples include cardiac (in the heart), intravenous (into a vein) and urine (to collect urine, e.g. Foley) catheters. A thin flexible cardiac catheter is inserted into the chambers of the heart and associated blood vessels, either via the femoral artery in the groin or the radial artery in the wrist. The catheter is inserted using a long guidewire and moved towards the heart. Once the catheter is in position the guidewire is removed. The cardiologist can view the progress of the catheter on a video screen and may insert a further device or contrast medium (a type of dye) through the catheter to treat a specific condition or provide further visualization. This procedure is usually performed using a local anesthetic that is injected into the skin at the point of entry (wrist/groin) to numb the insertion area.

A summary of some examples of common medical and diagnostic procedures performed in hospitals and clinics is given in Table 3.2.

Surgical procedures

Surgical procedures are generally performed by a surgical team in a dedicated operating room. The basic surgical team consists of experts in operative procedure, pain management and overall or specific patient care. The surgical team have the responsibility to care for the patient during the peri-operative period which includes the pre-, intra- and post-operative management of the patient from preparation for the surgical procedure, surgery itself and through to discharge. Peri-operative care is therefore considered to include care given to a patient before, during and after surgery, and is referred to as pre-, intra- and post-operative care:
- Pre-operative care is the preparation and management of a patient prior to surgery. It can include both physical and psychological preparation.
- Intra-operative care is the management of the patient during the operative procedure whilst in the operating room. The intra-operative period begins when the patient is transferred onto the theatre table in the operating room and ends when the patient is transferred to the recovery area. During this period the patient may be anesthetized, prepped and draped, and the operation is performed.
- Post-operative care is the management of the patient after the procedure until discharge.

Table 3.2 Common medical and diagnostic procedures.

Procedure	Explanation
Blood transfusion	Blood previously taken from a patient or from another person (donor) is administered directly into a patient via an intravenous catheter.
Coronary angiogram	Using a cardiac catheter, this procedure shows up the structure of the coronary arteries to detect any narrowing or damage. A doctor inserts a small catheter (diameter of 2–3 mm) through the skin into an artery (in the groin or the arm), which is guided, with the assistance of a fluoroscope (a special X-ray viewing instrument), to the coronary arteries. A small amount of radiographic contrast (an iodine solution), which is easily visualized with X-ray images is injected into each coronary artery. The X-ray images that are produced are referred to as an angiogram.
Percutaneous transluminal coronary angioplasty (PTCA) or Percutaneous coronary intervention (PCI)	An angioplasty is a non-surgical procedure that involves the insertion of a small balloon catheter into an artery in the groin (femoral) or arm (brachial), which is advanced past the narrowing in the coronary artery. The balloon is then inflated to enlarge the narrowing in the artery. As part of this procedure, a stent (a stainless steel wire-mesh design) can be inserted into the coronary artery to assist in keeping it open; during a PCI the balloon (angioplasty) is removed, but the stent remains in the artery to keep it open. If successful, PCI can relieve chest pain and improve the prognosis of individuals with unstable angina, minimizing the risk of a heart attack without having the patient having open heart coronary artery by-pass graft (CABG) surgery.
Atherectomy	An atherectomy is the removal of plaque usually from the coronary vessels.
Electrocardiogram (EKG)	An electrocardiogram (EKG) is usually the first and most simple test used to diagnose any coronary artery disease (CAD). It is a non-invasive test used to measure underlying heart conditions by measuring the electrical activity of the heart by positioning leads around the heart and on the arms and legs in standard locations. Information about the electrical activity of the heart is recorded on a screen.
Pacemaker insertion	A pacemaker is a small device that controls the heart (cardiac) rhythm using electrical impulses. A battery operated pacemaker is placed in the chest or abdomen through a small incision.
Computerized axial tomography (CAT) scan	A CAT scan produces a computer generated image of the structures within the body, to assist in diagnosing tumors, fractures, bony growth, and infections in the organs and tissues of the body. Data from multiple X-ray images is converted into pictures on a computer screen.
Magnetic resonance imaging (MRI) scan	An MRI scan is a radiology technique using magnetism, radio waves and a computer to produce images of internal body structures. The MRI scanner looks like a long tube (into which the body is placed) which is surrounded by a giant circular magnet. The magnet creates a strong magnetic field that is used to produce a very faint signal from the various parts of the body. These are detected by the scanner and processed by a computer to give an image. It can be used to detect small structural differences throughout the body.
Ultrasonography (sonography) and echocardiography	Ultrasonography (an "ultrasound") is a radiological technique using high-frequency sound waves to produce images of the structures within the body. Echocardiography uses ultrasound to visualize the heart. There are several types. During transthoracic procedures a transducer that transmits high frequency sound waves (ultrasound) is placed on the chest; these sound waves bounce off the heart structures, producing images and sounds that can detect heart damage and disease. In trans-esophageal echocardiogram (TEE) the transducer is inserted through the esophagus for the same purpose, but placed closer to the heart allowing for a clearer picture. A further example is a stress echocardiogram, being performed prior to and just after exercise in order to measure the motion of the heart's walls and pumping action when stressed.
Chemotherapy	This is the use of toxic chemicals (drugs) for treating disease. Antibiotic chemotherapy is used to treat bacterial infection (see Chapter 5). Cancer chemotherapy uses low concentrations of highly toxic drugs that may reduce or destroy fast growing and abnormal human tissue (such as in the cause of "tumor" or cancer development). In the treatment of cancer, chemotherapy can cure (no signs of the disease) or control (reducing the size of a tumor) the disease. Chemotherapy may be administered intravenously (through a vein), orally (by mouth), by injection, topically (applied to the skin), intra-arterially (directly into the artery that is feeding the cancer) or intraperitoneal (directly into the peritoneal cavity; Chapter 2). To allow multiple administration of the drug, often a catheter is surgically placed, or a port placed under the skin and connected to a large vein.
Dialysis	Dialysis is the movement of fluids and chemicals across a semi-permeable (selective) membrane. Medically, dialysis is used to correct fluid and electrolyte imbalances and removing waste products.

(continued)

Table 3.2 (*cont'd*).

Procedure	Explanation
	It replaces kidney function (see the section on the urinary system in Chapter 2) by artificially filtering and cleansing the blood of excess fluid, minerals and wastes. There are two main types of dialysis: haemodialysis and peritoneal dialysis. During haemodialysis the blood is removed from a patient and circulated through a dialysis machine, where the dialysis takes place and the blood is returned to the patient. Peritoneal dialysis uses the patient's own body tissues (peritoneal cavity) to act as a filter. A "dialysis catheter" is inserted through the abdominal wall into the abdominal cavity. Dialysis fluid ("dialysate") is infused into the abdominal cavity, allowed to exchange (dialyse) in the body and then removed.
Pap smear	A medical sampling procedure in which a sample of cells is removed from a woman's cervix (the bottom end of the uterus) and sent for microscopy in order to detect pre-malignant (before-cancer) or malignant (cancer) changes.
Biopsy	A biopsy is the removal of a sample of tissue from the body for diagnostic/examination purposes. A biopsy may be performed in a theatre, clinic or doctor's surgery by needle aspiration, or a suspected lump of tissue may be partially or completely removed (lumpectomy) for examination and/or treatment. Examples include a breast or liver biopsy. Sometimes special, re-usable devices are used to take a biopsy, such as with a laparoscope (Chapter 4, in the section on Endoscopy).
Apheresis	Apheresis is a medical procedure that involves removing whole blood from a donor or patient and separating or selectively removing individual components so that one particular component can be removed. The procedure involves passing the blood from the person through a machine and then back into the patient. For example, plasmapheresis is the removal of blood plasma (a colorless watery fluid of the blood in which the various blood cells are carried; see Chapter 2, section on the cardiovascular system).
Lumbar puncture (LP)	A sampling procedure used to diagnose or even treat diseases associated with the cerebrospinal fluid (CSF; see Chapter 2, section on nervous system). In some cases, the CSF is removed to decrease spinal fluid pressure in patients.
Collagen injections	Collagen injections are cosmetic injections used to give the skin a plumper, smoother appearance.
Acupuncture	A commonly used alternative medicine procedure, to theoretically rebalance patterns of energy flow ("Qi") through the body that are essential for health. Any disruption of Qi is believed to be responsible for disease. The most common procedure involves penetration of the skin by thin, solid, metallic needles for manual/electrical stimulation of acupuncture points.
Amniocentesis	Amniocentesis is a non-surgical procedure, where a sample of fluid is removed from the amniotic sac (fluid-filled structure inside the pregnant uterus within which the baby lives) for analysis. Fluid is removed by placing a long needle, often guided using ultrasound imaging, through the abdominal wall into amniotic sac.
Bone marrow aspiration	A medical procedure used to withdraw bone marrow, the blood-forming portion of certain bones (Chapter 2, in the section on the skeletal system). A special needle is inserted into the hip bone or sternum (chest bone) to withdraw a sample.
Restoration of dental caries	Caries is any kind of progressive bone, including teeth, decay/damage over time. Dental caries is therefore tooth decay caused by bacteria in the mouth. During a routine procedure, a dentist uses a drill, air abrasion instrument or laser to remove the decayed areas of the tooth. Once the decay has been removed, the tooth is prepared for filling by cleaning the cavity of bacteria and debris, and then restored using a "filling". If the tooth has extensive decay or if there is a risk of infection or injury to the tooth's pulp, this may require a more serious surgical intervention by extraction (removal of the tooth) and endodontic therapy (known as a "root canal"). A root canal involves the removal of the outer and lower tooth, which can be reconstructed with a replacement, artificial tooth (including the outer "crown").
Endotracheal intubation	Medical procedure to assist breathing, where a tube is inserted through the mouth into the trachea (the large airway from the mouth to the lungs). The endotracheal tube artificially opens a passage through the upper airway allowing air to pass freely to and from the lungs. Can be connected to a mechanical ventilator to provide artificial respiration. The tube is inserted through a device known as a laryngoscope, which allows the practitioner to see the upper portion of the trachea, just below the vocal cords.

The basic make-up of any surgical team will depend on the type of surgery to be performed (discipline), the precise procedures (complexity, etc.), and the location and the type of anesthesia (the induced loss of pain) that will be used. The team may include surgeons, anesthesiologists, and nursing and technical staff who are trained in general surgery or in a particular surgical specialty. Complicated specialized surgeries require larger teams. Minimally invasive procedures (using a variety of endoscope types) often require specialized expertise and high levels of technical knowledge; these procedures use highly specialized but smaller teams, create smaller wounds, resulting in less trauma which leads to quicker healing, but often require more operating time.

Surgical team members

Surgical team members can include a few or many qualified persons, depending on the complexity of the surgical procedure. These generally include the surgeon, an anesthesiologist and various nursing staff.

The surgeon generally leads the surgical team and is responsible for performing the surgery in an effective and safe manner. Surgeons are qualified doctors who have undergone further intensive training in surgical procedures.

The anesthesiologist is responsible for ensuring the safety of the patient and reducing the stress of the operation, including pain relief. Anesthesiologists are qualified physicians with advanced training in anesthesia, which can be defined as the induced or controlled loss of sensing pain. Anesthesia may or may not be associated with falling asleep (loss of consciousness); examples include local and general anesthesia, referring to methods used to render part of the body free from pain (but remaining conscious) and putting the patient "to sleep" (unconscious and loss of pain) respectively. Anesthesiologists are therefore directly or indirectly involved in all three stages of surgery (pre-operative, operative and post-operative) due to their focus on pain management and patient safety before, during and after surgery. An anesthetist is often a registered professional nurse who is trained to administer anesthetics and supports the anesthesiologists.

Nursing staff are an important part of the surgical team. Nursing staff are involved in care, assistance and pain management throughout the peri-operative period. Specific nursing staff will include the scrub and circulating nurse. The scrub nurse is a professionally qualified nurse who prepares the set-up and assists the surgeon by passing instruments, sutures, etc., during surgery. A circulating nurse is also professionally registered and is free to support the surgery team to include obtaining any

supplies, supporting the anesthesiologist/anesthetist and assisting the scrub nurse.

Surgical techniques

There are many different surgical techniques that may be used depending on the type of surgery to be performed, available equipment, the surgeon or patient's preference and the patient's anatomy or physiological condition at the time. A summary of the major different types is given in Table 3.3.

Surgical disciplines and common procedures

There are a number of different surgical specialities or disciplines generally classified depending on the areas of the body that the procedures may be performed on, for example the brain, stomach, liver, intestines, appendix, breasts, heart, etc. Depending on the capabilities and specialties of any facility and the associated staff, a number of common procedures may be performed. The most common surgical specialities include:

• General surgery – general surgeons operate on almost any part of the body. They confirm the diagnoses provided by primary care or emergency physicians, then perform the necessary procedures to correct or alleviate the problem. If a specialized procedure is involved they will often refer the patient to a relevant specialist.

• Cardiothoracic surgery – this is a common surgical specialty and often with very high demands. The cardiothoracic surgical team treats pathological conditions within the chest, including the heart and its valves, the lung, esophagus, and chest wall and blood vessels.

• Neurosurgery – neurosurgical teams specialize in surgery of the nervous system, including the brain, spine and peripheral nervous system, and their supporting structures.

• Oral and maxillofacial surgery – maxillary facial surgical teams deal with surgical problems of the head and neck, that is, the ears, sinuses, mouth, pharynx, jaw, and other structures of the head and neck.

• Reconstructive and plastic surgery – performs surgery on abnormal structures of the body due to injury, birth defects, infection, tumors, or disease. They also perform cosmetic surgery to improve a patient's appearance.

• Transplantation – specializes in specific organ transplant techniques, such as heart and heart-lung transplants, liver transplants and kidney/pancreas transplants. These highly intricate surgeries require very advanced training and technological support.

• Urology and renal transplantation – deals with the kidneys, kidney stones, bladder, urethra and ureters and coordinate with transplant team members.

Table 3.3 Various types of surgical techniques.

Technique	Explanation
Open surgery	Procedures that require a large incision to access the relevant area of skin and tissues to allow the surgeon direct access to the internal structures or organs involved, for example the removal or repair of an internal organ, such as a gall bladder.
Laser surgery	Involves the use of a laser allowing the surgeon to precisely cut tissue instead of using a physical knife (scalpel) or similar surgical instruments. An example is LASIK (laser-assisted *in situ* keratomileusis) surgery, a special type of laser-assisted eye surgery for correcting eyesight.
Microsurgery	Involves the use of an operating microscope positioned above a small incision, allowing the surgeon to visualize small structures.
Robotic surgery	Makes use of a surgical robot that controls the surgical instrumentation, by indirect or voice activation, under the direction of the surgeon.
Minimally invasive surgery (MIS)	A surgical technique that requires a minimum or limited number of incisions. Minimally invasive surgery involves smaller incisions to the skin to insert specially designed instruments into a body cavity or structure. The surgeon can see into the body through the use of associated devices, with the advantages of reducing the risks of infection, promoting rapid healing and cosmetically leaving smaller scars. Further modern forms of MIS include procedures that enter the body through natural orifices such as the alimentary canal and the belly-button (navel, "umbilicus").
Reconstructive surgery	Involves reconstruction of an injured, mutilated or deformed part of the body (including the teeth in dental surgery).
Cosmetic surgery	Performed to improve the appearance of an otherwise normal surface structure of the body.
Transplant surgery	Replacement of an organ or body part by removing the diseased organ and replacing it with a donated healthy organ.
Tattooing	A tattoo is a marking made by inserting indelible ink into the dermis layer of the skin.

• Gastrointestinal surgery – the team specializes in problems of the digestive tract (stomach, bowels, liver and gall bladder).

• Vascular surgery – diagnosis and treatment of arterial and venous disorders such as aneurysms, lower extremity revascularization and other problems.

• Pediatric surgery – specially trained to perform procedures on infants and children. They work closely with specially trained anesthesiologists, and are experts in childhood diseases of the head, neck, chest and abdomen, with training in birth defects and injuries.

A range of other types of surgical procedures are given in Table 3.4.

Introduction to endoscopic procedures

Endoscopy is one of the fastest growing areas of medical and surgical procedures used in hospitals and clinics. Endoscopy refers to any procedure using a device (known as an endoscope) to look inside the body, for medical, diagnostic and surgical reasons. These devices are traditionally sub-classified into two types of devices, known as rigid and flexible endoscopes (Figure 3.2).

This refers to their design, where rigid devices are constructed of rigid materials and flexible devices are designed to be more supple; these are discussed in more detail in Chapter 4. They can be designed to allow for direct viewing through an eye-piece on the endoscope (as shown for the rigid devices in Figure 3.2) as well as through a video system viewing images on a monitor (a flexible video-endoscope is shown in Figure 3.2). They are particularly used for diagnosis (direct visualization as well as internal sample collection, e.g. using biopsy forceps and aspiration needles) and/or for surgical techniques. Endoscopic procedures can be defined based on the area of the body they are performed, with specific types of devices designed for use in these areas (Table 3.5).

Endoscopy clearly has many benefits to the patient and medical/surgical staff. They allow many procedures (medical, diagnostic and surgical) to be performed that would otherwise require complicated and long surgery,

Table 3.4 Examples of specific surgical procedures.

Procedure	Explanation
Appendectomy	Surgical removal of the appendix, a small appendage that branches off the large intestine.
Cesarean section	Surgical delivery of a baby through an incision in the mother's abdomen and uterus.
Cholecystectomy	Surgical removal of the gall bladder because it is infected, cancerous or has an accumulation of gall stones.
Coronary artery by-pass	Involves grafting (surgically taking a portion of living tissue from one part of an individual to another part, or from one individual to another) of veins or arteries, taken from the leg or chest, from the aorta to the coronary artery, in order to by-pass vessels that are blocked.
Wound debridement	Surgical removal of foreign material and/or dead, damaged, or infected tissue from a wound or burn in order to facilitate effective healing.
Skin grafting	Detaching healthy skin from one part of the body to repair areas of lost or damaged skin in another part of the body. Usually performed when the wound is too large to be repaired by stitching or natural healing.
Hemorrhoidectomy	Removal of hemorrhoids in the lower rectum or anus.
Hysterectomy	Surgical removal of a woman's uterus (womb). This may be performed either through an abdominal incision or vaginally, and may or may not include the removal of Fallopian tubes and ovaries.
Inguinal hernia repair	Inguinal hernias are usually found in men and are protrusions of part of the intestine into the muscles of the groin. These can be surgically repaired.
Mastectomy	Removal of all or part of the breast, usually performed to treat breast cancer.
Partial colectomy	The removal of part of the large intestine (colon) to treat cancer or ulcerative colitis.
Prostatectomy	Is the removal of all or part of the prostate gland in males, which surrounds the neck of the bladder. A prostatectomy may be performed for an enlarged or cancerous prostate. Can be done as a minimally invasive procedure (using a rigid cystoscope) or as an open procedure.
Adeno-tonsillectomy	Removal of the adenoids and/or tonsils, generally due to chronic infection.
Tracheotomy (tracheostomy)	A tracheotomy is a surgically created opening in the trachea (the breathing tube). It is kept open with a hollow tube called a tracheostomy tube. They are performed to by-pass an obstructed upper airway that prevents oxygen from reaching the lungs, to clean and remove secretions from the airway or to deliver oxygen directly to the lungs. Commonly performed in an intensive care unit, emergency room or operating theatre during emergency situations or on very ill patients.
Arthroplasty	The surgical reconstruction or replacement of a joint.
Amputation	This involves cutting off a body part, usually a limb or digit. Re-plantation involves reattaching a severed body part.
Surgical endoscopy	The use of specific types of devices (endoscopes) and accessories through tiny incisions, called portals, to allow the surgeon to visualize and operate within a patient. A form of minimally invasive surgery used for a variety of procedures, including appendectomies, gall bladder surgery, oopherectomy, repair of shoulder and knee ligaments, etc.
Restoration of dental caries	Dental caries is progressive tooth decay and can be minor or serious. Serious cases may require surgical intervention by extraction (removal of the tooth) and endodontic therapy (known as a "root canal"). A root canal involves the removal of the outer and lower tooth, which can be reconstructed with a replacement, artificial tooth (including the outer "crown").
Tattooing	A tattoo is a puncture wound made by penetrating the skin with a needle and injecting ink into the area, usually creating some sort of design. What makes tattoos so long-lasting is that the ink is injected into the dermis, which is the lower layer of skin (see Figure 2.11). A tattoo machine is a handheld electric instrument that uses a re-usable or disposable handle and disposable needle system. On one end is a sterilized needle, which is attached to tubes that contain ink. A foot switch is used to turn the machine on and off, which moves the needle in and out while driving the ink into the skin.

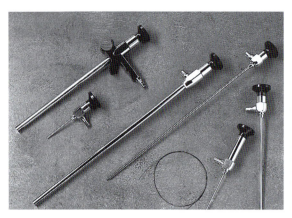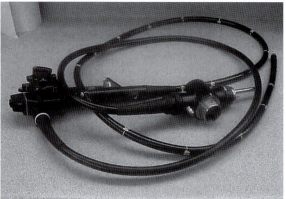

Figure 3.2 Examples of rigid (left) and flexible (right) endoscopes used for endoscopic procedures (endoscopy).

Table 3.5 Examples of various types of endoscopic procedures.

Procedure	Explanation
Arthroscopy	An arthroscope is inserted into a joint to examine or treat the interior of the joint.
Bronchoscopy	Bronchoscopy is a procedure performed to inspect the respiratory system including the lungs, larynx (voice box), vocal cord, trachea and bronchi. Lung tissue can be biopsied and lung contents can be sampled using a variety of methods (such as by aspiration or washing) through the bronchoscope. Bronchoscopes are commonly flexible in design, but may also be rigid.
Colonoscopy	Visualization of the colon by inserting a flexible device (colonoscope) through the anus and into the colon. Typically used for diagnosis (e.g. causes of bleeding and colon cancer screening), but also for some surgical techniques. Samples of the colon can be removed for further analysis using specific accessories such a biopsy forceps.
Cystoscopy	Examination of the urinary tract. A cystoscope is inserted through the urethra to examine the urethra and bladder cavity.
Endscopic retrograde cholangiopancreatography (ERCP)	Using a duodenoscope inserted through the mouth and through the upper digestive system particularly for investigations and procedures in the duodenum (between the stomach and small intestine), including the bile duct (connecting the liver/gall bladder to the duodenum)
Gastroscopy	Flexible gastroscope is inserted through the mouth into the upper digestive system to visually inspect the lining of the esophagus, stomach and upper duodenum. It is also possible to perform minor procedures (polpectomy) and take tissue samples via a gastroscope.
Hysteroscopy	Examination of the vagina and uterus. Introduction of a hysteroscope through the vagina.
Laparoscopy	A laparoscope is inserted through a small incision and used to visualize a surgical procedure in the abdominal cavity using other devices (as an example of MIS, minimally invasive surgery). The procedure is performed with other instruments inserted through additional incisions in the abdominal wall, to include inspection (for diagnostic purposes) and surgical removal (e.g. ovaries and Fallopian tubes in women).
Laryngoscopy	A laryngoscope is inserted through the mouth into the oropharynx to inspect the larynx and to assist with intubation.
Sigmoidoscopy	A sigmoidoscope is introduced into the anus to examine the rectum and the lower part of the large intestine (known as the sigmoid colon).

allowing greater flexibility to doctors and surgeons. Most of these procedures also provide rapid and more detailed visualization of many parts of the body. For the patient's benefit, endoscopic procedures can have little or no invasiveness (allowing for rapid recovery), have limited associated discomfort and are associated with little or no scarring. Advances are continuing in the development of new and even more complicated devices and procedures, such as those involved with robotic surgery and with more surgical procedures being performed through natural body offices (belly-button, mouth, anus, etc.) using flexible or rigid endoscopic systems (e.g. natural orifice transluminal endoscopic surgery or NOTES).

The operating/procedure room

Medical procedures, due to their nature and range, can be conducted in a variety of settings, ranging from at home, general practice doctor office, clinics, dedicated hospitals rooms, etc. Some of these procedures require specialized instruments (such as MRIs and dialysis machines) and are therefore limited to where the equipment is available; but with technological advances in both medical and diagnostic equipment, even complex instrumentation is becoming more widely available, being miniaturized and mobile. Surgical and critical medical procedures pose an increased risk of infection and other complications to the patient; for this reason, these procedures are usually conducted in specifically designed and dedicated areas. These include various designs of operating and dedicated procedure rooms. An operating room (OR/"theatre") is usually a purpose built, enclosed area with ample space to accommodate the patient, surgical staff and equipment.

The area is primarily designed to accommodate any defined surgical procedures and reduce contamination risks, but also other patient/staff considerations (such as patient dignity, access to equipment/supplies, etc.). They should be easy to maintain and clean, with limited and controlled access (including automatically closing doors, no open windows and a controlled humidified, cool temperature). Most modern operating rooms are designed with specialized air handling systems that maintain the temperature/humidity (for staff and equipment), keep the area under a positive pressure (slightly pressurized, to keep out contamination), filter the incoming air (to remove microorganisms and other particles) and control the flow of air in the room to reduce any cross-contamination risks. In addition, the OR may also have a back-up electricity supply to ensure an uninterrupted power supply in case of a black-out/power outage. Furniture, fittings and equipment should be limited to the minimum required for the types of surgery that are conducted in the area. Standard equipment consists of the operating table, anesthetic delivery unit, theatre (surgical) lights, cardiac monitor, diathermy machine, suction, oxygen and various other gasses. In addition, there are trolleys to set instruments on. The room is usually well lit with overhead surgical lights that do not shadow, and may have in addition viewing screens, monitors and other specialized equipment. Typical designs and equipment for operating rooms are further discussed in the next section.

Operating room set-up

Each theatre should have an adjacent preparation (or "scrub") room or have access to a scrub area common to a few theatres. It is designed to allow staff to prepare to enter the operating room (theatre), but is also used for storage and pre-warming (in a warming cabinet) of supplies used during surgery (including fluids, blankets, sterile surgical supplies, etc.). The scrub area is usually adjacent to (outside) the theatre, and is equipped with a double sink and antiseptics available for staff for surgical hand washing (surgical "scrubbing"; Chapter 9, section on antiseptics; Figure 3.3). This area is therefore used for hand washing and gowning-up (wearing dedicated gowns, clothing and footwear) before entering the aseptic ("sterile") OR area.

Once in the operating room, some of the typical equipment found in the area is shown in Figure 3.4.

Central to any operating room is the surgical table (on which the patient is placed), which can range in complexity from a simple table to a fully adjustable surgical table that can be raised, lowered and tilted in any direction to meet the need of the surgeon and surgical procedure. Directly overhead is an adjustable surgical table light that allows for direct illumination of the surgical area and is usually designed to minimize shadowing and any heat build-up during surgery. In many cases, dedicated sterile light handle covers are used to allow the surgeon to adjust the light position aseptically during surgery. Modern designs of surgical lights and tables may be voice controlled, to allow easy, non-touch access to control features of the equipment.

As most surgical procedures are performed under anesthesia (to take away pain), an anesthetic delivery unit and cart is usually placed at the head of the operating table. This allows the anesthesiologist/anesthetist to work in an area that minimally affects the surgical staff but with direct access to monitor the patient's health during surgery.

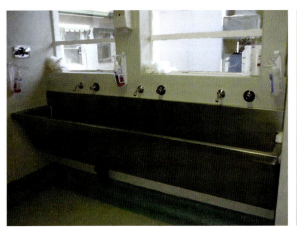 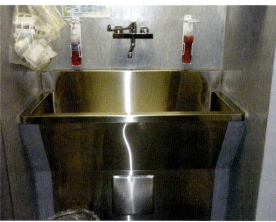

Figure 3.3 A typical scrub area, showing sinks and available antiseptics for hand washing prior to entering the operating room.

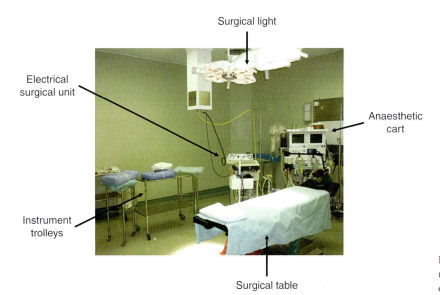

Surgical light

Electrical surgical unit

Anaesthetic cart

Instrument trolleys

Surgical table

Figure 3.4 A typical operating room design with room equipment highlighted.

Depending on the complexity of the procedure being performed, a number of moveable stainless steel instrument trolleys or "back tables" and "mayo" (device/ instrument stands) are available. These are used to lay out and position instruments before, during and after surgical use by the scrub sister and/or other support staff. Other movable equipment may include waste disposal carts/trolleys with disposable bags.

An electro-surgical unit that is used to control bleeding is usually available and placed on the side of the table. This uses an electric current to cut, coagulate and desiccate (dry) tissues, particularly to reduce blood loss during surgery.

As discussed in the introduction, most modern operating rooms are designed with specialized air handling systems. These are not just designed to maintain the area as a comfortable environment (for temperature and humidity), but also to reduce the risks of microbial contamination from the air in the room. Operating rooms are usually under positive air pressure relative to the surrounding corridors/areas, forcing air out of the room and minimizing any "dirty" air flowing into the room. The internal air is constantly being replaced, such as at ~20–25 changes per hour of high-efficiency particulate air (HEPA). This is generated by passing the air through HEPA filters mounted on the

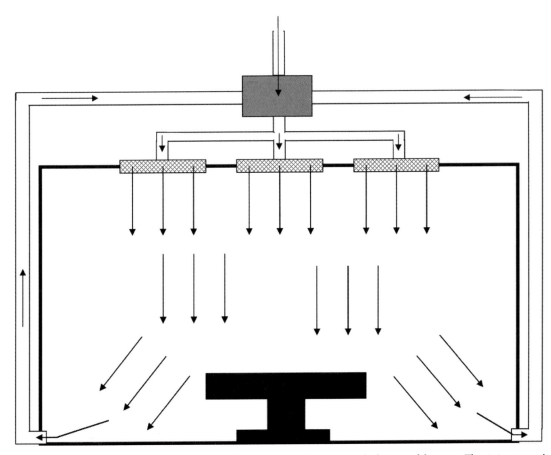

Figure 3.5 An air handling system, showing the flow of air (as arrows) through the room in a downwards motion from entry at the top of the room (gray box at the top), through a dedicated air handling system, through HEPA filters (three shown) on entry into the room and air returning to the system at the bottom of the room. The air is constantly being passed through the filters that remove bacteria/fungi, providing a clean flow of air over the patient area (representation of a surgical table shown in the center, in black).

incoming air in the ceiling; these filters are designed to remove most bacteria and fungi (typically larger than ~0.2 μm in diameter). The air currents in the room provide a downward stream of air through the room (especially around the patient) and are taken out at floor level (Figure 3.5). The principle of controlling the pressure and quality of air can be applied to any controlled environment (often referred to as "clean") procedure room or area, such as in laboratories, pharmacies, intensive care units and reprocessing areas, etc.

Principles of aseptic (or "sterile") technique

Any medical or surgical procedure should be performed using an aseptic technique, and particularly within designated operating rooms. Aseptic technique refers to practices and procedures to prevent microbial contamination and to maintain an essentially "sterile" or "clean" area. This is an important concept in that it helps minimize any risks of contamination and therefore the development of infection following a medical or, particularly, a surgical procedure. Aseptic technique is practiced in many ways in pre-, intra- and post-operative procedures including pre-surgical scrubbing, gowning and wearing sterile gloves, the design of air handling systems within the operating room, use of sterilized surgical devices, etc. The set-up of an operating room for a procedure follows the same aseptic technique practices. An aseptic (or "sterile") field is established in the operating room and separated from the unsterile area, such as contaminated areas and equipment. Only sterile instruments are used when performing an aseptic technique and these

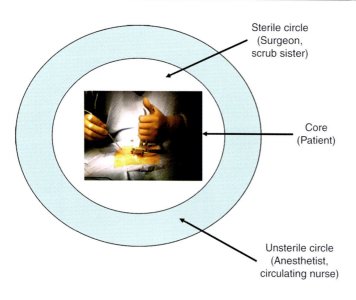

Sterile circle
(Surgeon,
scrub sister)

Core
(Patient)

Unsterile circle
(Anesthetist,
circulating nurse)

Figure 3.6 The three areas of a restrictive procedure room.

instruments must all be re-sterilized once they have been used or become contaminated (i.e. handled in an unsterile manner, or allowed to touch an unsterile surface).

Important aspects of aseptic technique are the divisions of working areas around and within operating rooms. These areas are traditionally divided into three working areas:

- Unrestricted
  - General area outside the operating room complex
  - Street clothing is worn
  - Patient receiving area, changing rooms, office
- Semi-restricted
  - Mid-way between an unrestricted and restricted area
  - Restricted to authorized personnel only
  - Theatre attire must be worn
  - Operating Room complex passages/corridors, reprocessing area (if present)
- Restricted
  - Where procedures are performed
  - Authorized personnel only
  - Scrub area, procedure room, sterile supplies stores

The actual restricted procedure room is further subdivided into three areas (Figure 3.6):

- The core or centre is the patient, on whom the procedure is being performed.
- The "sterile" circle is the area directly around the patient where the person/people (surgeon, scrub nurse, etc.) are operating using sterile instruments.
- The unsterile area where associated support staff (i.e. anesthesiologist, circulating nurse, etc.) are performing their duties within the procedure room.

Pre-operative procedures

Pre-operative care is the preparation and management of a patient prior to surgery. It can include both the physical and psychological preparation of the patient, including reviewing medical history, checking for any allergies, skin disinfection, physical/medical examination, etc. In parallel, the surgical staff are preparing to receive and operate on a patient in the operating room.

When "setting up" for a procedure, before the full surgical team are present, a scrub sister will begin to open the sterile items following specific aseptic guidelines. Any devices within packages or containers will be checked to ascertain that they have been sterilized (e.g. for a re-usable device that the sterilization chemical indicators have changed color on correct exposure to a sterilization process), have not been tampered with and that the packaging is intact. If the scrub sister is satisfied that the sterile barrier has not been compromised, before opening the package it must be positioned on a clean, dry, usually covered, flat surface at the level of the sterile field (Figure 3.7).

The external seal or tape is then removed and the top layer of wrap is unfolded (note: sterile packages are usually double-wrapped; Chapter 10, see the section on selection of packing materials). If using a rigid container the container is placed on a solid, clean surface, and checked that it is sealed and dry and that any filters are correctly in place; the lid is then removed according to the manufacturer's recommendations, making sure there is no contact between the lid and the inner rim or any part inside the container.

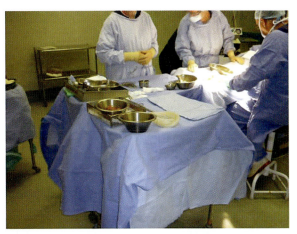

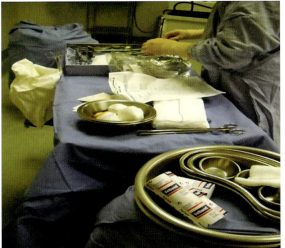
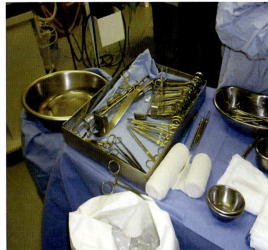

Figure 3.7 Setting up for a surgical procedure within the operating room.

Following surgical hand washing, the remaining sterile layer can be unwrapped or the inner trays removed from the container, taking care not to touch the sides of the containers. The scrub nurse will then check any in-pack sterilization indicators and that all instruments are present for the procedure.

All staff entering the operating area should at least wear surgical scrubs and surgical masks that cover all hair, including sideburns, and neckline as well as covering the nose and mouth. Jewellery, nail polish or artificial nails should not be worn. Sterile surgical gowns should be worn over surgical scrubs by all staff working within the sterile circle and participating directly in the procedure. Water repellent surgical gowns or aprons should be worn for procedures at high risk of blood contamination.

Surgical hand scrubbing should be performed by all staff prior to entering the sterile area and participating in the procedure. As an additional precaution, staff working in the sterile circle should wear at least one pair of sterile surgical gloves, with double gloving being recommended for procedures with a high risk of puncture, such as orthopaedics. Gloves should be changed immediately after any accidental puncture during a procedure.

Intra-operative procedures

The patient is the "core" or centre of the sterile area. This will also include any theatre staff directly involved in the procedure wearing sterile surgical attire, the operating table, other accessory equipment and any furniture that is covered with sterile drapes such as trolleys and stands.

The patient will also be fully covered with sterile drapes or other such materials; no part is uncovered except the operating field and areas needed for the administration and maintenance of anesthesia and fluids.

It is generally recommended that anyone working in the sterile circle must adhere to sterile or aseptic techniques using only sterile items, such as instrument sets, drapes, sponges, etc. Strictly speaking, gowned and gloved personnel directly involved with procedures are only considered sterile on their front and from the chest down to the level of the patient. Self-gowning and gloving should be done from a separate sterile area on the outskirts of the sterile ring. Sterile personnel must always keep their hands within sight, in the front of the body and below shoulder height. Sterile personnel should always face the sterile area. Generally the scrub sister, surgeon and surgeon's assistant work within this area. In addition, only the tops of the sterile draped table, instrument trolley and mayo stand are considered sterile. All items used within the sterile area should be sterile. Once a sterile drape has been placed in this area it should not be moved as this may compromise the sterile field. Sterile personnel may only touch sterile items or areas and may not leave the sterile area. Items are brought to the sterile area by "non-sterile" personnel, such as the circulating nurse. Sterile items should be opened and presented so that the scrub nurse can safely take the item avoiding any contact with the wrap or peel pack or the item can be opened and carefully placed onto the sterile field. Peel packs, for example, are opened by separating the seal halfway open, folding the top down half way, before presenting the contents.

While assisting "sterile" personnel, unsterile personnel remain in the unsterile area and avoid crossing into or between sterile areas. The circulating nurse assists with room preparation, opening of sterile instruments, opening of packs and collecting supplies. The anesthesiologist/anesthetist deals with the patient's airway. Neither generally come into contact with the sterile operative area or sterile area.

Surgical items should not be dropped onto the sterile field as they may fall off the sterile field or could cause other items to be displaced, contaminating the sterile field. In some situations, a device may be inadvertently dropped on the floor during a procedure; in such situations, the level of potential contamination may be low but is still considered significant. It is best that the device is replaced with alternative, sterilized devices. As an alternative, a "flash" sterilization process can be employed (Chapter 11). These are generally steam sterilization processes, specifically developed for rapid, flash treatment to reduce any surface contamination risks; sterilization cycles in these cases are developed for non-wrapped devices, where the device is placed directly into the sterilizer, exposed and quickly removed to proceed with the surgical process. This is usually performed in a sterilizer located in an adjacent area to, or even within, the operating room. Flash sterilization should not be considered as a replacement for normal decontamination and sterilization processes (in particular for wrapped devices), as they are generally not designed for such applications.

Post-operative procedures

Similar to pre-operative procedures, there are a series of procedures performed post-surgery to ensure the well-being of the patient. On completion of the actual procedure, but typically before the surgical opening is closed ("sutured"), the scrub sister should check that all instruments, sponges or any other items used during the surgery are present. If everything is accounted for, any healthcare contaminated waste and heavily soiled items will be segregated at the point of use (Chapter 7). Soiled sponges and any biological contaminants are directly discarded as per hospital policy on handling heathcare contaminated waste. Particular attention should be paid to the correct handling of disposable sharp devices, such as scalpel blades. Sharps are usually disposed into specific sharps containers. This can include any single-use tips, such as an electrosurgical tip being removed from its handle. All disposable scalpel blades are safely removed from their handles using a hemostat or a needle holder, and discarded.

Soiled instruments should be placed into containers for transport to a reprocessing area outside the operating room. Practices at this stage can vary from hospital to hospital, but it is generally good practice that devices are not allowed to dry on transport and storage, prior to reprocessing; this is discussed in further detail in Chapter 8, as an important part of the decontamination cycle. Any linens should also be separated. These can include single-use, disposal materials that are directly disposed of as healthcare waste, or linens that are collected and reprocessed as hospital laundry (Chapter 15, section on surgical and medical laundry). A hospital policy should be in place to describe the containerization and transport of contaminated equipment/linens to any applicable reprocessing area(s).

All horizontal surfaces and surgical furniture, such as tables and trolleys, are recommended to be cleaned/surface disinfected between procedures. At the end of a theatre "list" (series of procedures in a row) the entire surgical area is typically also cleaned and disinfected (Chapter 9, in the section on antiseptics). In some cases, operating rooms are closed to further procedures for longer periods of time while the area is disinfected. Care should be taken to review any manufacturer's instructions provided with surface/environmental disinfectants; in general, cleaning should be performed first, but can be combined with disinfection depending on the product claims and instructions. Chemicals (cleaner and disinfects) should never be mixed (unless specified) and, if required, should always be prepared according to manufacturers' instructions.

4 Instrumentation

Introduction

Hippocrates, considered by many to be the father of medicine, is believed to have said, "what cannot be cured with medicaments is cured by the knife, what the knife cannot cure is cured with the searing iron, and whatever this cannot cure must be considered incurable". Today, in the 21st century medicine offers us innumerable modern treatment medications, diagnostic and therapeutic instruments and devices to cure the sick by medical and surgical means. There is evidence that surgical instruments and devices have been used for thousands of years (Figure 4.1).

Archaeologists have discovered primitive knives that would have been used for surgical procedures as early as 5000 BC. Rough trephines,(instruments used to cut out a round piece of the skull) for performing round craniotomies (surgical opening of the skull) have been discovered and associated with Neolithic (2500 BC) sites in many places; it is believed that they were used by shamans to release evil spirits and to alleviate headaches and head trauma associated infections from war-inflicted wounds. Surgeons and physicians in India have used sophisticated surgical instruments since ancient times. Sushruta (circa 500 BC) was probably the most important surgeon in ancient history, often known as the "father of surgery". In his text *Sushruta Samhita* he described over 120 surgical instruments, 300 surgical procedures and classified human surgery into eight categories. Surgeons and physicians in Greece and Rome developed many instruments made from bronze, iron and silver, such as scalpels, lancets, curettes, catheters, tweezers, specula, trephines, forceps, probes, dilators, tubes, surgical knives, etc.

The first instruments were certainly made by men that made armour and cutlery, but some were also made by other metal workers such as silversmiths. Instrument making only became a modern profession in the 18th century. The invention of more advanced surgical instruments was directly linked to the discovery of anesthesia and modern sterile techniques. These developments allowed the penetration of the previously forbidden body cavities, namely the skull, the thorax and the abdomen. Due to the increased severity of war-inflicted wounds by shot, shrapnel and cannon, amputation sets were more widely described and used.

During the 19th century and first decades of the 20th century an explosion of new instruments occurred, with hundreds of new surgical procedures being developed. New materials, such as stainless steel, chrome, titanium and vanadium were available for the manufacturing of these instruments. The invention of stainless steel in 1913, by English metallurgist Harry Brearly, brought about perhaps the greatest change to the manufacture of surgical instruments. Whilst working on a project to improve rifle barrels, Brearly accidentally discovered that adding chromium to low carbon steel gives it stain resistance.

Precision instruments were developed for neurosurgery, microsurgery, ophthalmology, etc., in the second half of the 20th century. Energy-based power tools were also developed, such as diathermy, ultrasound and surgical tools for endoscopic surgery. Advances were made from the 1950s with new types of rigid and flexible endoscopes that could be used for direct observation within the body for diagnostic, therapeutic and surgical procedures. New and ever changing surgical techniques and advances create a continual need for new technology as well as for the introduction of entirely new instruments; finally, now, in the 21st century we see the more widespread use of surgical robots and advances in minimally-invasive surgery (MIS; Chapter 3).

Today there are more than 5000 surgical instrument types available that perform at least one essential

A Practical Guide to Decontamination in Healthcare, First Edition. Gerald McDonnell and Denise Sheard.
© 2012 Gerald McDonnell and Denise Sheard. Published 2012 by Blackwell Publishing Ltd.

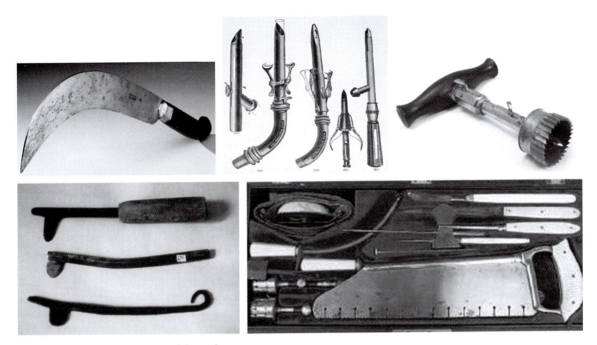

Figure 4.1 Examples of older surgical device designs.

function, such as cutting, holding or clamping, retracting, observing, draining, injecting, sealing, ligating and measuring (see the section on surgical instrument types and descriptions). Most surgical instruments are made from stainless steel. Other metals, such as titanium, copper, aluminum, chromium, vanadium, molybdenum and even a certain amount of silver and gold are also used. In addition, various types of plastics and instruments that are made of a mixture of these material types are available. In this chapter various types of instrumentation are discussed; the terms "instrument" and "device" are used interchangeably to describe any inanimate object that is used for medical, diagnostic or surgical procedures. In some countries these terms are used specifically from a legal point of view, such as the term "medical device".

Single-use and re-use instrumentation definition

Instruments and devices can be classified in a variety of ways, such as for what purpose they are used, materials of construction and the risk of contamination/infection transmission to a patient (Chapter 5, in the section on an introduction to infection prevention and control). An important classification to consider in this section is if the device is designed for single use or re-use (multiple use). A re-usable device, is a device that has been designed to be used again and again, with particular attention being paid to the correct, recommended procedures to ensure that the device is safely handled and/or reprocessed between patients (e.g. according to the Spaulding classification, Chapter 1, section on Spaulding classification). In such cases, there it is the responsibility of the manufacturer of the device to provide detailed instructions on how this needs to be done. A useful international standard that describes the manufacturer's requirement for safely reprocessing a re-usable device between patients is ISO 17664 *Sterilization of medical devices – information to be provided by the manufacturer for the processing of resterilizable medical devices*. This standard outlines what should be required for critical devices, to be sterilized, but equally applies in its content to other devices requiring between patient or routine reprocessing. This includes, but is not limited to:

• The manufacturer and their contact information
• Device description
• Any appropriate warnings on the use or limitations of decontamination, such as minimum number of sharp edges, limited number of re-uses, temperature or chemical restrictions, etc.

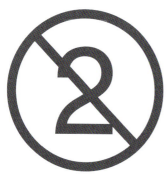

Figure 4.2 The internationally recognized symbol for a single-use device.

• Any instructions on handling at point of use and transport
• Instructions on preparation for decontamination, including disassembly
• Cleaning and disinfection instructions, manual and automated
• Drying, if applicable
• Any maintenance, inspection and testing instructions
• Sterilization, including packaging if applicable
• Instructions for use and/or storage

A single-use device can be simply defined as a device that has been designed and provided by a manufacturer to be used on a single patient. Note, that under this definition the device may be used multiple times on the same patient, although this may depend on the design of the device and the instructions given by the manufacturer on how it should be safely used. The internationally recognized symbol that designates a single-use device is shown in Figure 4.2.

A single-use device has not been designed to be reprocessed, although in many parts of the world healthcare facilities will decide to reprocess such devices and allow them to the used on other patients. The decision to reprocess a single-use device should not be taken lightly. In some countries, re-use of single-use devices is considered illegal, while in others it is accepted if the correct procedures are used to ensure that the device is safely reprocessed without adding any additional risk to another patient/user. Although the benefits may appear to be reducing costs and environmental considerations (less waste for incineration or other disposal), risks will include damage (seen and unseen) to the device (which can lead to adverse patient effects), toxicity and infection concerns (also adding patient risks), and legal considerations. Any decisions regarding the reprocessing of single-use devices should be taken at the highest level of any healthcare facility, in collaboration with infection prevention/control and written approval by management. This subject is considered in further detail in Chapter 15, on single use devices.

Materials used in the manufacture of instruments

Over the ages, surgical and medical instruments have been made from many different types of materials; copper, brass, silver, tin, plastic, etc. The most commonly used material today is stainless steel, although the surfaces of such instruments may be finished in different ways depending on the use of instrument (e.g. highly polished or dull, nickel, gold or silver plated). Steel is an alloy, a further chemical term used to describe a mixture of metals (mixed together by heating at high temperatures). Steel is an alloy of iron mixed with mostly carbon (in a typical range of 0.02–2.2%), but also sometimes other metals (such as manganese). These are mixed with iron to give strength, as hardening chemicals. Other examples of alloys, which may also be used to manufacture instruments, include bronze (a mixture of copper and tin) and brass (an alloy of copper and zinc). Stainless steel has a further metal added to steel, being chromium (e.g. at 5–30%) to make the steel more resistant to surface damage (corrosion). High-grade, low-rusting stainless steel has been widely used because it is strong, hard, resistant to heat and resistant to corrosion. Corrosion is damage to any metal due to the effects of chemicals (including oxygen, in a process known as oxidation that forms oxides such as ferric oxide, Fe_2O_3 more commonly known as rust). Despite this, even with the use of high grades of stainless steel, over time/use and especially when not correctly cared for, instruments will corrode or be otherwise damaged, causing a variety of problems, including perforation (pitting), loss of strength, degradation of appearance, breakage and accumulation of chemical (scale or rust) deposits that can lead to adverse patient outcomes. The various types of stainless steel are made up of a combination of basic elements (Chapter 6): predominantly iron, carbon and chromium, but also silicon, nickel, nitrogen, molybdenum, titanium, aluminum, niobium, copper, nitrogen, sulfur, phosphorus, selenium and manganese. Properties of the final stainless steel alloy/compound are tailored by varying the amounts of these elements.

There are over 80 types of stainless steel manufactured, but only about a dozen of them are widely used for making surgical instruments in particular. The choice of steel is determined according to the desired physical properties (such as flexibility, hardness, tensile strength and malleability). Some types of steel can be "hardened" (made more hard wearing), others cannot, depending primarily on the carbon content of the steel. The most common forms of stainless steel are known as the 300 series (or austenitic). This is typically an alloy of iron, carbon (e.g. 0.15%), chromium (16%) and nickel/manganese. "Surgical" stainless steel grades are usually considered easier to clean, disinfect and sterilize, as well as being stronger and corrosion resistant. Examples include 304 (contains iron with <0.08% carbon, 17–20% chromium, 8–11% nickel, <2% manganese, <1% silicon, <0.045% phosphorous and <0.03% sulfur) and 316L (essentially the same but with a lower <0.03% carbon level), where L denotes a lower carbon level, and 2–3% molybdenum. The higher percentage of chromium gives the metal its scratch and corrosion resistance. The chromium also combines with oxygen in the atmosphere to form a thin, invisible layer of chrome-containing oxide (a chemical molecule, Chapter 6), called a "passive" film or layer. If the metal is cut or scratched and the passive layer is disrupted, this can allow the formation of rust (ferric oxide) or the regeneration of the chrome-containing oxide that recovers the exposed surface and protects it from further oxidative corrosion of the iron. The nickel provides a smooth and polished finish. The molybdenum gives greater hardness, and helps to maintain a cutting edge.

Other widely used metals and molecules include titanium, tungsten carbide, copper, aluminum, chromium, vanadium, molybdenum, and even a certain amount of silver and gold. Titanium is widely used in the manufacture of implants used to repair fractures, for example plates and screws. Titanium has a proven high biocompatibility property, which means that body tissue will adhere to, but not react adversely to, it. Titanium is also used in the manufacture of microsurgical instruments, where its light weight is an important factor in avoiding surgeon fatigue. Tungsten carbide is an alloy of tungsten and carbon used in the manufacture of needle holders, scissors, pin cutters, pliers and wire tighteners, because it is harder than the steel used in needles, pins and wires, resulting in instruments with exceptional durability. Usually the tungsten carbide is soldered or welded to the jaws or working ends of instruments.

Some lightweight instrument parts and cases are manufactured from aluminum, which has often been treated with an electrochemical process, called anodization (therefore referred to as "anodized" aluminum). This process forms an oxide layer on the surface of the aluminum which offers good corrosion resistance. The oxide layer can also be colored with pigments/dyes. Aluminum is often used for manufacturing orthopedic devices, as it is lighter than stainless steel.

A range of plastics are used in the manufacture of medical and surgical devices. Plastics are complex chemical (organic, carbon-containing) molecules. Some are naturally occurring, but most modern plastics used for devices are artificially manufactured. Plastic examples include nylon, polystyrene, polypropylene, polycarbonate, polyvinyl chloride (PVC) and polyethylene. Most of these more rigid plastics are specially formulated to withstand high temperatures (such as polytetrafluoroethylene (PTFE, also known as "Teflon"), polyethylene terephtalate (PET) and ultra high molecular weight polyethylene (UHMWPE)), while others will not (e.g. polyurethane and low-density polyethylene, LDPE). This is an important consideration in the reprocessing cycle as some devices can be heat-disinfected or sterilized, while others will be restricted to only low-temperature chemical treatment methods (Chapters 9 and 11).

It is not unusual to see a variety of materials being used for the manufacture of medical and surgical devices, depending on their required purposes. This can be very complicated considering the range of materials (metals, alloys, plastics, glass, adhesives, electrical components, etc.) that can be used, their various grades or methods of generating these grades, and various surface finishes. Such flexibility in the choice of materials gives the widest range of options for a device designer to meet the needs of surgeons, doctors and patients. Given the range of materials that can be used, it is important to consider all instructions provided by the manufacturer (see the section on single-use and re-use instrumentation definition) of these devices to ensure that the various materials are not damaged (or have limited damage) over time and re-use.

Device manufacturers and suppliers

Introduction and quality standards

In the simplest terms, the manufacturer is responsible for making the device to a defined quality standard. Defining "quality" can be difficult depending on your perspectives and expectations, but a reasonable definition is the provision of a product or service to a defined, consistent standard. It is not always the case that the same company designs, manufactures and provides/sells a device to a healthcare institution. If there is a single company or a range of companies involved in the process, they all have responsibilities to provide the device in a safe and effective manner for its intended use. In general, this will apply to those involved in designing and making the product but also those directly involved in selling or providing it in a given geographic region (e.g. in the European Union or a specific country like India). It is also important to note that by definition in some regions of the world, a reprocessing department may also be considered a "manufacturer" because it takes a device and renders it fit for use in or on another patient; therefore, many of the quality requirements on those that make the device may also be applicable to those reprocessing the device for patient use.

An important quality requirement for any manufacturer is having a quality management system (QMS), being a documented organizational structure and with the relevant procedures, processes and resources needed to implement quality within an organization. International standards are available that define these requirements. For example, ISO 9001 *Quality management systems – requirements*, defines these requirements for any type of organization, while ISO 13485 *Medical devices – quality management systems – requirements for regulatory purposes* is more specific to those requirements for medical devices. ISO 13485, for example, provides guidance to develop, implement and maintain a quality system, with emphasis on having this correctly documented, supported by management and correctly resourced. This standard has become the minimum quality requirement for medical device manufacturers worldwide. Compliance to this standard should be initially and periodically verified by an approved ("accredited") third party such as organizations like BSI Group and TÜV; the relevant ISO standard is assessed and, if satisfactory, a certificate confirming that the organization complies with the requirements of the standard is issued. An important aspect to such a quality system is to reduce the risk of something going wrong. Risk analysis with any product, process or service is therefore a further aspect of quality management. Guidance on risk management is provided in further medical device-related standards such as ISO 14971 *Medical devices – application of risk management to medical devices*. This standard provides guidance on all aspects of risk management; determining the safety of a medical device throughout its life cycle is considered by the manufacturer.

Further discussion on quality management and associated standards for reprocessing departments is given in Chapter 14, in the section on quality management.

Manufacturing process

Every instrument starts out as an idea, followed by a series of steps to design the device and ensure that it is fit for purpose. A variety of processes can then be used, based on the design, to manufacturer the device. It is outside the scope of this book to describe all of these processes, but some detail is given below regarding typical manufacturing processes for metal surgical devices.

The first step is common metal device manufacturing processes that are known as "hot forging", "cold forging" or laser cutting. These are all used to make the basic device design, known as a "blank". During hot forging, pre-cut pieces of stainless steel or other metal bars are heated to very high temperatures and shaped/forged under the weight of a giant drop forge weighing many tons. The quality of the forgings is critical, as errors or poor quality cannot be corrected later in the process. Cold-forged blanks are made out of sheet metals or bars. Instead of being shaped under heat, they are shaped/forged using the force of hammers. Laser cutters are also used to cut out or mill the desired shaped device and particularly for precision instruments.

Once the instrument manufacturer has verified the quality of the blanks to be used, the next step in the process is milling and/or turning. In the case of surgical forceps, this process is used to create the basic shape of the box lock, jaws and ratchets of the device (see the section on Basic everyday instruments).

Once all the parts are made the instrument may need to be assembled. On a two-part instrument there is generally a male and a female part, which is assembled depending on the type of hinge use. A typical forceps has a box lock, which is created by widening the female part under heat and inserting the male part; the hinge can then be secured with a pin or screw. At this point the shape of the metal is still quite rough and will need to be filed and ground into its final shape.

Now that the instrument is in its final shape it will generally need to be further tempered or hardened. This is necessary to make the instruments hard enough to withstand the rigors of their usage. The stainless steel is heated to a very high temperature and then cooled until it has reached the required hardness; this is a crucial part of the manufacture. If the steel is too soft, it will wear out or bend prematurely; if the steel is too hard, it will be brittle and break too easily. The correct hardness is usually defined and tested as part of quality control, for example being measured in units called Rockwell Hardness (HRC). A typical hardness range for a needle holder without tungsten carbide inserts is HRC 40–48. For scissors, the hardness may range be HRC 50–58.

When the correct hardness has been attained the manufacturer will typically need to further fine tune the shape and mechanism of the instrument. All unwanted sharp edges, burrs, etc., are removed. Scissors and other cutting instruments are sharpened and adjusted. It is at this point that an instrument is transformed from a piece of stainless steel into the precision instrument a surgeon will rely on. Once this is completed the instrument is polished in order to create a homogeneous surface which is a key element in rendering the instrument more corrosion resistant. Most instruments have a silk matte or satin finish that reduces glare in the operating room. Finally the instruments may be electro-polished. This process chemically removes foreign substances and makes the surface even more corrosion resistant, creating a thin protective layer, known as passive or passivation layer. If properly cared for during use, these passive layers can actually protect the device over time, ensuring the longevity of the instruments.

Instrument marking

Instruments can be marked with a variety of symbols, labels or unique identification codes. These are usually limited and minimal (especially on any part of the device that would enter a patient), but can include manufacturer's names, logos, device model and/or serial numbers. Any instrument markings should preferably only be done at the time of manufacture by the manufacturer. These may be visible (e.g. color coating and model numbers) or invisible (e.g. a code inserted into the device and detected using a specific sensor). Unique identification codes (UICs) are numerical or alpha-numerical codes that are defined through a coding system for the identification of a specific device on the market. Unique identification codes are becoming more widely used in and on medical devices, either as provided in the device design (by the manufacturer) or with/on a device at the site of use (by healthcare staff or a third party). Examples of these labelling systems include those that are visible and read directly by the eye, bar codes, two-dimensional data matrix and radio-frequency identification devices (RFIDs). Examples are shown in Figure 4.3. At the time of writing, there are international efforts to harmonize the coding systems used with medical devices; an example is

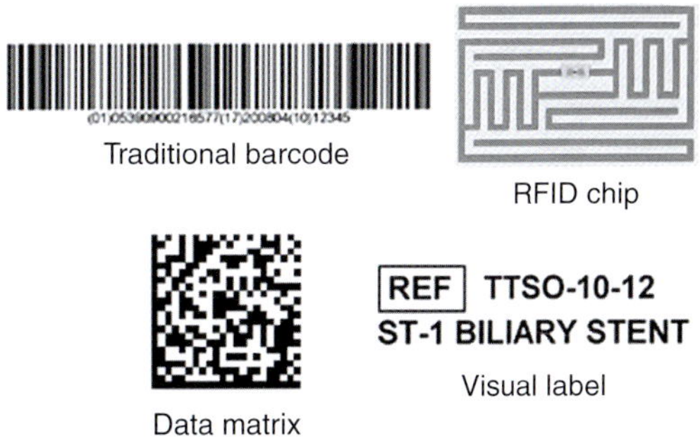

Traditional barcode

RFID chip

Data matrix

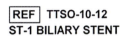

Visual label

Figure 4.3 Examples of labeling systems used with medical devices/instruments. Similar systems are used to label instrument sets (a set of instruments for a particular procedure).

the GS1 identification standards that are used for tracking and identifying products worldwide.

Although it is not generally recommended by manufacturers, instruments are often directly labelled post-manufacture. This can include the use of engraving, laser marking, indelible (water-insoluble) markers, adhesive tapes, etc. Such procedures may provide problems; unapproved engraving can damage the surface of the device (in the case of stainless steel leading to removal of the passivation layer and corrosion), while other labels/tapes may present problems to staff and patients during surgical or medical use. Labels and tapes should never be placed on areas of the instrument that are directly handled by staff or used directly in/on a patient; they can pose an infection risk (during reprocessing) and can become dislodged/introduced into a patient during a procedure. Etching, laser marking or other similar marking methods should also be done in collaboration with the device manufacturer to limit any safety risks.

Today, individual device marking/labeling systems are not in widespread use, but are commonly observed internationally using a variety of systems. In contrast, various labeling systems used to identify surgical and medical instrument sets are widely used for tracking and traceability purposes (Chapter 14).

Surgical instrument types and descriptions

Instruments range from basic forceps to delicate micro-surgical instruments to air/battery powered drills and complex endoscopic equipment. They have a variety of different angles, curves, lengths, tip lengths, sizes and

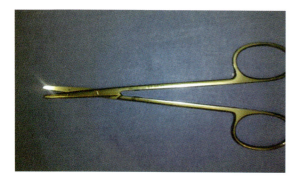

Figure 4.4 A pair of surgical scissors.

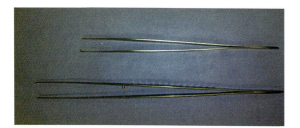

Figure 4.5 Examples of dissecting forceps.

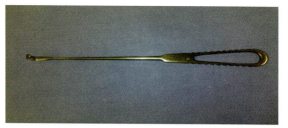

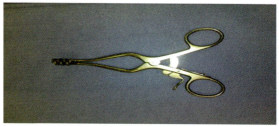

Figure 4.6 Examples of retractors, showing handheld (top) and self-retaining (bottom) designs.

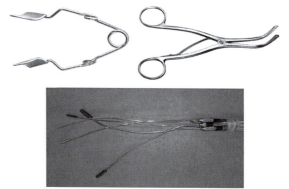

Figure 4.7 Dilator examples.

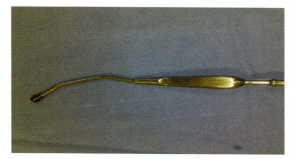

Figure 4.8 A suction nozzle.

serrations which are necessary to accommodate the difference types of procedures and anatomical structures as well as the surgeon's or medical staff's preferences.

Surgical instruments are designed to be minimal in design, cause as little damage as possible and are generally named either according to the action they perform (e.g. scalpel), the name of the inventor (e.g. "Mayo" forceps), or the kind of surgery it is used for (e.g. osteotome). They can be classified in a variety of ways, including type of surgery, handheld or robotic, powered or non-powered, etc. In this section some of the most commonly encountered surgical instruments are described, based on their surgical use.

Basic, everyday instruments

Some of the most common surgical instruments used are briefly described in this section. Scalpel or a pair of scissors (Figure 4.4) are the instruments of choice to cut or separate skin, fat, fascia, muscles, etc. Dissecting forceps (Figure 4.5) are used to hold, clamp, or pull tissue, or to stop bleeding. A handheld or self retaining retractor (Figure 4.6) is used to hold backhhold back the edges of a skin opening, wound or cavity. Dilators are used to keep open (or wider) a natural opening or orifice ("dilated") to inspect various body cavities (Figure 4.7). A suction nozzle (Figure 4.8) attached to a suction source within the operating room, is used to suction fluids (such as blood) from cavities during procedures. A needle holder (Figure 4.9) is used to hold a suturing needle for closing wounds ("anastamosis") and for other procedures (such as removing scalpel blades from BP handles).

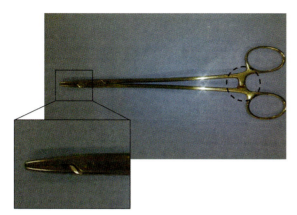

Figure 4.9 A needle holder; note the tip of the device (expanded) and the clamping mechanism or ratchet (circled, similar to a hemostat; see the section on instruments used for clamping and occluding).

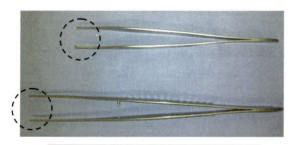

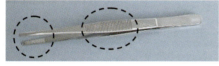

Figure 4.10 Examples of serrated instruments.

Some instruments have serrations or "teeth" at their ends to strengthen the grip on body tissues or elsewhere along the device to aid the surgeon in holding the device (Figure 4.10). These may be coarse or fine, run lengthways or crossways; run the length or only part of the blade, be curved or straight, long or short. A ratchet allows a surgeon to control their grasp or vary the tension they are applying through the instrument. Ratchets vary in size and strength, with some having a self-retaining clasp at the handle for ease of use.

A common term that is used in many of these instruments is referred to as the "joint". The joint is the junction of the instrument that allows the working (patient) end to be open and closed (Figure 4.11). There are various types of joints, including:

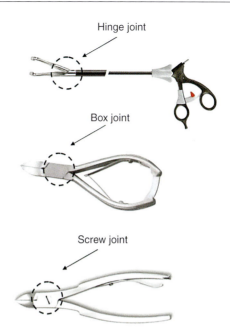

Hinge joint

Box joint

Screw joint

Figure 4.11 Various types of joints on instruments.

• Hinge joint: the shaft of the device is stable and only the end of the device ("jaw") moves, either one or both jaws.
• Box joint: a box joint is fused in the factory and cannot be taken apart for repairs. A joint pin is electrically fused during manufacturing through the outer elements of the hinge before the hardening step; this strengthens the joint and therefore the instrument. Even if the pin fractures during use, the fused box hinge prevents broken-off parts of the pin from falling out of the instrument and into the patient.
• Screw joint: a screw joint is used on instruments that can be sharpened as it allows the instrument to be completely disassembled to ensure effective sharpening, for example scissors, some bone nibblers, some bone cutters, etc.

Instrument classification

Surgical instruments can be classified in a variety of ways, but are considered in further detail in this chapter based on their surgical use. The most frequently used instruments are considered further, but this section is not exhaustive of the range of traditional and new types of devices in surgical use. These are defined as being used for:

• Cutting and dissecting
  ◦ Scalpels
  ◦ Knives

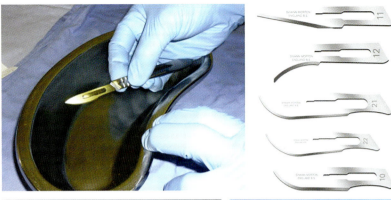

Figure 4.12 A scalpel blade and associated BP handle (top left). Also shown are examples of various different types of scalpel blades (top right), BP handles (3, 4, 7; bottom left) and an example of a disposable scalpel blade remover.

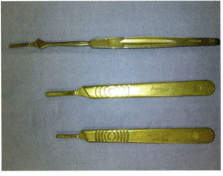

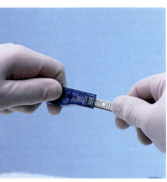

- ○ Scissors
- ○ Bone cutting
- ○ Other sharp dissectors
- ○ Blunt dissectors
- • Grasping and holding
  - ○ Delicate forceps
  - ○ Adson/Gillies forceps
  - ○ Bayonet forceps
  - ○ Strong-toothed forceps
  - ○ Debakey forceps
  - ○ Diathermy forceps
  - ○ Lane tissue forceps
  - ○ Babcocks
  - ○ Vulselm
  - ○ Bone holders
- • Clamping and occluding
  - ○ Hemostatic forceps
  - ○ Crushing clamps
  - ○ Vascular clamps
- • Exposing and retracting
  - ○ Handheld retractors
  - ○ Malleable retractors
  - ○ Hooks
  - ○ Self-retainers

- • Suturing or stapling
  - ○ Needle holders
  - ○ Clip appliers
- • Viewing
  - ○ Speculums
  - ○ Rigid and flexible endoscopes
- • Suction irrigation/aspiration
- • Dilation
- • Measuring
- • Powered tools
- • Other miscellaneous instruments
  - ○ Mallet
  - ○ Pressure cuffs
  - ○ Thermometers

Consideration is also given to some of the unique devices used for microsurgery, dentistry and tattooing.

Instruments for cutting and dissecting

A scalpel is a very sharp blade used for surgery (Figure 4.12). Scalpel blades are loaded or mounted onto BP handles. The blades are available in various shapes and sizes, and the blades used will depend on where and how the surgeon needs to cut. For example, a general surgeon will make a skin incision into the abdomen using a 21 or a

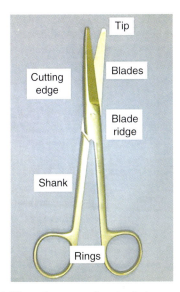

Figure 4.13 The various parts of a pair of scissors.

20 blade. A plastic surgeon will make an incision on the face using a 15 blade. Different shapes and sizes of scalpels fit onto different sizes of BP handles. BP handles are also available in various shapes, lengths and sizes (Figure 4.12). Size 3, 4 and 7 BP handles are commonly used. For example, a 15 and an 11 blade will fit onto a size 7 BP handle.

Scissors are probably one of the most common cutting tools, both for tissues but also for various other accessories during a procedure (e.g. sutures, bandages, etc.). The various parts of a pair of surgical scissors are shown in Figure 4.13.

A variety of scissor types are used surgically, known by names such as Mayo, McIndoe, Metzenbaum, Littler and Potts (Figure 4.14). There are two types of Mayo scissors: curved and straight. Curved scissors are used for dissecting tough tissues and tend to be used by orthopedic surgeons and gynecologists. Mayo straight scissors are used mostly to cut sutures and dressings.

McIndoe and Metzenbaum scissors are used for fine dissection and tend to be used by general and vascular

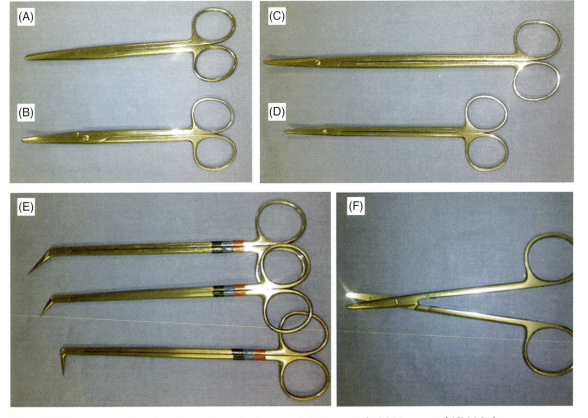

Figure 4.14 Various types of surgical scissors. Examples shown are (A) Mayo straight (B) Mayo curved (C) McIndoe (D) Metzenbaum (E) Littler (F) Potts scissors.

surgeons. Littler scissors are fine dissecting scissors used by plastic surgeons and hand surgeons. Potts angled scissors are used to make incisions into vessels, and are therefore commonly used by vascular and general surgeons. Potts scissors are available in various angles (Figure 4.14 (E)).

There are many types of instruments that are able to cut through bone and cartilage (bone cutters). They are commonly used by neurosurgeons, orthopedic and plastic surgeons. An example is bone rongeurs that are also known as bone "nibblers" (Figure 4.15). The term "ronguer" is derived from a French word meaning "to nibble". Nibblers can be single or double action (depending on the hinge mechanism).

Other, simpler instruments with no moving parts are also used on bone, including periosteal elevators, chisels, osteotomes, gouges, mallets and curettes (Figure 4.16). Periosteal (e.g. Freer) elevators are used for scrapping and elevating the periosteum (a tough membrane material that covers bone) away from the surface of the bone. Normally this procedure is performed prior to the surgeon either cutting or drilling the bone. Osteotomes are designed to cut bone, chisels to shave and shape bone in one plane or level, and gouges are used to shave bone into a curved surface. Osteotomes are used for splitting bone and they have a gradual bevel (or slant) on both sides (Figure 4.16). Chisels have a bevel on one side which provides a controlled direction cut by using the bevel. Chisels are

used for chipping pieces of bones away. These instruments may be curved or straight and are available in a variety of widths. Handles may be flat, square, hexagonal or round.

Other types of sharp dissectors include various types of biopsy forceps, punches, curettes and snares (Figure 4.17). A snare is a loop of wire that is put around a pedicle of tissue to dissect it, such as in the case of a tonsil snare. The snare is

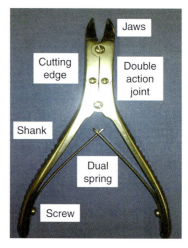

Figure 4.15 A double-action bone cutter (also known as a rongeur or nibbler).

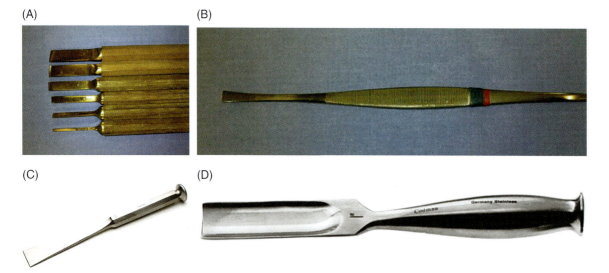

Figure 4.16 Other types of instruments used to cut into or from bone (A) osteotomes (B) a Freer periosteal elevator (C) chisel (D) bone gouge.

(A)

(B)

(C)

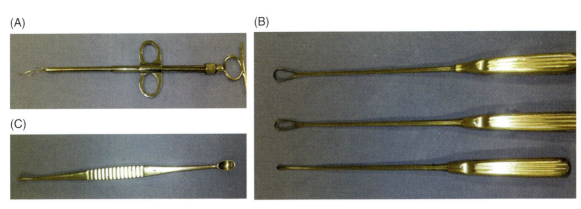

Figure 4.17 Other types of sharp dissectors (A) a tonsil snare (B) types of uterine curettes (C) Volkmann spoon/curette.

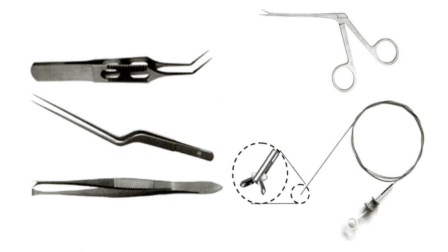

Figure 4.18 Various types of forceps. A close-up of a biopsy forceps is shown on the bottom right.

looped around the tonsil and pulled tight; the wire cuts through the tissue as it pulls back into the instrument to extract the tissue. A curette removes tissue by scraping it away. As examples, uterine curettes can have a sharp or a blunter tip; they are available in different sizes depending on the volume of tissue that is required to be scraped out of the uterus. Another example is a Volkmann bone curette (also known as a Volkmann spoon) and is used in many different types of surgery. Blunt dissection (tissue separation, without cutting) is also desired during some surgical procedures and can be done using a scalpel handle, the blunt side of a scissor blade or a "swab on a stick" (for example swab loaded on to a Kocher's forceps (see next section).

Instruments used for grasping and holding

Tissue is grasped and held in place for the surgeon to work on it using a variety of forceps, such as when inspecting, cutting (e.g. in the case of a biopsy forceps) or even suturing (stitching). The specific type of forceps that the surgeon will select will depend on the type of tissue or surgical material they need to grasp or hold (Figure 4.18).

Delicate or fine forceps are used on delicate tissues such as during eye or certain types of plastic surgery. Forceps are often named after their inventors, with examples being Adson, Gillies and Kocher's forceps (Figure 4.19). Adson forceps are often used by surgeons when suturing the skin (closing a wound using stitches/sutures) following a surgical procedure; they can include toothed or non-toothed types and are generally fine tipped, short forceps. Gillies forceps are also commonly used when suturing the skin. The tip is relatively fine, but this forceps is slightly longer than an Adson. A Kocher's forceps is also a heavy toothed instrument normally used for clamping or holding tissue, but also other materials

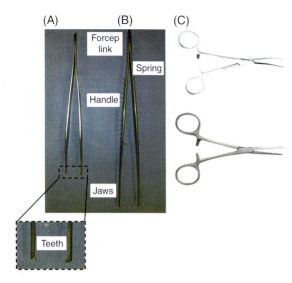

Figure 4.19 Adson (A) Gillies (B) and Kocher's (C) curve shown over straight example) forceps.

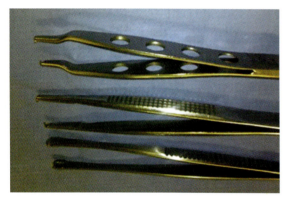

Figure 4.20 Russian, Lane and Jean forceps (shown from top to bottom respectively).

used during surgery. It is used in many disciplines including orthopedics, general surgery and gynecology.

Various types of strong toothed forceps are used by orthopedic surgeons and gynecologists when grasping large chunks of tissue. Examples of strong toothed forceps include Russian, Lane and Jean forceps (Figure 4.20). A Russian forceps, for example, is considered less traumatic when used surgically than other toothed forceps and is used by some gynecologists when suturing (stitching) tissue.

Bayonet forceps, as they are shaped like a knife used on the end of a rifle), are normally used in small surgical spaces (Figure 4.21); they are angled so that the surgeon can see around the forceps into the space. Bayonet-shaped forceps are used in neurosurgery and ear nose and throat surgery.

An example of a "diathermy" forceps is shown in Figure 4.22, with a further example in Figure 4.23. Diathermy forceps are used to cauterize (burn or freeze) blood vessels, in order to stop bleeding quickly; "diathermy" specifically refers to the local production of heat at the tip of the forceps. These types of forceps are available in various lengths and have various shaped tips at the working (patient) ends. An electric source is connected at the surgeon end of the instrument for heating purposes. Diathermy forceps are covered with insulation (usually a plastic coating) to protect the surgeon while in use. Examples of various commonly used types of forceps are shown in Figure 4.23.

Lane tissue forceps are used to grasp tough tissues. They are often used in orthopedics and gynecology. Babcock forceps are designed to fit around a specific structure. This forceps is designed to cause minimal or no damage to tissue and is used in various disciplines (e.g. to grasp the appendix). Vulselm forceps are used to grasp the cervix when doing a dilation and curettage

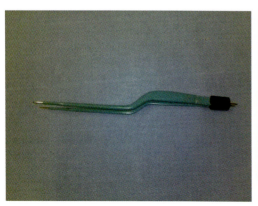

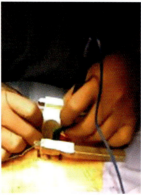

Figure 4.21 Bayonet-shaped diathermy forceps (left) and being used in a procedure (right).

(surgery to remove tissue), or a vaginal hysterectomy. It is a strong toothed forceps. Green Armytage forceps are used during Cesarean sections to grasp the uterus. It can be used to clamp the bleeding vessels of the uterus.

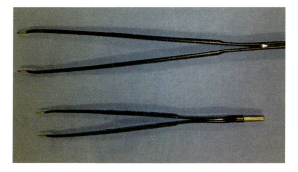

Figure 4.22 Long and short, non-toothed diathermy forceps.

Bone holder forceps (Figure 4.24) are specific types of heavy grasping forceps used to stabilize bone tissue, especially when reducing a fracture (fixing a broken bone, where "broken" is the same as "fracture", to its pre-injury position).

A further example is the Wrigley's forceps that is used to assist with the delivery of a newborn baby (Figure 4.25). The forceps is applied gently around the baby's head, allowing the safe delivery of the baby. There are different types and designs of delivery forceps. Wrigley's are most often used during a Cesarean section.

In addition to holding and manipulating tissues, certain types of forceps are used to hold various objects that assist in a surgical procedure. Sponge or swab holding forceps are examples (Figure 4.26). These are used to grasp swabs or sponges immersed in an antiseptic to disinfect the skin (pre-operative preparative; Chapter 3, in

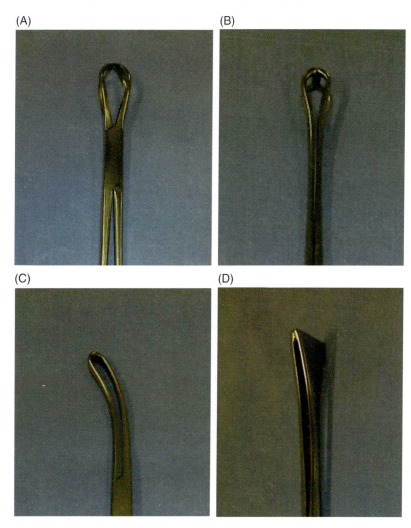

Figure 4.23 Other types of forceps, with their patient-end tips shown (A) Lane tissue (B) Babcock (C) Vulselm (D) Green Armytage forceps.

the section on surgical procedures) just prior to the surgeon making an incision.

Common types of towel clips are used to secure items and drapes within the sterile field (Figure 4.27). As reusable devices, they are often forgotten post-surgery and mistakenly thrown away with disposable drapes.

Instruments used for clamping and occluding

These types of instruments are used to apply pressure to a structure, clamp a structure or to close or block a passage ("occlude", as in the case of hemostats and their use on blood vessels). Some will crush tissue and others are non-crushing.

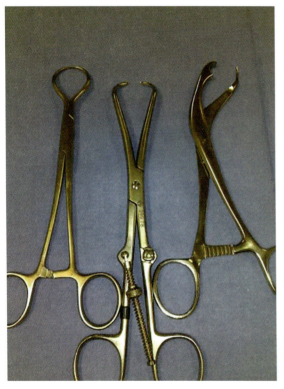

Figure 4.24 Various types of bone holder forceps.

The type of instrument used will depend on the patient's anatomy, the type of operation, the location of the surgical site and the surgeon. The various parts of a typical clamping/occluding device are shown in Figure 4.28.

Hemostatic forceps are clamps designed to stop a blood vessel from bleeding (Figure 4.29). They normally have serrations (grooves in the surface) on both jaws. The serrations can run across the jaws or down the length of the jaws. There are a number of different types of these forceps, and each instrument is designed to clamp blood vessels and tissue in different areas of the body.

An example of a crushing clamp, where the serrations run down the length of the instrument, is a Maingot (Figure 4.30). It is used to clamp the uterine pedicle during a hysterectomy (surgical removal of the uterus); the forceps are placed straight either side of the uterus (womb) and used to clamp down on the associated blood vessels.

Other types of clamps include various types of blood vessel ("vascular") clamps. There are two types of vascular clamps, those that partially occlude and those that totally occlude. Vascular clamps have different jaw designs that include (Figure 4.31):
• Cooley type jaws, having a double row of finely serrated teeth arranged in opposing rows.
• DeBakey type jaws have two rows of finely serrated teeth on one blade and one row on the opposing blade to provide a triangular grip.
• Dardick type jaws have a three or two vascular teeth configuration, and a flatter more flexible blade.

Instruments used for exposing and retracting

Retraction refers to pulling or holding back. Retractors are crucial instruments for providing adequate working space and visualization of the operative site for the surgeon, by keeping an incision through the skin open and exposing underlying tissue. Equal forces of traction (grip or pulling power) and counter-traction are actually needed to hold the incision open correctly; damage may result from mismatched retractors causing tissue healing problems.

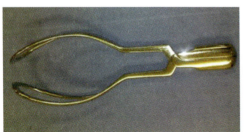

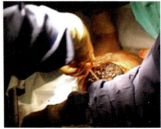

Figure 4.25 Wrigley's forceps and its use during childbirth.

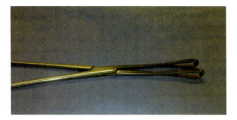

Figure 4.26 Sponge/swab holding forceps.

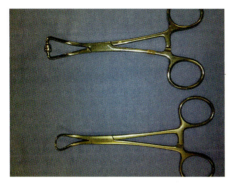

Figure 4.27 Backhaus towel clamp (above) has a blunt tip and is ideal to use to secure a disposable drape. Linen drapes are often secured with the pointed tip towel clamp (below).

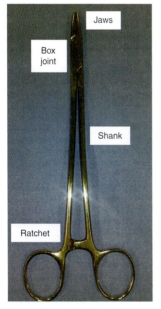

Figure 4.28 Various parts of a needle holder, shown as an example. The jaws shown are typically made of tungsten carbide, while the ratchet is designed to allow a locking-and-release mechanism. Needle holders grasp suture needles.

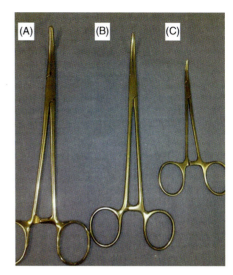

Figure 4.29 Various types of hemostatic forceps ("hemostats") (A) Artery (B) Birkett (C) Mosquito.

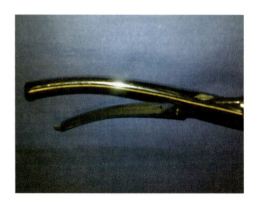

Figure 4.30 The patient end of a Maingot clamp.

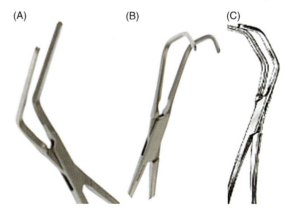

Figure 4.31 Examples of vascular clamps, with types of jaws shown (A) Cooley type (B) DeBakey type (C) Dardick type.

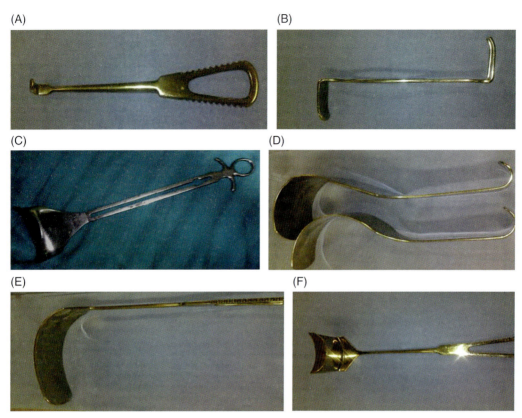

Figure 4.32 Various types of retractors (A) Langenbeck (B) Czerny (C) Doyen (D) Deaver (E) Kelly (F) Morris.

Handheld retractors are designed to hold open a wound or to pull structures (such as internal organs) aside so the surgeon can reach the various internal anatomies (Figure 4.32). The Langenbeck retractor was designed by German surgeon Bernhard von Langenbeck, originally for urological procedures. Today it is used for plastics, general and urological procedures. Other examples of widely used retractor designs are known as the Czerny and Doyens. Deaver, Kelly and Morris retractors are particularly used in abdominal surgery. These are handheld retractors which are normally held by the surgeon's assistant.

Malleable retractors can be bent into whatever shape is required. They are made from different materials and can be used anywhere in the body, particularly with soft tissues such as in the abdomen or even the mouth. They are available in different shapes, widths and lengths (Figure 4.33). Simple hooks are also used for retraction (Figure 4.34). Hooks can be sharp or blunt, single or double. They are often used to retract skin, nerves and tendons. Self-retaining retractor designs are also used. These are retractors that can

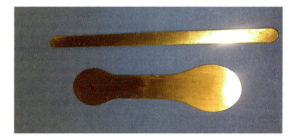

Figure 4.33 Malleable copper retractors used in the mouth.

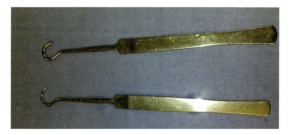

Figure 4.34 Blunt (top) and sharp (bottom) hooks.

(A)

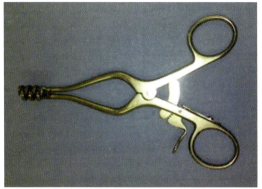

(B)

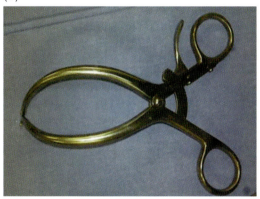

(C)

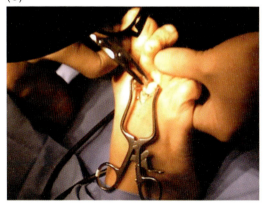

Figure 4.35 Examples of various types of self-retaining retractors (A) Weitlaner (B) Gelpi (C) self-retainer (in surgical use).

be placed into a wound to spread and hold it open on its own, in contrast to the handheld retractors discussed above. There are a variety of shapes and sizes of self-retainers all used in different areas of the body (Figure 4.35).

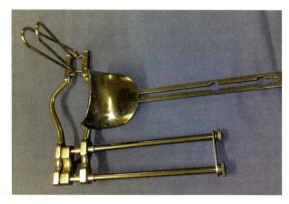

Figure 4.36 A Balfour retractor (left) with screws attached and associated with a Doyen retractor (on the right).

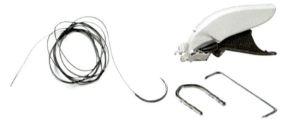

Figure 4.37 A needle and suture (left), used for suturing, and staples with a surgical stapler.

A final example of a commonly used retractor is the Balfour retractor, which is used to keep an abdominal wound open. It can be used on its own or with the Doyens retractor, which attaches to the Balfour (Figure 4.36). The Doyens is normally used in conjunction with the Balfour when doing surgery on organs in the pelvic cavity. The Balfour typically has three screws that are loosened and tightened during surgery (note, a concern as these can be easily lost during reprocessing or even surgical use!). The Doyens retractor can also be used on its own as a hand-held retractor (Figure 4.36).

Instruments used for suturing or stapling

Suturing and stapling are two methods used to close ("ligate") a wound or cut in a tissue. Suturing (stitching) is done using a needle and suture material (thread made of materials such as silk, nylon and polypropylene), while stapling uses a U-shaped piece of wire (Figure 4.37).

Different devices are used to assist with suturing and stapling. Common examples are needle holders, used during suturing. Needle holders are designed to be used with curved suture needles (Figure 4.38). They lock the needle in a manner that allows the surgeon to push the needle and associated suture through the tissue. Needle holders are available in many different lengths and have different types of tips (Figure 4.38). They are designed to be used with specific needle and suture sizes. The tips of the holder can be thick or thin, they can have tungsten carbide inserts, and the pattern on the jaw can vary. Tungsten carbide is much stiffer than steel so it grips the needle well and does not wear out as quickly as steel.

Staplers (or clip appliers) are used to insert staples (clips; Figure 4.39). Ligaclips are examples of commonly used staples in general and vascular surgery. They can be

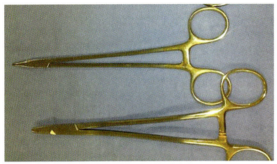

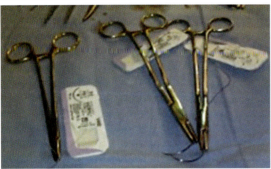

Figure 4.38 Types of needle holders. Debakey (top) and Thompson-Walker (bottom, with needles/sutures).

used to clip any tissue. There are different types and sizes of clips (depending on what type of tissue is being stapled), and these are also available as disposable items. The correct clip applier must be used with the correct clip. They often have color-coded ring handles, where the color on the applicator will match up with the color of the packaging of the clip.

Instruments used for general viewing

Speculums are retracting instruments that are used during operations or examinations on the external openings of the body, including the ear, mouth, eye, nostril, rectum and vagina. Their shape generally corresponds to where and how they are used, with examples shown in Figure 4.40.

More complicated and penetrating types of viewing instruments are known as endoscopes. These can be generally considered as being rigid or flexible in design (Chapter 3, in the section on introduction to endoscopic procedures and Figure 3.2). These are considered further in the section on Endoscopy, as they are both used for viewing, diagnostic and surgical procedures.

Instruments used for suction and aspiration

Various types of tubular suction devices are used to connect to a vacuum source to aspirate (suck up) various body fluids (such as blood) or other liquids that can be present during the surgical procedure. There are many shapes and sizes of suction devices, again each designed to be used in specific areas of the body and to suck up different volumes of fluid (Figure 4.41).

The Yankauer suction nozzle was originally designed to be used by the surgeon when operating on the throat, but it is now often used for abdominal surgery as it has a large bore to suck away fluid. A pool suction nozzle is designed with a cover to stop any soft tissues (such as the intestines) being accidentally sucked up into the tube,

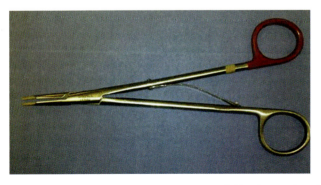

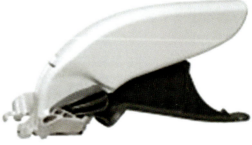

Figure 4.39 Staplers, including a LigaClip applier (left) and surgical stapler (right).

Figure 4.40 Speculum types (A) nasal (B) vaginal and (C) anal.

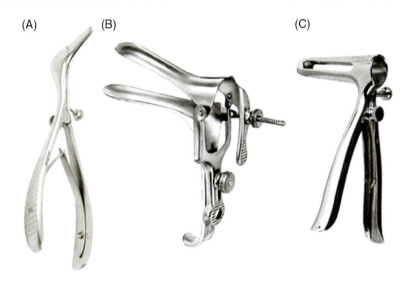

(A) (B) (C)

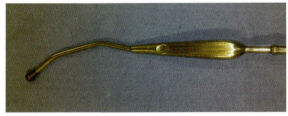
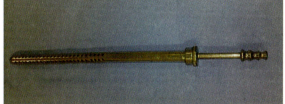

Figure 4.41 Two common types of suction-associated devices. Yankauer (left) and Pool (right) suction nozzles.

thus causing damage. It is very useful when sucking up large volumes of fluid in the abdomen.

Similar instruments are used to irrigate a wound or area under surgery, such as a simple syringe/needle or more complicated systems such as those in flexible endoscopes (see the section on endoscopy) and dental water line units.

Instruments used for dilation

Dilators are used to enlarge or open up various orifices or ducts during surgery (Figure 4.42). The tissue is expanded by starting with a smaller size and then increasing to wider sizes until the surgeon is satisfied that the anatomy has been dilated enough.

Instruments used for measuring or positioning

Various instruments can be used for measuring during surgical procedures, such as simple rulers, trial sizes, depth gauges and calipers. A depth gauge (Figure 4.43), for example, is used to measure the length of a hole drilled into bone so the surgeon knows what length of screw to insert during an orthopedic procedure. A caliper is a device used

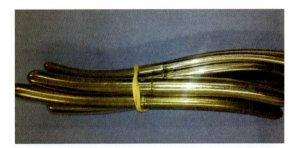

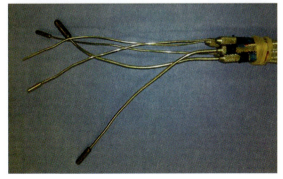

Figure 4.42 Examples of dilators used in surgery. Sets of Hegar uterine (top) and Bakes gall duct (bottom) dilators shown.

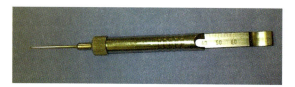

Figure 4.43 A surgical depth gauge.

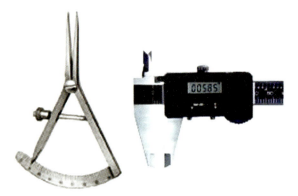

Figure 4.44 Examples of manual (left) and digital (right) calipers.

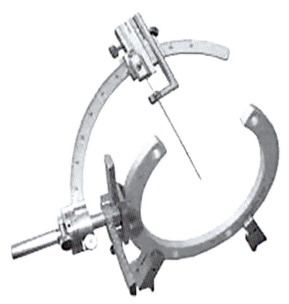

Figure 4.45 An example of a frame-type device used on the head for stereotactic surgery.

to measure the distance between two sides of an object (Figure 4.44).

In addition, various devices are used for surgical positioning, with one of the more advanced examples being instruments used in stereotactic surgery (Figure 4.45). This makes use of a computer-based locating system to identify and operate on relatively small targets inside the body, such as in the brain. These and similar procedures can also be assisted with X-ray or tomography computer systems to directly visualize the target tissue.

Powered instruments/tools

Powered devices can operate on electricity, battery or high pressure air. They can often be complex instruments, associated with a variety of accessories, and it is very important to follow the manufacturer's instructions carefully when disassembling, reassembling and particularly cleaning these instruments. Examples are shown in Figure 4.46.

Other miscellaneous surgical instruments

There are many other miscellaneous types of devices that are used for surgery. Examples are mallets that are generally used in orthopedics to hammer with (into bone). There are various sizes and types of mallets, with heavy mallets being used for strong, hard bones (Figure 4.47). Another example is a chisel (used with a hammer).

Other types of surgical devices include surgical bone screws and bone plates used in orthopedic surgery (Figure 4.48). These are often provided in sets, as a mixture of single-use (e.g. screws and pins) and re-usable (e.g. forceps, depth gauges, etc.) devices, and are also frequently on loan to a hospital or clinic for use. Although some of the devices provided in the set are single use, the surgeon will only use a number of these during a procedure, while the remaining are reprocessed, along with the other re-usable devices. They provide much debate in reprocessing circles, as they do provide a mixture of single and multiple devices, are often heavy sets (as typical of many orthopedic sets) and are passed from hospital to hospital.

Microsurgery

Microsurgery is a general term used for surgery that is done with the aid of a microscope. A microscope is a device used to magnify, by a series of lenses, an area of the body or indeed any small object to view its structure. Microsurgery is used extensively in plastic (reconstructive) surgery as well as neurosurgical, ophthalmological and cardiovascular surgery. The procedures done with a microscope include re-plantation (re-attachment of a part of the body), transplantation (transfer of one tissue/organ/body part from one subject to another) and LASIK eye surgery. These specialty procedures often require the

Figure 4.46 Examples of powered instruments and tools. Orthopedic power tools (left) and the use of an Ansback drill during a surgical procedure (right) is shown.

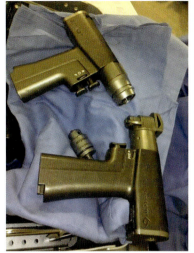
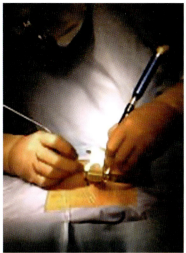

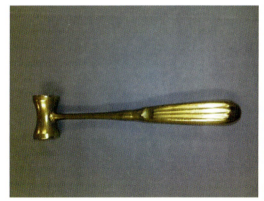
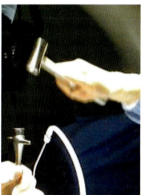

Figure 4.47 A surgical mallet (left) and being used during orthopedic surgery (right).

most delicate and complicated surgical instrumentation, to allow access and manipulation of small tissues and organs. These include electro-surgical bipolar forceps, Frazier suction tubes, aneurysm clip appliers, curettes and cranial clamps and screws. Examples of these instruments are shown in Figure 4.49.

Micro-instruments are designed to be used when operating whilst looking through a microscope and are specially designed so that they do not obscure the surgeon's vision during such procedures. These are fine delicate instruments and must be handled with the utmost care.

Robotic surgery

Robotic (also known as robot or computer-assisted) surgery is a relatively new technology, used in many types of surgical procedures, that allows complicated precise and particularly minimally invasive surgery to take place. Surgery is done with the aid of a computer-controlled robot, where the surgeon can be within the sterile field (with the robot), remotely from the patient (outside the sterile field) or even in the absence of a surgeon (the robot conducts the procedure on its own). An early example of robotic-assisted surgery was the AESOP (automated endoscopic system for optimal positioning), consisting of a robotic arm controlled by the surgeon's voice commands to manipulate an endoscopic camera and was first developed with the US army (Figure 4.50).

Another example is the SRI Green Telepresence Surgery system, which has since been optimized and reintroduced as the multi-armed da Vinci surgical system. Further recent examples include the multi-armed Zeus system and two-armed ARTEMIS system. All of these systems are remotely controlled by the surgeon, allowing for greater surgical precision. Both the Zeus and da Vinci system are comprehensive master-slave surgical robots with multiple arms operated by the surgeon remotely from a console with

(A)

(B)

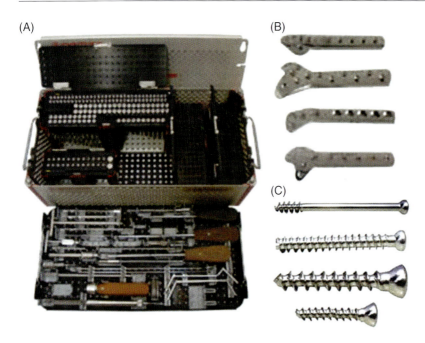

Figure 4.48 Example of a mixture of single-use and re-usable devices, in this case an orthopedic instrument and screw set (A) the instrument set (B) bone plates (C) orthopedic screws.

(C)

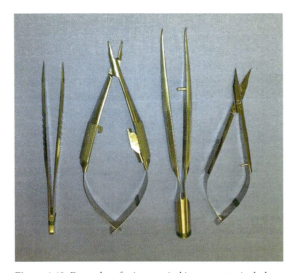

Figure 4.49 Examples of microsurgical instruments, include needle holder, tying forceps and scissors.

video assisted visualization and computer enhancement. The devices used as part of these procedures are sophisticated robotic assisted endoscopes and accessories designed for minimally invasive procedures that treat a range of conditions. These include bladder, prostate and colorectal cancer, coronary artery disease, kidney disorders and uterine fibroids. Further consideration of endoscopic devices is given in the section on endoscopy.

Devices used in dental surgery

There are typically three different sets of instruments used in oral and maxillofacial surgery clinics: (1) simple extraction sets, (2) surgical extraction sets and (3) biopsy sets. Other instruments will include those used for minor procedures, observation and probing, such as dental mirrors, suture scissors, forceps, suction tips, etc. An example of a typical extraction set is shown in Figure 4.51.

Examples of some specific dental devices are shown in Figure 4.52. Many of these devices are similar to those used in general surgery, described in the preceding sections, such as retractors, probes and forceps. An example is a dental syringe that is used to inject local anesthetic (usually provided in a glass cartridge) into a patient.

Tattooing

Although tattooing is conducted in a wide variety of non-clinical settings, many of the devices or instruments that are used for these procedures are considered critical as they may penetrate the skin and may come into contact with the blood. A typical example is a re-usable tattoo gun, with an example given in Figure 4.53. The gun handle and other associated parts of the device may be disposable or re-usable.

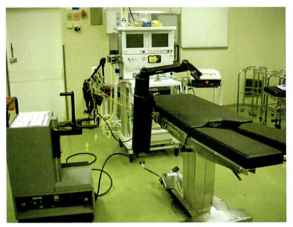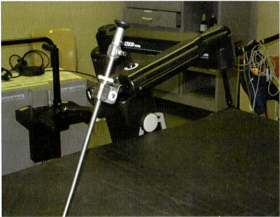

Figure 4.50 AESOP (automated endoscopic system for optimal positioning) robotic system. On the left is a surgical table with robotic arm attached, and on the right a close up of the arm holding a rigid endoscope.

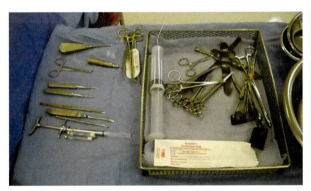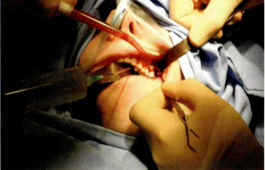

Figure 4.51 An example of a dental extraction (wisdom tooth) instrument set (left) and procedure (right). Note, in the procedure, a suction tube (top left), syringe (bottom left), retractor (top right) and probe (bottom right).

Endoscopy

Some basic types of internal viewing devices were introduced in the section on instruments for general viewing, but more complicated types are known as endoscopes. "Endoscope" is derived from two Greek words, *endon* meaning inside and *skopeo* or *skopo*, which is an old verb meaning look into or through something very thoroughly. These can be generally considered as being rigid or flexible in design (Chapter 3, in the section on introduction to endoscopic procedures; Figure 3.2). They are internally made up of fiber optic bundles or lenses with an eyepiece at one end, and a lens at the other for viewing purposes. This allows surgeons to look inside their patients in order to directly view, diagnose and/or perform surgery through a small incision (known as "keyhole" or minimally invasive surgery), causing

minimal trauma to the patient. These are extremely delicate instruments and must be handled with care.

Being "flexible" or "rigid" refers to their design, where rigid devices are constructed of rigid (inflexible) materials and flexible devices are designed to be more supple (in particular those parts that are placed into the patient). They can be designed to allow for direct viewing through an eye-piece on the endoscope (as shown for the rigid devices in Figure 3.2) as well as through a video system viewing images on a monitor (a flexible video-endoscope is shown in Figure 3.2, where part of the device is introduced into the patient, part is attached to a control and supply system and a central part is held and managed by the operator). The various types of endoscopic procedures are defined, based on the area of the body where they are performed, such as arthroscopes (inserted into a joint for

(A)

(B)

(C)   (D)

(E)

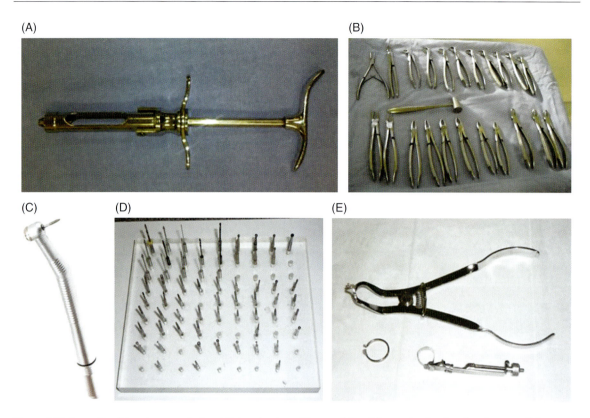

Figure 4.52 Examples of dental surgery devices (A) dental syringe (B) a set of dental forceps (with a dental mallet centrally) (C) a dental drill (D) a range of drill bots and burrs (E) matrix band and holder.

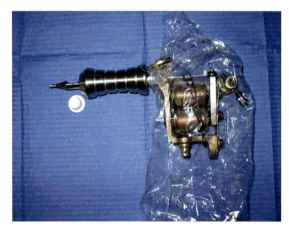

Figure 4.53 A tattooing gun and handle.

examination or visualization for treatment), broncho-scopes (used in the respiratory system including the lungs, larynx (voice box), vocal cord, trachea, and bron-chi), laparoscopes (for visualization during surgical

procedures in the abdominal cavity) and colonoscopes (for procedures in the colon, inserted through the anus; Chapter 3, in the section on introduction to endoscopic procedures, Table 3.5).

Examples of rigid endoscopes are shown in Figure 4.54. Common rigid endoscopes include those used for joint (arthroscopes), abdominal, gynecology (laparo-scopes), chest (thoracoscopes), bladder (cystoscopes) and ENT (rhinoscope) surgery.

Rigid endoscopes have the following basic compo-nents:

• A solid metal tube, with an optical lens at one end (patient end) and eyepiece (surgeon end) at the other. The surgeon uses the eyepiece to look inside joints and body cavities to diagnose or perform surgical procedures. Rigid endoscopes do not generally bend.

• A series of internal glass lenses comprising of precisely-aligned lenses and spacers that form an optical chain. The optical chain transfers the image being viewed directly to the eye of the surgeon or to a video monitor. The optical

(A)

(B)

(C)

(D)

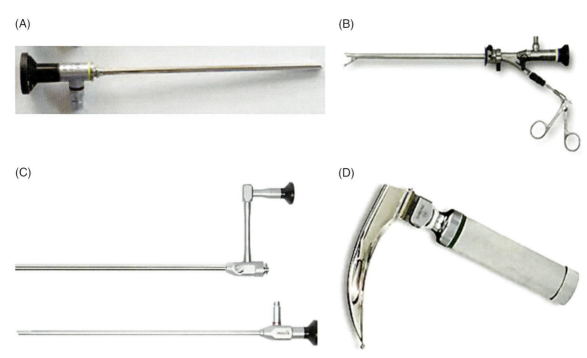

Figure 4.54 Types of rigid endoscopes (A) arthroscope (B) cystoscope, with an associated device (C) two types of laproscopes (D) laryngoscope.

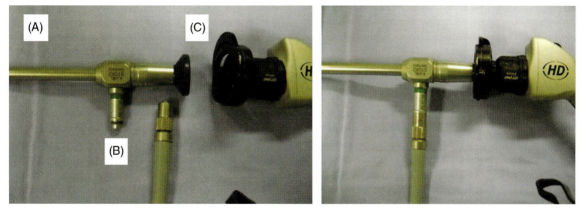

Figure 4.55 Example of assembly of a rigid endoscope (surgeon end shown). On the left disassembled and on the right assembled (A) rigid endoscope (B) light cable (and attachment site, light post, on the device) (C) camera (attaches to the device eyepiece).

element of a rigid scope is called a telescope. They are often used in conjunction with a camera system, which allows the surgeon to view a greatly magnified image. The camera head fits over the eyepiece and the image is transmitted via a camera cable to the processor and displayed on a monitor (Figure 4.55).

• A fiber optic light post and system. Light is delivered throughout the endoscope through fiber optic bundles, which are situated around the outside of the lens housing.
• Bridges and adapters connect to the telescope and cannula (lumen) opening (if present), and allow for the introduction of accessories (e.g. Figure 4.55 (B)) and

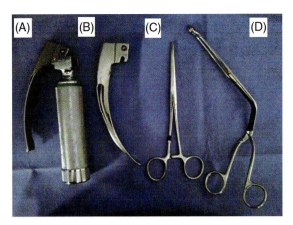

Figure 4.56 A typical laryngoscopy set (A) the laryngoscope (B) laryngoscope blade (C) artery forcep (D) McGills forcep.

the application of electrosurgical energy to resect or coagulate tissue.

Rigid laryngoscopes are one of the most commonly used rigid endoscopes and are used to expose and view the larynx to facilitate endotracheal intubation (Figure 4.56).

These endoscopes have a fiber-optic disposable or re-usable blade that is available in different sizes, may be curved or straight and connects to the laryngoscope's handle. They do not generally have any associated channels. Channels in rigid endoscopes, or within associated devices utilized as part of the procedure (such as trocars), are used for the placement of accessory instruments (such as forceps) and are often used when doing certain types of endoscopic procedures like arthroscopies or laparo-scopies (with an example given in Figure 5.54).

Many of the types of rigid endoscopes are also available in flexible form, based on where they are used (such as cystoscopes and bronchoscopes). Flexible devices are often preferred in allowing the devices to be flexed and bend when introduced into the patient, as well as for viewing and manipulation during the surgical or medical procedure. This is important in introducing the endo-scope into natural orifices of the body, such as the mouth (for gastroscopy and bronchoscopy) and the anus (during colonoscopy). Descriptions of the various types of endos-copy procedures are given in Chapter 3, in the section entitled introduction to endoscopic procedures (summa-rized in Table 3.5). Examples of various types of flexible endoscopes are shown in Figure 4.57.

In general, flexible endoscopes have much longer chan-nels and, similar to rigid endoscopes, are supported with either a plastic or glass fiber bundles that allow direct visu-alization or convey an image to a camera plus additional

fibers to provide light. They are designed for inspection, sampling (e.g. taking a biopsy) and even more recently surgical procedures in the bronchial tree (bronchoscopy), lower bowel (sigmoidoscopy), upper bowel (colonos-copy), stomach (gastroscopy), and urethra/bladder (cys-toscopy). Flexible endoscopes are particularly useful for viewing the inside of stomach, duodenum and intestines, where the endoscope may have to pass a long distance into the body, and around the twists and curves of the alimen-tary canal (Chapter 3, section on introduction to endo-scopic procedures). Rhinolaryngoscopes, for example, are used to diagnose and evaluate the normal physiological and pathologic conditions of the nose and larynx.

Despite their appearance, flexible endoscopes are extremely complicated and very fragile. The main, work-ing parts of a flexible endoscope are shown in Figure 4.58.

Flexible endoscopes also have the following basic components:

• A control handle/head that allows control of the device by the surgeon or other operator (Figure 4.59). Control buttons are provided to activate air/fluid/suction chan-nels on flexible scopes, and ports for placement of acces-sory instruments. Within the head are the fiber optic fibers arranged around one or more of the lumens that run elsewhere through the device.

• A viewing and optical system. Flexible endoscopes can be further sub-divided into two types: fiberscopes and videoscopes (Figure 4.59). Fiberscopes have an eyepiece for the surgeon to look directly through the device; some fiberscopes have the option of fixing a camera over the eyepiece to transmit a picture to a separate screen (for viewing of capture). A videoscope does not have an eye-piece as the image is transmitted directly to a video screen.

• A light source (connected to the control head via the light guide cable) to assist in inspecting internal areas. The light source connectors vary in design depending on the manufacturers and connect to a light source. Light is transmitted by optical fibers. The light guide connector end may also allow connection to air, water and suction sources, as well as to a video system.

• An insertion tube (also known as the body or shaft), containing internal lumens and fiber optics/cables. This also includes various parts (coils, etc.) that allow the device to be angulated during the procedure (particularly at the distal tip end). All these components are enclosed in an insulated jacket.

• An internal series of lumens (or channels). The device may have up to five separate and/or interconnected lumens, such as the suction/biopsy, air/water and elevator guide wire ("alberan") lumens. The biopsy port allows

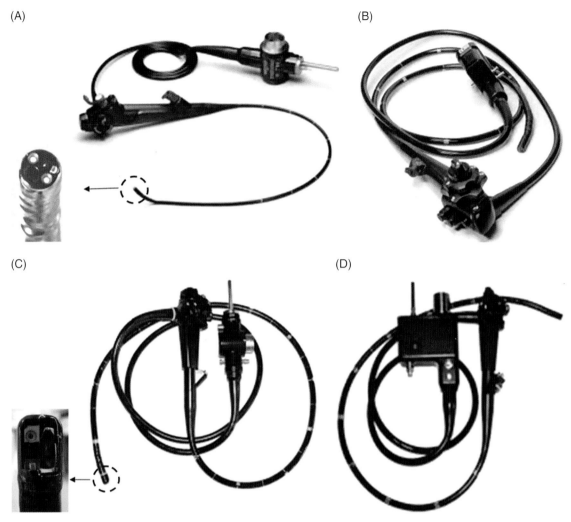

(A)

(B)

(C)

(D)

Figure 4.57 Types of flexible endoscopes. All devices shown are video-endoscopes (A) bronchoscope (with a view of the end of the scope showing the end of a channel and light source) (B) colonoscope (C) duodenoscope (with a view of the side-viewing end of the scope) (D) gastroscope.

entry into the suction/biopsy channel for placing an accessory device (biopsy forceps, see section on instruments for cutting and dissecting) through the channel and into the patient during a procedure. The suction channel is used to suction away water and debris. The water and air channels are used to introduce water or air, respectively to enhance visualization; these channels can be combined or separate.

Flexible endoscopes are becoming even more complicated as they become used in a wider array of medical and surgical situations. Once used for simple diagnostic purposes, flexible endoscopes are now being used for more elaborate procedures. Examples are endoscopic ultrasound procedures, where the flexible endoscope includes a small ultrasound device at the distal tip, which when introduced into the alimentary canal (through the mouth or anus) is used to visualize the digestive tract in greater detail, but also adjacent organs in the body. Further advances include the use of flexible endoscopes through natural orifices (mouth, anus, bellybutton, etc.) for surgery, known as NOTES (natural orifice transluminal endoscopic surgery) and other similar terms. In such cases, the flexible endoscope and associated accessories have been modified to allow for their microsurgical use.

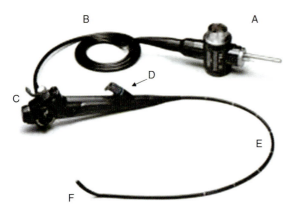

Figure 4.58 The main working parts of a flexible endoscope (A) light guide connector (the device can include air and/or air/water connectors, attachment to a light source/video system, suction system and even other gas supply systems such as carbon dioxide) (B) light guide cable (C) control body (allows the surgeon to hold and control the device, including various ports and valves) (D) a biopsy port (if present, allows accessories to be inserted through the device and into the patient to take a sample or biopsy) (E) the insert tube and at its end (F) the distal tip (including a section known as the bending rubber, which can be controlled by the surgeon during a procedure).

In many cases, flexible and rigid endoscopes use a variety of other devices/instruments during a procedure, with the endoscope used for visualization and sometimes access to internal tissues (Figure 4.60). These include separate devices used as part of the procedure, such as light and suction source instruments, trocars, forceps (see the section on instruments for cutting and dissecting), catheters, electrodes, etc.; others are specific parts of the device, such as valves used with flexible endoscopes. These accessories to the procedure may be re-usable or single use (disposable), and may vary in size, configuration and intended use. In many cases, the shafts of these devices and accessories are constructed of thin metal tubing due to size constraints; these can become easily dented or bent and should be handled carefully. Re-usable accessories, just like the endoscopes themselves should be checked thoroughly for function and integrity before and after each use. It is important to note that the endoscope itself and many of the associated accessories require similar levels of reprocessing, with the exception of any part that has no direct contact or risk of contact with the patient during a procedure or a device that is used on only one patient (single use).

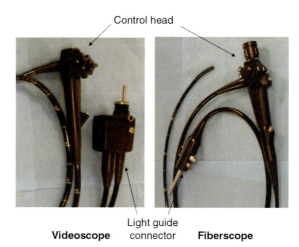

Videoscope   Light guide connector   **Fiberscope**

Figure 4.59 Examples of control heads and light guide connectors of flexible video and fiberscopes.

Miscellaneous devices used medically

There are various types of generally, non-critical medical devices that are used for basic patient monitoring and/or diagnosis (with examples shown in Figure 4.61). A number of common examples are discussed in this section.

Blood pressure (BP) monitors

A blood pressure monitor is a non-invasive blood pressure measuring device. There are various types of blood pressure apparatus: the older mercury gravity manometer and more modern gauge or electronic monitors. The most widely used devices (Figure 4.61) consist of an arm cuff connected to a source of pressure (manual or automated) and a pressure gauge (manual or digital).

Reflex hammer

A reflex hammer is a medical instrument to test deep muscle-tendon reflexes There are several types of hammers, usually constructed to resemble a metal disk, that have a rubber bumper attached to them, attached to a stem with a tapered edge that may be used to test reflexes, for example by scratching the underside of the foot.

Medical thermometers

Medical thermometers are used to measure body temperature. There are several, external places on the body where temperatures can be measured and many different types of thermometers (Figure 4.61). An oral thermometer is used in mouth and under the tongue, or

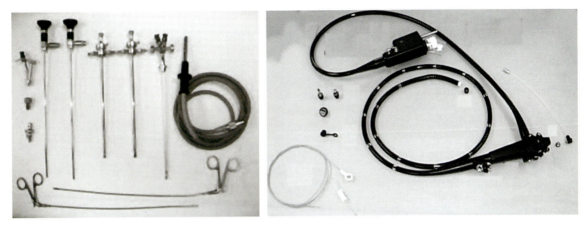

Figure 4.60 Sets of endoscopes used in procedures. A cystoscopic procedure (cystoscopy; left) and flexible endoscopy (right, showing biopsy forceps on the left of the picture) set of devices.

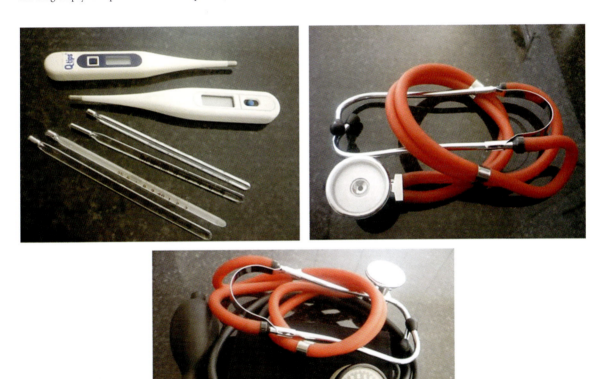

Figure 4.61 Examples of commonly used devices for routine medical use. These are thermometers (top left), a stethoscope (top right) and a manual blood pressure monitor (bottom).

in the crease of the armpit. A rectal thermometer is similar to an oral thermometer, but differs in that the metal bulb on the end is wider. An ear thermometer is a digital device designed to fit into the ear canal. The most commonly used thermometer is made of glass, with a narrow metal bulb at the end with a small ball of mercury or colored (red) alcohol inside it. There is a temperature range on the side where the temperature is registered. The mercury/alcohol rises as the temperature rises. Most thermometers come in both Fahrenheit and Celsius scales. Digital varieties of both the oral and rectal thermometers are also available. Thermometers are generally provided with a disposable plastic sheath that covers the end to take a temperature.

Stethoscopes

A stethoscope is used to listen to sounds produced inside the body. It is used primarily to listen to the lungs, heart and intestinal tract. It is also used to listen to blood flow in certain areas and heart sounds of developing fetuses in pregnant women. Stethoscopes vary in their design and material. Most are made of Y-shaped rubber tubing comprised of two flexible rubber tubes running from a valve to the earpieces (Figure 5.72). The valve also connects the tubes to a "chestpiece", allowing sound to enter the device at one end, which can be either bell-shaped or a flat disk for higher frequencies, and then travel up the tubes and through to the earpieces. Most modern stethoscopes are designed for use with both ears. Single stethoscopes are designed for use with one ear and differential stethoscopes allow the comparisons of sounds at two different body sites. Electronic stethoscopes, which electronically amplify tones, are also available.

5 Microbiology and infection control/prevention

Introduction

Microbiology is the study of microscopic organisms ("microorganisms"). *Mikros* is the Greek word for small and therefore microbiology is the study of small, living forms. It is a wide-ranging science, including many types of organisms that can be beneficial as well as detrimental to our lives and health. In this chapter we are particularly concerned with those microorganisms that can do us harm and cause ill-health or disease. A "disease" is a disorder of the structure or function of the body and is usually associated with specific signs and symptoms. An "infection" is a type of disease caused by microorganisms, which are collectively referred to as "pathogens" or disease-causing microorganisms. Examples of some of the prominent pathogens (or pathogenic microorganisms) are given in Table 5.1. An infection occurs when a pathogen is allowed to grow on or within a host (e.g. the human body) possibly leading to detrimental effects (or "disease"). It is important to note that many microorganisms can live on and in the body with no ill effects and in some cases are important to the structure and function of the body.

"Infection prevention and control" is the discipline that *prevents* the spread of infectious agents and also *controls* their *further spread* in case of an "outbreak" which is a sudden increase in the numbers of cases of an infection putting others in the vicinity at risk. Proper cleaning, disinfection and sterilization of re-usable medical devices are essential for effective infection prevention and control in healthcare settings.

Microorganism types

The microbial world: an introduction
The microbial world is very diverse and only briefly described in this section. In Chapter 2 in the introductory section, the various different types of cells and their components that make up the human body were discussed. In general, similar structures make up the microbial world, but they are not directly visible to us and require a microscope (a magnification instrument) to observe them. For example, if you measure across the head of a pin it is about 1 mm in diameter and the end of a human hair about ten times less (0.1 mm); you can just about see these with the human eye and then you can estimate that the average number of cells or microorganisms across the head of a pin could be:

- 100 human cells (~0.01 mm per cell)
- 100 yeast cells (~0.01 mm per cell)
- 1000 bacteria (~0.001 mm per cell)
- 100,000 small viruses (~0.00001 mm per virus)

These individual organisms vary in size and structure. Some, are multicellular, similar to humans, where different cell types join together to make up the various parts (organs) of the organism. These include the helminths and are commonly known as microscopic "worms". Others are unicellular (single, individual cells) but of the same essential structure as a human cell (known as "eukaryotes", including fungi and protozoa) or a different and smaller type of cell structure (known as "prokaryotes" such as bacteria). It was thought for many years that cell structures, although varied, were the basis of "life". But microbiology also includes viable but non-cellular forms such as viruses and prions that are more simply composed of molecules such as nucleic acids and proteins. In the following sections, each of these classes of microorganisms is considered in further detail. It should be noted that microbiology is a progressive science, with new types of microorganisms being discovered continually. Their description, classification and our knowledge of the types of diseases they can cause is an area of ongoing research.

A Practical Guide to Decontamination in Healthcare, First Edition. Gerald McDonnell and Denise Sheard.
© 2012 Gerald McDonnell and Denise Sheard. Published 2012 by Blackwell Publishing Ltd.

Table 5.1 Examples of microbial pathogens and their associated diseases.

Microorganism type	Microorganism	Associated disease(s)[1]
Prion[2]	PrP^{Sc}	Creutzfeld-Jakob disease (CJD) and variant CJD (vCJD), diseases particularly associated with the nervous system and loss of brain functions.
Viruses	Hepatitis B	Hepatitis, an inflammation leading to liver damage and possibly liver cancer.
	Human immunodeficiency virus (HIV)	Primary cause of acquired immunodeficiency syndrome (AIDS), a disease affecting the immune system, with increased vulnerability to other infections.
	Norovirus (previously called the "Norwalk agent")	Acute infection (also known as gastric flu, tummy bug and stomach flu) of the gut leading to diarrhea and vomiting.
Bacteria[3]	*Staphylococcus aureus*	Causes skin (and wound), gastrointestinal and respiratory tract infections. MRSA (for methicillin-resistant *S. aureus*) is a type of *S. aureus* that has developed resistance to certain types of antibiotics.
	Escherichia coli	While it is a normal inhabitant of the gut, certain strains can cause severe infections of the intestinal and urinary tracts.
	Mycobacterium tuberculosis	Tuberculosis, mainly a disease of the respiratory tract, but can also infect other parts of the body.
Fungi	*Aspergillus niger* or *braziliensis*	Causes mainly respiratory tract infections ("aspergillosis").
	Candida albicans	Candidiasis, infections of the skin, mucous membranes and blood.
Protozoa	*Cryptosporidium parvum*	Cryptosporidiosis, a form of acute diarrhea.
	Acanthamoeba castellanii	Infections of the skin and eyes (keratitis).
	Plasmodium falciparum	Malaria, a disease of red blood cells and the liver.
Helminths ("parasitic worms")	*Wuchereria bancrofti*	Elephantiasis, where worms get lodged in the blood or lymphatic systems.
	Ascaris lumbricoides	Ascariasis, infection of the lung and intestine (often associated with poor hygiene).

[1] For information on the structure and functions of the various systems of the human body, refer to Chapter 2.
[2] Prions are not strictly considered as "living", but are often considered under microbiology as they are transmissible and infectious like other microorganisms.
[3] The scientific names of all organisms including microorganisms are written either in italics or underlined, such as *Staphylococcus aureus* or Staphylococcus aureus. The exception to this are viruses.

Prions and other infectious proteins

Prions are widely accepted to be infectious proteins. Proteins are one of the major biochemical molecules that make up life (see Chapter 2); they play an important role in the structure and function of cellular and non-cellular life. In cells, they are constantly being made, used for specific functions and then broken down. In certain types of diseases, proteins appear to accumulate and therefore precipitate in various organs of the body. In prion-associated diseases the protein is known as PrP^{C}, which is a normal protein found in human and animal cells. The protein appears to play a role in the normal functions of neurons (as part of the nervous system). Like other proteins, it is made and broken down over time, but in rare cases it changes its shape into a form (known as PrP^{res}) that is not degraded by the cell (Figure 5.1). In such cases, PrP^{res} can induce normal PrP^{C} to also change shape and then together accumulate in the cells, leading to cell damage/death and the appearance of the disease. These effects are seen particularly in the nervous system (see Chapter 2), where the dead nerve cells are not replaced. Over time, the cumulative damage to the nervous system causes gradual and irreversible loss of body functions and eventually death. The exact reasons for the changes in protein shape are not known, but in about 10% of cases there is a genetic cause and certain

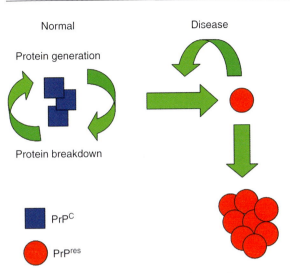

Normal   Disease

Protein generation

Protein breakdown

PrP^C

PrP^{res}

Figure 5.1 The prion theory. The accumulation and precipitation of protein leads to the development of disease.

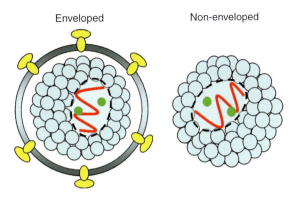

Enveloped   Non-enveloped

Figure 5.2 The basic structure of viruses. Viruses display a wide range of structures but can be classified into two types, enveloped and non-enveloped. In non-enveloped viruses the central nucleic acid (often associated with proteins) is surrounded by a capsid (protein) structure that is unique to the specific virus type/strain. This basic structure is the same for enveloped viruses, but surrounded by an external, lipid-based envelope.

prion-based diseases can therefore be inherited. The remaining 90% of cases appear sporadically and randomly with no known cause.

Prions are unusual infectious agents as they appear to be composed of protein alone and without any detectable DNA or RNA, unlike other types of life forms. They were previously called "slow viruses", but are now known to be quite distinct from viruses in composition and structure. For these reasons they are not strictly considered as "living", but are self-promoting and infectious. Research is continuing to further define the nature of these agents as it appears that other factors that are yet to be defined are involved in the initiation and progression of protein precipitation/deposition and therefore disease.

Prions are implicated in a group of rare diseases known as transmissible spongiform encephalopathies (TSEs). These include the animal diseases scrapie (in sheep) and bovine spongiform encephalopathy (BSE) (in cattle), human diseases such as Creutzfeld-Jakob disease (CJD) and a similar disease known as variant CJD (vCJD). Variant CJD in humans has been known to be due to the same agent as BSE in cattle. These diseases, once diagnosed, are always progressive, invariably fatal and with no known treatments. Prion diseases are transmissible via injection, ingestion and transplantation of contaminated nervous tissues (such as the brain) and through improperly decontaminated re-usable devices such as those in brain surgery. Prions are generally highly resistant to common chemical and physical methods of disinfection and sterilization. There is suspicion that prion-like

misfolded and precipitated proteins may also be the cause of other diseases such as Alzheimer's disease.

Viruses

Viruses are sub-microscopic and relatively simple forms of life that are obligate parasites. While they do not resemble any typical prokaryotic or eukaryotic cell, they possess typical structural features of their own and vary in size and shape. A typical viral particle (virion) consists of an internal DNA or RNA-genome surrounded by a protective protein shell or "capsid". Certain types of viruses contain a second lipid-containing coat or "envelope". Viruses with only the capsid are termed "naked", non-enveloped or "hydrophilic". The other category is termed "enveloped" or "hydrophobic" (Figure 5.2). In general, enveloped viruses are less stable to environmental conditions and also more susceptible to chemical and physical agents when compared to the non-enveloped ones.

This classification is generally used to differentiate between virus types and used as a guide to their resistance to various chemical and physical disinfection/sterilization methods. Non-enveloped viruses consist of an inner compartment that holds the DNA or RNA (the nucleic acid specific for that virus type), but can also include various types of structural or other associated proteins. This is surrounded by a protein coat (known as a capsid), also unique to the virus type, which can protect the virus from damage. Although these structures may sound relatively fragile, they are the opposite and the most difficult

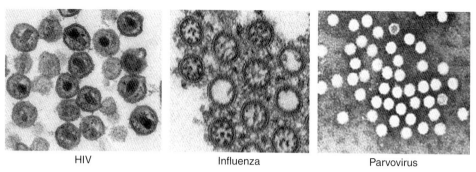

HIV   Influenza   Parvovirus

Figure 5.3 Examples of the variety of viral structures. These examples are not shown to scale and special (electron) microscopes are used in order to directly observe them, due to their small size.

viruses to inactivate. Examples include the poxviruses, parvoviruses, rotaviruses and coxsackieviruses. Enveloped viruses have the same essential structure as that described for the non-enveloped types but also have at least an additional, external envelope that is lipid based and can contain various types of proteins. For some enveloped viruses, these proteins can play important roles in how the viruses attack and take over host cells. A common example is influenza virus, a member of the orthomyxovirus family. Influenza virus causes a respiratory disease known as flu, with typical symptoms including fatigue (feeling tired), headache, fever (increased temperature) and cough. These viruses have been associated with various pandemics ("avian flu", Spanish flu and "swine flu"); a pandemic is an infectious disease that spreads worldwide and affects many people over a wide geographic region, as opposed to an epidemic that would occur in a smaller region/area. These viruses are classified based on two types of surface proteins that are involved in infecting human cells: H for haemagglutinin and N for neuraminidase, therefore being classified such as influenza H1N1 or H5N1. Other examples of enveloped viruses include human immunodeficiency virus (HIV, a type of "retrovirus" that causes AIDS, acquired immunodeficiency syndrome), hepatitis B virus, Ebola virus, herpesviruses and measles virus. Because the external envelope structure plays an important role in the ability of such viruses to infect cells, damage to these structures can prevent the virus from causing disease and for that reason they are actually found to be much more sensitive to inactivation. This can often cause confusion, as viruses such as HIV are widely known to be particularly difficult to treat in infected patients but are actually considered relatively easy to inactivate on exposed surfaces (even

by drying alone under some conditions). At the same time, these viruses are most often associated with various types of human fluids such as mucus and blood that can prevent them from contacting a disinfection or sterilization method; this is an important perspective not only for safe decontamination of these viruses but all other microorganisms and an important concept in decontamination practices.

In some classification systems, a third group of viruses can also be differentiated, based on having moderate resistance to disinfection/sterilization, essentially being non-enveloped although having features similar to enveloped viruses and presenting greater resistance to enveloped viruses, but less than other non-enveloped viruses. Important examples are the adenoviruses, which can cause a variety of conditions such as respiratory, eye and intestinal (diarrheal) diseases.

Examples of the various different structures of viruses are shown in Figure 5.3. They can range in diameter from ~20 nm (e.g. parvoviruses and polio virus) to ~400 nm (typical of the poxviruses such as vaccinia). Different types of viruses can infect (and therefore can cause disease) a wide variety of cell types, including human, animal and plant cells as well as bacteria. For example, viruses that live in bacteria are known as bacteriophages; these are used for various laboratory investigations (e.g. to test disinfectants as they are considered difficult to inactivate) and have even been used as alternatives to antibiotics to treat bacterial infections. Some of the most widely known human diseases caused by viruses are summarized in Table 5.2. It is interesting to note that in addition to diseases typically associated with virus infections, such as inflammation, tissue damage, etc., some viruses have also been associated with cancer; examples include specific types of human

Table 5.2 Examples of human diseases caused by viruses.

Virus name	Family	Type	Associated diseases
Human Immunodeficiency Virus (HIV)	Retroviridae	Enveloped	AIDS (acquired immunodeficiency disease)
Influenza virus	Orthomyxoviridae	Enveloped	Influenza ("flu")
Varicella zoster virus	Herpesviridae	Enveloped	Chicken pox, shingles
Hepatitis B virus	Hepadnaviridae	Enveloped	Hepatitis
Measles virus	Paramyxoviridae	Enveloped	Measles
Adenovirus	Adenoviridae	Non-enveloped	Pharyngitis, conjunctivitis
Papillomavirus	Papillomaviridae	Non-enveloped	Warts, cervical cancer
Parvovirus	Parvoviridae	Non-enveloped	Fifth disease
Poliovirus	Picornaviridae	Non-enveloped	Poliomyelitis

papillomaviruses (HPVs) that are the most common cause of cervical cancer in women (and can be routinely monitored during a procedure known as a Pap smear).

In addition to being enveloped or non-enveloped, viruses are often classified and named based on other criteria such as the type of nucleic acid (DNA or RNA), the shape of the virus and type of disease they cause. An example is a series of viruses that are the most common cause of liver inflammation (the reaction of the liver to infection or damage), known as the "hepatitis" viruses. These are recognized by their alphabetic names such as hepatitis A, B, C, D and E. Although all these viruses have similar names they do vary in their effects during an infection and are also structurally distinct. For example, hepatitis A is a non-enveloped virus (therefore considered highly resistant to disinfection), while hepatitis B and C are both enveloped (and therefore more sensitive to disinfection).

Further consideration of hepatitis B virus and HIV virus should be given here as they are both known to be transmitted through blood and other body tissues; for this reason, they are often referred to as blood-borne pathogens and are an important consideration for anyone working with patient-contaminated materials such as re-usable devices. Not only can HIV and hepatitis B be transmitted through blood, but other examples include viruses such as hepatitis C and viral hemorrhagic fevers (e.g. Ebola virus), as well as other types of microorganisms (bacteria, protozoa and fungi). These diseases are transmissible and healthcare workers have a significant risk of being infected when not taking the correct precautions. Therefore, an important principle in infection

prevention and control and in decontamination practices is to regard all blood (or indeed any body fluid/tissue) as potentially infectious. Standard precautions are required in these cases to minimize disease transmission; in device decontamination these include the use of personal protective equipment (PPE) and vaccination (immunization). Personal protective equipment consists of clothing and/or equipment worn to protect a worker from spillages, splashing, etc. Typical examples include the use of gloves, eye protection and face masks.

Vaccination (or immunization) refers to taking a vaccine to reduce the risk of developing a disease. One of the most important findings in microbiology was that previous exposure to a given type of pathogen could render a person "immune" from infection and disease to any subsequent exposure to the same or closely related pathogens. A simple solution was to prepare samples of the pathogen (or parts thereof) that were damaged or dead; these are referred to as vaccines, and when introduced into us allow our bodies to generate a resistance to those agents as part of our immune system (Chapter 2). Vaccines are now available for a wide range, including viral, diseases. This includes the MMR vaccine for measles, mumps and rubella. They are unique to specific microorganisms and in some cases are specific to certain strains of virus types (as in the case of seasonal flu vaccines). Healthcare workers are also recommended to take a hepatitis B vaccine (usually given over a course of three injections) that is widely available. This is considered a very effective and safe vaccine, but it can only protect against hepatitis B and not other viruses such as HIV. It is important to note that these practices do not completely prevent disease transmission or progression, but when used correctly can reduce this risk to a safe level. Further consideration to infection prevention and control, and standard precautions is given later in the chapter.

Viral diseases can often be difficult to threat, as they generally require specific identification in order to recommend specific drugs for the type of virus implicated. Examples of anti-viral drugs include oseltamivir (commonly known as Tamiflu) specifically against influenza viruses and ribavirin more generally used to treat a wide range of RNA-containing viruses such as measles, mumps and hepatitis C viruses. Viruses can develop resistance to such drugs over time, rendering the drug ineffective against the new form of the virus; this is a common concept in the treatment of all microbial diseases and considered in more detail under the section on bacteria, below.

Bacteria

Bacteria (in singular form, bacterium) are a class of microorganisms that have a prokaryotic, unicellular (one-celled) structure. They are probably the most studied area of microbiology. They are classified in many ways, such as by their appearance when examined under a microscope (e.g. shapes, staining characteristics), how they grow (e.g. biochemical reactions, ability to use oxygen (or not) to grow) or various structural characteristics (lipids and more recently by their genetic nature). Their basic structure is shown in Figure 5.4, but similar to viruses they present with a wide range of structures, shapes and sizes, which even change as they grow.

As an example, bacteria are often classified as being "Gram positive" or "Gram negative". This is based on a very simple staining method; stains are essentially dyes or pigments that are used to visualize bacteria (and other types of microorganisms) under the microscope. The Gram staining method is an example of such a method, which was actually described by Hans Christian Gram, a Danish scientist, in 1884. The method is able to differentiate between two types of bacteria, based on the outer, cell wall structure (Figure 5.4). In Gram positive bacteria, the cell wall is composed mostly (up to 90% in some cases) of a net-like structure known as peptidoglycan (a polysaccharide-peptide structure). In Gram negative bacteria this is quite different, consisting of a small layer of peptidoglycan (~10%), an area known as the periplasmic space and an outer lipid membrane structure. In the staining method, two dyes are used first (crystal violet followed by iodine to give a purple color) that stain the peptidoglycan layer and then followed by a quick alcohol

wash that can remove the dyes; Gram positive bacteria will retain most of the dyes but Gram negative bacteria will lose it quickly (are "destained"). The final step is to restain the bacteria with another dye (safranin or fuchsin) that will color them pink or light red. Overall, when examined under a microscope, the Gram positive bacteria will appear purple and the Gram negative pink/red. It is at this stage that bacteria can also be examined for their shapes: cocci (circular), rods (bacilli) or spirals as the main examples. In this way bacteria are often referred to as "Gram positive rods", "Gram negative cocci", etc. This is, however, an oversimplification as the staining method can vary depending on the person performing the procedure, the exact method used, how they are examined under the microscope and even the bacteria themselves (e.g. if they are freshly grown, as microbiologists would say "cultured", or an older culture). Some bacteria are actually known to be Gram variable, meaning that some individual cells will stain purple while others in the same group look pink. Similarly, many types of bacteria will show a variety of shapes when stained (known as pleomorphic, meaning of different shapes/sizes).

Bacteria also vary in their requirements for growth and multiplication. An example previously mentioned, being their ability to grow only in the presence of air ("aerobic"), in the absence ("anaerobic") and under both conditions ("facultative"). Some bacteria can grow under what we would refer to as extreme conditions (e.g. less than 4°C, higher than 50°C or in the presence of high concentrations of salts), under conditions with little nutrients (e.g. types of bacteria from the genus *Pseudomonas* can grow in high purity water systems with minimal available nutrients) and, similar to viruses, only in other cells (e.g. the genus *Rickettsia* and *Chlamydia* grow in human cells).

When bacteria find themselves in the right environment, including the right nutrients, temperatures, etc., they can begin to divide and multiply. They do this by a process known as binary fission, where one cell divides to give two identical "daughter" cells. Under optimum conditions for that bacteria type, this process can happen very quickly (e.g. for *Escherichia coli* this can be ~20–30 minutes) or very slowly (*Mycobacterium tuberculosis* can take up to 15–24 hours!). In the case of *Escherichia coli*, one bacterium alone can rapidly multiply to give thousands in only a number of hours under the right conditions. They will continue to multiply until these optimal conditions are no longer available. At this stage bacteria can demonstrate a wide range of reactions that help them survive. These include slowing down multiplication rate and metabolism to conserve energy,

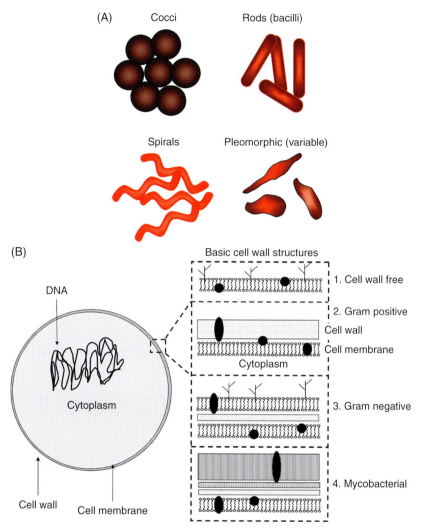

Figure 5.4 The basic structure of bacteria. (A) Examples of bacterial shapes. (B) Representation of a typical bacterial cell is shown on the left, consisting of the interior cytoplasm (the genetic material DNA is shown), surrounded by a cell membrane and an outermost cell wall. A cross-section of various types of cell wall structures are shown on the left, highlighting the cell membrane and cell wall in the Gram positive example. In this case the majority of the cell wall is made up of peptidoglycan (a peptide-polysaccharide), but also exists as a smaller section in Gram negative and mycobacterial cell walls but not in cell-wall free bacteria.

production of various types of enzymes and chemicals to protect them from damage and scavenge resources, the production of surface structures that make them mobile and the production of external protective mechanisms. As an example of a protective structure, many bacteria produce what is referred to as a capsule structure, which is a protein or carbohydrate-based (polysaccharide) structure that is formed over the bacteria to protect it and therefore help it to survive. Capsules can prevent drying (that can kill a lot of bacteria), prevent the interaction of chemicals (such as drugs and disinfectants) and also protect bacteria from the human body's defence mechanisms (the immune system, as described in Chapter 2). Bacterial communities can also protect themselves in a similar way by producing what is known as a *biofilm* (discussed in more detail later in this section).

Probably the most extreme change that has been described in bacteria in relation to adverse environmental

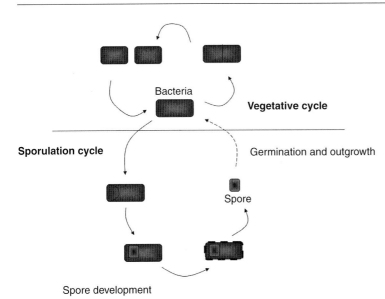

Figure 5.5 An overview of the sporulation process in bacteria.

conditions is a process known as sporulation. This is a remarkable process, where an actively growing cell decides to fundamentally change its structure to produce a dormant form of itself. These dormant forms are known as "spores" (or more correctly in bacteria as "endospores" due to the method in which they are produced, from within the original cell; *endo* for internal). They are not only just dormant (non-metabolizing or non-active) forms of bacteria, but have been radically changed in structure to make them highly resistant to various types of chemicals and physical inactivation methods. It is for this reason that they are considered one of the hardest types of microorganism structures to kill and are used to test sterilization methods. Only certain types of bacteria have been described that produce spores, with typical examples being bacteria belonging to the groups known as *Geobacillus, Bacillus* and *Clostridium*. Not all spores are the same in structure or in resistance to inactivation. For example, spores of the bacteria *Geobacillus stearothermophilus* are very heat-resistant, requiring temperatures in excess of 120°C for inactivation; they are also highly resistant to most types, but not all chemicals. Notable exceptions are the spores of *Bacillus atrophaeus* that are less resistant to wet heat, but more resistant to ethylene oxide (a gas used for sterilization). Spores of *Clostridium* are generally much more sensitive to heat and chemicals than those of *Bacillus* or *Geobacillus*. Due to their high resistance to disinfection and sterilization, the spores (endospores) formed from these types of bacteria are used to develop and routinely test sterilization

methods. Examples include the use of *Geobacillus stearothermophilus* for steam and hydrogen peroxide gas sterilization processes and *Bacillus atrophaeus* spores in ethylene oxide sterilizers. These are further discussed in Chapters 11 and 14. It is worthwhile considering the sporulation process in bacteria in further detail, as a remarkable example what bacteria are capable of (Figure 5.5).

During vegetative growth, the bacterial cell is continually sensing its environment and will adapt its growth rate and metabolism. When these conditions become limited, the bacteria decide to sporulate (produce a spore). During the process the cell commits itself totally to this process, producing only one spore for each bacterium cell. During development, part of the cell is separated with a complete copy of the DNA molecule and various layers are built around the spore to protect it. The internal compartment of the spore is further dried out and different types of chemicals and proteins are deposited. Their function is to protect the DNA from damage, but also to provide nutrients later when the spore decides to grow again. Sporulation is considered complete when the final spore is released from the cell and the cell dies. Bacterial spores can survive for years, if not decades in some cases, in dormant form. This can include extremes of temperatures, dryness and the presence of chemicals at concentrations that would normally kill vegetative cells. They are in a dormant stage but monitor their environment from any changes that will allow them to re-grow again. When these conditions are favorable, including temperature, presence of nutrients, etc., the spore re-activates. Reactivation is in two phases, known as germination and outgrowth, to provide a vegetative cell identical to the original cell that made the spore, which can then proceed to multiply as before in the vegetative cycle (Figure 5.5).

Although bacteria are unicellular, they commonly live together as groups of their own type (as they have multiplied together) and/or with other microorganisms. The way they grow and multiply alone often ensures that they are connected if not in very close proximity with each other. There are various terms used to describe these populations of bacteria, such as biofilms and microbiomes. A microbiome is a relatively recent term in microbiology that describes a population of microorganisms in a given environment. Examples of microbiomes include within the oral cavity (mouth), the lower intestine and the skin, all populated by various types of bacteria and other microorganisms that co-exist together. There is much evidence that these communities of microorganism are beneficial to us, for example by preventing other bacteria from attacking us to cause infection and their importance is an area of active research.

A biofilm is defined as communities of microorganisms (either single or multiple types) that have developed on or with surfaces. These can include various types of water or liquid contact hard surfaces (such as water pipes and indwelling catheters that are often used in hospitalized patients). Bacterial biofilms have been particularly well studied, with notable examples of *Pseudomonas aeruginosa, Staphylococcus aureus, Staphylococcus epidermidis, Mycobacterium* species (e.g. *M. fortuitum*) and *Legionella pneumophila*. Biofilms are also caused by fungi, with an important example being *Candida albicans* (fungi are discussed later in this chapter). Biofilms can have a negative impact, causing a variety of effects such as pipework damage ("biocorrosion"), blockages and, more importantly for our discussion, bacterial infections. Biofilms are often the source of bacterial contamination and infections from indwelling medical devices, devices that remain within us for extended periods of time such as contact lenses, catheters in the blood system and urinary tract, and implants or prostheses (an artificial replacement for a body part such as a hip or joint). Other sources include water, water handling systems or medical devices that use water, which when not maintained correctly can quickly become overgrown by biofilms. Such biofilms are a concern as they are hard to remove from surfaces and difficult to disinfectant/sterilize. They form at or on surfaces by a series of steps (Figure 5.6). First, the bacteria will attach or be associated with the surface and

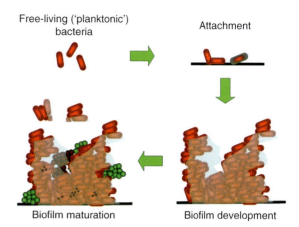

Figure 5.6 Biofilm development: free-living bacteria attach or become associated with a surface, which allows them to begin to divide and develop a biofilm, with production of a polysaccharide-based matrix that protects them from the environment, including the effects of drugs, detergents (used in cleaning chemistries) and disinfectants. As the biofilm matures, other bacteria, protozoa and viruses can become associated, grow and even feed on the biofilm. Parts of the biofilm can become dissociated from the matrix, being released and free to form other biofilms.

begin to multiply; as they multiply and develop, the bacteria begin to produce a matrix not dissimilar to the capsule material described above, being polysaccharide in nature. This is often referred to as "slime" as it has that slimy appearance. A good example of this is along the surface of teeth, where the slime material is actually a biofilm of bacteria such as *Streptococcus mutans*. It is this structure that is difficult to remove from surfaces and protects the bacteria in the biofilm from attack by drugs, detergents and disinfectants. It is also in this form that bacteria can produce a variety of chemicals and enzymes that can damage surfaces. As the biofilm further matures, other bacteria, viruses and protozoa can become associated with the biofilm, growing/dividing within the matrix, surviving within it or even living off it (as a food source). This relationship between bacteria of various kinds and other microorganisms is an area of active research. Further, parts of the biofilm can become loose and dissociate from the original biofilm to develop elsewhere. Overall, biofilm can be a particular concern as a source of contamination and therefore infection in medical institutions, especially when related to water, fluids and other liquids. They are particularly resistant to chemical disinfection but also physical removal during cleaning, which can make these processes inefficient.

Table 5.3 Examples of human diseases caused by bacteria (pathogenic bacteria).

Bacteria name	Features	Associated diseases
Mycoplasma pneumoniae	Cell wall free, pleomorphic	Pneumonia (inflammation of the lung) and other respiratory diseases.
Chlamydia trachomatis	Gram negative cocci or rods; only grow inside host cells ("obligate intracellular pathogens")	Infections of the eye and genital tract. Other species can cause pneumonia such as C. pneumoniae.
Staphylococcus aureus	Gram positive cocci	Wound and surgical site infections; impetigo (a skin infection); toxic shock syndrome, gastroenteritis (inflammation of the stomach/intestines). Antibiotic-resistant forms, such as methicillin-resistant S. aureus (MRSA) are a particular concern as they are more difficult to treat due to their resistance to the drugs (antibiotics) used to control them.
Enterococcus faecium and Enterococcus faecalis	Gram positive cocci	They are commonly found as part of the normal types of bacteria in the human intestine, but can be infections such as in wounds and in the urinary tract. Some strains are also highly resistant to antibiotics, such as the vancomycin-resistant Enterococcus (VRE) strains.
Streptococcus pyogenes	Gram positive cocci	Pharyngitis ("strep sore throat"), impetigo, scarlet fever, otitis media (middle ear infection, "ear-ache" but also commonly caused by another species called S. pneumoniae, a common cause of bacterial pneumonia).
Clostridium difficile	Gram positive rods Clostridium species only grow in the absence of oxygen ("anaerobic")	Diarrhea and intestinal perforation (leaking of the intestine contents into the body). Other species can cause wound infections such as Cl. tetani (tetanus) and Cl. perfringens (gangrene).
Neisseria gonorrhoeae	Gram negative cocci	Gonorrhea (commonly referred to as "the clap") is a sexually transmitted disease shown by a discharge from the sex organs and can lead to a variety of complications. Was treated in the past with drugs such as penicillin, but many strains are now resistant to such antibiotics.
Enterobacteriaceae, such as Escherichia coli; Salmonella enterica and Klebsiella pneumoniae	A family of Gram negative rods	Many are often associated with diarrhea and gastrointestinal infection, such as Escherichia and Salmonella. E. coli is also a leading cause of urinary tract infections (UTIs) and meningitis (in neonates – young children). Sal. enterica causes typhoid ("enteric fever"), an aggressive gastrointestinal disease. Klebsiella pneumoniae and other species are common causes of infections in hospitals such as in wounds, pneumonia and urinary tract infections.
Pseudomonas aeruginosa	Gram negative rods	Can cause range of opportunistic infections (infections in individuals that are more susceptible than normal, e.g. due to an existing infection or damage to part of the body or being "immunodeficient", where the body's ability to fit an infection is compromised). Examples of infections include wound infections, pneumonia and urinary tract infections.
Mycobacterium tuberculosis	Gram positive rods; also referred to as "acid-fast" due to other staining methods used to differentiate them from other bacteria	Tuberculosis; there is another similar form known as "bovine" tuberculosis that can occur in humans and animals caused by Mycobacterium bovis.
Mycobacterium leprae	Gram positive, acid fast rods; do not grow under normal microbiology laboratory growth (culture) conditions and only in certain animals (armadillos)	Leprosy or Hansen's disease, which is a disease of the nerves (peripheral) but presents with skin lesions.
Corynebacterium diphtheriae	Gram positive rods, although have a cell wall similar to Mycobacterium, but are not acid-fast	Diphtheria, an upper respiratory tract disease associated with a sore throat and other complications. Once considered very common, the overall occurrence is low due to the diphtheria vaccine; the vaccine is usually given as part of a combined vaccine for three bacterial diseases, known as DPT, for C. diphtheriae, Bordetella pertussis (pertussis or whooping cough) and Cl. tetani (tetanus).

Examples of various types of disease-forming bacteria are given in Table 5.3. Bacteria are named based on various groups that are similar in structure and genetic type; the group (or what is specifically called the "genus") name is given first and the specific branch of the group (known as a species) is given next. The names of bacteria should always be italicized or underlined, such as is the case for *Mycobacterium tuberculosis* or <u>Staphylococcus</u> <u>aureus</u>. They can also be referred to as particular varieties (known as sub-species, strains, isolates or types). As an example, let's take *Staphylococcus aureus* (or *S. aureus* for short and often referred to as "*Staph. aureus*") as a well-known bacteria that can cause various types of diseases such as wound-infections, skin infections (carbuncles, pimples and impetigo), pneumonia and toxic shock syndrome. The genus is *Staphylococcus,* species *aureus*, and an example of a sub-species is *S. aureus subsp. aureus N315*. *S. aureus* Newman and ATCC 6538 are examples of strains or isolates. American Type Culture Collection (ATCC) refers to a culture collection of microorganisms, from which various types of bacteria and other microorganisms can be purchased; these strains are often considered as standard strains and are often specified in various antimicrobial test methods for disinfectant testing purposes. Other examples of culture collections include the United Kingdom National Culture Collection (UKNCC), China Center for Type Culture Collection (CCTCC), Collection de L'Institut Pasteur (CIP) and All-Russian Collection of Microorganisms (VKM). A very common series of strains are known as MRSA strains for "<u>methicillin</u>-<u>resistant</u> <u>Staphylococcus</u> <u>aureus</u>" referring to strains of *S. aureus* that have developed resistance to some drugs (antibiotics) that used to be used to kill these types of bacteria. More on antibiotics later in this section.

What makes certain types of bacteria good for us, while others are bad and can cause disease? Even similar types of bacteria can cause different types of effects or diseases. Remember that not all bacteria can or want to do harm to a host (human, animal, plant or other organism). The ability to cause disease is based on two considerations: the host and the bacteria (or any other microorganism for that matter). There are many factors that can influence this relationship. Host factors include the patient age, their health, genetic predispositions, if they are on certain types of drugs, if they have an existing disease, use of devices in parts of the body (such as in the urinary tract and through the skin into the bloodstream), etc. Examples of the effects of drugs or medications include antibiotics (as they are often used to treat an infection they may also kill many of the other bacteria

that may be preventing infection from other microorganisms), chemotherapeutic agents (e.g. for cancer treatment) and immunosuppressive drugs. In all these cases, patients on these drugs can be more susceptible to getting infections. Patients can be immunocompromised due to existing bacterial, viral or other infections; HIV has already been discussed as a virus (see previous section) that affects the human immune system causing it not to work well and predisposes an infected individual to a variety of bacterial, fungal and other infections that they would normally be able to fight off (leading to AIDS). In hospital environments, considering the function of hospitals to treat people with injuries, illness and disease, it should be no surprise that these patients will be more susceptible to infections.

Epidemiology is the study of the various factors that affect the health, illness and disease in such populations. This not only applies to infectious diseases, but also other illnesses such as cancer and the influence of various other factors on public health (such as smoking, eating habits, etc). Epidemiology often studies the rates of diseases and in the study of infectious diseases there are two commonly used rates relating to morbidity and mortality. Morbidity refers to a disease or illness, where the morbidity rate is the number of cases of a particular disease in a population over time. Mortality refers to death due to an illness or disease, where the mortality rate is the rate of death from a particular disease/illness in a population over time. The study of epidemiology is closely linked with the practice of infection prevention and control, which is considered later in this chapter.

The other consideration is the bacterium (or microorganism) itself. In this regard, two terms that are useful to define are pathogenicity and virulence. They both refer to the ability of a microorganism to cause disease. A pathogen is a disease-causing microorganism and virulence is a measure of how aggressive a pathogen is to be able to cause disease. Some bacteria can cause mild diseases even when present at high numbers, but others are more virulent even when present at low numbers. A measure of virulence is called the LD_{50} that can be defined as the dose of a microorganism that can be given to cause death in 50% of cases (usually determined in experimental animals and estimated for humans).

Pathogens can be considered over two extremes: those that always cause a disease (examples include bacteria like *Neisseria gonorrhoeae* and *Treponema palladium*, causing sexually transmitted diseases gonorrhea and syphilis, respectively) and those that only cause infections under special, opportunistic conditions ("opportunistic

Table 5.4 Various types of toxins produced from bacteria and their effects in humans.

Bacteria	Toxin(s)	Effects
Exotoxins		
Streptococcus pyogenes	Erythrogenic ("pyrogenic") toxin	Cause the red skin rash during scarlet fever, as well as fever and other complications during infection.
Escherichia coli	Variety of toxins including LT, ST, verotoxin and the shiga toxin	LT and ST cause intestinal cells to lose fluid/electrolytes, leading to diarrhea. LT is considered heat sensitive and ST is heat resistant. Verotoxin also leads to diarrhea, but by a different mechanism. The shiga toxin is produced by specific strains known as *E. coli* O157:H7, but the original source of the toxin is from *Shigella dysenteriae*. In both cases it prevents protein synthesis in cells, the effects of which leads to diarrhea and other effects.
Vibrio cholerae	Cholera toxin (Ctx)	Similar to the *E. coli* LT toxin it causes intestinal cells to lose fluid/electrolytes, leading to diarrhea.
Clostridium tetani	Tetanus toxin	Inhibits communication between nerve cells leading to paralysis.
Bacillus cereus	Emetic toxin (ETE), diarrheagenic enterotoxin* (Nhe) and hemolytic enterotoxin* (HBL).	The emetic toxin (which is heat stable) causes vomiting, being the first sign of disease. This is followed by the diarrheal toxins Nhe and HBL (both heat sensitive) due to the loss of fluids from intestinal cells.
Clostridium difficile	Toxin A/Toxin B	Causes intestinal cells to die, leading to bloody diarrhea.
Corynebacterium diphtheriae	Diphtheria toxin (Dtx)	Inhibition of protein synthesis leading to cell death.
Endotoxins		
Gram negative bacteria such as *Neisseria meningitidis, E.coli* and *Pseudomonas aeruginosa*	Endotoxin or lipopolysaccharide (LPS)	This molecule is an important part of the structure of the outer membrane of Gram negative bacteria. They can be released (in small amounts) during growth of the bacteria, but more importantly when they are damaged or killed. Endotoxins are very heat stable (even by boiling or by steam). They are toxic by stimulating the immune system leading to a variety of effects, including fever (increased body temperature), changes in blood cells, shock and even death (depending on the level).

* The term enterotoxin is often used to describe an exotoxin that is produced by bacteria and has an effect in the intestine.

pathogens"). In the first case these bacteria may be considered aggressive pathogens that cause disease on contact, over time, with humans or animals. Opportunistic bacterial pathogens are actually considered poor pathogens, rarely if ever causing disease in healthy persons, but under the right situations (such as in sick patients) can cause disease. An example in *Staphylococcus epidermidis* that is actually found as a major component to the normal bacteria that live on the skin, but in a patient that is immuno-compromised it is often implicated in infection, particularly when related to skin or mucous membrane contact such as with indwelling catheters. More bacterial pathogens are considered to be between these extremes and are referred to as facultative pathogens; important examples are

Escherichia coli and *Staphylococcus aureus*, and this can vary depending on the specific strain. The capability to cause disease is due to having various types of virulent factors that contribute to allowing microorganisms to invade humans (e.g. through the lungs, intestine or skin), evade the immune system and damage the host.

One of the most important virulence factors in bacteria is the production of toxins. Toxins are various types of proteins or polysaccharides that are produced or released from bacteria that have a direct toxic effect in the body. Examples are given in Table 5.4. There are two main types: exotoxins, which are produced and released by the bacteria, and endotoxins, which are a structural component of the outer, cell wall structure of Gram negative bacteria. Exotoxins, depending on their structure,

Table 5.5 Examples of the groups/types of antibiotics.

Antibiotic group*	Examples
β-lactams and cephalosporins	Penicillin, flucloxacillin, amoxicillin, methicillin. Cephalosporins are closely related to the β-lactams and include ceftazidime.
Glycopeptides	Vancomycin, teicoplanin.
Aminoglycosides	Streptomycin, kanamycin, neomycin.
Quinolones, fluoroquinolones	Nalidixic acid, ciprofloxacin.

*Antibiotic groups are usually classified based on their chemical structure. They often have official names as well as commercial/trade names. Many antibiotics are naturally occurring, such as penicillin that is isolated from the fungus *Penicillium chrysogenum*; others have been chemically synthesized.

have been shown to have a variety of effects that cause host cell damage and death; the disease effects that we see include rashes on the skin, vomiting, paralysis and diarrhea (Table 5.4). Most exotoxins are proteins. In some cases, where the toxin is no longer produced the bacteria are no longer pathogenic. Also, some of these toxins are heat stable, so even though the bacteria are inactivated by heat their toxins can remain in water or on a surface to elicit their toxic effects. Endotoxins are different in that they are part of the outer cell wall structure of Gram negative bacteria such as *E. coli* and *Pseudomonas*. Endotoxins are also known as lipopolysaccharide (LPS) due to their structure being based on lipid and polysaccharide. As a structural part of the bacteria, they are not generally released by bacteria to have an effect on an infected person, but when the cell is damaged or is killed (due to the effects of the body's immune system, antibiotics or disinfectants/sterilants) endotoxins can be released at high levels with dramatic effects. Endotoxin causes a cascade reaction in the immune system, leading to fever and more serious effects (depending on the dose), such as organ failure and even death. They are particularly heat resistant (even to boiling or steam sterilization).

In addition to toxins, other virulence factors include the production of enzymes (urease, collagenase, lipases as examples), production of capsules or biofilms (as protective mechanisms), ability to bind and penetrate host cells or structures associated with cells (e.g. collagen) and ability to survive within cells for extended times (e.g. *Mycobacterium tuberculosis*). A further interesting virulence factor of importance today is the ability of bacteria to develop resistance to antibiotics. Antibiotics are a group of drugs that kill or inhibit the growth of bacteria;

this is an important definition, as antibiotics are only generally effective against bacteria and should not be used for other purposes such as to treat viral infections! Since the first antibiotic was discovered (penicillin in 1928), they have become widely used both to prevent bacterial infections (as in the case with the practice of giving antibiotics before invasive surgery, referred to an antibiotic prophylaxis) and to treat them. In many cases they have actually become abused, such as not being used correctly (at the right dose for the right amount of time), being used with diseases that are actually caused by viruses or as growth promoters in animal feeds. Examples of some of the most widely used antibiotics today to treat bacterial diseases are given in Table 5.5.

Antibiotics have very specific mechanisms of action against bacteria. As an example, the β-lactams such as penicillin and methicillin inhibit the ability of bacteria to produce the structure of peptidoglycan, a major part of the cell wall structure (Figure 5.4). This is important because the effects are specific to the target bacteria and not human cells (e.g. human cells do not have peptidoglycan), antibiotics can be used to treat infections at low doses within the body without any significant toxic effects (in most cases) against human/animal cells. Naturally, penicillin itself is not equally effective against all types of bacteria, being particularly effective against Gram positive bacteria; the development of other β-lactams such ampicillin and amoxicillin had much greater activity against Gram negative bacteria despite having similar structures. This is a natural phenomenon, where the normal structure of bacteria does not allow access of the antibiotic to its site of activity or has other means of making them insusceptible to the antibiotic. Mycobacteria are an example of this, where specific antibiotics have been identified or developed as being specifically effective against mycobacteria due to their natural resistance to other antibiotics, predominantly due to their unique cell wall structure (Figure 5.4). Bacteria can be very resilient and as antibiotics are used (or abused) they can develop mechanisms of resistance to antibiotics with dramatic consequences. This is not surprising as their mechanisms are so specific that bacteria can use a variety of ways to overcome their effects, for example they can change the structure of the antibiotic target so that it no longer reacts with the drug, produce enzymes that break down the antibiotic so that it is no longer effective and they can use specific proteins that act as cellular pumps to expel the antibiotic to where it needs to be present to have its effect. In some cases these are unique mechanisms that have been developed by specific bacterial strains and in others the factors responsible for resistance can be transferred to other bacteria, even different genus and species. In all these cases, the ability to survive the presence of the antibiotic allows the strain to survive even in the presence of antibiotics, an important virulence factor, and therefore cause disease more readily in patients. Well-cited examples of antibiotic resistance bacteria include: methicillin-resistant *Staphylococcus aureus* (MRSA, despite the name is resistant to the β-lactams and cephalosporins and a leading cause of healthcare-acquired infections); vancomycin resistant *Enterococcus* (*Enterococcus* are naturally resistant to many antibiotics and vancomycin is often used to treat enterococcal infections); multi-drug (MDR-TB) and even extensively drug resistant (XDR-TB) *Mycobacterium tuberculosis* (resistant to many and even most of the specific antibiotics that are used to treat mycobacterial infections); carbapenem-resistant Enterobacteriaceae (CRE) such as *Klebsiella pneumoniae* (CRKP); and *Escherichia coli* (CREC), which are often associated with high rates of morbidity and mortality.

As a final consideration, there is also a large, separate group of microorganisms that are considered prokaryotes and are similar to bacteria, but are actually quite distinct. They are known as the archaea and include a wide variety of groups and types. Examples include genus such as *Halobacterium*, *Methanococcus* and *Thermococcus*. They have been of interest scientifically as they have been identified to live and grow in a variety of extreme environments on earth, such as hot springs, where humans and other forms of organisms could not survive. Interestingly they have rarely been associated with human or animal disease, and so are not further considered here, but there is speculation on potential links to disease.

Fungi

Fungi are a group of cell-based microorganism, but have a different basic cell structure to prokaryotes (such as bacteria) and are known as eukaryotes. Eukaryotes (or eukaryotic cells) are larger and more structurally organized cells than prokaryotes, like bacteria. They include fungi, protozoa, helminth, human, animal and plant cells, but their exact structure and how they are organized internally or together will vary significantly. Fungi are a large collection of microorganisms that are found everywhere in the environment (air, food, water, surfaces, etc.); they are therefore widely found as surface contaminants (e.g. in dust and in the air). Despite their diversity, it is estimated that we have only truly identified less than one-tenth of the various types of fungi that are present in the world. From a medical perspective, most fungi are not known as serious pathogens, but many are opportunistic or facultative pathogens (see the previous section for discussion on pathogenicity). They are, however, often associated with product spoilage (such as in foods or liquids) and are widely used for industrial purposes (such as for making bread, cheese, wine and a source of drugs like antibiotics, while large growth forms such as mushrooms are themselves edible fungi). Specific examples include the yeast known as Baker's or Brewer's yeast that is officially called *Saccharomyces cerevisiae*, *Rhizopus stolonifer* as type of mold that is also known a black bread mold due to its common furry black growth on bread and *Penicillium roqueforti* which is the "blue" in blue cheese. Fungi are therefore officially named in a similar way to bacteria, with the genus followed by species name always in italics or underlined (*Saccharomyces cerevisiae* or Saccharomyces cerevisiae); various sub-species and strain types/numbers can also be defined after the genus/species name similar to bacteria. Macroscopic and microscopic examples of fungal structures are shown in Figure 5.7. As stated before, the cells are more organized intracellularly (as typical eukaryotes) and are surrounded by a fungal cell wall; the basic fungal cell wall structure is similar to that of bacteria, consisting of an inner cell membrane attached to an outer cell wall, but the cell wall consists of various types of polysaccharide, with internal fibrils of cellulose or chitin that gives the cell wall a rigid structure. These structures are generally more resistant to inactivation than bacteria.

Fungi are classified into two groups based on how they grow: filamentous fungi (also known as molds) and unicellular forms (known as yeasts). Filamentous fungi typically grow together as long filaments (lines of cells), while yeasts are generally unicellular (grow as individual

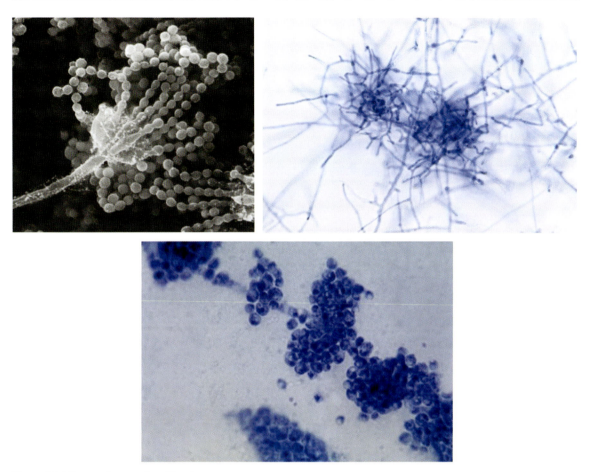

Figure 5.7 Microscopic examples of fungi.

cells; Figure 5.7); some fungi are found to present in both ways when examined (known as "dimorphic") and depending on the conditions they are exposed to during growth.

Fungi reproduce in three ways, depending on the specific species of fungi: vegetative spores, and by the production of asexual and/or sexual spores. Similar to bacteria, they can grow vegetatively by cell division. For molds, when the cells divide they may not separate and form the long, filamentous lines of cells (called hyphae); these filaments form a loose net-like structure typical of mold growth on surfaces (known as mycelia). Most yeast divide by binary fission (like bacteria, to give two identical cells) and/or by budding where a small part of the cell "buds" off to form a small cell. *Candida* is an example of typical dimorphic yeast that can grow vegetatively in both ways (as filaments or as one cell forms). In addition to vegetative growth, fungi also reproduce by producing spores, but in mechanisms quite different to those

described in bacteria. Spores can be produced in two ways: sexual and asexual. Asexual spores are produced directly from fungal cells by budding and generally develop together in specialized structures typical of the fungal type (e.g. within conidia or sporangia). Sexual spores are produced when two cell types of the same fungus, known as male and female forms, join together and develop to make the dormant spore forms. These spores can also be contained within specialized structures (such as ascospores within an ascus); these structures are often used microscopically to identify the type of fungus under laboratory conditions. Overall, little is known about the actual structure of the various types of fungal spores that have been described, but they are generally considered more resistant than vegetative fungi and less resistant than bacterial spores; the ascospores of *Aspergillus*, as an example, are widely considered as one of the most resistant forms of fungi to disinfection.

Table 5.6 Fungal pathogens and respective diseases.

Fungus type	Diseases
Molds	
Aspergillus fumigatus	Aspergillosis that includes symptoms such as cough, chest pain, breathlessness and fever. Many allergic reactions (with similar symptoms) are due to reactions with fungal spores including *Aspergillus*.
Mucor indicus	Mucormycosis is used to describe disease caused by fungi such as *Mucor* and *Rhizopus*. Disease is most often associated with the lungs, sinuses and sometimes in serious cases the brain. These infections are generally only encountered in immunocompromised hosts.
Trichophyton rubrum	Commonly known as a dermatophyte (as well as other *Trichophyton*, *Microsporum* and *Epidermophyton* species) as they are often implicated in skin and nail infections in animals and humans. Examples include athlete's foot (medically referred to as tinea pedis) and ringworm (dermatophytosis). Athlete's foot is an itchy, scaling infection in particular seen between the toes.
Stachybotrys chartarum	A green-black mold often associated with buildings that have been flooded, allowing the mold to grow. Often referred to as "sick-building" syndrome, associated with a series of symptoms similar to allergies, including irritation of the eyes, nose and throat, but also leading to other complications.
Yeasts	
Candida albicans	By far the most common fungal infection in humans, in particular in immunocompromised or hospitalized patients. Infections are particularly associated with the oral and genital cavities, often referred to as thrush. More serious infections (where the yeast becomes disseminated around the body) are frequently reported in hospitalized patients. Diseases are generally known as candidiasis.
Cryptococcus neoformans	Cryptococcosis, most commonly as lung-based infection, but similar to other fungi; can lead to a variety of serious effects in immunocompromised patients.
Histoplasma capsulatum	Infections often in the lungs, but symptoms/health effects can vary and be disseminated.

Fungi have been traditionally classified based on how they grow on culture media in the laboratory and how they appear microscopically (including the types of spores and they way they are produced); more recently, classification systems have been studied based on genetic techniques.

Fungal infections in humans can be rather common, such as thrush in the oral or genital cavities and athlete's foot/ringworm as skin-based infections. Serious infections of their own accord in healthy individuals are rare, but can be particularly severe in immunocompromised or sick patients. Typical examples of pathogenic fungi and their associated diseases are given in Table 5.6. *Candida albicans* is an important example that normally can be found in the oral or genital cavities with no ill effects, but in some cases can lead to mild infections such as thrush; it can lead to more serious infections in immunocompromised individuals, such as blood infections, where *C. albicans* and other *Candida* species are leading causes of bloodstream and urinary tract infections in hospitalized patients. Other fungal species that are often implicated in infections, particularly in hospitalized patients, include *Aspergillus* and *Cryptococcus*, while in the general population infections and complications due to molds such as *Trichophyton* (also known as tinea infections) and *Stachybotrys* are common (Table 5.6).

Fungi can cause disease due to the many pathogenic or virulence factors similar to bacteria (as described in the section on bacteria). Examples include the production of toxins, known as mycotoxins, the presence of protective capsules on their external surface, their ability to be able to survive and spread through the environment, cell surface binding capabilities, immune system interference, and their intrinsic resistance to disinfection and even biofilm formation. Mycotoxins are produced by many types of molds and not considered as potent (dangerous) as some bacterial toxins; despite this they can have significant health effects. It is widely known, for example, that some mushrooms are poisonous when eaten, due to the presence of these toxins, and in many countries the levels of mycotoxins in foods are required to be controlled. Other mycotoxin examples include the aflatoxins (in *Aspergillus* species, some of which are carcinogenic, referring to their ability to cause cancer in humans/animals), ochratoxins and citrinins.

There are a variety of drugs that can be used to treat fungal infections, generally known as antifungal drugs. They are mostly quite specific in their activity against fungi, and in some cases only to specific types of fungi, due to specific targets in fungal structures (such as the production of specific molecules for their cell walls). Examples include amphotericin B and terbinafine. Similar to antibiotics and bacteria, the use of these drugs has also lead to the development of resistance in some fungi with similar clinical implications (requirements to use higher concentrations that are often toxic to patients or inability to control the infection).

Protozoa

Protozoa are a further group of unicellular (one-celled) eukaryotic microorganisms, but as distinct from fungi. Protozoa and another group of eukaryotes known as the helminths (see the following section) are often referred to as "parasites", although strictly speaking a parasite is actually defined as any microorganism able to live on and cause damage to its host (human, animal, plant, microorganism, etc.). Similar to fungi, they are considered abundant, but many species remain to be described (as well as any potential health effects). They can be found in a variety of environmental sources, and are often associated particularly with water and even in the air. They are further sub-divided into four groups: the sporozoans, ciliates, amoeba and flagellates, based on their microscopic structures. Overall, protozoa have not been as widely studied as bacteria and have been even less studied from a disinfection point of view. A summary of some of the more important protozoal pathogens and their associated diseases in given is Table 5.7. Some of the more important pathogens in this group include *Plasmodium falciparum* (the cause of malaria), *Cryptosporidium parvum* and *Giardia lamblia*

Table 5.7 Protozoa and associated diseases.

Protozoa type	Diseases
Sporozoans	
Cryptosporidium parvum	Cryptosporidiosis. Most often transmitted through contaminated water, even in cases where the water has been disinfected (e.g. chlorinated) due to the resistance to the oocyst form of the protozoa to chemical disinfection treatments. Disease most commonly presents with diarrhea, although can lead to other complications in immunocompromised patients.
Plasmodium falciparum	Malaria, a widespread disease in tropical and sub-tropical regions of the world, carried from person to person by female mosquitoes (a type of fly) through infected blood. Malaria is a leading cause of disease and death worldwide; other species of *Plasmodium* also cause milder forms of the same disease. It is a disease of the blood, affecting particularly the red blood cells, where typical signs of the disease include anaemia (low levels of red blood cell, that limits the carriage of oxygen through the blood) and repeated cycles of coldness followed by fever, shaking (known as "rigor") and sweating; in severe cases this can lead to coma (loss of consciousness similar to a deep sleep) and death.
Ciliates	
Balantidium coli	Balantidiasis, a diarrheal disease, which is often transmitted through pigs (in many cases where it shows no ill effects but causes disease in humans), via contaminated water or foods.
Amoeba	
Acanthameoba castellanii	Diseases include eye infections (amoebic keratitis) and encephalitis (inflammation of the brain). It is generally considered an opportunistic pathogen.
Flagellates	
Giardia lamblia	Giardiasis, a disease of the lower intestine in human but also other animals and birds. Disease outbreaks are commonly associated with contaminated water and foods (e.g. where the foods are rinsed with water). The disease usually presents with diarrhea, often explosive, but is generally short-lived.
Trypanosoma brucei (also known as *T. gambiense*)	Sleeping sickness (African trypanosomiasis), a common disease in Africa that presents as fever, swollen lymph nodes, confusion, and periods of fatigue/tiredness and the opposite, insomnia. The protozoa is transmitted through flies (specifically tsetse flies), and human contact (e.g. blood transmission).

(important causes of diarrheal disease) and *Acanthamoeba* species (eye infections). As can been seen from these names, protozoa are classified and designated in a similar mechanism to bacteria and fungi (see sections on bacteria and fungi, respectively). Many protozoal diseases are often associated with poor water quality, transmitted through contaminated water or through flies (such as *Trypanosoma brucei*, a flagellate causing a disease known as sleeping sickness that is transferred through tsetse flies and commonly described in sub-Saharan Africa). Note: in this case the tsetse fly is considered as a "vector" for the microorganism, where a vector can be any living agent (human, animal, fly, microorganism, etc.) that transmits an infection. Vectors are commonly used to describe various types of flies/insects that transmit infection, including the mosquito as a vector for the malaria parasite, *Plasmodium falciparum*. In a similar way, any disease that is transmitted by an animal is known as a zoonosis or zoonotic disease, such as rabies (the rabies virus in dogs and other animals), anthrax (the bacteria *Bacillus anthracis* in cattle)

and toxoplasmosis (the protozoa *Toxoplasma gondii* through contaminated meat or cats feces).

Protozoa present with a variety of vegetative (actively growing) forms, including what are known as trophozoites (e.g. sporozoites (Figure 5.8)). They reproduce in a variety of ways depending on the specific type, including by binary fission and by other sexual/asexual mechanisms. These vegetative structures can vary in sensitivity to disinfection, due to their individual structures and various protective mechanisms, but of particular note is their ability to form dormant, resistant forms of themselves that are known as cysts or oocysts. Examples of cyst-forming protozoa include *Giardia* and *Acanthameoba* species, while *Cryptosporidium* and *Plasmodium* species produce what are known as oocysts. These structures can survive various extreme environmental conditions such as drying and the presence of chemical disinfectants, allowing them to be disseminated through water and the air. *Cryptosporidium* oocysts have been particularly described as being highly resistant to chemical disinfection, surviving even high

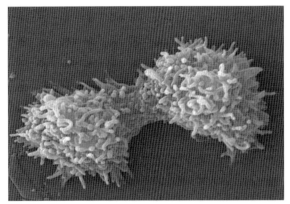
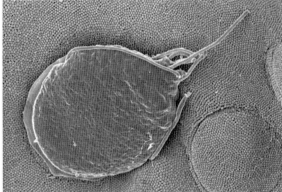
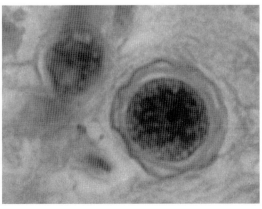

Figure 5.8 Examples of various types of protozoa structures.

concentrations of chlorine used for the preparation of potable (drinking) water.

Protozoal infections can be controlled or prevented by various types of drugs, such as chloroquine (against malaria) and, interestingly certain types of antibacterial drugs (antibiotics) such as metroniadazole and tetracycline. Chloroquine is often prescribed to prevent malaria transmission (medically this is an example of prophylaxis, which is defined as a measure taken to prevent a disease or infection), although in recent years there has been increasing reports of *Plasmodium* strains showing resistance to this drug.

Helminths

Bacteria, fungi and protozoa are all unicellular microorganisms, where each individual cell has the ability to grow alone or to develop into communities, but retain the ability to grow on their own. Helminths (also known as parasitic worms) are multicellular, eukaryotic microorganisms. They are similar to animals and humans in that they have an organized cell structure of various organs and systems not dissimilar to those describes in animals/humans; these structures are required for survival. Other examples of multicellular organisms are the arthropods, such as flies, fleas and lice. Externally, helminths are surrounded by a tough layer, known as a tegument or cuticle (equivalent to skin in animals/humans but more protein-based), with internal organization such as digestive systems (including intestines), reproductive (testes and ovaries), attachment organs and even primitive brain organs. They can be further subdivided into three groups based on their structures (Figure 5.9): tapeworms (cestodes), flukes (trematodes) and

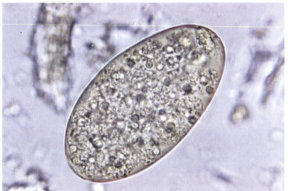
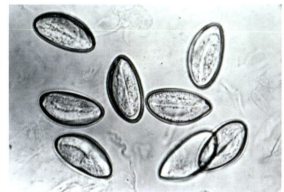
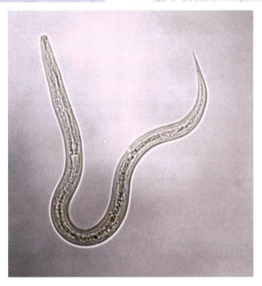

Figure 5.9 Examples of various types of helminth structures. They grow in life cycles that can show various different structural forms during the cycle such as eggs/cysts (dormant forms), larvae and worms/flukes (the adult forms).

roundworms (nematodes). The tapeworms and flukes are often grouped together as platyhelminths, due to their flat structures, while the nematodes are more rounded, thread-like structures. Similar to protozoa, it is believed that only a small proportion of the various types of helminths that exist have been described. Although many require microscopy to observe them (especially when in egg or cyst form), others can be very visible by normal sight, as in the case of some of the larger worms in this group; examples include the adult, worm forms (called giant roundworms) of *Ascaris lumbricoides* that can grow up to typical lengths of 35 mm and up to 4 mm in thickness! They are often associated with water, food (especially meat) and environmental surface contamination.

They develop in life cycles, where they grow through different physical stages: an adult form (worms/flukes), larvae (that can have various stages) and eggs/cyst (dormant forms). *A. lumbricoides*, for example, is introduced into humans via the oral route and in its egg form can survive the acidic conditions in the stomach; on passing through the duodenum (the part of the digestive system between the stomach and the small intestine) the egg can then produce a larvae that can attach to the intestine wall and enter the blood system. Interestingly, the larvae are carried to the heart, liver and eventually the lungs to develop; they can then be re-introduced into the intestine (by coughing and swallowing) where they can mature in adult worms to produce new eggs in the intestine that get released into the environment through the digestive system. During disease, typical symptoms can include vomiting, diarrhea and coughing, but more serious effects can lead to significant disease presentation. The eggs can actually survive for many years in the environment until introduced into a new host. The eggs/cysts are produced sexually in helminths; they have male and female forms, although the worms themselves can be considered "bisexual" (developing into specific male or female forms, reproducing between two worms) or hermaphroditic (both male and female systems, and reproduction in the same worm).

Similar to protozoa, the various structures and protective mechanisms of helminth eggs/cysts have not been described in detail, but they appear to have protective lipid, protein and polysaccharide (e.g. chitin) layers that help them resist not only drying and, to a certain extent heat, but also various types of chemicals such as those used for disinfection. They are parasites as they live on animals and humans, and can be present asymptomatically (not causing any obvious symptoms, which is a benefit to the host and the parasite) but can also cause damage to their hosts (often intestinal related diseases/

Table 5.8 Helminths and associated diseases.

Helminth type	Diseases
Wuchereria bancrofti	Elephantiasis, a roundworm (nematode) infection that is spread by the mosquito. The disease is also known as lymphatic filariasis, where the worms become lodged in the lymphatic systems (typically in the legs) leading to a build up of fluid, causing the limbs to swell. It is a common disease in tropical and sub-tropical areas.
Schistosoma mansoni	Schistosomiasis (also known as bilharzia) is a common trematode (fluke) disease in Asia, Africa and South America associated with contaminated water (as water snails are an important host in addition to humans). This species of *Schistosoma* causes an intestinal disease. Infected humans present with various signs, such as abdominal pain and diarrhea.
Enterobius vermicularis	Enterobiasis (or pinworm/threadworm infection) is usually associated with itching in the anal area and is particularly prevalent in children. These nematodes are usually transmitted in egg form by hands, food, or water contamination. Not considered a serious pathogen.
Ascaris lumbricoides	Ascariasis, the most common helminth infection in humans. These roundworms can grow up to 35 cm in length, found in the intestine and known as giant worms. They can cause serious disease and even death in immunocompromised humans, causing a variety of effects, such as associated with the intestinal tract (vomiting, diarrhea) and other systems (such as the lungs and coughing).
Taenia saginata	The beef tapeworm causes taeniasis in humans and is transmitted through infected meat (beef). These worms can grow up to 5 meters in length. Infections are generally asymptomatic (no obvious symptoms), although more serious complications can occur when they proliferate, such as constipation, abdominal pain, and diarrhea.

symptoms; Table 5.8). Examples include diseases, such as schistosomiasis often associated with contaminated water, leading to intestinal disease and elephantiasis, a disease of the lymphatic system (Table 5.8). In many case, immunocompromised patients can often have more serious helminth diseases that can even lead to patient death.

Investigations of and medical treatments with helminth infections are limited, with most serious diseases being seen in various parts of Africa, South America and Asia. Emphasis is on preventing helminth transmission, usually by improving water quality or removing vectors for the helminths (such as water snails to prevent *Schistosoma* transmission). Infections can be treated during de-worming methods to aid in expelling the worms, by injuring or killing them; examples of such drugs include ivermectin and praziquantel. Interestingly, although often considered controversial, helminths are actually used therapeutically to help in the control of immune system-related disorders (such as inflammatory bowel disease, asthma, eczema and hay fever). The theory is that helminth infections help the immune system react correctly (prevent over-reaction) on exposure to agents such as pollen and dust that trigger such disorders.

An introduction to infection prevention and control

Public health is an important subject to all of us, individually, to our families and to the communities in which we live. As a science, the study of public health may be defined as preventing disease, prolonging life and promoting health. Within this definition, a disease may be defined as any effect that impairs/harms the body's normal function and therefore has an effect on our health (mild, moderate or even severe). Diseases can be infectious (such as those caused by bacteria and viruses) or non-infectious diseases (such as with certain types of cancer, effects of drug abuse, stress, chemicals, etc.). Examples of public health efforts to reduce disease in populations include improving drinking water quality (chemical and microbiological), campaigns to stop smoking (due to the associated risks of cancer and other health effects), washing of hands and good waste collection and disposal/treatment. As we experience in our daily lives, these efforts can have significant effects on our health and well-being, ranging from major efforts with a population (water treatment, waste control), but also be affected by our own choices and practices (washing our hands and deciding whether or not to smoke).

Epidemiology is part of the science of public health, being the study of the factors involved in disease and the control of such diseases. Specialists in this area are known as epidemiologists and they investigate the rates of various diseases in populations as well as the effects of preventative measures in reducing these rates. It allows scientists to recommend various "evidence-based" practices that have been shown to have a significant impact in reducing the rates of diseases.

The analysis and control of infectious diseases is an important part of this study; it not only affects public life but has an even greater implication in certain groups where the risks are higher, such as in the younger, older, infirm, those in hospital or with underlining diseases. Infection prevention and control (also commonly referred to as "infection control") is the discipline concerned with preventing the spread of microorganisms and the infections they can cause; it is therefore a branch of epidemiology, both in scientific investigations as well as in its practical application. It can include how diseases are spread, prevented, controlled and treated. It is useful to distinguish between "prevention" and "control". Prevention strategies are employed to prevent the disease from spreading from one person to another, from one part of our body to another, from animals/insects, from air and from surfaces; examples include the washing of hands (antisepsis) and surface disinfection. It can also include measures that prevent the disease even if the microorganism is transmitted, which is the concept behind vaccination. Vaccination is defined as the intentional introduction of microorganisms (usually modified or parts of the microorganism) into the body to allow the development of immunity (or resistance) to the development of infection with that microorganism; it is discussed in further detail in this section.

Control strategies may be differentiated as those used to control the infection when it has happened, with a typical example being the use of anti-infective drugs such as antibiotics and preventing transmission to others by isolating infected patients. It is important to note that these practices are not only important to a patient but also to those caring for or visiting the patient. These definitions are, of course, not strict as sometimes the same practices are used in both cases, for prevention and control, depending on the situation. In addition to these measures, infection prevention and control personnel are also involved in many other aspects such as investigating the sources of infection outbreaks, managing outbreaks and studying the effects of various preventative and/or control measures. Experts in this area may be known by a variety of terms, such as

surfaces (importantly, high-touch surfaces), aerosols (e.g. cough) or even the air itself, and re-usable medical devices. Other sources include foods, water and animals/insects. These sources are not unique to healthcare facilities and actually apply to our daily lives, with many of these risks being reduced by practical public health measures (see the following section). Remember, the risks of infection are higher in many healthcare facilities because the patient may be more open to developing an infection (immunocompromised), such as with other illnesses, various therapies for other diseases (e.g. chemotherapy for cancer) and wounds due to injury or surgical procedures. As the patient can be contaminated by a variety of sources, the patient can also be the source of contamination to other patients, facility staff and visitors.

The role of infection prevention and control

The primary role of infection prevention and control is to put procedures and practices in place to reduce the risks of microbial, in particular pathogen, transmission. This is not only directed at reducing the risks to patients, but is equally important for the protection of facility staff and visitors. It is therefore a quality standard for any facility and, like any quality standard, requires constant support and maintenance.

The overall responsibility for infection prevention and control at any facility is the hospital manager, director or management team. Infection control and prevention should interact closely with the various facility departments and their staff, ranging from operating rooms, wards, decontamination facilities and staff, waste disposal, facility maintenance, pharmacy and even finance. It is important to point out that infections are not only a significant cause of morbidity (disease cases) and mortality (death due to diseases) in healthcare, causing distress to patients and their families, but can also lead to considerable costs due to increased hospital stay, additional treatments required, specialized patient handling, repeated surgery, etc. This can be avoided by ensuring practical and active infection control and prevention measures.

The organization of infection control and prevention within a facility will vary in size, depending on the facility. It can range from a single individual (typical of small clinics and practices) to large infection control teams (especially in larger hospital groups). What is recommended is that responsibility is designated for establishing, maintaining and ensuring the practice of various policies and procedures. Designated staff can typically involve specialists such as infection control nurses, epidemiologists, consultant microbiologists, infection control officers, decontamination department managers, etc. Their expertise can include infectious diseases, medical microbiology, nursing, prescription practices and infection prevention/control practices. In larger facilities it is typical to have a designated infection control team and/or committee, with the head of such groups being represented at the upper levels of hospital management. It is important to remember, particularly in healthcare facilities, that *everyone* is responsible for ensuring that these are safely applied and not only those that are in direct contact with a patient. The best procedures and practices can be in place but if they are not adhered to they will have no impact; success is dependent on people and their training. Examples of the various different procedures and practices that are employed are further discussed in the following section, with particular emphasis on the reprocessing of re-usable devices wherever they are used in a facility.

While the primary role of infection prevention and control practitioners is to put procedures and practices in place to minimize microbial transmission, their day-to-day roles will include:

- Ensuring facilities and equipment are available to staff and patients (e.g. washer-disinfectors, sterilizers and hand washing facilities).
- Ensuring that policies and procedures are being followed.
- Advising on any infection concerns within the facility.
- Updating procedures and guidelines as required by clinical practice.
- Monitoring the rates of infections (surveillance) and identifying any problems (e.g. outbreaks). In this case, an infection outbreak may be defined as an occurrence of a disease (infection) at a higher rate than would otherwise be expected at a particular time and place. Outbreaks of infections may be within a small group at a single facility or can impact on thousands of people across the world. They may also be referred to as epidemics (affecting a particular region, such as part of a country, or of a continent, including a number of countries) or pandemics where it spreads across the world. Examples include the outbreak of a bacterial or viral disease in a hospital leading to ward closures and the 2009 swine flu pandemic. Infection prevention and control specialists can play an important role in ensuring that any infection outbreaks that occur are rapidly investigated and controlled.
- Monitoring the correct use of anti-infective chemicals (e.g. antibiotics) used to control infections (either as preventative or treatment measures).

Infection control and prevention strategies

As stated above, infection prevention and control specialists are responsible for establishing policies and practices to reduce the risks of infection and cross-infection. Specific measures that are generally part of this goal are summarized in Table 5.9.

This is not an exclusive list, but includes most of the important interventions that involve various decontamination methods, such as cleaning, disinfection and sterilization. Other examples can include the prudent use of antimicrobials (such as antibiotics) and correct patient handling procedures. A familiar example should be hand disinfection, a practice that is often cited to be one of the most significant yet simple ways to reduce microorganism transmission. The skin, and particularly the hands, is naturally colonized with a variety of resident and transient microorganisms (see Chapter 2) and it is the carriage of various types of microbial pathogens that causes the most concern in healthcare workers and the transmission of contamination. Reducing the level of microbial contamination is an important infection control and prevention strategy to reduce the risk to patients and staff. Hand disinfection (a form of antisepsis, or disinfection of the skin or mucous membranes) can include hand washing (using water and soaps, including antimicrobial soaps) and hand rubbing (that do not use water, typical examples including 60–80% alcohol-based products that are rubbed into the skin and allowed to dry). Hand or skin disinfection can be used routinely for personal hygiene (e.g. before eating or after using the toilet, where non-antimicrobial soap and water is actually sufficient) but also in clinical practice before and after patient contact (e.g. by nurses and doctors tending to a patient, including before surgery), handling instruments that have been used or before they are used on patients or in preparation of an area of skin for incision during a surgical procedure (referred to as part of pre-operative preparation). While compliance with hand washing prior to surgical intervention is considered high, it may be surprising to note that compliance to general hand disinfection practices in caring for patients is less. Studies have shown that this can vary from 16 to 81% compliance; these rates may often be lower in non-patient contact areas, but may be important to personal health, as is particularly the case in decontamination areas. It is also important to note that hand washing or hand rubbing are often not done correctly, to ensure that all areas of the hands are correctly cleaned (Figure 5.11).

Further examples that will be familiar are the use of gloves, disinfecting surfaces and the use of specialized air handling or isolation rooms. Gloves are widely used to prevent a physical barrier, not only to microorganisms but also in handling of chemicals (e.g. during manual cleaning or disinfection practices). Gloves are designed for different uses and typical examples in clinical practice are:

• Vinyl (PVC, polyvinyl chloride) gloves are used for general low-risk or housekeeping activities.
• Natural rubber (latex) gloves can be used for high (microbial) risks such as handling blood or blood spills,

Table 5.9 Examples of infection control and prevention measures.

Sources of contamination	Infection prevention and control measures
Re-usable devices/instruments	Cleaning, disinfection, sterilization. Methods to prevent needle or sharp injuries. Correct handling (insertion, maintenance and removal) of catheters.
Droplet/air/gas	Isolation rooms and associated precautions, air handling system including filtration, masks, eye protection, wound protection.
Soiled textiles, liquids and various single-use instruments (e.g. needles, sharps, etc.)	Cleaning, disinfection, sterilization. Examples include laundry cleaning and disinfection, waste disposal and incineration.
Environmental surfaces, such as tables, chairs and bed-rails	Cleaning, disinfection.
Hands and skin	Hand washing (with water), hand rubbing (without water), gloves.
Food	Hand washing, glove use, correct storage and handling.
Water	Disinfection (or the water and/or water lines), filtration.
Animals/insects	Limit or exclude contact, de-infestation (e.g. spraying) and pest control.

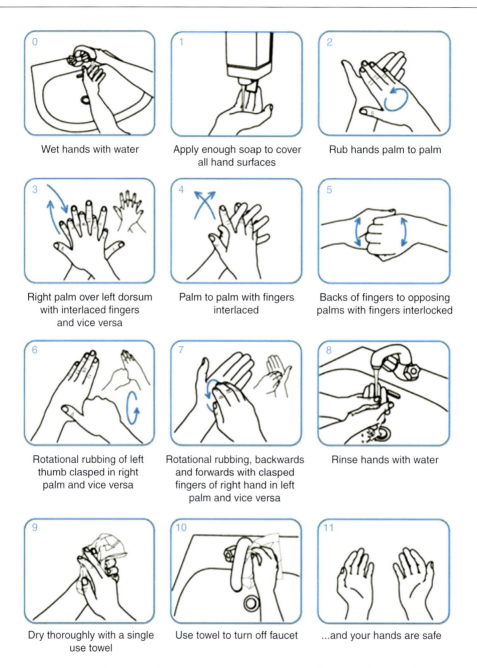

Figure 5.11 A recommended hand washing technique with water to ensure that it is done correctly. Note: when using a hand rubbing (alcohol-based) product, steps 2–7 should be followed as water is not necessary.

but are also commonly associated with allergic reactions that can even be severe in some cases (latex allergy).
• Nitrile (acrylonitrile) gloves can provide good biological and chemical barrier functions and are often used as a safer alternative to latex or when using chemicals.

• Neoprene (polychloroprene) gloves are also generally used due to their good biological and chemical barrier capabilities.
These can also be provided as sterile gloves (provided pre-packaged and sterilized, generally for use directly on

a patient, e.g. during surgery) or non-sterile, as well as powdered or non-powdered. In instrument cleaning (manual) applications it is generally recommended that gloves should be worn with chemical and microbial barrier properties (such as natural rubber, nitrile or neoprene gloves), but other types of gloves may be recommended for particular applications, such as the handling of certain types of chemicals (e.g. chemical resistant gloves such as heavy duty neoprene coated gloves) and for handling hot surfaces (e.g. autoclave gauntlets made out chemical polymers known as aromatic polyamides that are thermal resistant).

Surface disinfection is widely used to reduce the levels of microorganisms that may be present on a surface, be they work areas, patient contact surface or re-usable surgical instruments. Examples of surface disinfectants include alcohols, bleach solutions (preparation of sodium hypochlorite that releases chlorine, an efficient antimicrobial chemical), iodophors (that provide iodine) and products containing a variety of other antimicrobials (such as phenolics and quaternary ammonium compounds). These antimicrobial chemicals are also known as microbicides and are considered in further detail in Chapter 6.

It is typical for all of these strategies to be used together in a hospital or clinical situation. None of them on their own will completely reduce the risk of cross-contamination to a patient or member of staff. An example is in the surgical theatre, where the surgical instruments are provided sterilized, surgeons and staff usually follow strict routines for hand washing and use of pre-sterilized gloves, an air handling system is employed to keep the microbial population in the air low (e.g. using air filters such as HEPA, high efficiency particle air, filters), various surfaces are frequently disinfected and the patient is prepared by skin disinfection and the use of gowns. It is equally the case that if one of these practices is compromised, such as rigorously washing the hands, putting on gloves and then touching various contaminated surfaces prior to handling a patient that contamination can readily transfer and could cause an infection. With this in mind, a common term that is used in infection prevention and control practice is a "care bundle"; this refers to a collection of 3–6 infection control and prevention practices that are specified to be used collectively, reliably and continuously to significantly reduce the risk of infection. An example of a surgical site infection bundle, to reduce the risk of a patient getting an infection, could include ensuring:

• Correct skin preparation including skin disinfection and avoiding hair removal.

• Correct use and administration of prophylactic antibiotics, where a dose of antibiotics is given to a patient to reduce the risk of getting a bacterial infection.
• The patient's body temperature is maintained at normal throughout the operation (excluding certain types of procedure such as cardiac interventions).
• Correct hand washing and glove use in surgical staff.
• Correct device cleaning, disinfection and/or sterilization practices are in place.

As an example of a care bundle, these include a number of the strategies outlined in Table 5.9, but also the use of prophylactic antibiotics to prevent infections that could happen during or after the surgical procedure (e.g. from the skin, hands or even the surgical instrument) and correct peri-operative (the time during surgery) care of the patient.

A further important strategy in infection prevention and control, as well as for public health in general, is disease surveillance. Surveillance can be defined as the monitoring of the occurrence and distribution of infections within a facility, area or population. By surveying the rates of infection, strategies can be investigated to reduce infection rates, and outbreaks can be rapidly identified and steps taken to control the outbreak. The incidence rates of hospital acquired infection can vary widely, both due to methods of surveillance as well as the impact of various infection prevention and control strategies in place from hospital to hospital, area to area and country to county. Typical average rates worldwide may be in the range of 5–19% of admitted patients to hospitals who may present with a hospital-acquired infection. These can lead to significant costs, increased length of hospital stay, stress and further patient complications. These rates are quite significant considering that a further estimated average of 10% of these cases may lead to death. Therefore efforts to reduce the rates of hospital-associated infections in a hospital and targeting areas for reducing these rates is an important strategy for infection prevention and control staff.

Reprocessing role in infection control and prevention

Decontamination personnel play an important role in infection prevention and control strategies, specifically in reducing the risk of surgical site infections (SSIs) and device associated infections (DAIs). These infections can occur by the introduction of microorganisms in the use of various types of instruments and devices used for various patient procedures, including endoscopic investigations and surgery. Device associated infections can be defined as being always associated with a device and its use on a patient as the source of infection. In general, from epidemiology investigations, DAIs are considered relatively low and are infrequently reported in medical literature; despite this, there are many examples of infections and infection outbreaks that have been linked to the inadequate cleaning, disinfection and/or sterilization of a variety of instruments. It is clear that in the majority of cases this can be associated with the improper practice of cleaning, disinfection and/or sterilization as defined in international standards and guidelines. At this time, it is generally agreed that many cases of infection are never reported or adequately investigated, so while these rates may be considered low they remain significant and, most importantly, preventable. Surgical site infections may be due to the use of a device (and therefore may be also DAIs), but not always; other sources of infection may be from the patient's skin, contamination following a surgical procedure of a wound (e.g. from contaminated gloves or hands) or from the environment (e.g. present in the air). In many of these cases it is often difficult to identify a cause and investigators rarely have the time to investigate these cases in full detail.

The infection prevention role of a decontamination associate should be considered in two parts: protecting themselves and co-workers, and protecting the patient.

Protect yourself and co-workers

In any infection prevention and control consideration, the objective is to reduce a known risk of cross-contamination. It is important that these risks should be reduced to those working in decontamination facilities. Remember, as discussed earlier, microorganisms can be everywhere and you will not see them. In clinical use, it is good practice to handle any contaminated surface (whether contamination is visual or not) as if they pose a risk to your health. To reduce any risks, a series of personal protective equipment (known as PPE) can be used, that are based on the various strategies outlined earlier. These are summarized in Table 5.10.

It is common for a number of these preventative measures to be applied together, in particular in areas with higher risks, as is the case with manual cleaning. The exact policies on the use of PPE will vary from hospital to hospital, and further guidance is given on the recommended minimum requirements in further chapters of this book. Many of these protective methods not only apply to microbial risks, but equally to chemical risks (Chapter 6). There are two further points that should be considered:

• Personal protective equipment should be provided by an employer and is recommended for your personal protection. Do not underestimate its value or its impact on your health. If any recommended PPE method is difficult to use

Table 5.10 Examples of personal protective equipment (PPE) that can be used to reduce the risks of microbial cross contamination.

Personal protective equipment (PPE)	Risk reduction
Gloves	Prevent hand contamination that could lead to cross-contamination or direct penetration through the skin or associated wound. Heavy duty gloves may protect the hands from accidental sharp object risks. Objects that pose a risk to glove tearing (e.g. jewellery) should be avoided.
Hand washing or hand rinsing	Reduce the risk of hand contamination in a cleaning area (e.g. on touching a contaminated surface) or cross-contamination on handling instruments after they have been reprocessed. General good personal hygiene.
General surface disinfection	Reduce the levels of microbial contaminants on a surface in high-risk areas, such as around a manual cleaning sink.
Instrument cleaning/disinfection	Reduce the levels of microbial contaminants on surfaces to make them safe for handling/packaging for further sterilization.
Face masks	Reduce inhalation or swallowing risks from air or droplets generated during manual cleaning.
Protective/safety glasses or goggles	Reduce the risks of introduction of microorganisms (and chemicals) into the eyes from air or water droplets generated during manual cleaning.
Aprons, overalls	Protects clothing from contamination that could be transferred outside a designated area and even to the home.

correctly or causes pain/discomfort, it is important that this is not ignored and is highlighted to management and/or a policy is reviewed. In most parts of the world it is a legal requirement to provide a safe working environment and is an important part of any decontamination facility.

• Personal protective equipment is only as good as the person using it. Correct training on the use of PPE is essential and should be periodically reviewed. As an example, face masks will only be effective if used over the face, and eye glasses or safety goggles will only provide partial protection is they do not fit well or do not have side shields.

Protect the patient

The primary purpose of any decontamination or reprocessing facility is to ensure that a re-usable device is safely returned for further clinical use (Chapter 1). The instrument or device can be heavily or lightly contaminated with microorganisms and the various steps of cleaning, disinfection and/or sterilization are designed to reduced the risks of transferring these organisms to another person to a minimum (if not to an absolute) level. The various processes and practices associated with cleaning, disinfection and sterilization are outlined in further detail in this book. It is sufficient to highlight at this point that any lapses or failures in these practices can have a significant and often dramatic effect on subsequent patients. It is the duty of every decontamination associate, staff and management, to ensure that this does not occur.

Establish a policy, and ensure it is followed

Decontamination practices can vary from place to place, depending on facility, regional and even cultural requirements. This variability is acceptable, but in each case the facility should have a written policy of what is expected to be done. The policy should reflect the established practices that are expected to be performed and therefore should be clearly and practically written. Such policies make it clear to management and staff what is expected and safe for the patient; individual modifications to the policy (e.g. skipping a step, fast-tracking, etc.) are unacceptable unless approved by an authorized manager and should always be documented. Documenting such situations is a simple and effective way of ensuring that a change in hospital policy has been authorized and that those authorizing such a change are held responsible for it. Once a policy is in place it can then be periodically reviewed and modified as required by changing guidelines/standards, hospital management and infection prevention/control needs. Remember, the presence of a decontamination policy itself does not mean that the policy is being faithfully applied in a facility; training and frequent re-training is essential to ensure that staff are aware of the policy and understand how to conduct their job safely and effectively.

6 Chemistry and physics

Introduction

Chemistry is the study of chemicals and chemical reactions. It is the basis for all living and non-living things, including forms of life (humans, animals, plants, microorganisms, etc.), surfaces we touch and see, and the air around us. In chemistry living and non-living things are referred to as "matter". As described in Chapter 2, the human body is an encyclopedia, with chemistry and the essential elements of chemistry (the "elements") providing the words or essential building blocks for the various body structures (Table 6.1). These same elements, although a larger range of them, make up or are the source all non-living materials around us: air, water, radioactivity, rocks, etc., including the world itself and indeed the universe as we know it. In this section we consider in further detail the basics of chemistry, as it is essential for our understanding of how cleaning, disinfection and sterilization work. The study of chemistry is closely linked to physics, which is the study of matter (or nature) and how it behaves. This includes concepts such as energy, the structure of elements/atoms, radiation (including light), temperature, pressure, etc.; these are also basic concepts that are considered further in this chapter.

The elements (also known as atoms) are the essential building blocks of chemistry. They can be further subdivided into other parts (such as electrons, protons and neutrons), but this is beyond the scope of this book and it is not necessary to consider further, apart from mentioning that electrons and protons also make up electricity. Based on these simple structures, there are 94 naturally occurring elements in the world (but when other unstable elements are considered there are over 100) that have been described and these are generally organized, based on their complexity, into what is known as the periodic table (Figure 6.1). Examples include carbon (C), oxygen (O) and nitrogen (N); they can be referred by their full name (e.g. gold and silver) or their abbreviated name/symbol (e.g. Au and Ag, respectively).

These elements can exist on their own (e.g. gold, silver) or combine together to form molecules (e.g. H_2O, the chemical symbol of water, made up of two hydrogens and one oxygen). A molecule is therefore made up of two or more atoms with the following examples: O_2 (oxygen molecule, being made up of two atoms of oxygen), N_2 (nitrogen molecule), and NaCl (sodium chloride, table salt). NaCl is a stable molecule, but when it is dissolved into water (by mixing it) it does sub-divide into its elemental forms as "charged particles" that are known as ions: the ions of NaCl are Na^+ (a cation, as it has a positive charge) and Cl^- (an anion, as it has a negative charge); ions are often unstable and can be very reactive. In the introduction to anatomy (Chapter 2, introductory section), we discussed the fact that only six types of elements make up the different molecules that form life: carbon (C), hydrogen (H), nitrogen (N), oxygen (O), sulfur (S) and phosphorus (P). But there is a much wider variety used naturally in nature and artificially. Examples include a group of antimicrobial chemicals that are known as the halogens and include chlorine (Cl) and iodine (I); further examples are synthetic polymers (these are long molecules) that are widely used plastics such as nylon and polystyrene, and molecules like "ferric" oxide (Fe_2O_3 commonly known as rust, where Fe is the symbol for iron) and calcium carbonate ($CaCO_3$, a major component of water hardness or "scale").

The study of chemistry can be further sub-divided into various disciplines. A common example is called organic chemistry that considers any molecule that is based on carbon with the other discipline, inorganic chemistry, considering all non-carbon based chemistry. This simple

A Practical Guide to Decontamination in Healthcare, First Edition. Gerald McDonnell and Denise Sheard.
© 2012 Gerald McDonnell and Denise Sheard. Published 2012 by Blackwell Publishing Ltd.

Table 6.1 Chemistry is the basis of living and non-living materials (known as "matter"), with the elements forming the essential building blocks. In this case the structure of the body is broken down to these elements in an analogy to an encyclopaedia.

Structures	Encyclopaedia analogy	Examples
Systems	Volume/section	Nervous, respiratory, digestive and cardiovascular systems
Organs	Chapters	Stomach, heart, kidney, liver, brain
Tissues	Sub-chapters	Epithelial, muscular, nervous, connective tissues
Cells	Paragraphs	Nerve, muscle, skin, blood cells
Molecules	Words	Water (H_2O), proteins, carbohydrates, lipids, nucleic acids
Atoms/elements	Letters	Carbon (C), hydrogen (H), oxygen (O), nitrogen (N)

differentiation is useful, but strictly speaking does not mean that all carbon containing chemistries are "organic" and all non-carbon are "inorganic"; however, these are exceptions and a simple example includes a group of chemicals known as carbonates, such as calcium carbonate ($CaCO_3$) and sodium carbonate (Na_2CO_3), which are considered as inorganic (as they do not contain carbon with hydrogen). Biochemistry can be considered part of organic chemistry as life is carbon-based and biochemists specifically study the chemical processes and structures in living organisms. Other branches of chemistry may include pharmacology (the study of chemical drugs) and radiochemistry (the study of radioactive materials). It is interesting to note that radioactivity is produced from special types of elements known as radioactive isotopes: these are unstable elements (naturally occurring or artificially generated) that release radiation over time to become more stable. Although a detailed understanding of radioactivity and its properties is not necessary, it is important to note that radioactivity is often used for medical procedures (nuclear medicine). Examples include the use of radioactive isotopes for medical imaging (to view internal parts of the body, such as during positron emission tomography (PET)) and for cancer radiotherapy. Widely used radioactive isotopes include technetium (99m), Iodine (123 and 131) and Thallium (201). In some cases these may require special consideration in device decontamination (Chapter 13, in the section on types of workplace safety hazards).

Solids, liquids, gases and plasmas

The most commonly known states of matter are solids, liquids and gases (but we will also discuss the so-called fourth state of matter, being plasma). All molecules can assume various different states depending on the energy provided; an example of energy is thermal energy (measured by temperature) and electromagnetic energy (e.g. from ultraviolet (UV), X-ray or gamma (γ) radiation). Temperature is an important source of energy, used not only to increase how quickly chemical reactions work (e.g. for cleaning and disinfection applications with chemicals) but also as a reliable method on its own for disinfection (e.g. hot water over 65°C) and sterilization (in the form of steam but also dry heat). Let us consider the effect of temperature on a common molecule: water (H_2O; Figure 6.2).

The three forms shown are ice (solid), water (liquid) and steam (gas). Solids will have a defined (or maintain their own) shape (in the case of water, ice crystals), liquids adopt the shape in which they are put (e.g. in a glass) and gases have essentially no shape (not restrained). Water likes to be in a liquid form, an essential component for life and covering over 70% of the world's surface. The liquid form is generally present under ambient conditions of temperature and pressure, atmospheric pressure; the influence of pressure is considered in further detail later in this section. If the temperature of water is reduced below 0°C ("degrees Celsius") or 32°F ("degrees Fahrenheit") it forms a solid, ice. The freezing (liquid to solid) or melting (solid to liquid) point of water is therefore 0°C. (Note: for conversion between various different methods of measure temperature, see the section on common chemical measurement methods.) If the temperature is increased (above 100°C or 212°F) it forms a gas, steam. Therefore, the boiling (liquid to gas) or condensation (gas to liquid) point of steam is 100°C, under normal atmospheric pressure conditions. In this case, steam is also referred to as a "vapor", where a vapor is a gas but can readily return to being a liquid (e.g. by reducing the temperature). As shown in Figure 6.2, true steam (as a gas) is

Figure 6.1 The periodic table of elements.

Key:

6	Atomic number (The number of protons)
C	Element symbol
Carbon	Element name
12.0107	Atomic mass (The number of protons and neutrons)

Labels: Alkali metals · Alkaline earth metals · Transition metals · Non-metals · Metals · Halogens · Noble gases · Not metal, gas · Groups · Periods

Periodic table of elements:

Period	1A	2A	3B	4B	5B	6B	7B	8B	8B	8B	1B	2B	3A	4A	5A	6A	7A	0
1	1 H Hydrogen 1.00794																	2 He Helium 4.003
2	3 Li Lithium 6.941	4 Be Beryllium 9.012182											5 B Boron 10.811	6 C Carbon 12.0107	7 N Nitrogen 14.00674	8 O Oxygen 15.9994	9 F Fluorine 18.9984032	10 Ne Neon 20.1797
3	11 Na Sodium 22.989770	12 Mg Magnesium 24.3050											13 Al Aluminum 26.981538	14 Si Silicon 28.0855	15 P Phosphorus 30.973761	16 S Sulfur 32.066	17 Cl Chlorine 35.4527	18 Ar Argon 39.948
4	19 K Potassium 39.0983	20 Ca Calcium 40.078	21 Sc Scandium 44.955910	22 Ti Titanium 47.867	23 V Vanadium 50.9415	24 Cr Chromium 51.9961	25 Mn Manganese 54.938049	26 Fe Iron 55.845	27 Co Cobalt 58.933200	28 Ni Nickel 58.6934	29 Cu Copper 63.546	30 Zn Zinc 65.39	31 Ga Gallium 69.723	32 Ge Germanium 72.61	33 As Arsenic 74.92160	34 Se Selenium 78.96	35 Br Bromine 79.904	36 Kr Krypton 83.80
5	37 Rb Rubidium 85.4678	38 Sr Strontium 87.62	39 Y Yttrium 88.90585	40 Zr Zirconium 91.224	41 Nb Niobium 92.90638	42 Mo Molybdenum 95.94	43 Tc Technetium (98)	44 Ru Ruthenium 101.07	45 Rh Rhodium 102.90550	46 Pd Palladium 106.42	47 Ag Silver 107.8682	48 Cd Cadmium 112.411	49 In Indium 114.818	50 Sn Tin 118.710	51 Sb Antimony 121.760	52 Te Tellurium 127.60	53 I Iodine 126.90447	54 Xe Xenon 131.29
6	55 Cs Cesium 132.90545	56 Ba Barium 137.327	57 La Lanthanum 138.9055	72 Hf Hafnium 178.49	73 Ta Tantalum 180.9479	74 W Tungsten 183.84	75 Re Rhenium 186.207	76 Os Osmium 190.23	77 Ir Iridium 192.217	78 Pt Platinum 195.078	79 Au Gold 196.96655	80 Hg Mercury 200.59	81 Tl Thallium 204.3833	82 Pb Lead 207.2	83 Bi Bismuth 208.98038	84 Po Polonium (209)	85 At Astatine (210)	86 Rn Radon (222)
7	87 Fr Francium (223)	88 Ra Radium (226)	89 Ac Actinium (227)	104 Rf Rutherfordium (261)	105 Db Dubnium (262)	106 Sg Seaborgium (263)	107 Bh Bohrium (262)	108 Hs Hassium (265)	109 Mt Meitnerium (266)	110 (269)	111 (272)	112 (277)	113	114				

Lanthanides:

58 Ce Cerium 140.116	59 Pr Praseodymium 140.90765	60 Nd Neodymium 144.24	61 Pm Promethium (145)	62 Sm Samarium 150.36	63 Eu Europium 151.964	64 Gd Gadolinium 157.25	65 Tb Terbium 158.92534	66 Dy Dysprosium 162.50	67 Ho Holmium 164.93032	68 Er Erbium 167.26	69 Tm Thulium 168.93421	70 Yb Ytterbium 173.04	71 Lu Lutetium 174.967

Actinides:

90 Th Thorium 232.0381	91 Pa Protactinium 231.03588	92 U Uranium 238.0289	93 Np Neptunium (237)	94 Pu Plutonium (244)	95 Am Americium (243)	96 Cm Curium (247)	97 Bk Berkelium (247)	98 Cf Californium (251)	99 Es Einsteinium (252)	100 Fm Fermium (257)	101 Md Mendelevium (258)	102 No Nobelium (259)	103 Lr Lawrencium (262)

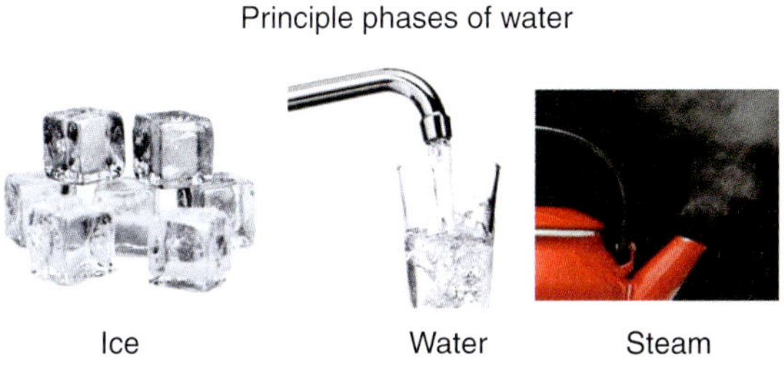

Principle phases of water

Ice   Water   Steam

Figure 6.2 The three principle forms or phases of water commonly found. As energy increases (e.g. by temperature), the phase changes from one to another (i.e. from ice to water to steam). Note, contrary to common belief, true steam (as a gas) is invisible (note just at the point of exiting the kettle), but what is generally seen is "condensed" steam, a mixture of steam (gas) and water (liquid). This is an important concept in considering steam sterilization (Chapter 11, see the section on steam (moist heat) sterilization).

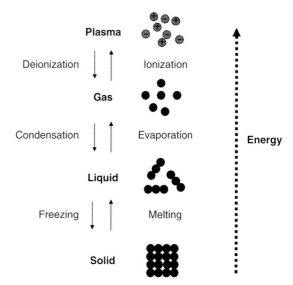

Figure 6.3 Phase (or state) changes of matter. As energy increases the phases change from solids to liquids, gases and plasmas, and vice versa. Various other terms to describe these changes in phase can be given, for example evaporation can also be described as vaporization or boiling, and in some cases a phase can be skipped, such as in a phase change known as sublimation a solid can go directly into a gas. Note: the release of energy during the condensation of steam (gas) to water (liquid) is responsible for the antimicrobial efficiency of steam sterilization (Chapter 11, in the section on steam (moist heat) sterilization).

invisible (note at the point of exiting the kettle) but what is generally seen is actually "condensed" steam, a mixture of steam (gas) and water (liquid). This is an important concept in considering steam sterilization (Chapter 11, in the section on steam (moist heat) sterilization). Other examples of water in a mixture of gas and liquid forms that are visible are fog, mist and clouds. Another example of a liquid that forms a gas or vapor is hydrogen peroxide, also used as a liquid and a gas/vapor for disinfection and sterilization (Chapters 9 and 11). Similarly, all other forms of matter can form similar phases depending on their chemistry. As an example, carbon dioxide (CO_2, not to be mistaken for CO, carbon monoxide a poisonous gas) forms a gas under normal, ambient conditions (temperature and pressure); CO_2 is breathed out through our lungs as a waste product from the body. For CO_2 to form a solid the temperature has to be reduced to −78°C. The associated words used to describe the conversion between the different phases of matter are summarized in Figure 6.3.

In discussing solids, liquids and gases above, constant reference was made to "ambient" conditions of temperature and pressure. This is important and it is the basis of one of the groups of "laws" of chemistry: the gas laws. The gas laws define relationships between the volume, temperature, pressure and concentration (the amount) of a gas. Examples include Boyle's Law (the specific relationship between the pressure and volume of a gas) and Charles' Law (the specific relationship between the temperature and volume of a gas). They can be all be defined mathematically, but in simple terms if you have a fixed amount (concentration) of any gas in a fixed volume (the

area or space in which the gas is contained), there is a direct relationship between the temperature and the pressure: as the temperature increases the pressure decreases and vice versa. Pressure refers to a force applied to a surface. A high pressure suggests a greater force, while a low pressure is less force. Pressure is measured in a variety of ways, but specifically as the force applied to a specific size of a surface (e.g. psi: pressure per square inch, mmHg: millimetres of mercury, where the pressure applied acts on mercury in a confined area, atm: atmospheres, and the correct international measurement of pressure is the Pa: Pascal; for more discussion on weights and measure see the section on common chemical measurement methods). Therefore, if we consider water further, at atmospheric pressure (sea level) at about 100,000 Pa (also given as 100 kPa, where k is kilo or 1000) water is a liquid between 0 and 100°C, below which it forms ice and above which it forms steam. But if the pressure is changed, so do these ranges (Figure 6.4).

At lower pressures, also referred to as being under a vacuum (where the lower the pressure the "deeper" the

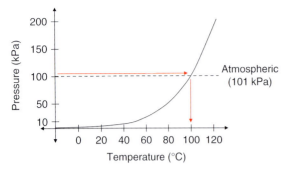

Figure 6.4 The relationship between temperature and pressure. The relationship shown is specifically for water and would vary in temperature/pressure ranges depending the molecule or matter being considered. The line in the graph represents the point at which gas (steam) is made at a given temperature and pressure; an example is given in red, where at 101 kPa pressure (which is atmospheric pressure at sea level) steam will form at 100°C. At lower pressures, steam is formed at lower temperatures and at higher pressure steam forms at higher temperatures.

vacuum), steam is formed at lower temperatures and at higher pressure (under pressure) steam is formed at higher temperatures. For example in Figure 6.4 for water, at 101 kPa pressure (which is atmospheric pressure at sea level) steam will form at 100°C, but at about 47 kPa steam forms at 80°C and similarly at about 200 kPa steam forms at 120°C. In this way, higher temperatures can be achieved with steam as the pressure increases, which is the basis for a steam sterilization process (Chapter 11).

Finally, let us consider plasma. A plasma is essentially a gas that has been further energized (or ionized; Figure 6.3). In its true form, the gas is energized to break apart the molecules, which make up the gas, into sub-parts (ions and other reactive species), which basically makes the molecules and elements unstable. Therefore, if water (H_2O) is used as an example; as the energy is increased, ice (H_2O in a solid form) will turn to water (H_2O in liquid form), then steam (H_2O in gas form) then into water plasma (essentially H and O, although the various species formed will vary to include OH, OH^-, O_2^- and H^+). When the energy used to make the plasma is removed, the elements will rapidly recombine to form the starting gas (e.g. H_2O) but also other molecules (O_3: ozone and H_2O_2: hydrogen peroxide) may form as well as releasing energy (e.g. released as UV light; see the section on light and radiation and the electromagnetic spectrum).

Mixtures, formulations and solutions

Solids, liquids and gases can range in their chemical composition; they can be used on their own (e.g. pure water) or as mixtures. A mixture may be defined as a combination of two or more chemicals into one. The air is an example of a mixture of gases, consisting of approximately (in chemistry is shown as the symbol ~) 78% nitrogen, 21% oxygen and a range of other gases at much lower amounts (e.g. carbon dioxide, CO_2). It is not, however, as simple as that, with various other components present, such as water and various particles (e.g. dust, pollen and microorganisms). Important examples of liquid and solid mixtures that are used in reprocessing are the various types of cleaning or disinfection formulations. A formulation is a mixture and can be further defined as a combination of ingredients, including active and inert ingredients, into a product for its intended use. An example of the various chemicals used in such liquid formulations and the reason for their use are given in Table 6.2.

It was stated in the opening of this section that solids, liquids and gases can range in their chemical composition, with some, like pure water (just containing H_2O), being used on their own. It is important to note that water is rarely pure, but is actually found to have a range of different chemical, microbial and other contaminants (Table 6.3; water is discussed in further detail Chapter 15).

Many chemicals "dissolve" into water to give a homogeneous (or uniform) mixture that is known as a "solution". As an example, consider a glass of water and then adding common salt (NaCl) into it: the salt will dissolve into the water to give a solution of salt in water. A solution is therefore a homogeneous mixture of two or more chemicals into one. In our example of salt in water, as you continue to add more salt you will eventually reach a point that the water cannot take (or dissolve) any further salt (this is referred to being saturated or "full"). If you increase the temperature more salt can be dissolved, but this will fall out of solution as you reduce the heat; similarly if you boil the water, the water is removed as steam and the salt will be left behind. Also note, that in the example of water, there are other components that are not dissolved (not in solution), but are just floating (or "suspended") in the water (Table 6.3).

You are correct to conclude that the terms mixtures, formulations and solutions are often used interchangeably to mean similar things, but they do have different chemical definitions.

Table 6.2 Various different chemical components used in formulations used for cleaning and disinfection.

Chemical type	Examples[1]	Formulation use
Water	—	Dissolving other chemicals (for this purpose, water is considered chemically as a "solvent".
Surfactants	Ionic surfactants, amphophilic surfactants	Aid in dissolving and dispersing materials such as soil, including lipids that do not mix with water. Assist in cleaning and can have some antimicrobial activity.
Chelating agents (or chelants)	EDTA, DTPA, NTA	Bind elements (in particular "heavy" metals) such as calcium and iron. By binding they cannot react and can therefore optimize activity (including soil breakdown and damage/inhibiting effects when present in water).
Solvents	Water, alcohols	Dissolving other chemicals or materials.
Bases	NaOH, KOH	Make solutions more alkaline and also breakdown organic materials (basic hydrolysis).
Acids	Acetic acid, citric acid	Make solutions more acidic and also dissolve inorganic materials.
Corrosion inhibitors	Hexamine, Benzotriazole	Protect against corrosion (damage) on surfaces.
Biocides	QACs, phenolics, glutaraldehyde, hydrogen peroxide	Biocides are antimicrobial chemicals and are used to kill (in disinfectants/sterilants) or inhibit (preserve, as preservatives) microorganisms. Some may also be used for hydrolysis (soil breakdown).
Enzymes	Proteases, lipases	To break down organic molecules such as proteins and lipids (enzymatic hydrolysis; see the section on cleaning chemistries).

[1] Note: specific chemicals can be given different names (official, trade, descriptive, etc.) and it is usual to abbreviate them to make them easier to refer to. An example is the chemical EDTA, which stands for ethylenediaminetetraacetic acid but also edetic acid and Hampene or Versene.

Table 6.3 Examples of various common components that can be found in water. Some components are dissolved (or in solution) with water, while others are suspended (floating in or on water).

Component	Examples
Water	Pure water (H_2O)
Dissolved components	
Inorganic materials	Calcium (Ca), magnesium (Mg), chlorine (Cl_2)/chloride (Cl^-), silicates (molecules with SiO_4^{-4}), sodium (Na), nitrates (molecules with NO_3^-), iron (Fe)
Organic materials	Pesticides and herbicides, for example trihalomethanes, trichlorethylene, and polychlorinated biphenyls (PCBs)
Gases	Oxygen (O_2), carbon dioxide (CO_2)
Suspended components	
Inorganic materials	Calcium carbonate ($CaCO_2$), clay, silt, silica
Organic materials	Endotoxins, proteins, fats, oil
Microorganisms	Bacteria, viruses, protozoa

Weights, measures and other physical considerations

Units of measurement are used to define quantity (amounts) in chemistry, physics, mathematics and the sciences in general. We use them in our daily lives, with examples being weights, volumes and lengths. Some of the more important units are described briefly in this section.

A variety of methods of measurement are used, with the two major systems being imperial and metric. Imperial system units of measurement include pounds (lbs) and inches, while equivalent units in the metric system are grams (g) and meters (m). Most countries around the world have adopted the International System of Units (SI) as their official units of measurement, which is based on the metric system. Exceptions, today, are the United States, where imperial measurements are still widely used and in the UK, where the SI system has been adopted but is used in parallel with the imperial system. For the purpose of simplification, the SI units are used throughout the book, but reference is given to the imperial system (or other widely used units) when considered applicable. In this section, units of measurements from the two systems are introduced. In addition, to convert from one unit to another, some mathematical conversion factors are given, but these are not exclusive and may be more readily converted using many of the Internet-based conversion sites (such as www.onlineconversion.com).

The basic, metric units of measurement are summarized in Table 6.4. It is quite a long list, although there are some that we will use more frequently than others, such as those for temperature (C or K/°C or °K), weights (grams, g) volumes (liters, L), and pressures (pascals, Pa).

One of benefits of the metric system is that it is based on factors of 10. In the system a prefix can be placed before the unit to make it more practical to write or describe. A summary of some of the most widely used prefixes is given in Table 6.5.

These prefixes are based on multiples or divisions of 10 and include terms such as kilo- (e.g. kilogram or kg) and centi- (e.g. centimetre, cm). For example 1 kg is equal to 1000 g (also written mathematically as 10^3g; counting the

Table 6.4 The SI (metric) units of measurements and other units commonly used.

Quantity	Unit		Other measures
	Name	Symbol[1]	
Area	square metre	m^2	Acre, square-foot
Chemical amount[2]	mole	mol	
Flow (of volume)[3]	cubic meters/second	m^3/s	Gallons per hour, cubic feet per minute
Frequency	hertz	Hz	
Length	metre (meter)	m	Foot, inch, mile
Mass/weight	gram	g	Ounce, pound, ton
Power	watt	W	Horsepower, calorie per second, BTU/min
Pressure	pascal	Pa	Bar, atmosphere (atm), millimeters of mercury (mmHg), Torr, pounds per square inch (psi)
Speed	meters/second	m/s	Miles per hour, knot
Temperature[4]	kelvin	K	Celsius (C), Fahrenheit (F)
Time[5]	second	s	
Volume	cubic metre or litre	m^3 or L	Cubic inch, gallon, pint, ounce, teaspoon

[1] Any capitalized units are done so on purpose and are correctly written as such.
[2] Chemists consider the "amount" of a chemical as different to its weight or volume, referring to "moles" of a chemical.
[3] The symbol '/' in this context is referred to as meaning "per", as in cubic meters per second.
[4] Kelvin (K) is used but not as widely as Celsius (C) or Fahrenheit (F). Note that in both cases they are often referred to as "degrees" of that unit (°F or °C).
[5] The second is the SI unit, but unlike other SI measures, it follows the traditional convention of 60 seconds in a minute (min), 60 minutes in an hour (hr) and 24 hours in a day.

Table 6.5 Commonly used prefixes in the SI/metric system for units of measurement. For example 1 kg is equal to 1000 g but also written mathematically as 10^3 g; counting the number of zeros and where 10^0 is 1, 10^1 is 10, etc. Also, in divisions of these units, counting the number of decimal places (or numbers after 0.) 10^{-1} is 0.1, 10^{-2} is 0.01, etc. Therefore 10^{-2} g is 0.01 g and 10^{-3} g is 0.001 g.

Prefix symbol[1]	Name	Factor	Example
Unit multiples			
k	kilo-	10^3, thousand	kg, kilogram
M	mega-	10^6, million	Mm, megameter
G	giga-	10^9, billion	GL, gigalitre
Unit divisions			
c	centi-	10^{-2}, hundredth	cm, centimetre
m	milli-	10^{-3}, thousandth	mm, millimetre
μ	micro-	10^{-6}, millionth	μg, microgram

[1] Any capitalized units are done so on purpose and are correctly written as such.

number of zeros and where 10^0 is 1, 10^1 is 10, etc., and where 10^{-1} is 0.1 (in some countries given as 0,1), 10^{-2} is 0.01, etc. Note: such mathematical terms are also used widely in microbiology, where 10^6 is one million or 1,000,000 of, say, a bacteria or virus population. The more correct term is 1×10^6, where 2×10^6 will be 2 million and 10×10^6 is 10 million or correctly written as 1×10^7.

A further benefit of SI units is that they are standardized internationally; for example in older systems some weights and measures could vary in their specific quantity depending on the country of origin (for example the US and UK gallon or ounce are different measures/weights). Thankfully it is now normal process for product suppliers providing instructions on weights and measures to give any local and widely used units in addition to the metric/SI units, to minimize any misunderstanding.

Some common conversion factors are provided in Table 6.6 for reference.

As a final consideration, let us look briefly at dilution and dissolution. Diluting is mixing a concentrated liquid product with water to give the right product concentration for a given application (e.g. for cleaning or disinfection). In chemical use it is important that the instructions of diluting a product are closely followed to prevent waste of the product (where too much is used for the application), where damage can occur (again, if too much product is used) or that the product is not going to be effective (too little product is used or "under-dilution"). Instructions are normally given on a product label and/or instructions as a certain volume or weight of a product mixed with a volume/weight of water. Examples include:

g/L: weight of the product (liquid or solid) into a liter of water. For example, 1 g/L (one gram per liter) is 1 g in a final volume of a liter of water, which is the same as 50 g/50 L if making up a final desired volume of 50 L).

mL/L: volume of the product in a volume (liter) of water. For example, 10 m L/L is made up by taking 10 mL of the product and adding water until you make one L (i.e. 10 mL product + 990 mL water).

%: percent, being a weight or volume in 100 mL of water, such as 1% is one mL in a final volume of 100 mL (i.e. one mL adding 99 mL water). In this case, it is common to see terms such as v/v and w/v, referring to volume in a volume or weight in a volume. As an example, 1% v/v would mean measuring a volume of 1 mL and adding 99 mL of water; in the case of w/v the weight of a product is added to water to give a final volume of 100 mL.

In all cases it is important that the product is well mixed to ensure it is diluted correctly. Dissolution is where a solid product is added to water. In certain situations a product is given in two parts, being mixed together (sometimes or not including water) for the desired product; in these cases the chemical product may require a reaction time to be ready for use and will always require adequate mixing to ensure the product is correctly prepared. Overall, it can be quite complicated, but remember these rules: follow the written manufacturer's instructions on how to prepare chemistries for their desired use and if you do not understand the instructions ask for assistance.

Table 6.6 Common units of measurement conversion factors. They can be used to convert between units of measurement but if you are unsure it is important to check with an expert or use simple conversion systems online.

Measurement	Conversion factor
Length	1 foot (international) = 1/3 yard = 12 inches = 0.305 m. 1 m = 100 cm = 1000 mm.
Weight	1 stone = 14 pounds (lbs) = 6.35 kg 1 ounce (US) = 28 g 1 kg = 1000 g
Pressure	1 Torr = 1 mmHg = 133.3 Pa 1 psi = 6.89 kPa; 1 atm = 101 kPa; 1 bar = 100 kPa 1 kPa = 1000 Pa Note: atmospheric pressure (at sea level) is ~101.3 kPa = 1 atm = 760 Torr or mmHg = 1 bar
Temperature	1°C = 33.8°F = 274 K. But unlike the other factors, you cannot simply multiply to get the correct conversion. To convert between the two major units (C and F) use: °C = (°F-32)/1.8 °F = °C × 1.8 = 32
Volume (of liquid)[1]	1 gallon (imperial) = 160 fluid ounces = 4.546 L 1 gallon (US) = 128 fluid ounces = 3.785 L 1 L = 1000 mL = 1000 cm³ (therefore 1 mL = 1 cm³)

[1] Note: the conversion of the volume of liquid using non-metric units may be different depending on being the volume of a solid/liquid, or on where you live (e.g. a "gallon" in the US can be a dry or liquid gallon and both are different to the imperial gallon).

The pH scale: defining acids and bases

Chemists can use a variety of ways to study and analyse various different types of chemicals and solutions. One such measurement is known as pH, which is a measure of how acidic or alkaline a liquid or solution is. The strict chemical understanding of pH is that it is a measure of the hydrogen ion (H^+) concentration in a solution, but this is not considered further. The pH scale ranges from 0 to 14 (Figure 6.5) and all liquids will fall somewhere on this scale. The mid-range of the scale is at 7, at which a liquid is considered "neutral", while the more acidic the lower the number ("strong acid") and the more alkaline (or basic) the higher the number ("strong alkali/base").

An example of a neutral liquid is drinking water (if it is correctly provided) which is generally in the neutral range (pH 6–8). Another is blood that is generally at and maintained at a pH of about 7.4 (this can also be referred to as being slightly alkaline). As liquids are measured to be more acidic (<6) or alkaline/basic (>8), they are considered more aggressive. Some common types of acids are vinegar (which is actually a dilute or watered-down version of an acid known as acetic acid, which has the chemical formula

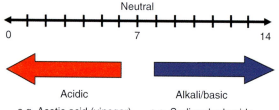

Figure 6.5 The pH scale. Note: it is correct to write the p in lower case and the H in upper case. Neutral is to the centre (pH 6–8) of the range, with acids to the left (<6) and alkali (or bases; >8) to the right. At lower levels of pH, liquids are considered more acidic and high levels of pH they are considered more alkaline/basic.

CH_3COOH or also written as $C_2H_4O_2$), orange juice and lemon juice. Hydrochloric acid (HCl) is produced by the body in the stomach, which gives the stomach contents an acidic pH to aid in the digestive process (see Chapter 2). Examples of alkaline liquids are bleach solutions (a mixture of a chemical known as sodium hypochlorite, NaOCl, in water) and many liquid soaps and detergents. It should be noted that the difference, for example, between a solution of pH 6 and pH 5 is larger than it seems because it is what is referre d to as a "log" scale. A log scale means that for every 1 unit increase or decrease in pH the actual scale is 10 times different; therefore an acid at pH 2 is 10 times more acidic than at pH 3 and 100 times at a pH of 4.

Acids and bases are used for a variety of decontamination purposes, including cleaning, disinfection and sterilization; however, it is unusual to see them used as just pure acids or bases. Examples of a pure acid solution would be mixtures of hydrochloric acid, citric acid or peracetic acid. These acids will be particularly good at dissolving inorganic salts (e.g. calcium carbonate, a major component of water hardness or "scale"; Chapter 15, section on water quality and purity) and peracetic acid is an efficacy antimicrobial chemical (see Chapter 9, in the section on peroxygens). Although they could all be used for cleaning and disinfection purposes, they would also be considered damaging to many device materials. It is for these reasons that they are used in combination with other chemicals in formulation, which are designed to give the benefit of the acid but minimize the negative effects. Similarly, alkalines such as sodium hydroxide (NaOH) and potassium hydroxide (KOH) are extremely good for breaking down and removing organic materials from surfaces, therefore would be efficient cleaners (in removing blood and other materials from surfaces after surgical procedures); but they are also considered aggressive and are optimally used in formulation for the same reasons. Another common use of pH in formulation is to help other chemicals be efficient for their desired use. An example mentioned above is in bleach solutions; bleach is a mixture of sodium hypochlorite in water, where the hypochlorite provides or releases chlorine for its antimicrobial properties. Another example is the use of peracetic acid for its antimicrobial purposes, where although the pH or a per-acetic acid solution on its own is very low (<pH 2), in typical disinfectants and sterilants they will be closer to neutral pH; in this way they are less aggressive on surfaces, but still are effective at killing microorganisms. A common term used to describe this is a "buffer", where a buffer is itself a type of chemistry that is used to control the pH to its desired level.

The pH of a solution can be conveniently measured using pH paper (that changes color when placed into the solution and is compared to a color chart to match the pre-defined pH level) or using handheld probes (Figure 6.6). As a note, the pH can vary depending on the temperature; therefore it is common for pH measurement to be conducted at ambient temperature (~20°C) or that the temperature is stated with the pH measurement.

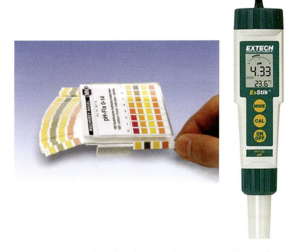

Figure 6.6 Examples of methods used to measure pH. On the left is an example of pH paper and its associated color chart (where the color developed on placing the paper into the solution is matched to the chart) and a pH probe, which is placed into the solution and gives a digital read-out of the pH.

Other common chemical measurement methods

As mentioned earlier, chemists can use a variety of techniques to study and analyse various types of chemicals and solutions. These techniques help them determine what types ("qualitative") and how much ("quantitative") of various chemicals are present in a given sample of a gas, liquid or solid. Therefore, as an example, in a chemical analysis of a water sample one could say qualitatively that there was carbon and chlorine present, but quantitatively there was 240 mg/L and 20 mg/L, respectively. Analytical chemistry is the use of these techniques to study chemical composition. A number of further examples of these methods are discussed in brief below, with particular emphasis on methods you may come across in use in, or being conducted for, a reprocessing department.

An introduction to sampling

A sample is simply a small amount of any solid, liquid or gas taken for analysis (e.g. a water sample). There are two important considerations in sampling that should be understood. The first is that the analysis of a sample is only as good as the person taking or collecting the sample; if, for example, a water sample is taken in a dirty bottle (remembering that chemical dirt may or may not be visible to the eye) it can be contaminated and give a wrong result when analyzed. The second is that any sample taken is only representative at the time it was taken. A typical example is with water: most facilities will have two sources of water, hot and cold, and the chemical quality of both can change even over a day, and considerably over a year.

Titration

This is a quantitative method to determine the concentration of a chemical/type of chemistry in a sample. It is also known as "volumetric analysis". In a typical titration a defined, known chemical (a "reagent", as it reacts) is added to the sample being analyzed to react with it (e.g. to change its pH, which can give a color change in the presence of a dye not dissimilar to those used for pH measurements, see the section on the pH scale: defining acids and bases). By then adding a measured amount of another chemical, in this example to change to pH to a certain point to allow a color change, the final amount of this chemical added is related to the original amount of the chemical being analyzed. Examples of the use of titrations in water analysis include the measurement of water hardness and chlorine levels (Figure 6.7).

Conductivity

This is a quantitative method used to measure the ability to conduct electricity (specifically electrical conductivity or EC, as can also refer to heat or even sound conductivity).

It is measured in microSiemens per centimeter ($\mu Si/m$ or $\mu Si\ m^2$), but is often also give as millimhos per centimetre (mmho/cm). It is a simple, but indirect, method for estimating the amount of various types of charged contaminants in a sample (particularly metals such as iron, copper and silver, and other elements like chlorine and silicates). A good example is the conductivity of water, where the higher the measured conductivity the greater the level of charged chemical present. An example of a conductivity meter is given in Figure 6.8. Conductivity is often directly compared to another analysis method, TDS for total dissolved solids (see the next section).

Total dissolved solids

This is the measurement of all organic and inorganic substances in a liquid. A simple way of thinking about this is to take a water sample and boil off all the water, with whatever remains being the total dissolved solids (TDS). This will include various elements (calcium, iron), suspended molecules (phosphates, nitrates) and other materials. It is therefore a measure of all chemicals in a sample (given as mg/L) and can be estimated in relation to electrical conductivity as the more chemicals present the

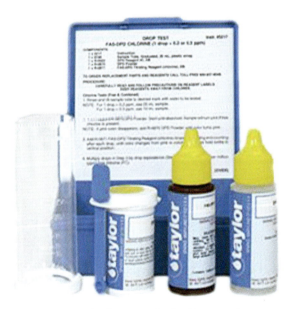

Figure 6.7 Example of a titration kit for chlorine analysis.

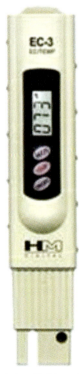

Figure 6.8 Example of a handheld conductivity meter.

greater the conductivity. It is typical for a conductivity probe to be used to estimate both conductivity (in μSi/m) and TDS (in mg/L).

Total organic carbon

In its simplest terms, this is the measure of the amount of organic carbon present in a sample. It is generally used to estimate the quality of a sample, in particular water cleanliness and for surface cleaning evaluation. Carbon molecules are the basis for any type of human, plant, animal and even microbial contamination, but also other chemistries that can be present, such as herbicides, detergents and some disinfectants (e.g. phenols and aldehydes). Note: total organic carbon (TOC) only gives the total amount of organic carbon present, but no further information on the exact types present.

Inductively coupled plasma mass spectrometry

This is commonly known as ICP analysis. Measurements such as conductivity and total organic carbon are gross estimates of chemicals that can be present and are not very specific. Inductively coupled plasma mass

spectrometry (ICP-MS) analysis is an example of a very specific measurement method. It is capable of determining the types and amounts of chemicals present in a sample even at extremely low concentrations. It is beyond the scope of this book to describe the exact method, but it includes preparing the sample and then introducing this into a specific machine for the analysis.

Light, radiation and the electromagnetic spectrum

A branch of chemistry and physics is the study of light. Light is more than what we see, which is known as 'visible' or white light. In technical terms, it refers to the electromagnetic spectrum (Figure 6.9).

Various forms of light are used for antimicrobial purposes including microwaves and infrared (IR), both as methods of heating, and ultraviolet (UV), X-rays and γ-rays (that can be directly antimicrobial due to their higher energy levels; Figure 6.9). Microwaves, IR and UV can be used indirectly or directly as disinfection methods in hospitals and other clinical facilities. X-rays

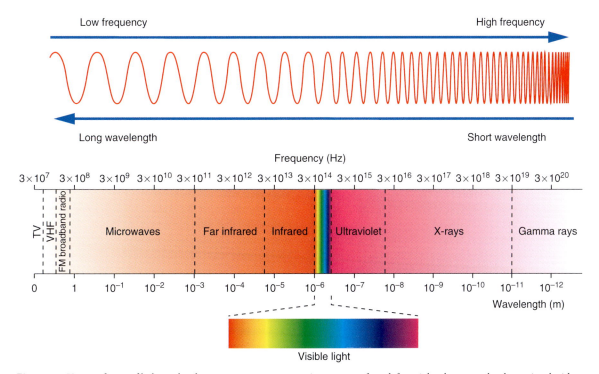

Figure 6.9 Various forms of light or the electromagnetic spectrum. As you move from left to right, the energy level associated with the type of light (or "frequency") increases. The shorter the wavelength, the greater the energy.

and γ-rays are not commonly or practically used in such facilities for such applications, but are used for industrial disinfection/sterilization (e.g. for single-use devices that are provided pre-sterilized to a hospital); as antimicrobial technologies, they are not considered further in this book.

Safety considerations

Various types of chemicals are used in clinical facilities, including those for cleaning, disinfection and sterilization. They are designed to disturb, disrupt, remove, damage and even kill the various materials (or soils) that remain on a device surface from patients after surgical, medical or dental use. It should therefore not come as any surprise that these chemicals can and usually are dangerous to your health, as we are made up of the same types of basic molecules. As a general statement, all chemicals can do you harm under the right conditions. Some of these are obvious, such as strong acids and alkalis (see the section on the pH scale: defining acids and bases) can give a direct, quick and even serious burn when placed on the skin. Others will be more subtle, with some extreme cases leading to increased allergic reactions (sensitization), toxic effects or damage over time and carcinogenicity ("cancer-causing", where a carcinogen is a cancer-causing agent/chemical). Even chemicals we take for granted can lead to problems, for example common table salt (NaCl) when taken at high doses in your diet can be damaging to your health. The lesson we learn from this discussion is to respect the use of chemicals and take the necessary precautions to limit your exposure to them.

In considering chemical safety, there are at least three considerations:
• Personal safety
• Patient safety, that can be associated with chemicals remaining on a device surface (e.g. not being rinsed away) or that could damage the device
• Environmental safety, which is becoming a growing concern internationally

Personal safety is the responsibility for each employee by ensuring that chemicals are correctly handled, but also the responsibility of supervisors/managers to ensure that their employees are aware of any safety risks and have been given the correct training and equipment to minimize those risks. Note: this may not only apply to those working in a given area but also to visitors in the area, as many chemical accidents happen to those in the vicinity of someone using a chemical.

There are four steps to consider in establishing and maintaining good and safe personal safety practices when using chemicals:
• Identify and understand the chemical risks in a given area. Good sources are product labels, material safety data sheets, etc.
• Decide what precautions are necessary (e.g. ventilation, eye or face protection, monitoring systems).
• Introduce and train on any procedures or control mechanisms to prevent or control exposure.
• Ensure that procedures/measures are used and are maintained (e.g. by auditing).

For each chemical product, it is good practice (if not a legal requirement in most countries) for safety information to be provided with the product. This is usually provided with the product label; note that a product label can include what is physically written on the product (the attached label) but also any other accessory information such as additional instructions for use, the material safety data sheets (MSDS) and technical literature.

The label (in all its parts) is an excellent source of information, but many pay little attention to the detail provided. It can provide information on how the product should be used (e.g. correct dilution or not diluted but ready for use), any safety risks/symbols, storage and disposal considerations and any immediate steps (or first aid) that can be taken on exposure (e.g. eye/skin contact or accidental swallowing). As labeling standards vary from country to country, the label itself may not actually provide all the correct safety information; in these cases it is recommended to request further information from the supplier or even to change suppliers. Internationally, for example, there is a series of standardized warning symbols that can be used to recognize certain health risks associated with the product (Figure 6.10).

In general, the most effective ways to reduce the risks associated with any chemical in use is to provide training, use personal protective equipment (PPE) and to periodically audit that safety practices are being following in a department. Training is the first step, to allow any chemical user to understand their risks, that they appreciate how PPE or other safety precautions can reduce those risks. Personal protective equipment includes equipment such as gloves, safety glasses or goggles, face shields and disposable aprons (Figure 6.11; see Chapter 13). Note, for example, that safety glasses are usually designed to protect the eyes from splashes from the front as well as from the sides.

The final step is safety auditing; auditing can be defined as an evaluation or review of practices based on established procedures. When safety policies and procedures are put

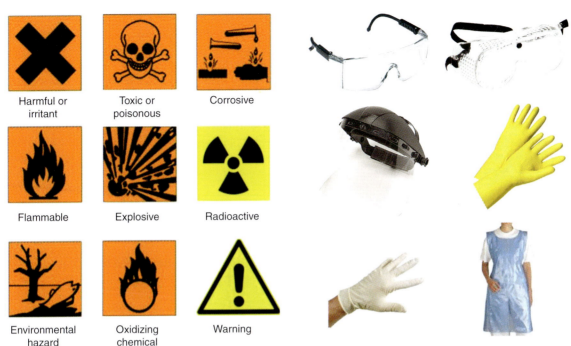

Figure 6.10 Some examples of widely used internationally standardized chemical safety warning symbols.

(Figure 6.10 labels:)
Harmful or irritant
Toxic or poisonous
Corrosive
Flammable
Explosive
Radioactive
Environmental hazard
Oxidizing chemical
Warning

Figure 6.11 Various types of PPE, personal protective equipment.

in place it is important to review over time that they are being followed. Audits can be defined at intervals, in cases where they are expected or, more beneficially, unexpected; they help establish that safety is important in a given area and that staff/management are committed to it.

Specific chemicals may require further and even tighter controls. Examples include the use of various types of gases such as ethylene oxide (for sterilization; see Chapter 11) or aldehyde-based liquid disinfectants like glutaraldehyde (see Chapter 9). Ethylene oxide gas, for example, is considered flammable/explosive at concentrations of ~3% gas in air, can be lethal at 800 ppm and is considered a carcinogen (cancer causing) over time. For this reason, reasonably tight controls and monitoring systems are strongly suggested for use in areas using the gas for sterilization.

In addition to personal safety, there are chemical risks to patients and to the environment. Patient chemical risks should be minimized by correct use and removal of chemicals used for reprocessing or maintaining the device. Patient risks will include direct or indirect safety concerns. A direct concern is where a chemical is mistakenly used and left on a device prior to the use in/on a patient; in these cases, toxic effects can be observed in the patient, leading

to health consequences. Examples can include overuse of the chemical (e.g. not diluted correctly) and inadequate rinsing (to remove the chemical after use). Many chemical disinfectants, for example, require multiple cycles of water rinsing (sometimes up to 5–6 rinses in fresh water, each time) to adequately remove toxic residues of the chemistry. Indirect effects are due to damage by the chemical to the device; this damage, over time, can lead to problems in the safe use of the instrument on a patient.

Environmental safety on the use of chemicals is a growing concern internationally, with many countries internationally putting restrictions on the types of chemicals that can be used. The main concern is regarding those chemicals that are not easily broken down in the environment and can therefore lead to accumulation in environmental sources (such as water, the air and plants/animals).

How to choose and use a chemical product

In deciding to use any chemical or chemical-containing product, there should always be three considerations: safety, compatibility and efficacy. Safety has been addressed in the section on safety considerations, to include safety for the person using the chemical, for the patient and for the environment. Compatibility, referring to the ability of the chemical to be used on a device and the materials it can be made of without any significant damage, can be considered as a further safety requirement, but is separately discussed in this section.

Device compatibility is an important aspect: a chemical has little benefit if it is used for its intended purpose but also damages/destroys the device! This can be a difficult area to address as it may vary depending on the chemical, its formulation, temperature or even pressure used. Equally, it can vary depending on the various types of metals, plastics, glass, adhesives, etc., used in a device. Compatibility (or more specifically the opposite being incompatibility) can be obvious to the eye but can equally not be and only build up over time. If plastics or adhesives are thermo-sensitive (sensitive to heat) they will obviously damage the device if heat disinfected or particularly steam sterilized to render them unfit for future use. An example includes the rusting of stainless steel devices (formed from the reaction of iron, which is present in stainless steel, with oxygen, to form a red-brown color, chemically known as ferric oxides); rusting is due to initial damage (scratching, wear and tear) on the device surface that allows for oxygen to react with exposed iron to initiate rusting, which leads to corrosion of the device. Note: the physical signs of rusting can be removed (see Chapter 15) but not the underlying damage. Device and chemical/process manufacturers are a good source of information regarding device compatibility with various devices.

Efficacy (or effectiveness for a given task) is the main reason a chemical product is used, for cleaning, disinfection, sterilization or other use (e.g. lubrication that allows the devices to be correctly used). It is important to remember that chemical products vary considerably in formulation, despite even having similar main, active ingredients; therefore close inspection should be made on product claims to ensure they are correctly used and fit for purpose. For example, it would not be good practice to use an antiseptic product that has been developed and labeled for use on the skin (e.g. chlorhexidine and iodine-based products used for surgical hand washing prior to surgery by operating room staff) to be used for cleaning of the devices following their use in a surgical procedure. Equally, the presence of the chemical or chemical product alone may not ensure efficacy if it is not used with the right process conditions: time, temperature,

concentration, etc. These conditions should be defined by the product manufacturer and specified in the labeling provided with the product.

Although safety, compatibility and efficacy are essential to consider, there are other requirements, many of which may be specific to each facility depending on their local, regional and/or country-specific requirements. These include that a chemical product has been registered or approved for use in a given country or regional area, that the product is cost effective and whether it can be routinely used for a given application (e.g. reasonable contact time). All these considerations are clearly important in choosing the right chemical product for various stages in device reprocessing.

Introduction to cleaning and accessory chemistries

Cleaning is the removal of contamination (or "soil") from an item to the extent necessary for its further processing and its intended subsequent use. It is usually enabled using a cleaning chemistry, in addition to physical and other process effects such as spraying, brushing, flushing, temperature control, etc. Further, detailed consideration is given to cleaning in Chapter 8. In this section a brief introduction is made to the types of chemistries that are used for cleaning, as well as different types of accessory chemicals (e.g. for lubrication or to aid in drying) that are used during reprocessing.

Patient soil

The target for cleaning is the removal of patient soil, which can be made up of a variety of components, including organic and inorganic materials from the patient or used during the procedure (e.g. gels, lubricants, cements, etc.; Table 6.7).

Classification of cleaning chemistries

Cleaning chemistries can be classified in two main ways: based on the main types of active chemicals that are present and/or how they are used during reprocessing. First and foremost, cleaning chemistries are formulations and therefore are mixtures of chemistries for their intended use. They can include main active ingredients such as enzymes, alkalis and acids, but also other components that combine together to aid in the cleaning process.

Let's first consider the classification based on how they are used. These are given generally and can often cross over, where the same product can be used for transport,

Table 6.7 Examples of various components of soil found on devices following use on/in patients.

Organic materials	Inorganic materials
Blood, mucus, feces, urine	Salts, such as NaCl
Tissues, such as those in skin, muscles, etc.	Metals, including iron
Proteins, carbohyrates, lipids/ fats, lipopolysaccharides[1]	Other elements and molecules, such as calcium and iodine
Microorganisms such as bacteria, viruses and fungi	Cements (used in orthopaedic procedures)
Gels and lubricants	

[1] A lipopolysaccharide is a molecule that includes a lipid ("lipo") and polysaccharide (carbohydrate) part.

manual or pre-cleaning and automated cleaning. They can be described as being used or designed for:
• Storage and transport: these can include liquids, foam or gel-based products that limit soil on devices from drying while being transported to a defined area for reprocessing. In addition to preventing drying, they may also inhibit the growth of bacteria and fungi, protect the device from damage (due to the presence of soil) and initiate the cleaning process.
• Pre-cleaning or manual cleaning: used directly at the point of use (e.g. at or adjacent to a surgical site) or in a defined area for reprocessing for manual cleaning, usually in a sink or basin. These are often used in ultrasonic baths to aid in the ultrasonic cleaning process (Chapter 8).
• Automated cleaning: used in a washer or washer-disinfector machine (Chapter 8) for cleaning.
• Accessory cleaning: specific chemistries used to remove certain soil components, such as acid cleaners to remove rusting or dissolve water hardness accumulation, or used for a particular accessory application such as neutralization (where some high alkaline products used for cleaning need to be neutralized back to a neutral pH, despite being drained and rinsed), lubrication (applied particularly to moving parts to allow the device to operate correctly and smoothly) and drying aids (to speed up the drying process following cleaning-disinfection).
As stated earlier, patient soil can include a variety of complex materials such as blood, various tissues, lipids/fats, proteins, etc. These can be difficult to remove by water

alone, as only some will be water soluble or immiscible ("hydrophilic", meaning water loving) while others will be water insoluble ("hydrophobic", meaning water hating). Cleaning chemistries provide different ways to aid in the removal of such soils when used in combination with the right cleaning process conditions (in particular heat and time). These include:
• Hydrolysis: the breakdown of larger molecules into smaller molecules that are easier to remove by cleaning. Hydrolysis can be achieved in some cases by heat alone, but is most effective in cleaning processes by the use of acids, bases and various types of enzymes (see the section on enyme-based cleaners).
• Solubility: the ability to be dissolved (or go into solution; see the section on mixtures, formulations and solutions). The chemical being dissolved is called the "solute" and it is being dissolved into the "solvent". Water, for example, is a great solvent for many chemicals such as salt (NaCl, the solute).
• Wetting: the ability to spread over a surface. By wetting, a cleaning product is able to contact a greater surface area and improve interaction with surfaces/materials that may be hydrophobic ("water hating"). Surfactants (see the section on mixtures, formulations and solutions) are both good wetting and emulsification agents.
• Emulsification: a substance/liquid to be dispersed (in small, fine droplets) within another liquid. This allows for soils to be mixed with water that would normally be repelled by water (such as a lipid in water emulsion). They are dispersed (suspended) not dissolved (solubilized).
• Dispersion: for one component to be mixed with another (but not dissolved). Examples include emulsions/emulsification.
• Chelation: bind elements (in particular "heavy" metals such as calcium and iron; see the section on mixtures, formulations and solutions). Such heavy metals can interfere with the cleaning process and have other negative effects on device surfaces.
Other chemicals that can be found in cleaning chemistry formulations are considered in the section on mixtures, formulations and solutions.
Cleaning chemicals can also be classified based on the types of chemistry, or indeed the main mechanisms of hydrolysis, that are used for their cleaning activity. They are:
• Enzyme-based chemistries
• Non-enzyme-based, including acid, neutral or alkaline/basic chemistries
It is important to note that these terms are not exclusive; enzymatic chemistries can range from being used at acid,

neutral or alkaline conditions. Also, a cleaning formulation can include further mixtures, where, for example, enzymes may be present as one mechanism but also a non-enzyme based hydrolysis mechanism may be in place as a separate mechanism.

Enzyme-based cleaners

In Chapter 2 (see introductory section) the four basic types of molecules that make up the structures of the variety of cells found in our bodies were discussed: proteins, lipids, carbohydrates and nucleic acids. Proteins are particularly important because they not only play an important role in the structure of cells but also the function of them. A group of proteins involved in these functions are known as "enzymes". An enzyme is a protein molecule that speeds up a chemical reaction (but is not changed in the process); they are therefore examples of being catalysts, which is any chemical that can speed up a chemical

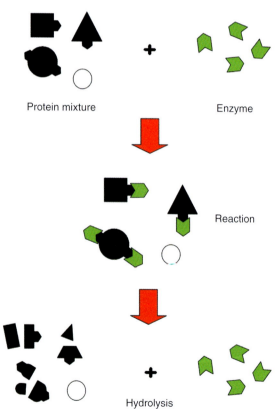

Figure 6.12 The mechanism of action of enzymes. Note: target molecules (e.g. proteins or lipids) are only broken down if they react with the enzyme and the enzyme remains unchanged after the reaction.

reaction. Enzymes are therefore often referred to as biological catalysts. They are responsible for making and breaking down various different parts of the cell over time, including the variety of proteins, lipids, carbohydrates and nucleic acids that exist. For example, when we eat food, it is the variety of enzymes (as well as chemicals) found in the digestive tract (Chapter 2) that break down the food into smaller parts that then allow the body to adsorb this into the blood system for use around the body. It is the ability of some of these enzymes to break down these molecules (that are known as "substrates") that makes them useful for cleaning purposes. A description of how enzymes work is given in Figure 6.12.

For an enzyme to act it first has to be able to recognize a target on the molecule; this target is called an active site. When the enzyme binds, it causes a breakdown in the structure of the molecule, releasing the enzyme. The enzyme remains unchanged (and can proceed to react with other molecules), while the original substrate is broken down into fragments. Some enzymes are very specific in how they work, only being effective against some types of target molecules 'substrates', while others have a wider range of activity. Generally those with a broader range of activity are used for cleaning purposes.

Enzymes are further classified depending on the types of molecules that they target. Some of the more common types are given in Table 6.8. In general, they are named by adding the suffix "–ase" to the type of substrate they attack, such as proteases refer to enzymes that attack proteins and lipases attack lipids. In the case of proteases; you are correct to notice that these enzymes are proteins themselves but break down other types of proteins! This

Table 6.8 Various types and examples of enzymes commonly used for cleaning purposes.

Enzyme type	Target substrate[1]	Example
Protease	Protein	Alcalase, savinase, properase
Carbohydrases		
Amylase	Amylose, a type of carbohydrate	α-amylase, purastar
Cellulase	Cellulose, a types of carbohydrate found in plants	Fungal cellulose, Cellusoft
Lipase	Lipids	Lipolase, Lizyme-P

[1] The "substrate" is the material that an enzyme acts on.

is due to differences in their structure. It is also important that although the enzymes such as proteases and lipases used in cleaning applications can often react with a wide range of substrates, there may be many types of proteins and lipids that are not affected by these enzymes (as shown in Figure 6.12). Enzymes are also given commercial names by companies that manufacturer them as well as official names that describe their types of enzymatic functions.

As biological catalysts, enzymes are not only specific in their mechanisms of action but their optimal activity is very dependent on how they are used, with specific variables such as:

• Contact time and enzyme concentration (or right amount/quantity of enzyme). They need to be present and the time to penetrate and react with soils to be effective.

• Temperature: enzymes are very sensitive to the effects of temperature, with each type of enzyme having an optimum range in which they work best. Lower temperatures would make them less efficient, higher temperatures stop them from working.

• Other conditions are required for them to be "active", such as the correct pH range (acid, alkaline or neutral conditions). The exact range will be specific to the type of enzyme.

Non-enzyme-based cleaners

Non-enzymatic cleaning formulations can be used on a variety of other chemical methods to remove and/or hydrolyze soils. These various components have been discussed in the section on classification of cleaning chemistries. Chemicals that hydrolyze soils when used correctly in formulation can include oxidizing agents (e.g. sodium hypochlorite, a source of chlorine, hydrogen peroxide and peracetic acid), acids, alkalis and other specific chemicals (such as urea). In general, unlike enzymes, these chemical agents are considered less specific in their mechanisms of action. Oxidizing agents are not widely used for cleaning applications in healthcare facilities but have been used successfully in some parts of the world. More commonly used chemicals are acids and alkalis/ bases. Acids and bases have been previously discussed in the section on the pH scale: defining acids and bases. Their specific applications as a cleaning mechanism are further discussed in this section.

Acid-based cleaners are considered as having a pH of <7 and can be considered as being moderately acidic (pH 4–7) or strongly acidic (pH <4). They are used for the removal (dissolution) of inorganic materials such as various types of salts. Specific examples include the removal of hardness (such as calcium carbonate, $CaCO_3$;

"descaling") or rust (ferric oxide, FeO_2) deposits that can build up or form on instrument, washer-disinfector, sink and steam sterilizer surfaces. Acid cleaners are also used as neutralizers following cleaning with some types of high alkaline cleaners, where high alkaline conditions are returned to a neutral pH before proceeding with further reprocessing.

Alkaline/basic chemistries are formulated to have pH levels of >7, ranging from being moderately alkaline (pH 7–10) to being highly alkaline (pH 10–14). They are particularly effective at removing organic materials, including proteins and lipids, from surfaces. A variety of types of alkalis can be used in these products and they work by both assisting in the removal as well as the hydrolysis of soils. In general, the higher the pH the more aggressive the product will be on surface and soil removal, but this is not always the case and will depend on the product label. Moderate and high alkaline products are widely used for manual and particularly automated cleaning processes.

Other types of chemicals are used for cleaning purposes, to aid in the physical removal of soil from a surface although without necessarily causing hydrolysis on the soil. They include various types of detergents and solvents, as examples of solubilization/dispersion/emulsification agents. Others are used to control the effects of bad quality water (such as chelating agents) that ensure the formulation is effective. As stated before, these are used in combination with or without hydrolysis chemicals in cleaning formulations.

Introduction to antimicrobial (disinfection/sterilization) chemistries

A wide variety of chemicals are used for their antimicrobial purposes. Many of these are used as drugs (or anti-infectives) to treat infections in or on patients, such as antibiotics (these are specific drugs against bacteria and some types of fungi), anti-fungal and anti-viral drugs. An even wider range of chemicals are used for antiseptic, disinfection and sterilization applications; these are commonly known as "biocides", "microbiocides" or even types of pesticides (a pest being another term to include microorganisms). They are used due to their ability to inhibit (–static activity, such as bacteriostatic and fungistatic) and/or kill (–cidal, such as bactericidal and viricidal) various types of microorganism. The science of microbiology has already been discussed in Chapter 5, and includes various types of infectious/disease-causing agents such as prions, viruses, bacteria, fungi, protozoa and helminths. This section will discuss the various types and uses of chemical biocides in microbial control.

Classification of biocides

Biocides can be classified based on their primary mechanisms of action (i.e. how they kill microorganisms), their specific chemical type and how they are used in healthcare applications. A summary of their primary mechanisms of action and chemical types are given in Table 6.9.

The basic chemical types include groups of elements known as the "halogens", with examples including chlorine and iodine, and molecules such as the aldehydes, alcohols, phenolics and peroxygens. These chemicals are rarely used on their own, but more commonly as parts of liquid, gel or foam formulated products (such as liquid disinfectants) and/or as part of defined processes (e.g. gases used for disinfection and/or sterilization such as ethylene oxide, hydrogen peroxide and formaldehyde). For most of these biocides it is unknown exactly how they work against microorganisms, but they may be considered as being generally toxic/damaging to microorganisms. Some, such as the surfactants (in particular a

Table 6.9 Examples of the basic types of chemicals (biocides) used for antimicrobial purposes. These are classified based on their major mechanisms of action against microorganisms and their chemical type.

Mechanism of action	Chemical types	Examples
Structure disruption	Surfactants	QACs[1], anionics
	Biguanides	Chlorhexidine, PHMB[2]
	Metals	Copper, silver
Oxidizing agents	Halogens	Chlorine, iodine
	Peroxygens	Peracetic acid, hydrogen peroxide, chlorine dioxide, ozone
Cross-linking/ coagulating agents	Aldehydes	Glutaraldehyde, formaldehyde, ortho-phthaldehyde (OPA)
	Alkylating agent	Ethylene oxide
	Phenolics	Phenolics, triclosan
	Alcohols	Ethanol, isopropanol

[1] QACs: quaternary ammonium compounds.
[2] PHMB: polyhexamethylbiguanides (PHMB).

group of biocides known as quaternary ammonium compounds, QACs or also known as QUATs) specifically target the cell membranes (Chapter 5) of bacteria and fungi, leading to disruption of their structure and function. Others, such as glutaraldehyde and formaldehyde, react with various proteins found on the surface of microorganism and can cause them to "cross-link", therefore losing their essential functions. These examples are simplified in that each individual type of biocide will range in its ability to inactivate microorganisms. Consider, for example, the QACs: there are many different types of QACs and other types of surfactants that are available and range in their antimicrobial activities; they are often used in combination with each other and/or with other types of biocides to give maximum antimicrobial effects. Further, the activity of a biocide on its own can be dramatically enhanced (or even the opposite, made worse!) by various different formulation effects (see the section on mixtures, formulations and solutions). This discussion highlights that the antimicrobial activity of any antiseptic, disinfectant or sterilant will not only be based on the biocide or biocides present, but on the overall activity tested with the product or process. It will also be based on how the product/process is used and controlled, as discussed in the section on how to choose and use a chemical product.

The various types of microorganisms were discussed in Chapter 5; they range in sizes, shape, surface structure, etc. As introduced in Chapter 1 (see the section on the decontamination process), microorganisms range in their resistance to inactivation by physical (e.g. with steam) or chemical means (Figure 6.13).

Further discussion of Figure 6.13 is required. First, this list is only given as an example and will vary depending on the type of biocide or biocidal process. It is generally considered that bacterial spores are the most resistant to biocides and that mycobacteria are some of the more resistant forms of vegetative bacteria (see Chapter 5, the section on bacteria). Viruses also range in biocide resistance, with the non-enveloped viruses (such as polio and parvoviruses) being highly resistant and the enveloped viruses (hepatitis B and HIV) being very sensitive to disinfection (Figure 6.13 and Chapter 5, in the section on bacteria). Second, it should not be taken for granted that if antimicrobial activity is shown for one type of microorganism (e.g. bacterial spores) that all other types of microorganisms listed under this type will be sensitive to the same disinfectant; in some cases this will be true and in others it may not. Third, this list is given as an estimate and does not reflect other factors that may affect the

	Microorganism types	Examples
More difficult to kill ↑ **Less difficult to kill**	Bacterial spores	*Geobacillus stearothermophilus, Bacillus atrophaeus, Bacillus cereus, Clostridium difficile*
	Mycobacteria	*Mycobacterium tuberculosis, Mycobacterium avium, Mycobacterium leprae, Mycobacterium chelonae*
	Non-enveloped viruses	Poliovirus, papillomavirus, parvovirus, Rhinoviruses (common cold)
	Fungi	*Trichophyton, Aspergillus, Candida albicans*
	Gram negative bacteria	*Pseudomonas, Escherichia coli, Salmonella, Acinetobacter baumannii, Klebsiella pneumoniae*
	Gram positive bacteria	*Staphylococcus aureus, Streptococcus pyogenes, Enterococcus*
	Enveloped viruses	Human immunodeficiency virus (HIV), herpes virus, hepatitis B virus, influenza virus

	Microorganism types	Examples
More difficult to kill ↑ **Less difficult to kill**	Prions	Creutzfeldt-Jacob disease (CJD), Scrapie
	<u>Dormant microorganisms</u> Bacterial spores Protozoal oocysts/cysts Helminth eggs	*Geobacillus stearothermophilus, Clostridium difficile* *Cryptosporidium, Giardia* *Ascaris, Schistosoma*
	Mycobacteria	*Mycobacterium tuberculosis, Mycobacterium avium*
	Small, Non-enveloped viruses	Poliovirus, papillomavirus, parvovirus, Rhinoviruses (common cold)
	Dormant fungi (Spores)	*Aspergillus, Penicillium*
	Helminths Protozoa	*Cryptosporidium, Giardia* *Ascaris, Schistosoma*
	<u>Fungi</u> Molds Yeasts	*Aspergillus, Penicillium* *Candida*
	Gram negative bacteria	*Pseudomonas, Escherichia coli, Acinetobacter*
	Large non-enveloped viruses	*Adenovirus*
	Gram positive bacteria	*Staphylococcus aureus, Streptococcus pyogenes*
	Enveloped viruses	Human immunodeficiency virus (HIV), influenza virus

Figure 6.13 Resistance levels of microorganisms to inactivation. Traditionally, the list of microorganisms is often given as in the upper section, but the lower section is an extended list that has been updated based on microbiology research. Note that this is only given as a guide: it will vary depending on the product/process being considered.

Table 6.10 Classification and examples of various types of biocides based on how they are used. Note: the range of biocides that can be used for each application are not exclusive, for example some antiseptics are also used for disinfection and vice versa.

Biocide application	Definition	Biocide examples
Antisepsis	Reduction or inhibition of microorganisms on the skin or mucous membranes	Alcohols, iodine, chlorhexidine, triclosan
Disinfection	Antimicrobial reduction of microorganisms	Alcohols, chlorine, hydrogen peroxide, peracetic acid, glutaraldehyde
Preservation	Prevent the multiplication of microorganisms	Acids, formaldehyde, phenolics
Sterilization	Defined process used to render an item completely free from viable microorganisms	Ethylene oxide, formaldehyde, hydrogen peroxide, ozone

resistance of any microorganism to a chemical biocide, such as the clumping of microorganisms and presence of soil/interfering substances that protect them from the biocide. These and other factors will also affect the ability of disinfectant to be effective.

Biocides may also be classified based on how they are used. In healthcare applications these are defined as antisepsis, disinfection and sterilization. A brief summary of these applications is given in Table 6.10 and these are discussed in further detail later in the final sections of this chapter.

In considering their practical use, biocides are often restricted to certain applications. For example, not all biocides could be used as antiseptics (on the skin and mucous membranes) in that they need to be effective against certain types of microorganisms (e.g. bacteria and enveloped viruses), but at the same time cause minimal damage or irritation to the skin; examples of biocides used in antiseptics include triclosan, chlorhexidine, iodine and various types of alcohols. A much wider range of biocides are used for disinfectant purposes, particularly when used on the variety of surface materials (metals, plastics, etc.). These include alcohols, aldehydes and oxidizing agents. These biocides and biocidal products will range in activity and are often sub-divided into three types: low, intermediate and high-level disinfectants (Figure 6.14).

As illustrated in Figure 6.14, low-level disinfectants are generally effective against enveloped viruses and various forms of vegetative bacteria. Intermediate-level disinfectants are effective against a wider range, including fungi, non-enveloped viruses and mycobacteria. High-level disinfectants are effective against all these microorganisms, including bacterial spores (although for sporicidal activity this may require longer contact time and/or

special exposure conditions). In all cases, these are true to their definition as disinfectants: to reduce the level of microorganisms to a safe level. Other terms, such as fumigants, pasteurizers and sanitizers are considered as disinfectants; in many countries these terms are defined for particular applications and/or to be able to kill certain types of microorganisms. In some cases following disinfection there may be no viable microorganisms present, but in other there may be; complete inactivation of all and every type of microorganism is not assured. The final, higher level of inactivation is sterilization, as the complete inactivation of all microorganisms. Sterilization provides the highest level of assurance. In practical application, sterilization can only be achieved with a limited number of biocides that have been shown to inactivate all types of disease-causing microorganisms. These include biocides, such as ethylene oxide, formaldehyde and hydrogen peroxide, all used for sterilization in gas form.

Antiseptics

Antisepsis is the reduction or inhibition of microorganisms on the skin or mucous membranes. Products used as antiseptics are known as antiseptics, but also by a variety of other terms such as hand washes, hand rubs, antimicrobial soaps, pre-operative preparations, surgical scrubs, tinctures and mouthwashes.

Hand hygiene is seen as one of the simplest yet most effective methods of reducing the transmission of microorganisms in healthcare facilities. They are sub-classified in a variety of ways to include:

• Products that are used with or without water. Examples include antimicrobial soaps that are used to wash the hands or skin with water and those that are simply applied or rubbed into and left on the hands or skin. Examples of

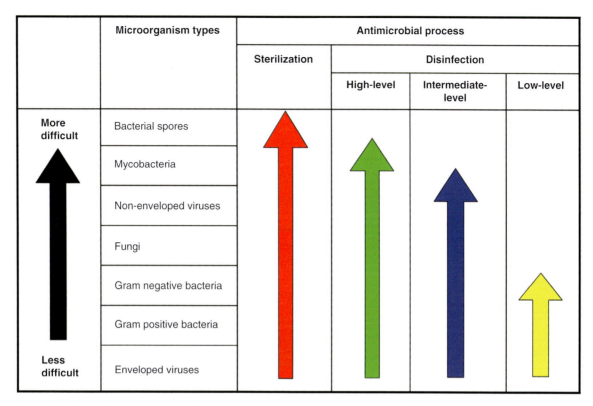

Figure 6.14 The definition of various levels of disinfectants, based on their activity against different types of microorganisms.

rub-in or leave-on antiseptics include alcohol-based gels and foams, antiseptic creams and mouthwashes.

• Products used for defined healthcare. Examples include antiseptic hand washes/hand rubs (also known as hygienic hand disinfectants and healthcare personal hand washes) for routine use in facilities, pre-operative preparations (used to disinfect the skin prior to a surgical procedure, such as antiseptics based on iodine and chlorhexidine), surgical scrubs (used to disinfect the hands of surgeons and other peri-operative personnel prior to surgery, particularly iodine and chlorhexidine- based products) and for wound treatment (e.g. iodine and hydrogen peroxide). In many countries, specific tests are required to ensure that they meet specific efficacy requirements for these particular purposes.

• Types of antimicrobial biocides that are used in the product, such as triclosan, iodine, alcohols, chlorhexidine and even combinations thereof.

A summary of the most widely used biocides in antiseptics is given in Table 6.11, but it is important to highlight that products containing these biocides can range considerably in antimicrobial activity.

In decontamination facilities we are primarily concerned with the use of hand washes or hand rubs to reduce the risk of carrying contamination out from a cleaning area (e.g. on touching a contaminated surface) or on handling instruments (recontamination) after they have been reprocessed. Good hand hygiene in these cases will particularly reduce these risks to our own and the patient's health.

In considering antiseptics, there are three important considerations: efficacy within a typical time of application, how gentle they are on the hands and that antiseptics are used correctly. The typical time taken to disinfect the hands, for example, is 5–10 seconds, with a typical time for surgical scrub being three minutes. These products should therefore be designed to provide maximum efficacy within the minimum recommended (and practical) application time. Antimicrobial hand washing products (with water) in such situations can have the added advantage of the physical removal of various microorganisms from the skin by the washing process alone, in addition to any antimicrobial effect. Irritation on the use of antiseptics is a common complaint, with the majority of healthcare workers reporting problem at some time.

Table 6.11 Major types of biocides used in antiseptic products. Note, the specific antimicrobial efficacy and any negative effects will vary from product to product[1]. Most antiseptics are considered low to intermediate level disinfectants (see section on Antiseptics).

Biocides	Antimicrobial effects[1]	Negative effects[1]	Comments
Alcohols; ethanol, isopropanol (IPA) and n-propanol	Bacteria, fungi, some viruses, mycobacteria	Can cause skin drying and irritation	Hand rubbing products. Typical recommended concentrations are at 60–80% alcohol. Products often use chemicals to prevent the alcohol from drying too quickly, therefore increasing its activity. Effects can vary depending on the alcohol used and type of fungi/virus in particular.
Chlorhexidine (CHG)	Bacteria, mycobacteria and some viruses (particularly enveloped) Inhibits fungi	Irritation has been reported	Used for skin washing and in combination with alcohols as a skin rub. Can remain on the skin following washing to give a residual activity (prevent growth of bacteria). Often used for high-risk applications such as surgical scrubs.
Iodine and iodophors	Bacteria, fungi, viruses, mycobacteria	Irritation has been reported and can cause staining	Iodine in alcohol (tinctures) is rarely used today. Iodophors (e.g. PVPI) are iodine-releasing agents that release active iodine on demand.
Triclosan	Bacteria (particular Gram positive) and some viruses (enveloped). Inhibits the growth of fungi and mycobacteria	Environmental stability	Widely used due to its low irritation but is more limited in its antimicrobial activity (product-specific).

[1] Refer to the product manufacturer regarding specific product claims on efficacy, safety and irritation.

Having a product that is rapidly effective, but at the same time non-irritating is a difficult balance given the disadvantages of the various types of biocides that can be used for antisepsis (Table 6.11). In general, if a product is, or even perceived to be, irritating it will not be used; therefore the choice of an acceptable antiseptic product to staff is an important decision to any healthcare facility. Finally, the correct antiseptic technique is important, as highlighted in Chapter 5, in the section on infection control and prevention strategies, to ensure that the product can be effective all over the surfaces of the hands.

Disinfectants, including preservatives

Disinfection is the antimicrobial reduction of microorganisms and the various levels of disinfection (high, intermediate and low) have been defined. Disinfectants are used to disinfect water, the air and various surfaces, including work areas, patient contact surface or re-usable surgical instruments. A further use of biocides is for preservation, to prevent the multiplication of microorganisms in products or even water (an example is the use of chlorine for water disinfection). Preservatives, as biocides, are widely used in products such as in liquids and other formulated products, including cleaning chemistries and antiseptics themselves. In such cases they may not, and are not intended to, inactivate microorganisms, but will prevent the growth of bacteria (bacteriostatic) and fungi (fungistatic), which are often associated with product spoilage. Examples of such biocides include a group of biocides known as the parabens, alcohols and the QACs.

There is a wide variety of biocides used for various disinfection purposes. They are also classified in a number of different ways including:

• Type of chemical biocide (e.g. aldehyde and phenolic-based).

• How they are provided for use (e.g. concentrates, liquids, solids or even gases).

• How they are used in healthcare facilities (such as device/instrument disinfection and general surface disinfection).

Some of the most widely used biocides for disinfection in healthcare facilities are summarized in Table 6.12 with

Table 6.12 Major types of biocides used in disinfectant products. Note, the specific antimicrobial efficacy and any negative effects will vary from product to product[1].

Biocides	Antimicrobial effects[1]	Negative effects[1]	Comments
Alcohols; ethanol and isopropanol (IPA)	Bacteria, fungi, some viruses, mycobacteria, some cyst forms.	Flammability risks. Can be damaging to some surfaces.	General surface and device disinfectant (usually low and intermediate level) in the 60–90% alcohol range. Fast drying, used for disinfection and drying applications. Efficacy against fungi and viruses can vary. Not effective against bacterial spores.
Aldehydes: glutaraldehyde, orthophthaldehyde (OPA) and formaldehyde	Bacteria, fungi, viruses, most mycobacteria and bacterial spores.	Difficult to rinse away residues prior to patient use. Only use in areas with correct ventilation due to toxic risks. Strong odor and irritating. OPA can cause surface staining.	Widely used for high level disinfection of flexible endoscopes and other devices. Glutaraldehyde is significantly more effective against bacterial spores than OPA. Formaldehyde is generally only used in gas form and rarely for disinfection in healthcare.
Halogens: iodine and chlorine	Bacteria, fungi, viruses, mycobacteria, bacterial spores, protozoal cysts. In some cases prions.	Can be damaging on surfaces, particularly at higher concentrations on metals. Strong odor and irritating.	Can be used for rapid low, intermediate and high-level disinfection. Chlorine (as bleach or sodium hypochlorite solutions) is widely used for environmental surface and water disinfection. Not widely used on instruments/devices.
Peroxygens: hydrogen peroxide, peracetic acid, chlorine dioxide and ozone	Bacteria, fungi, viruses, bacterial spores, protozoal cysts. In some cases prions.	Can be damaging to some surfaces. Strong odor (particularly peracetic acid) and irritating.	Used as (or in) liquids and in gas form, for various levels of disinfection and in some cases sterilization, including environmental surfaces and on re-usable devices/instruments. Gas and liquid forms can differ in activity and safety characteristics.
Phenolics: cresols, 2-phenylphenol and 2-chlorophenol	Bacteria, fungi, viruses (especially enveloped and variable against non-enveloped).	Can be damaging to some surfaces. Often strong odor. Residue can have toxic effects.	Used for low and intermediate environmental disinfection, with little to no activity against dormant forms, including bacterial spores. Can be acid, neutral or alkaline in formulation.
Quaternary ammonium compounds (QACs or QUATS): cetrimide, benzalkonium chloride and cetylpyridinium chloride	Bactericidal (particularly Gram positive bacteria and vary in activity against Gram negatives), enveloped viruses, some fungi and mycobacteria (some formulations).	In diluted products, water quality can affect activity. Can damage some surfaces.	Used for low and intermediate environmental disinfection, with little to no activity against dormant forms, including bacterial spores. Often used for combined cleaning and disinfection activity due to their surfactant nature.

[1] Refer to the product manufacturer regarding specific product claims on how they should be used, their efficacy, safety and irritation potential (see the section on How to choose and use a chemical product). Antimicrobial activity and negative effects can vary depending on how the biocide is used.

consideration of chemical type. Most of these are used in liquid form, including their direct use alone on surfaces (such as prepared concentrations of alcohols and hydrogen peroxide), but more commonly in formulation with other chemicals. These include bleach solutions (preparation of sodium hypochlorite that release chlorine, an efficient antimicrobial chemical), iodophors (that provide or "release" active iodine), phenolics, quaternary ammonium compounds, aldehydes (e.g. glutaraldehyde) and oxidizing agent-based formulations (such as those based on hydrogen peroxide, peracetic acid and chlorine dioxide). They can be provided in a variety of forms, such as concentrates or in dry form (that are diluted in water for use as recommended by the manufacturer), activated products (two components mixed to prepare the disinfectant for use), ready-to-use products (liquid disinfectants provided in spray bottles, for example, for immediate use requiring no activation or dilution) and biocide-impregnated wipes.

There are also a limited number of biocides that are used either on their own or as formulations for air/surface disinfection; these are known as fumigants (for fumigation), where the disinfectant is provided as a fog/mist or gas into a general area for disinfection. Examples of fumigants include hydrogen peroxide mists or gas/vapor, and formaldehyde gas processes. A further group of biocides are used to integrate into various surface materials, to provide "antimicrobial surfaces"; examples include the specific use of silver, triclosan and copper-containing materials.

Close attention should be paid to the instructions (label) provided with disinfection products to ensure optimal activity (including recommended dilutions and preparation methods when applicable, recommended contact times and how long they can be used for, "shelf-life") and to understand any safety risks in using the product. Some general considerations include:

• Only use disinfectants for their intended and labeled use, for example general surface disinfectant should not be used on patient instruments and vice versa.

• *All* chemical disinfectants will be negatively affected by the presence of soil, although some are considered more sensitive than others. These negative effects can include loss of activity, microbial protection (and therefore lack of activity) and fixing of patient material to surfaces.

• This will vary depending on the product formulation/process, biocide(s) being used, and the level, type and extent of soiling, as examples. As a general rule, disinfectants work better on cleaned surfaces compared to soiled surfaces, but some products are labelled to be used for combined cleaning (wiping) and disinfection.

• Always prepare and use disinfectants according to their label claims or to written instructions provided by a manufacturer. Failure to do so can lead to efficacy and safety risks. Consider, in particular, any recommended preparation method, handling procedures, exposure method and any limitations on how long they can be used (shelf-life).

• For diluted products, always use the correct and recommended dilution: higher or lower concentrated products can have more negative than positive effects.

• Never mix chemicals unless they are designed for mixing, the consequences can be quite serious including toxic gas formation and explosive risks.

• All disinfectant products can do harm to human health and all necessary precautions, in particular the use of PPE (see the section on safety considerations) and other safe handling recommendations should be used.

• If you are unsure about the efficacy and safety recommendations with a product, seek advice from someone in authority: it is better to be safe than sorry.

• In some applications, such as disinfecting instruments, it may be necessary to remove any residual disinfectant that is on or in the device prior to use on a patient. This is particularly true with the disinfection of instruments/devices (Chapter 9).

Further consideration is given to the classification of disinfectants for their specific healthcare (device) use. A useful and widely used classification is known as the Spaulding classification, named after E.H. Spaulding and developed during the 1950s–1960s. This classification is based on the risk of infection to a patient on the use (or re-use) of a device or indeed any surface. The greater the risk to a patient, the greater the level of antimicrobial activity that should be applied. The various different levels of biocidal activity have been introduced previously (summarized in Figure 6.14), being sterilization and high, intermediate and low-level disinfection. According to the Spaulding classification, they are recommended in the following situations (with examples given in Figure 6.15):

• Critical devices; these present the highest risk to a patient as they enter (or could enter) a normally "sterile" area of the body and therefore require sterilization (complete inactivation of all microorganisms). Sterile areas of the body include the bloodstream and the various internal organs (with the exception of the intestinal tract) and therefore sterilization is the standard applied to most surgical devices, be they single-use or re-usuable. Sterilization methods include steam, dry heat and chemical sterilization (Chapter 11);

• Semi-critical devices, being devices that may only contact mucous membranes or non-intact (broken) skin. Examples of such devices include laryngoscope blades, rectal speculums and some types of flexible endoscopes. At a minimum these devices should be subjected to high-level disinfection, which should eliminate most viruses, bacteria (particularly mycobacteria), fungi, and in some cases bacterial spores (although this may require long exposure times). Typical biocides widely used in high-level disinfectants include glutaraldehyde, ortho-phthaldehyde (OPA), hydrogen

Figure 6.15 Examples of typical critical, semi-critical and non-critical devices according to the Spaulding classification. It is important to note that the device classification may vary depending on its use on a patient; for example a normally non-critical device will be considered critical if for some reason it is used in a sterile area of the body (e.g. during many surgical procedures) and vice versa.

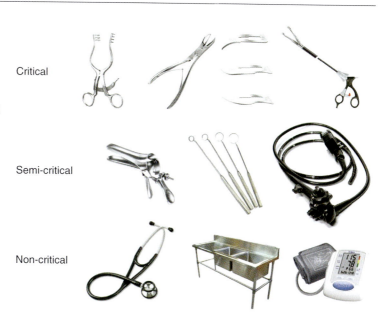

Critical

Semi-critical

Non-critical

peroxide, chlorine dioxide and peracetic acid. Note: in some countries the term "sterilant" is used and often in combination with high-level disinfectants; a sterilant should *not* be confused with sterilization. A sterilant, in these cases, should have the ability to kill all forms of microorganisms to particularly include bacterial spores and generally require longer contact times according to approved label claims. This is distinct to sterilization, being a defined and controlled process to provide sterility (see Chapters 9 and 11);

• Non-critical or low risk devices, where intact (non-broken) skin is contacted such as stethoscopes, sinks, general work surfaces, etc. It is recommended that such surfaces/devices be treated either with disinfectants that have a low or intermediate level of disinfection or even in some cases just by cleaning alone (to physically remove soil and microorganisms). Examples of biocides used in low/intermediate disinfectants are QACs, phenolics and alcohols.

Although this classification can in most cases be easily applied in a healthcare facility, it is good practice to establish and maintain a facility policy regarding disinfection-sterilization practices. This policy should be developed and maintained in close interaction with surgical, medical and particularly infection prevention/control staff. This is important not only in the classification of the various devices/instruments used in clinical practice but also in consideration of what types of disinfection-sterilization products/processes should be used in each case. A good source of information is the device manufacturer; it is good practice, and in many countries

a requirement, to provide detailed instructions on cleaning, disinfecting and (if required) sterilization of reusable devices (e.g. in conformance to ISO 17664 on information to be provided by the manufacturer for the processing of resterilizable medical devices). In some countries disinfection products require strict regulatory (governmental) approval before they are allowed to be used (e.g. in the USA by the Food and Drug Administration (FDA), for any disinfectant used on a device and by the Environmental Protection Agency (EPA), for any environmental disinfectant, and in Australia by the Therapeutic Goods Administration (TGA)); in other regions these are self-regulated by the companies that provide individual products (as in the case of the European Union). In all cases it is important that any disinfectant is chosen based on the efficacy and safety requirements of the facility (see Chapter 9).

Chemical sterilization

Unlike disinfectants, there are only a limited number of biocides used for sterilization applications. This is primarily due to the fact that the minimum criteria for sterilization is to be able to inactivate all forms of microbial life, including bacterial spores; only a limited number of biocides can be practically used for this purpose. In addition to being able to inactivate all microorganisms, chemical sterilization processes are also required to meet strict process definition requirements (such as sterility assurance levels, a concept further discussed in Chapter 11). At this time, it is sufficient to know that the ability to kill all microorganisms is only one of the starting requirements for a biocide to be used in a defined sterilization process. In addition to efficacy requirements, the other considerations of safety and compatibility should also be evaluated. In most cases, chemical sterilization is only recommended when steam sterilization cannot be used (e.g. with heat-sensitive devices or materials), but this is not in any way a rule. All systems are controlled under defined process control conditions, as required to be considered as sterilization processes. A brief summary of the major types of chemical sterilization processes is given in Table 6.13.

Table 6.13 Examples of sterilization processes using chemical biocides[1]. The exact process (times, temperatures, gas concentrations, etc.) and specific advantages/disadvantages will vary considerably depending on the product/sterilizer design. Each sterilization process/product should be considered individually (see Chapter 11).

Chemical	Typical process	Comments
Ethylene oxide (ETO or EO) Gas	Load humidified and heated (using low temperature steam[2]), gas distributed, held for an exposure time and then residual gas flushed ("aerated") from the chamber/load using pulses of low temperature steam.	Most loads require additional aeration following a cycle to ensure all gas residuals are removed. Processes are well described and the gas is very penetrating, but requires long exposure/aeration times. EO is toxic and explosive at low concentrations, requiring tight safety monitoring.
Hydrogen peroxide gas	Air/water is removed from the chamber/load under low pressure, load exposed to repeated phase of peroxide gas introduction, exposure and removal and then removed at low pressure.	Rapid cycle times, with loads ready for immediate use. Certain materials (e.g. liquids, paper) are restricted from use. Gas process is very penetrating. Peroxide gas is toxic, but has a good environmental profile.
Hydrogen peroxide gas plasma	Air is removed from the chamber/load under low pressure (sometimes with plasma generation assistance), load exposed to repeated phases of peroxide gas introduction, exposure and removal followed by plasma generation (to remove liquid/gas residues) and then aerated at low pressure (sometimes assisted by plasma generation).	Rapid cycle times, with loads ready for immediate use. Certain materials (e.g. liquids, paper) are restricted from use. Gas process can be penetrating. Peroxide gas is toxic, but has a good environmental profile.
Formaldehyde gas	Similar to EO, where load is pre-conditioned with steam (heating and humidity) and gas distribution, exposed for sterilization and then aerated using steam/low pressure pulses.	Most loads require additional aeration following a cycle to ensure gas residual removal. Processes are well described and the gas is very penetrating, but requires long exposure/aeration times. Gas is toxic and requires strict safety monitoring.
Ozone gas	Load is pre-conditioned humidity and ozone distribution, exposed to repeated phases of ozone gas introduction, exposure and removal under low pressure for sterilization and then aerated under low pressure.	Minimum chemical requirements (ozone made from oxygen and water). Cycle times are longer that peroxide but shorter than EO processes. Can be damaging to certain types of materials.
Peracetic acid liquid formulation	Devices exposed to a peracetic acid-based formulation at a specified temperature range and time, followed by water rinsing.	Rapid process. Can only be used for devices that can be immersed in water and devices should be used immediately after sterilization (no storage).

[1] There are other biocides (e.g. chlorine dioxide, other types of gas plasmas) that have been described for sterilization purposes but at the time of writing these where not commercially available.
[2] Low temperature steam is made by decreasing the pressure at which the steam is provided into the sterilization chamber; this is ruled by the gas laws and is the same concept that allows high temperature steam to be made under increased pressures.

Up to recent years, the most widely used systems were those based on ethylene oxide gas and, to a much smaller extent, formaldehyde gas. In both cases, the antimicrobial activity is optimized by ensuring that the load placed into the sterilizer is correctly humidified and heated prior to and during gas exposure. A variety and growing number of alternative chemical sterilization processes have been developed, such as those based on hydrogen peroxide gas (with or without the assistance of plasma generation), ozone gas or even liquid peracetic acid formulations (Table 6.13). These systems are described in further detail in Chapter 11.

7 Post-procedure handling, containment and transport

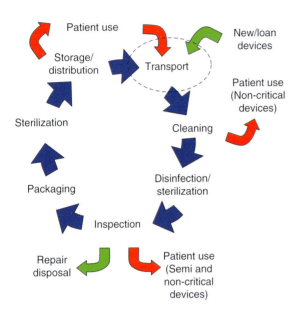

Introduction

Regardless of where a medical or surgical procedure is performed or how and where re-usable instruments are transferred for decontamination, the basic principles of reprocessing are universal. This includes the practices of cleaning, disinfection and/or sterilization. Preventing surgical and medical-related infections and cross-infections is a primary concern in any healthcare facility; this is essential in minimizing risks to staff, visitors and subsequent patients. A further concern is to ensure that these instruments are handled and transported safely, to minimize any risks of damage to them. Careful handling of medical and surgical instruments during and following a patient procedure is extremely important in prolonging the life of these instruments. Many are

obviously very sensitive to damage, such as endoscopes containing internal optics and electronics, but all instruments can be damaged by mis-handling, which can sometimes be seen and at other times may not be apparent until they are used again with another patient. All instruments should be protected from mechanical shock (being dropped, striking other instruments, etc.) and stress (bending, placed under heavier instruments, etc.). Staff should not drop or handle instruments roughly during procedures or while returning instruments to their trays at the end of a procedure. The tips of delicate and sharp medical devices should be protected at all times to avoid unnecessary damage or accidental injury to those handling them.

Therefore, the safe handling and transport of devices for decontamination following patient use is the responsibility of the staff involved with the procedure. In a surgical situation this is usually the peri-operative staff and specifically designated nursing personnel. In other situations it can be designated medical or dental staff. The first step in the cycle of decontamination is therefore preparation for and transport to a designated decontamination area. This chapter discusses the handling of instruments directly post-procedure and their subsequent safe transport. It is important to remember that many patient-used instruments can be contaminated with pathogenic microorganisms (particularly if blood or other body fluids/tissues are present), therefore such devices and associated materials should be considered as hazardous (bio-hazardous) to health. These risks, in addition to risks of injury and damage, should be considered during the post-procedure handling and any transport.

In some facilities, instruments will be handled and decontaminated by staff directly in the operating or procedure room. More often, and as recommended by most guidelines and standards worldwide, instruments are usually transported to a separate area to be reprocessed

A Practical Guide to Decontamination in Healthcare, First Edition. Gerald McDonnell and Denise Sheard.
© 2012 Gerald McDonnell and Denise Sheard. Published 2012 by Blackwell Publishing Ltd.

(often known as a "decontamination service"). These areas may be adjacent to the procedure area (e.g. a theatre sterile services unit, TSSU, or decontamination room/area), at a remote location within the hospital (e.g. a central sterile services department, CSSD) or even at a completely different facility (e.g. a "super-center" or off-site reprocessing center). In addition, pre-cleaning at or in close proximity to the procedure area will also be considered; at the time of writing there is no universally accepted recommendation regarding device pre-cleaning at the site of use, but the advantages and disadvantages of such procedures are discussed.

Post-procedure sorting

It is good practice post-procedure for all re-usable instruments to be sorted, separated and accounted for. This is important for a number of reasons:
• To ensure that all the devices are present and not mislaid during the procedure. It is not an uncommon occurence for smaller devices to remain in a patient following a procedure, with particular risks associated with surgical procedures.
• To keep the re-usable devices in designated sets for reprocessing together and subsequent re-use.
• To inspect the devices for any signs of damage, and make a note of any repair or disposal of devices for biomedical or designated decontamination staff.
• To allow a facility planning group to understand how many sets of particular devices are needed or available. This allows better control of any device inventory within a facility.
• To allow for traceability of individual devices or device sets in any case where infection control would desire to know on whom or with whom these devices have been used. This has become a particular concern and consideration in some parts of the world in the risks associated with certain types of transmissible diseases (e.g. CJD; Chapter 5, in the section on Prions and other infectious proteins and Chapter 15, in the section on Devices known or suspected to be contaminated with prion material).
Sorting is clearly a manual process and may be assisted using device checklists, not dissimilar to those used in decontamination facilities to check device sets arriving for decontamination or in preparing devices/device sets for sterilization (Chapter 10). Electronic tracking and traceability systems may also be used for this purpose, close to a surgical area or within a designated decontamination facility (further details on tracking and traceability systems are given in the section on tracking and traceability). Only trained personnel should sort contaminated items from any procedure areas.

Remember that during a procedure a variety of disposable materials, single-use devices, re-usable devices, linens/coverings and other materials (solids and liquids) may have been used (Figure 7.1). All materials and devices should be considered unsafe to handle without following standard precautions (assuming they are contaminated with infectious materials) and should be handled, collected and delivered by skilled trained staff wearing the appropriate protective clothing in accordance with relevant safety policies and procedures. It is recommended to always wash hands thoroughly after handling such used equipment – even if protective gloves have been worn during handling.

All re-usable instruments should be separated from soiled linens and disposable items at the point of use. It is considered good practice that these devices are then placed into leak-proof, puncture-resistant containers for transport, and clearly labelled as being biohazardous, to allow easy identification that the contents are contaminated. This includes all instruments, particularly within a set, whether they appear to be used or not, as they are all considered contaminated, and a possible source of microorganisms.

Particular care should be given in the handling of any sharp instruments, single use (disposable) or re-usable. As discussed in Chapter 4, in the section on Surgical instrument types and description, various types of sharp instruments are used for cutting and dissecting, including disposable needles and blades. Consideration should be given to safety and risks of sharp accidents, to the person responsible for sorting and also those subsequently involved or at risk of contact during transport and decontamination. This highlights the recommendation of using hard, puncture-resistant containers for transport. Therefore, any single-use sharps (e.g. blades and needles) should be removed and discarded on site. Care should be taken not to inadvertently discard any associated re-usable devices. In many cases, the blades or needles are single-use devices but are mounted onto re-usable holders or handles during use (e.g. "BP holders" with surgical blades). Disposable needles and blades must be removed and disposed of in appropriate puncture-resistant sharps containers at point of use, prior to transportation. It is the responsibility of the user or a designated assistant to remove all blades from re-usable handles so as not to endanger others. Examples of blade removal techniques are given in Figure 7.2.

Other general considerations on handling re-usable devices post procedure include:
• Arrange instruments to minimize any risks of damage to them or harm to staff. Instrument stacking, in particular placing heavier items on top of lighter instruments and

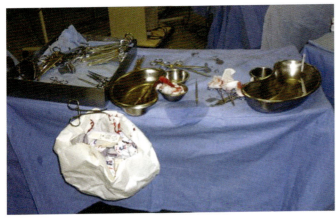

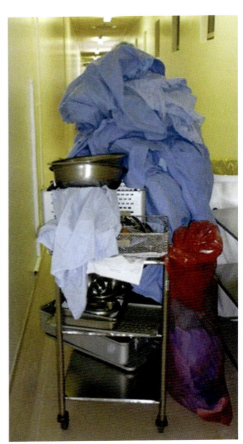

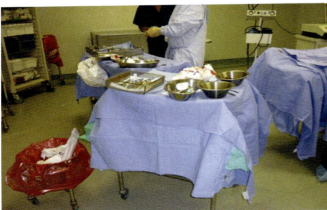

Figure 7.1 Typical range of disposal and re-usable items following a surgical procedure. The picture on the right is an unfortunate bad example of how devices and materials are not sorted or correctly transported for decontamination.

when transporting sensitive devices (such as endoscopes), should be avoided.
• Follow any manufacturers' guidelines regarding safety, disassembly and point-of-use pre-cleaning.
• Remove and dispose of any disposable parts or components.
• Remove and correctly discard any associated liquids used with the device as part of the procedure.
• Note and preferably inform any designated decontamination staff on damaged instruments requiring disposal or repair.

Re-usable linens remain widely used worldwide; they are also considered contaminated following many medical or surgical procedures. Therefore they should be treated in many ways like re-usable devices: separated, sorted and safely transported for decontamination (usually in a defined laundry facility, which may be part of or separate to a device decontamination site). Re-usable instruments

should *never* be washed with laundry items. Chemicals and processes used in laundry reprocessing may not be suitable for devices. Instruments that may become hidden in soiled linen can also injure unsuspecting laundry workers, may be inadvertently discarded as waste and may also cause damage to the linens.

Any single-use devices, liquids and materials (such as disposable drapes and linens) should be separately disposed of according to established policies at or near to the site of use. These are usually discarded directly into hazardous waste-bins or liquid-waste disposal containers (if known to be contaminated) and collected for incineration or other similar safe disposal policy. Particular consideration should be given to sharp materials.

Special consideration should also be given to the safe disposal or transport of materials (including devices) that have been used with radioactive or cytotoxic chemicals. Radioactive chemicals are often used for medical

(A)

(B)

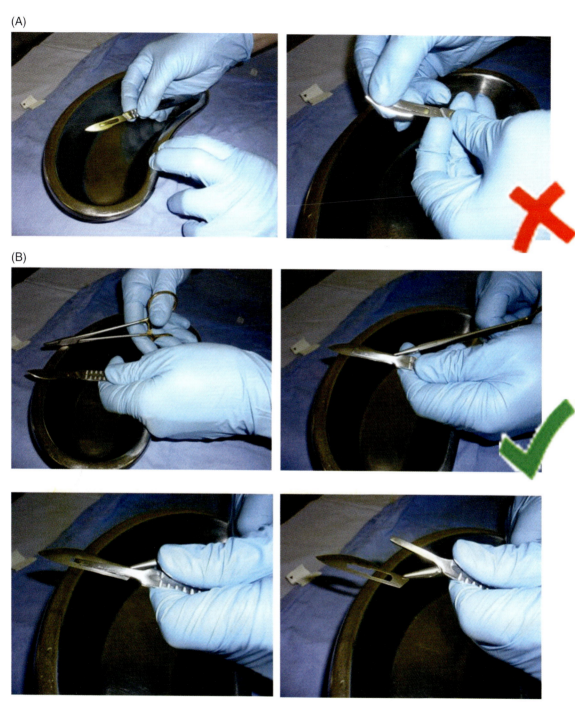

Figure 7.2 Correct disassembly and handling of single use blades from re-usable BP handles. (A) Do not remove the blades by hand. (B) Staff should be trained on the correct removal methods. An example is shown using a needle holder (other instruments or tools may also be safely used). Slide the blade up and away from the handle body allowing it to drop into a container and discard the blade according to facility sharp procedures.

procedures (nuclear medicine; Chapter 6, see the section on light, radiation and the electromagnetic spectrum). Examples include the use of radioactive isotopes for medical imaging and for cancer radiotherapy (see Chapter 3). Widely used radioactive chemicals ("isotopes") are technetium (99m), iodine (123 and 131) and thallium (201). Cytotoxic chemicals (or drugs) are chemicals used for medical purposes for the treatment of various conditions such as autoimmune diseases (e.g. arthritis) and cancer ("chemotherapy"); cytotoxic ("cell-toxic") refers to their ability to control the growth of or kill cells. Examples of cytotoxic drugs used for cancer chemotherapy include cisplatin, cyclophosphamide, doxorubicin and vincristine. Some of these chemicals are short-lived (degrading safely, naturally and quickly, e.g. over a few hours), while others are not. In both cases, special handling procedures may be required. In such situations, a facility policy should be in place to ensure that any wastes or reprocessing are handled safely to reduce any risks to staff or subsequent patients.

Other associated and fixed surfaces in the operating or procedure room area, particularly around the immediate patient-handling area (such as the surgical table, lights and trolleys), may have also become contaminated with blood or other tissues and materials during the procedure. In many cases these surfaces may be protected during a procedure with various protective coverings (e.g. operating room light handles and general surface coverings). These coverings should be routinely changed and discarded between patients. It is good practice for general surfaces, in particular those that have not been otherwise covered or may have become soiled, to be wiped down with a disinfectant between patient procedures. It is also common practice for certain procedure areas, including operating rooms and particularly frequently touched surfaces, to be wiped down with an appropriate disinfectant at the end of a working day; in certain circumstances, these areas may also be subjected to "deep" cleaning (including the use of disinfectants and/or fumigants, Chapter 9, in the section on Chemical Disinfectants).

Point of use cleaning

Following a procedure, instruments and equipment may be contaminated with a variety of materials such as blood, serum, skin, tissue debris, microorganisms, cements, saline, etc. These materials can pose health and safety risks, such as:
• Risks of infection and cross-contamination.
• Damage to instrument surfaces (e.g. salts can attack the surface of stainless steel to promote rusting).

• Damage to instrument operation (e.g. internal lumens or hinge joints may become blocked from soil drying/coagulation).
• Difficulty in subsequent cleaning, if the soil on instruments is allowed to dry.
It therefore makes practical sense that some pre-cleaning or pre-treatment of soiled devices is conducted at the site of medical/surgical use in order to minimize these risks (Figure 7.3). In some cases, point-of-use cleaning is specified by the device manufacturer as an essential step in reprocessing. The advantages and disadvantages of this practice are discussed further in the next section.

"Wet" and "dry" handling of instruments post-procedure

Traditionally, there have been essentially two recommendations regarding the safe handling of instruments post-patient procedure: these can be categorized as being "wet" vs "dry". Examples are shown in Figure 7.4.

In one case "dry" instruments are allowed to dry following use in a patient procedure and are transported to an area for safe handling under dry conditions. In the other case "wet" instruments are either cleaned (or at least rinsed) at the point of use to remove any visual soil prior to transporting to another area for further reprocessing or transported under wet or moist conditions to prevent instruments from drying prior to reprocessing. There are advantages and disadvantages of both recommendations. When soil on instruments is allowed to dry, this can reduce the risk of the multiplication of certain types of microorganisms (bacteria and fungi), but the soils (including proteins, lipids, etc.) can be subsequently difficult to remove and can damage the instrument functionally and structurally. If the soiling on instruments is maintained wet, the instruments will be less difficult to clean (and therefore decontaminate) and may not be damaged (if transported carefully); but equally, bacteria/fungi may be allowed to multiply (in particular on devices stored for extended periods before reprocessing), there may be increased costs in time/materials and spills/splashes of potentially infection material may occur on transport. As a compromise, some guidelines have recommended that visual soil should be removed at the point of use (by rinsing in water or by cleaning within close proximity to the patient procedure area). Whichever the procedure that is adopted by a facility, it is important to consider three basic concerns: safety of the instruments, safety of the subsequent patient and safety of those handling the devices. Any of these procedures can be used if these risks are carefully considered in any facility policy.

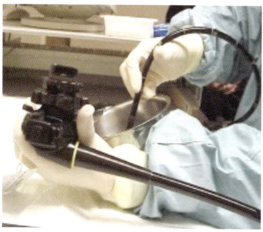
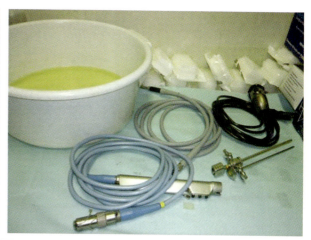
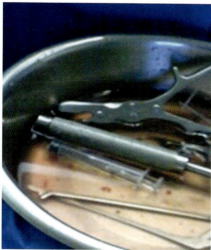
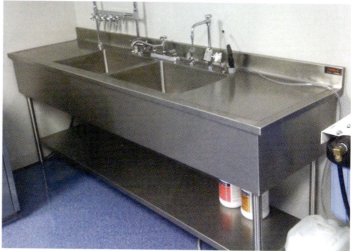

Figure 7.3 Examples of point-of-use pre-cleaning. At the top, a bedside procedure with a flexible endoscope (left, suctioning a cleaning solution through the internal lumens of the device) and a manual pre-cleaning set-up with a rigid endoscope set (right). Bottom, pre-cleaning a set of surgical instruments (left) and a pre-cleaning sink in an adjacent area/room (right).

Guidelines on point of use cleaning and/or preparation for transport

Point of use cleaning (pre-cleaning)

Contaminated instruments should be handled as little as possible at the point of use as staff are most at risk of infectious hazards when handling and separating contaminated instruments. Instruments are generally kept free of gross soil during a procedure to allow for their practical use (particularly in surgical procedures) and the decontamination process should begin as soon as possible following use. By removing gross soil at the point of use the efficiency and effectiveness of decontamination will be improved.

It is recommended that post-procedure cleaning is conducted at a separate, distinct site from, and preferably in an adjacent room to, the patient procedure area. A variety of cleaning chemistries or even water alone can be used, ensuring that they are prepared and maintained according to manufacturers' instructions; examples including enzymatic and non-enzymatic cleaning formulations. In some countries, cleaning chemistries that include some disinfection efficacy are also recommended; these are proposed to be used to reduce microbial (particularly bacteria and enveloped viruses) contamination and therefore personnel handling risks. With any products used, close attention to any labelling

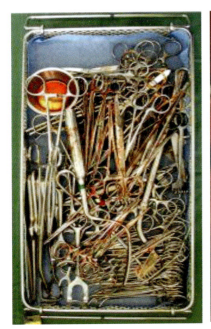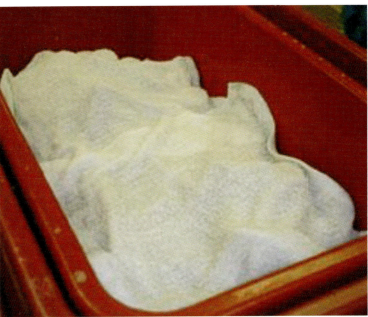

Figure 7.4 Examples of "wet" and "dry" procedures at the point of use prior to transport. On the left, a set of devices transported as soiled during a surgical procedure ("dry") and on the right an example of a "wet" transport procedure where the devices are maintained "wet" under a pre-moistened towel.

or other instructions is provided with the product to ensure that it is used optimally and safely (e.g. dilution, temperature, time, etc.). It is recommended that cleaning (or indeed any decontamination product) formulations are used that have been designed for use on medical or surgical instruments. Saline (note: saline is water with added salts, for patient use not for devices!), hand soaps, or surgical hand scrubs (such as iodine or chlorhexidine-containing products) should not be used to clean or immerse instruments because these chemicals may damage instruments, are not labeled or designed for such use or may cause other patient complications.

Cleaning formulations are recommended to be used as they will aid in the removal of various types of soils (Chapter 6, see the section on Classification of Cleaning Chemistries). Fresh water alone may be used, but should not be re-used; consideration should be given to the recommendations on the use of water and requirements for water quality (Chapter 15, see the section on Water quality and purity). Instruments should be immersed and can be cleaned with a variety of cleaning aids, such as sponges, cloths and brushes. It should be noted that abrasive materials and products (e.g. scouring pads) should not be used, as these can damage instruments. There are certain

types of soils (e.g. cements) that can be difficult to remove when dried; these should be removed prior to drying (or setting) if at all possible as they can only be subsequently removed by abrasive methods. For certain types of devices, pre-cleaning is recommended by the device manufacturers. An example is in the use of flexible endoscopes, where a bedside procedure is recommended. During this procedure, water or a cleaning formulation solution is flushed through the major channels of the device at the point of patient use of the device and prior to subsequent manual or automated cleaning (reprocessing of flexible endoscopes is considered in further detail in Chapter 8, see the section on Endoscopy).

Transport under dry conditions

If this procedure is adopted within a facility (in the absence of any pre-cleaning), it may be expected that damage to instruments will be observed over time and that cleaning requirements should be particularly rigorous at a remote area. Soil dried on the surface can cause damage to surfaces both structurally and functionally. These effects can be particularly rapid if devices are left in such a state for extended periods of time. For example, various types of patient soil can include salts that will attack the material surfaces of devices, particularly stainless steel, copper and brass. These effects can include premature rusting (see Chapters 6 and 15) and other corrosion effects that will limit the practical use of the device. These effects may be obvious or hidden, potentially causing a device to fail in operation during a subsequent patient procedure. Physical effects can include clogging of the device at various working parts or internal lumens. Consideration should be given to the recommendations on transport of instrumentation, as described in the following sections. Although transport of devices may limit the growth of microbial pathogens such as bacteria and fungi, many of microorganisms will be protected from these effects by the presence of soil components and will therefore continue to pose an infection or cross-contamination risk to those handling these devices. It is important to consider that just because an instrument is dry or may appear dry does it does not mean that it is safe for handling, and all standard precautions should be considered to reduce any risks to those handling these devices.

Transport under wet conditions

Transport under wet conditions can include a variety of procedures, such as the use of water, wet towels, sealed containers, use of chemicals (such as cleaning chemicals) or various types of products that have been designed for such purposes. In considering these practices, it is recommended that procedures are adopted that limit any handling risks, such as spillages and the overgrowth of microorganisms. Some bacteria can rapidly multiply, within 20–30 minutes, thereby creating a greater health risk to staff. It is therefore recommended that products that inhibit the growth of or even reduce the levels of microorganisms should be considered in these cases.

Examples of products used for safe transport include water, cleaning formulations, and various types of foam and gel-based products (see Figure 7.5). The optimum products should include the following features:
• Allow the instruments to be directly observed, in case any sharps are present. This will reduce any risks to those subsequently handling these devices.
• Prevent the drying of soil on instrument surfaces; note that any internal instrument lumens or channels will not readily dry out on transport due to the lack of air passage across these internal surfaces, therefore it is not necessary or practical to ensure that such surfaces are fully contacted with applicable products.

• Provide bacteriostatic and fungistatic activity (i.e. preventing the growth of bacteria and fungi respectively), although some products may provide different levels of bactericidal and fungicidal (i.e. killing these respective microorganisms) effects.
• Initiate the cleaning process during transport and prevent drying during elongated storage/transport times.
• Protect the devices from any damage on elongated storage/transport times.
• Should not inhibit any subsequent reprocessing steps (cleaning, disinfection and/or sterilization) or causing toxic risks to a following patient.
• Minimize any potential spillage risks that may give a risk to those handling the instruments or others on transport to another reprocessing area.

Transportation post-procedure

Contaminated items (single use or re-usable) should be contained post-procedure for transporting to a defined reprocessing area; containment during transport reduces the exposure of staff to contaminated materials. The removal of contaminated items from the procedure area should be performed safely and carefully to minimize exposure. It is considered good practice that the next patient procedure should not commence until all contaminated items are safely sorted, removed or discarded.

Materials for transport away from a patient procedure area can include re-usable instruments, re-usable materials (e.g. linens), and contaminated items for safe disposal (sharps, single-use devices, etc.) and, potentially, items to be discarded as non-clinical, normal waste. Procedures should be in place for how all these materials are transported. Materials requiring decontamination for re-use are our primary concern in this chapter.

As stated previously, re-usable devices should be placed into leak-proof, puncture-resistant containers for transport, and clearly labelled as being biohazardous to allow easy identification that the contents are contaminated (Figure 7.6).

Procedures should be in place to prevent contaminated devices requiring reprocessing from being accidentally mixed with decontaminated and single use devices being prepared for use in another procedure. Particular attention should be paid to the workflow within these areas, to prevent this from occurring (for discussion on the principles of separation of "clean" and "dirty" areas see Chapter 1, in the section on The design of a decontamination area).

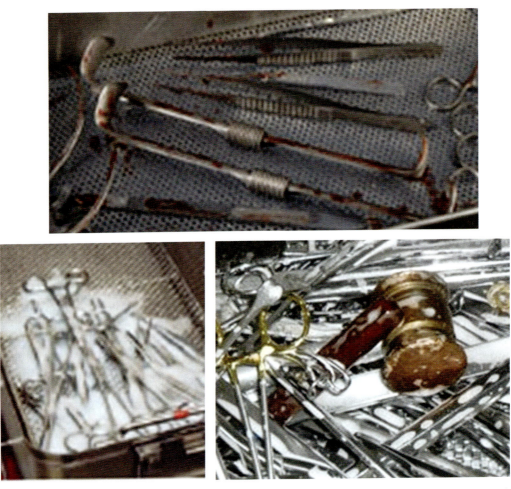

Figure 7.5 Examples of pre-cleaning and safe-transport products, as used on surgical instruments. A transparent gel (top), a foam (bottom left) and a liquid cleaning formulation (bottom right).

Contaminated devices can include those that have been used directly with a patient and those that may have been indirectly contaminated during handling, such as cart/trolleys, containers, etc. It is typical in surgical practices that a set of instruments is provided within a tray (in which they have been previously cleaned and sterilized) and the soiled set after a procedure is returned to the same tray. Similarly, transport systems such as trolleys may be used to transport clean instruments to a surgical area and then return them to a decontamination area/facility. These transport systems will also require routine reprocessing , either manually or in automated washer-disinfectors (see the section on Care of trolleys and containers).

Soiled instruments should ideally be transported, in closed trolleys, to a decontamination area for reprocessing as soon as possible after the procedure has been completed. If closed trolleys are not available, open trolleys/carts may be used but should be adequately covered (e.g. using unsoiled towels, wraps or other materials) to provide a degree of protection. In some cases, where the patient procedure room is in close proximity to the decontamination area, devices may carried directly by hand, keeping trays parallel with the floor (in order to avoid shifting of the instruments) and ensuring that soils or soiled materials are not allowed to spill or be dropped on transport. Even in such cases, it is still best practice to place the devices in

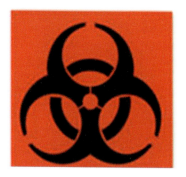

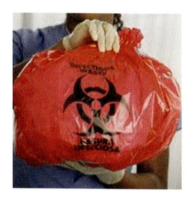
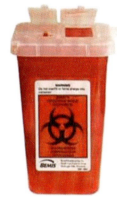
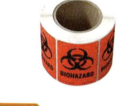
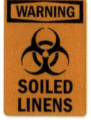
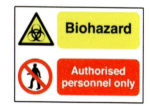

Figure 7.6 The internationally recognized symbol (top) for a biological- or "bio" hazard (may be presented in different colours, typically orange, red and yellow). Below are examples of a clinical waste bag and sharps container, with various examples of biohazard labels shown on the right.

a leak-proof and covered container. Such containers should not be overloaded, to avoid the risk of instrument damage and ensure that they are not too heavy for lifting (leading to risks of lifting/carrying-related strains and accidents).

Similar transport systems and procedure should be in place for any contaminated and re-usable linens, as well as for the transport of disposable, contaminated waste (to prevent accidental spillage, etc.).

Transportation systems

A variety of transport systems may be used to transfer contaminated instruments and instrument sets to a reprocessing area (Figure 7.7).

An instrument set may be comprised of an individual device needed for a simple or unique task, a tray of devices used for a specific procedure or a specialty set of multiple trays of instruments. A tray of instruments can range

from a few handheld devices to over a hundred different items. Therefore, there are various types of container systems that can be used, based on the facility needs.

Items may be transported manually by carrying the used instrument containers directly to a designated area or by using a designated transport system such as manual or motorized trolleys. Trolleys serve an important function in reducing the risk of injury to staff due to carrying an instrument tray (some of which can be heavy) from one point to another. Contaminated items should always be completely separated from clean/sterile items during transportation. It is important that a system is put into place to ensure that there is a distinction between soiled and reprocessed (clean/sterile) instruments, in order to ensure that soiled instruments are not mistakenly used on patients. The concept of clean and dirty separation (Chapter 1, see the section on Design of a decontamination area) does not only apply to the instruments

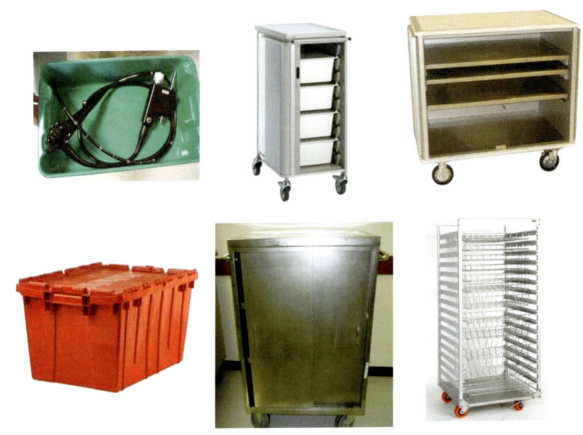

Figure 7.7 Examples of various types of transport systems. Shown are examples of open and closed container systems (left) and trolley systems.

themselves but also the transport aids such as containers and trolleys. Sterile or otherwise decontaminated items, in particular for critical and semi-critical procedures, should be transported in separate closed containers in clean dry conditions in a way that will not compromise their disinfected/sterilized state and provide a mechanical protection to prevent damage to the items or any associated packaging. Sterile packs, for example, should ideally be transported in closed solid walled containers, covered or enclosed trolleys with solid-bottom shelves.

A two-container or two-trolley clean and dirty system is always preferable, but not essential if effective safeguards are in place and monitored to prevent mix-ups. Similarly "open" trolley systems can be effectively used, where systems are in place to prevent mixing of dirty and clean instruments/materials, and the risk of public exposure to contaminated items is considered low (e.g. in a

staff-access only surgical facility with a defined, internal decontamination facility). Closed transport cart/trolleys should always be used for transporting of contaminated items between healthcare areas via other departments or for external transport.

Container and containment systems

There are various types of open and closed container systems available, these include trays, trolleys, impermeable bags, lidded bins and rigid container systems (Figure 7.7). Transport containers should protect both equipment and the handler from accidental contact during transit. Soiled items should be preferably placed into closed leak/splash proof containers. Remember, all patient soiled items (especially containing blood) should be considered biohazardous and correctly tagged or labeled as such, according to policy, as infectious. The ideal container/containment system should be:

• Easy to clean and disinfect, either manually or in an automated washer-disinfector.
• Specifically designed for transport of contaminated (and also disinfected/sterilized) items where greater protection than normal dust protection is required.
• Stable to prevent spilling or items from falling over or off any cart/trolley during transport.
• Closed to prevent contact with other healthcare personnel and patients in public areas leading to (or away from) any re-processing area.
• Covered, sealed and leak-proof to minimize contamination and soiling of any transport vehicle/person due to leakage of contaminated fluids.
• Carefully packed with lighter instruments on top of heavier instruments and to protect sharps and delicate devices from damage.

Specially colored, marked or labeled containers should be used for transporting soiled items. Red is usually the color of choice as it universally signals danger. Consideration should be given to any national, regional, local and/or facility regulations regarding the handling and transportation of biohazardous materials. These may be different within and between facilities.

Transport trolleys

In some cases, trolleys can be used as aids to transport instruments and materials to a defined reprocessing area. Distances between procedure and reprocessing areas can often be long and over multiple floors within larger institutions, restricting safe and practical transport. A variety of trolley systems can be used to aid in the transport of instrument sets from one area to another (Figure 7.7). They can generally be considered as being open or closed in design. They also range from being simple push-type trolleys, motorized trolleys and sophisticated, automated transport systems for a variety of supplies/materials around a facility.

Transport trolleys used for distribution of disinfected/sterilized items to users or for returning contaminated items from various sources within a facility to a processing area should be designed for handling and transporting items safely. All transport trolleys (motorized or manual) should be constructed from a material that allows for proper cleaning, this is particularly important if the trolley is transporting alternating decontaminated and contaminated items.

In order to avoid cross-contamination contaminated items should, where possible, be transported to a reprocessing area in a covered enclosed trolley/cart with a solid bottom shelf to prevent contamination of the floor from the trolley during transport. Preferably, items should be transported via a dedicated passage and/or lift that opens directly into or close to the reprocessing area. It is generally recommended that contaminated items are not transported through patient or general public areas; particular care should be taken in these cases to provide container and trolley system procedures that minimize any safety risks.

Only trained personnel wearing personnel protective equipment (PPE; Chapter 13), which includes at least protective gloves, should be involved with transporting. If potentially dealing with fluids where splashing could occur, safety goggles/visors and a facemask are also recommended. Particular care must be taken to prevent accidents whilst transporting; by either pulling or pushing the trolley, it is important to have a clear path of view in front and on either side of the trolley. For uncovered trolleys, it is better practice to transport by pulling so as to reduce the risk of contaminant/chemical exposure.

The trolley design should be stable and easy to maneuver with a combination of fixed and swivel wheels and ball bearings to maximize maneuverability. They should ideally have a handle to allow for easier and safer handling in narrow passages. For longer distance transport between areas, closed, lockable door trolleys are recommended. The trolley must be large enough for the amount of equipment being transported, but not too large to be difficult to maneuver. Items/containers should be placed securely in a flat position and should not extend beyond the edge of the any shelf or outside the trolley in any way. For the greatest flexibility, trolleys with adjustable-height shelves or a number of shelves may be considered. The trolley must at no stage be left unattended in an unsecured location.

External/road transport

When using off-site or outsourced reprocessing facilities particular care must be taken regarding the containment of contaminated items. Transport vehicles should be completely enclosed and allow for ease of loading and unloading. As in the case of every transport system, soiled items should be adequately separated from disinfected/sterilized items. For example, condensate may occur on plastic or metal surfaces that have been moved from an air-conditioned to non-conditioned environment. Extremes of temperature and humidity may also be a consideration (e.g. freezing).

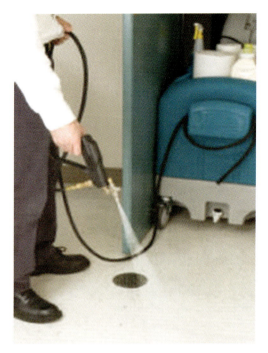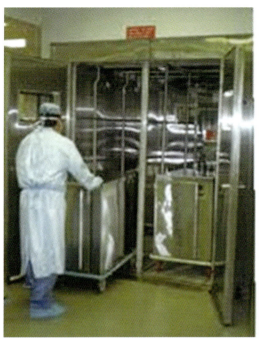

Figure 7.8 Examples of manual (left) and automated (right) systems for reprocessing trolleys and containers. The automated systems shown are commonly referred to as cart-washer or cart-washer-disinfectors.

As contaminated items are considered to be biohazardous, transport of such materials may be closely regulated by local, regional and national agencies. At a minimum, such items should be clearly marked as biohazardous and adequately contained (i.e. secure, tamper proof, leak-proof, sealed, rigid containers, trolleys or carts). Containers and trolleys/carts should be preferably locked and secured into position to prevent movement during transit. Transport vehicles should be designed to be routinely cleaned/disinfected on a regular basis.

General good practice dictates that personnel dealing with contaminated items are trained on how to handle items safely, including use of PPE and how to handle accidents such as spills (e.g. location and use of a biohazard spill kit).

Care of trolleys and containers

Trolleys and containers are recommended to be routinely decontaminated and preferably after each use. These are considered as non-critical items, but as they are potentially contaminated with biohazardous materials, they may need to be subjected to the same essential processes as those used to clean any other contaminated

medical devices. This is particularly important to protect staff and to prevent cross-contamination in situations where these same trolleys/containers are used to transport sterile or disinfected goods. This can be achieved manually or in automated cart/container systems (Figure 7.8); recommendations regarding the reprocessing and maintenance of hospital-designed trolleys/containers should be provided by their manufacturers.

In addition to reprocessing instructions, cart/trolley manufacturers' instructions should be provided and consulted regarding maintenance, such as lubrication of any hinge joints and wheel castors. Removal of debris and materials from trolley wheels will prevent jamming and difficulty with maneuvering over time. It is recommended that a maintenance schedule should be in place for washing and maintaining trolleys.

During the design of decontamination facilities, it is important to consider the use and reprocessing of containers, carts and trolleys. Designated unloading, reprocessing, cart storage and reloading areas are important to design into the workflow of these areas, not just the medical and surgical instruments themselves.

Manual reprocessing of transport systems

At a minimum, containers and various parts of the trolley (particularly shelving) should be wiped down with a hospital-grade disinfectant (to aid in cleaning and low-level disinfection) between each use. Typical disinfectants that can be used include at least low or intermediate-level disinfectants that are labeled for cleaning and disinfection (Chapter 9). Chlorine (or other halogen) based disinfectants (e.g. "bleach" or sodium hypochlorite solutions) are generally not recommended as they may lead to rusting and damage to carts/trolleys. More detailed and thorough cleaning of the inside and outside of the entire trolley is necessary periodically as blood and body fluids can seep into joints, seams, and under surfaces of shelving and doors. Procedures should be put in place to ensure workflow and/or physical separation of dirty and cleaned carts, trolleys and containers to avoid mix-ups.

To aid with trolley/cart manual cleaning, a wet-working area should be designated within the decontamination area. This can be equipped with a pressure washing system (spray gun) to allow for manual cleaning. These areas should be equipped with hot and cold water, and preferably with a spray gun allowing for automatic mixing of a cleaning chemistry/detergent with water and for water rinsing. A typical cycle will include washing (with detergent), rinsing and drying. Washed carts should be dried (generally manually) with lint-free cloths and may be aided by the use of 70% alcohol (assists in drying and provides a low level of disinfection).

Automated reprocessing of transport systems

It is preferable, in particular for medium or larger decontamination facilities, for automated systems to be use for reprocessing of transport systems. These include instrument washer-disinfectors and specifically designated cart-washers.

For instrument washer-disinfectors, specific cycles are usually defined to provide cleaning, rinsing and low to intermediate-level disinfection of containers by hot water (thermal disinfection); container systems may also be specifically designed to hold the medical/surgical instruments during cleaning-disinfection/sterilization and are therefore reprocessed in the same cycles as those instruments. The use of specific, shorter cycles is often preferred to maximize capacity for the use of the washer-disinfectors and efficiency of a reprocessing area.

Cart-washers (also referred to as cart-washer-disinfectors, cart "sanitizers", etc.) are larger sized washer-disinfectors for the reprocessing of carts and trolleys (Figure 7.8). These can also be used in combination for the reprocessing of containers and other non-critical items at the reprocessing facility (such as footwear, wheelchairs, etc.). A variety of reprocessing cycles can be defined in these washers in order to reduce time, energy and water consumption. For example, rinse water collected from one stage of a cycle may be collected and re-used for a subsequent stage of another cycle. A typical cycle includes pre-cleaning with water (to remove gross soil), cleaning with a detergent formulation, rinsing, disinfection (thermal or chemical), rinsing (if applicable) and drying. Thermal disinfection is the most common method, with a typical recommended cycle at 80°C for one minute, or equivalent (e.g. in accordance with ISO 15883, Washer-Disinfectors Parts 1 and Parts 6; Chapter 9, Automated cleaning); specific cycles range widely depending on the region or area in use and local requirements.

Tracking and traceability

Tracking and traceability should be considered an integral part of the reprocessing process. *Traceability* is the ability to verify the history, location, or application of an item by means of a documented recorded identification system. Traceability can only be achieved if the items are uniquely identified and relevant data about items is captured and recorded. This can be traditionally achieved manually by a paper-based system, but is increasingly being replaced by computer-based systems, including unique identifying codes provided on individual devices and with sets of devices. Today, most individual devices are not provided with unique identification codes and most tracking systems are used to track sets of surgical devices; this will change over time, with greater availability of tracking abilities with individual instruments.

A traceability or tracking system should be in place (in particular for medium to larger institutions) that records the progress of individual instruments or sets, through each stage of the reprocessing cycle (including clinical use and transport) and allow a retrospective reconstruction of the history of that set, including the patients on whom it was used. Tracking records that permit the verification that a set or re-usable devices have been through an approved reprocessing cycle (cleaning, disinfection and/ or sterilization) should be maintained; this can include details of each set, batch or load, date, cycle reference numbers, etc., which in the event of a recall or adverse patient incident would allow the devices to be investigated.

The tracking system may also be used to enable the identification of patients on whom the device/sets have been used as it is important that the relevant patients can be identified in the event of exposure to any potential health risk. It may also be used to control inventory, to understand the availability of devices and device sets for particular (especially surgical and endoscopic) procedures.

For an efficient system, the first requirement is to uniquely identify the items to be tracked by an identification system (manual or automated, e.g. manually recording a number/code or by bar coding). This can be done by either tracking the individual items or more commonly a set of devices. In computerized systems, such item identification can then be communicated to other members of the reprocessing and supply chain cycle. In some countries, it is recommended that devices within a set used in a patient procedure should remain, be tracked and reprocessed together; individual devices should not in this case be allowed to move from one set to another. In such cases, individual device tracking systems may be necessary. As most devices today are not provided with unique identification codes, facilities often consider and provide on-site marking and identification methods.

It is important, following transport from a site of surgical/medical use to a reprocessing area, that the instruments and all associated accessories (particularly parts associated with the devices that are re-used) have been received and accounted for. If items or parts are missing they will need to be located or replaced.

A more detailed discussion of tracking and traceability in device reprocessing is considered in Chapter 14 in the section on tracking and traceability.

8 Cleaning

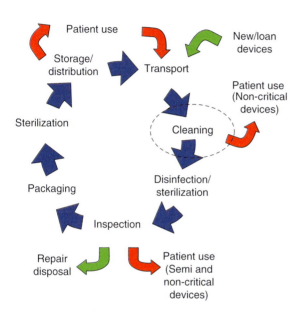

Introduction

Cleaning is the removal of contamination (or "soil") from an item to the extent necessary for its further processing and its intended subsequent use. The target for cleaning is the removal of patient and other soils, which can be made up of a variety of components, including organic and inorganic materials from the patient or used during the procedure (e.g. gels, lubricants, cements, etc., Table 8.1).

Cleaning may be the only required step in the reprocessing cycle to allow a device to be used (as in the case of some non-critical devices, for example; Chapter 1, in the section on Goals of Decontamination and the Spauldings Classification). For all re-usable instruments, cleaning is an essential prerequisite to ensure effective disinfection and/or sterilization as part of the decontamination cycle. The presence of organic and inorganic materials on devices can inhibit the contact with the surfaces of the device, of any disinfection or sterilization product or process which targets microbial cells, reducing their activity and effectiveness. The presence of soil can also lead to adverse reactions in patients, such as toxicity and immune reactions, as well as damage to device functioning. It is also a prerequisite for staff working in the decontamination facility to protect themselves from any contact with contamination when assembling and checking items in the cleaning area. Cleaning, therefore, should always be the first and is often considered the most important step in the reprocessing cycle.

Cleaning is a process that should produce an end result; unfortunately the result is subjective and not always easy to measure. The term "clean", in relation to medical/surgical device reprocessing, is not scientifically defined (to date) and is a relative concept that is difficult to define and measure. Clean may be loosely defined as being; "visibly free from dirt, stains, or impurities", a very subjective definition. In most healthcare situations, cleaning is currently considered adequate if the surface or device is visibly clean. This, however, is under debate. To the naked eye a device may appear soiled and then clean following a cleaning process; but if parts of the device are further magnified or tested in a laboratory for the presence of residual soil it may be present. It is also important to note that the presence of such low levels of soil may or may not have any patient risk or affect any subsequent disinfection/sterilization step. "Clean" may therefore have a visible, biochemical, chemical or even microbiological endpoint, but this remains to be internationally defined. Certain countries have defined requirements for testing and ensuring the efficacy of cleaning, by recommending defined test soils used to challenge a cleaning process and recommended endpoints (visibly clean and levels of protein below a

A Practical Guide to Decontamination in Healthcare, First Edition. Gerald McDonnell and Denise Sheard.
© 2012 Gerald McDonnell and Denise Sheard. Published 2012 by Blackwell Publishing Ltd.

Table 8.1 Examples of various components of soil found on devices following use on/in patients.

Organic materials	Inorganic materials
Blood, mucus, feces, urine	Salts, such as NaCl
Tissues, such as those in skin, muscles, bone, etc.	Metals, including iron
Proteins, carbohyrates, lipids/fats, lipopolysaccharides*	Other elements and molecules, such as calcium and iodine
Microorganisms such as bacteria, viruses and fungi	Cements (used in orthopedic procedures)
Gels and lubricants	Chemicals used on the skin or directly on the device pre-operatively or post-operatively

*A lipopolysacchaide is a molecule that includes a lipid ("lipo") and polysaccharide (carbohydrate) part.

defined level). It should also be understood that some body fluids may not be visible to the naked eye, including tears, pericardial fluid, synovial fluid, cerebrospinal fluid, etc.

The objective of the cleaning process is not only to safely clean the device or surface for further reprocessing and/or patient use, but at the same time to protect members of staff that could come into contact with such contaminated devices (e.g. in preparing them for further reprocessing). It is a common theme in healthcare facilities, throughout the world, that cleaning and decontamination should occur in a designated reprocessing area or facility. Note, as discussed in Chapter 6, pre-cleaning can often be conducted at the site of device use (e.g. in or in close proximity to a surgical theatre) or the cleaning process initiated before and even during transport to a reprocessing area. Cleaning can then be achieved manually (e.g. in a sink), semi-manually (using a machine to aid in or as part of the cleaning process) and automatically (using a washer-disinfector). A washer-disinfector is defined as a machine that cleans and disinfects devices and other articles; this definition, is applicable internationally in the context of medical, dental, pharmaceutical and veterinary practice. Automated cleaning is preferred to manual cleaning. The specifics of the cleaning process will depend on the instrument or device being reprocessed, ranging from simple to complicated and/or multi-part devices (Chapter 4). It is important to remember that it is the responsibility of the re-usable device manufacturer to provide detailed instructions, to users, on how to safely and effectively reprocess such devices, including cleaning. When such items are sold to a facility, in the absence of detailed instructions, they may be inadequately reprocessed, compromising patient safety and opening the hospital to litigation. Staff using any device in a healthcare facility

should have detailed training that will include its safe and proper use, as well as the correct reprocessing of the device, to include dismantling, cleaning, reassembly and subsequent disinfection/sterilization.

The key components required for cleaning are:
• A cleaning chemistry ("detergent", cleaning formulation) to break down, loosen and assist in removing the soil (proteins, lipids, etc.).
• Friction produced by mechanical action (manual or automated) to remove the soil.
• Water to aid in the process of removal and rinsing soil away.
If all three components are not present or sub-optimal, effective cleaning cannot take place; this presents a particular challenge in many countries where water and other resources are limited.

Receiving and sorting

The receiving and cleaning (dirty) area should be functionally separated from all other areas (e.g. packaging, sterilization or storage) of the reprocessing facility. Staff, must assume that all items arriving or returning to the reprocessing facility are contaminated; it is unacceptable to process only those instruments that are known or thought to have been in direct patient contact. All re-usable instruments and instrument trays opened in the clinical environment should be decontaminated between uses (Figure 8.1). This will include the devices and, in certain situations, the external surfaces of containers that have been touched by staff in the clinical area or have been in contact with body fluids. Examples include during surgery with handling by the scrub nurse, surgeon, circulating nurse or anyone else assisting with a surgical procedure.

Staff working in this area must be fully attired in recommended personal protective equipment (PPE). This is designed to reduce hazards, including microbiological (from patient soil), chemical (in particular with the cleaning chemistry) and sharp (device) risks. Personal protective equipment is therefore particularly important and should be mandatory (Figure 8.2). Care should be taken to ensure that staff are comfortable wearing PPE, that they comply with written protocols and are consistent in the way they behave when carrying out this activity. If this is uncomfortable

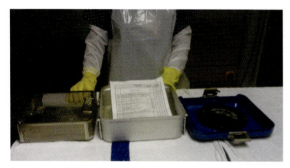

Figure 8.1 An example of a set of instruments, including container and trays being received into the decontamination area and prepared for sorting. Note: a device set checklist is shown (middle) as part of the facility tracking system (Chapter 14, see the section on tracking and traceability).

in any way, it is likely that they will not be efficiently used, despite the risks to health. Further, PPE should be inspected to be fit for purpose. An example is with gloves, that they should be immediately replaced if torn or otherwise compromised.

Recommended PPE for handling, sorting and cleaning will include:

• Face-protection: this can include a full face shield or separate eye and mouth protection. The eyes, nasal passages and mouth are the highest health risk areas. Facemasks can provide a certain level of protection. If mouth/nose masks are used, staff should be trained in the correct method to use these masks (ensuring that the mouth and nose are correctly protected). When used, safety glasses should have side-shields to prevent splashing from occurring from the sides. It is a useful training exercise to provide a new face mask or safety glasses to a staff member, allow them to do manual cleaning and then show them what is present on the glasses/face masks!

• Full-length waterproof gown or plastic apron, to protect clothing from splashes and spillages. Ideally separate clothing (including shoes) is provided to staff to be worn for sorting and cleaning of soiled devices. This will prevent the accidental contamination of personal clothing and transfer out of the cleaning area.

• Heavy duty gloves (e.g. nitrile gloves). These are usually longer gloves to cover the wrists and lower arm. It is

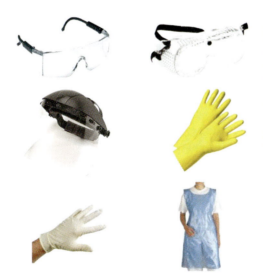

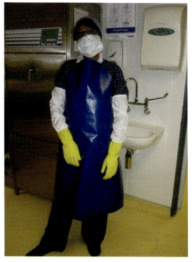

Figure 8.2 An example of typical personal protective equipment used during handling, sorting and cleaning of patient-soiled devices. On the left are safety glasses, face shields, gloves and an apron. In a typical example (right), the

lady is dressed in clothes specifically provided for staff in the receiving and cleaning area, with a protective apron and gloves (heavy duty), arm shields and face mask (disposable) and safety glasses.

recommended that jewellery and artificial nails are not used, as these can lead to glove damage. Jewellery may also be accidentally damaged during the manual cleaning process. Gloves may also be supported by arm protectors (as shown in Figure 8.2) that go further over the elbows;

• Other PPE should also be considered, such as hair/head protection and special foot protection (e.g. boots and protected footwear, such as steel-toed to minimize risks from dropping or spillage accidents).

Upon arrival in the decontamination area, all re-usable items should be removed from the transport cart/trolley and containers, sorted, checked and prepared for cleaning. Due diligence must be shown at all times when sorting and dealing with contaminated items. If not already conducted at the site of use, all waste materials and single use devices should be disposed of in accordance with the local waste policy (Chapter 13, in the section on Waste Management and Chapter 7, in the section on Post-procedure sorting) and any laundry items similarly sorted (see the section on laundry; Chapter 15).

Procedures should be in place to ensure that personnel safely handle re-usable devices and minimize any risks of accidental injury. Two important risks are accidental exposure to pathogenic microorganisms (via the hands, eyes, nose and mouth) and sharps-related injuries. Given the wide range of cutting, dissecting, injecting and other devices used (particularly surgically), sharps-related injuries are high risk and can be minimized. They can not only injure the skin but the consequences for cross-infection are high. Examples include safe removal, disposal of single use blades at the site of use (Chapter 7, Post-procedure sorting), ensuring technicians can directly see all devices in a set and consider using a sorting instrument tool (instead of using the hands directly to remove devices) for sorting (Figure 8.3).

The responsibility for the safe disposal of single use blades should be carried out by the user designated at site. If discovered in the sorting/cleaning area, this should immediately be reported to the line or facility manager as a failure of the user to comply with operational procedures, thereby putting staff health and safety at risk. In the event of a needlestick or sharp injury, the incident must be reported immediately and any facility policy implemented.

Medical and surgical instruments are generally delicate and should be handled accordingly; they should not be dropped, thrown into baskets or handled roughly as this can damage the instrument and affect its functionality. Sets/trays should be carefully checked against a contents list on receipt prior to washing and any missing or damaged items recorded and reported. Remedial action

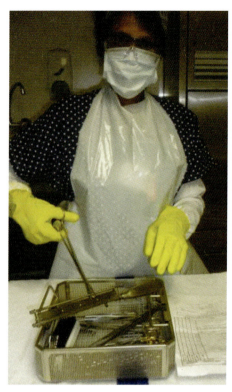

Figure 8.3 Safe sorting of surgical devices using a swab holder. Items are handled and sorted in accordance with any local policy. In this case, the instrument being used for handling is dedicated for this purpose and *not* an integral part of the set.

for missing or damaged equipment should be taken in accordance with the department's quality system. It is recommended that where there is more than one tray of devices (e.g. for hysterectomy and some orthopedic sets), such sets are sorted and organized into a limited number of numbered trays required for such procedures.

Certain items may need special attention and should be sorted accordingly; these include:

• Cannulated (lumened) instruments should be cleaned using a high pressure cleaning system or otherwise cleaned as specified by the manufacturer of the device. Consideration should be given to reducing any risks of staff exposure to aerosols that can be generated during cleaning. As an example, this can be minimized by cleaning the device under water.

• Non-immersible items – devices that cannot be immersed in water such as types of electrical drills must be cleaned according to the manufacturer's written instructions and protected from contamination wherever possible during the surgical procedure.

• Delicate items that have specialized cleaning procedures should be handled and cleaned as recommended by the manufacturer.

• Re-useable devices that are to be returned to a commercial provider for reprocessing must be accompanied with a contamination status certificate and be properly contained and labelled in accordance with any local requirement for the Transportation of dangerous goods (Chapter 7, transportation post-procedure).

• At the time of writing, high-risk devices that may be or are known or have been exposed to prions require separate consideration. Special precautions should be in place (where the device is used and in the decontamination area) in handling these devices, such as separate decontamination (including chemical and steam sterilization protocols) or incineration (Chapter 15, see the section on devices known or suspected to be contaminated with prion material). In some cases these devices may need to be isolated in accordance with any local policies. Protocols should be in place that instruct the staff member on the minimum requirements for reprocessing of each type of medical/surgical instrument. This is generally based on the Spaulding classification system, which defines critical, semi-critical and non-critical devices (Chapter 1, in the section on Goals of Decontamination and Spauldings Classification). As an example, dental equipment, such as extraction forceps, scalpel blades, bone chisels and surgical burs that may have penetrated soft tissue or bone during a procedure are classified as critical and should be thoroughly cleaned and sterilized after each use. Dental instruments that may accidentally penetrate oral soft tissue or bone (e.g. amalgam condensers, air-water syringes) are generally considered as semi-critical and must also be thoroughly cleaned and at least be high-level disinfected.

Consideration should also be given to the handling, reprocessing and storage of any transport containers and trolleys that are used in this area; this is discussed in more detail in Chapter 7, in the section on transportation post-procedure. Similarly, devices and device sets need to be entered into the tracking and traceability system in use by the facility (as discussed in Chapter 7, in the section on tracking and traceability and Chapter 14, in the section on materials management).

Disassembly and preparation for cleaning

If it is safe to do so, devices composed of more than one part or moving pieces should be opened and disassembled to the smallest part in order to expose all surfaces to the cleaning process (Figure 8.4). Before disassembly is considered, always refer to the manufacturer's guidelines, for device specific instructions and follow recommended procedures. These guidelines should specifically consider any disassembly instructions that are required to ensure adequate cleaning.

Surgical instruments, for example, may be divided into two groups, "simple" or "complex" (Chapter 4). Simple instruments, such as needle holders, scissors, handheld retractors, hemostats, etc., have simple moving parts, and articulation points, for example box locks, hinges or screw joints. These instruments are hardy and can usually pass through a manual and/or automated cleaning and decontamination process. Such simple instruments can become a greater challenge to clean if gross soil is allowed to remain and dry on the instruments for an extended time (as discussed in Chapter 7, in the section on Post-procedure sorting). Complex instruments may have multiple moving parts, be powered by electric motors, compressed gas (pneumatic), or batteries, have long cannula (lumens), etc. They will generally need special treatment, with close attention to detail provided according to the manufacturer's guidelines. Complex instruments usually require multiple steps to effectively disassemble and clean them, for example self-retaining retractors have multiple locking screws and securing ratchets that will need to be opened and retractor blades that will need to be removed to allow proper cleaning. Some of these complex instruments can only be cleaned manually, while others are recommended to be cleaned manually and then followed by automated cleaning. An example is with flexible endoscopes, where manual cleaning is recommended alone or in addition to automated cleaning. Endoscopes and other lumened devices provide a notable challenge, as the internal surfaces of such devices cannot be visually inspected (to check for cleaning efficacy) and, in many such cases, the presence, number and interconnections of lumens in these devices can be difficult to understand. Further, these devices can have an array of parts and accessories used as part of surgical/medical procedures (Chapter 4, in the section on Endoscopy). Some of these devices can be very heavily soiled due to their clinical use, such as colonoscopes. Unfortunate mistakes made in the cleaning and reprocessing of such devices are well published, in most cases due to their complexity and inadequate understanding of the steps required to safely reprocess. A further example is with delicate microsurgical instruments that normally need to be disassembled and are recommended to be hand washed and rinsed with water (usually high quality water due to the risks associated with

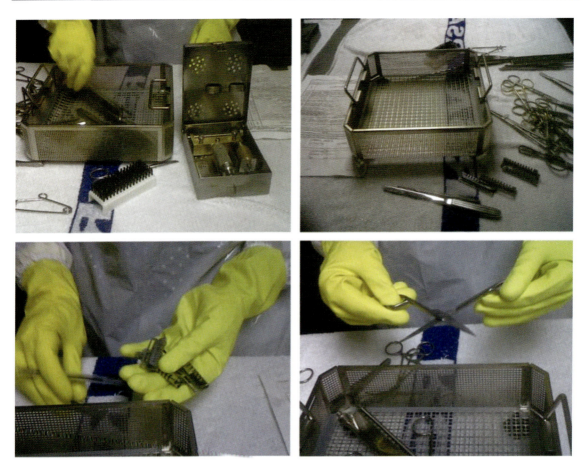

Figure 8.4 Disassembly and preparation for cleaning.

these types of devices; Chapter 15, in the section on Water Quality). Wherever possible these are protected and secured before being passed through an automated cleaning process.

Instruments used in orthopedic procedures present significant processing challenges for any reprocessing facility (Figure 8.5). Many such instruments require manual cleaning because bone, tissue and, in some cases, cement can become embedded in the instruments, for example drill bits and guides, cutting blocks, tibial keel punches and drills are among the instruments that often retain bone and tissue. It is important to note in this case that cement is a particular challenge to remove from a device surface when it has set; for this reason, it is recommended that cement should be removed at the site of use (e.g. in the surgical theatre) prior to it setting (becoming solid) and being transported (Chapter 7). Most orthopedic instrument trays contain many devices, being designed with multiple layers and containing large, medium and

very small devices. These are often provided by manufacturers as loan sets, moving from hospital to hospital (note: loan sets are further discussed in Chapter 15). Close inspection of manufacturers' reprocessing guidelines is essential. Reprocessing facility staff must understand how these device trays should be handled, disassembled and reprocessed. For example, they should ensure that tray lids are removed, all instruments should be removed (big and small), and some may require disassembly, before instruments are adequately cleaned. All pins, plates, screws and other parts (including implants or parts that are designed to remain in a patient) should be carefully inspected; this may require magnification and particular care following cleaning and prior to sterilization (Chapter 10). Overall, orthopedic instrument sets provide an example of a special challenge because of the size, weight and number of required trays, multiple layers of instruments, as well as the fact that they are usually

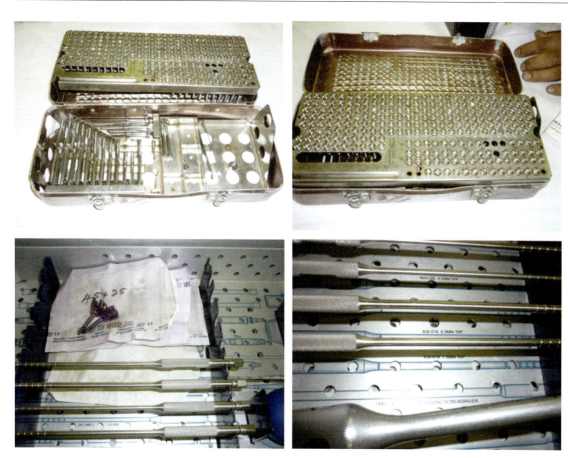

Figure 8.5 Examples of devices used in complex orthopedic sets.

loan sets. It is advisable to break down multi-layered trays onto single layered trays and companies providing these sets should be encouraged to provide them in this way so that they can be more easily handled and processed safely and effectively. Further consideration to loan devices/sets and implants is given in Chapter 15, in the section on loan devices, sets and implants.

Basic principles of cleaning

Cleaning is often considered the most important step in the decontamination cycle. If an item is not cleaned it will be unacceptable to use such a device medically or surgically for the following reasons:
• Visually, the use of a soiled device is unacceptable to staff and patients. Would you use a device on yourself if it was visually soiled with material from a previous person?

Foreign materials being left on or injected into a wound during surgery can lead to the need for further surgery and the patient being exposed to further risks.
• Microbiological and infection risk: microorganisms, particularly pathogens (disease-causing), can be present and can transfer to a patient. The presence of soil can compromise the effectiveness of disinfection and sterilization.
• Chemical toxicity risk: residual materials, despite the presence or absence of microorganisms, can lead to toxic reactions in patients and particularly in certain types of surgery such as ophthalmology. Certain types of "dead" bacteria release toxic substances that can also lead to adverse patient reactions (e.g. endotoxins, Chapter 5).
• Instrument damage: the presence of soil can damage the device, chemically (e.g. rusting, Chapter 7) and/or physically (e.g. loss of device function/operation).

Cleaning is an essential step, despite any further reprocessing and is often the only step used to reprocess devices (especially non-critical devices; Chapter 1). Cleaning can be attained using a variety of methods, including manual and automated cleaning. Right from the start, the appropriate cleaning method for a particular device will depend on its characteristics, and the manufacturer's instructions should always be first reviewed and considered in determining how a device is properly cleaned.

Consideration has previously been given to the chemical aspects of soils (Chapter 6, in the section on introduction to cleaning and accessory chemistries). Soil that remains on device surfaces following their use on a patient can contain a variety of organic and inorganic materials from the patient or others used during the procedure; these include blood, tissues and microorganisms. The amount and type of soil can vary depending on the medical/surgical procedure the devices have been used for and if any pre-cleaning has occurred (Chapter 3). Further, the devices may have dried soils present that are an even greater challenge to cleaning. As discussed in the introduction, the minimum expectation is to visually clean each individual device, with particular attention given to those devices or device parts that cannot be visually examined (such as lumened devices). Despite this, the required endpoints of cleaning (in order to claim or prove that a device can be called "clean") may require more detailed analysis, such as microbiological (e.g. levels of bacteria), biochemical (e.g. levels of protein) or chemical analysis (e.g. total organic carbon; see the introductory section and the section on troubleshooting cleaning problems). This analysis may need to be carried out on a regular basis and periodically reviewed to ensure that any sudden changes are investigated and the cause(s) resolved.

The key components required for cleaning have already been introduced as the cleaning chemistry, a method of friction and water. The various types of cleaning chemistries have been introduced in Chapter 6. They are classified based on their use and/or type of chemistry (e.g. enzymatic and non-enzymatic, such as alkalines). In all cases they are formulations, being combinations of ingredients, including active and inert ingredients, into a product for its intended use. In some cases, especially with manual cleaning, cleaning chemistries are often used that have additional, generally low-level, antimicrobial activity. Low-level disinfection is considered helpful to reduce staff handling risks during cleaning, but is not considered necessary as part of the reprocessing cycle (although it is recommended in certain countries).

Methods of friction include mechanical means to aid the cleaning process, which can be achieved by manual (e.g. hand washing or using brushes) and automated (e.g. spray, immersion and ultrasonic) methods. Water plays a particular role in aiding the cleaning process and in rinsing away soil, as well as any cleaning chemistry present on device surfaces prior to disinfection/sterilization. These essential components are considered in further detail in this chapter.

The cleaning process itself is actually a multi-step process, using these key components. A typical cleaning process (manual or automated) will include:
• Pre-rinsing or pre-washing (with water and/or with a cleaning chemistry). This is usually conducted at temperatures of less that 45°C (<45°C), in order to remove any gross soil that is present and ensure that soil is not fixed or clumped (due to higher temperatures). Fixing or clumping of soil components, such as proteins, can leave the device even more difficult to clean. Pre-rinsing may be conducted at (or near to) the site of patient use (Chapter 7), manually within a designated reprocessing area or in an automated washer-disinfector.
• Washing, with a cleaning chemistry used at the right concentration (dilution), temperature and recommended conditions by the manufacturer of the cleaning chemistry. This is the main stage of cleaning and the optimal conditions for this to occur should be recommended by the manufacturer (of the chemistry and/or the device being cleaned).
• Rinsing, with water to remove any residues of soil components and cleaning chemistry to render the device "clean" and ready for subsequent patient use or further reprocessing. This may require single or multiple rinses of water, depending on the chemistry type being used, device being reprocessed and the cleaning process being used.
Cleaning can be achieved by manual and/or automated processes. In manual cleaning, the devices are generally immersed into a sink or basin containing the cleaning chemistry at the right concentration and temperature.

Often, specific accessories are provided by the manufacturer or supplied locally to aid in this process; examples are lumen adapters, allowing a syringe to be attached to a device port and allowing flushing of internal lumens/surfaces. Care should be taken not to use any accessory (such as hard metal brushes and scouring pads) that could lead to device damage; if such an accessory is required to remove stubborn soils (e.g. cements), it is recommended that the soil is removed prior to hardening at the site of use. Metal brushes and scouring pads can

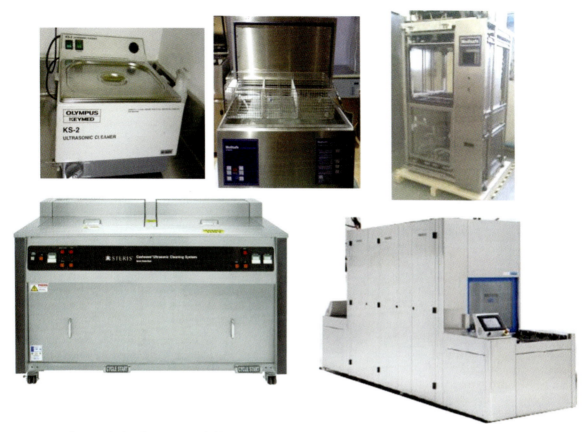

Figure 8.6 Ultrasonic baths of various sizes (left), used to aid in manual cleaning. Ultrasonics are also used in larger automated washer-disinfectors (single or as part of a multi-chamber washer), for pre-cleaning and/or automated cleaning processes (right).

significantly damage even metal surfaces (such as stainless steel, leading to damage to the passivation layer and provide opportunities for rust development; Chapter 10, Figure 10.6). A semi-automated cleaning process can include the use of an ultrasonic bath (Figure 8.6).

Ultrasonic baths come in a range of sizes, from table-top machines to free-standing baths, to integrated into washer-disinfectors and as a module in a tunnel or multi-chamber washer-disinfector (see below). These allow for devices to be immersed in a cleaning chemistry and cleaning aided by sonication, which is a process using ultrasonic (sound) waves to cause the disruption and removal of soil from surfaces (see the section on Immersion including ultrasonic cleaning). In some ultrasonic bath designs, lumen devices can be attached to flow ports designed to allow water and cleaning solutions to flow through the device and aid in cleaning. Fully automated cleaning processes can be conducted with various designs of the washers and washer-disinfectors (see the section on Automated

cleaning). These allow for the automated programming of standardized cleaning cycles, generally using immersion and particularly spray systems to clean and rinse devices.

The cleaning chemistry is an important part of the cleaning process. As introduced above and in Chapter 6 (in the section on introduction to cleaning and accessory chemistries), cleaning chemistries can be classified on how they are used and the main types of active chemistries that they use for cleaning (such as acids, alkalines and enzymes). It is important to highlight that a cleaning chemistry is a formulation of mixture of chemical for a desired purpose (in this case cleaning). A good cleaning chemistry should:
• Assist in the cleaning process.
• Protect the device from damage (e.g. from water or even the aggressive effects of the cleaning formulation itself).
• Be able to function in the presence of varying water qualities (e.g. presence of organic and/or inorganic contaminants, such as microorganisms and various chemicals; see the section on water quality).

Cleaning chemistry formulations can range significantly in their abilities in each of these areas and the benefits/ weaknesses of each product type should be closely considered. For example, neutral (~pH 7) formulations are good general cleaners but are generally not as efficient at organic soil removal as alkaline cleaners. Alkaline cleaners range significantly in pH (see the section on The pH scale: defining acids and bases, Chapter 6), from mild (pH 7–10) to highly (pH 10–14) alkaline; higher pH does not necessarily mean better cleaning or indeed that a product is more aggressive on a surface. It will essentially depend on the formulation of the product, where the manufacturer should be readily able to provide evidence to support claims of efficacy and safety. Equally, enzyme-containing formulations can also range significantly and the presence of enzymes alone should not be considered as being sufficient to remove certain types of soils; enzyme formulations are particularly variable in their activity. Acid cleaners, in contrast, are particularly used as "neutralizers" (following the use of an alkaline cleaner and to ensure that following cleaning the device surfaces are returned to a neutral pH) or specifically for the removal of rust or other inorganic contaminants (e.g. scaling; see Table 8.9). Overall, particular care should be taken to ensure that the cleaning chemistry being used is fit for purpose (designed for cleaning devices/instruments), and that instructions for use (including any benefits/limitations) provided by the manufacturer are closely reviewed. This may include reading the label (including what is provided on the detergent container or provided separately by the manufacturer), associated documentation and safety data sheets.

Choosing a cleaning chemistry is only the first step, as any cleaning formulation is only as good as the way it is used. We have already addressed the impact of the cleaning process itself in assisting cleaning (such as manual and automated cleaning method), but there are a number of key considerations to ensure that a product is used correctly and safely. These include:

• Product design: some products are designed specifically for manual, ultrasonic or automated cleaning, while others are designed to be used in all three applications. The choice may depend on the features/benefits of the product, as well as its aesthetic qualities (e.g. smell is often a concern in manual cleaning, to mask the odor associated with soil but at the same time not be irritating to those using the product).

• Product concentration: this refers to the amount of a chemistry that should be used. Instructions for use should provide details on how the product should be diluted in water (usually within a given range, such as 4 to 10 mL in 1 L water). For guidance on understanding weights and volumes in measuring, see Chapter 6, in the section on Weights, measures and other physical considerations. Over use of a product can lead to device damage, a requirement for additional rinsing (to remove chemistry residuals) and excessive foaming in manual or automated cleaning (where foam can prevent cleaning from occurring and even cause damage to automated cleaning systems). Foaming may be caused by two major factors: the cleaning chemistry itself and the presence of protein. The cleaning chemistry will contain various types of surfactants to assist cleaning (particularly removal and solubilization of soils) and foaming should therefore be expected. This is not always a negative sign, as in some cases foaming is used to optimize the effect of the product in cleaning, but excessive foaming can prevent the devices from being seen during manual cleaning and can prevent the mechanical actions in ultrasonic and automated (spray-type) washers. It can also be difficult to rinse water from a surface, requiring excessive rinsing. Protein foams when mixed with water; this can be from the cleaning product (e.g. enzymes are proteins) or from patient soil. Excessive foaming can be due to the fact that the instruments being cleaned are particularly heavily soiled. This may be overcome by doing pre-washing/rinsing. Under use of a product can lead to inadequate cleaning and device damage (e.g. if immersed in bad water quality).

• Washing temperature: temperature plays an important role in the activity of a product, sometimes positive and sometimes negative. All cleaning chemistries should be provided with recommended temperature conditions. As a general rule, the warmer the water is the more effective the cleaning action; similarly the higher the water temperature the greater the antimicrobial activity that may occur during cleaning (Chapter 6). However, this is not always the case. One example is that during pre-cleaning if higher temperatures (>45°C) are used then proteins and other soil components can become fixed onto surfaces and make them more difficult to clean. Another is that higher temperatures can cause the inactivation of enzymes present in some chemistries, thereby losing any enzymatic activity as part of the cleaning process; particularly close attention should be paid to the temperature ranges (upper and lower) recommended with enzymatic chemistries, as their optimal activities are very dependent on having the correct temperature.

• The quality of water: water is one of the most important ingredients for cleaning and is also widely used for disinfection/sterilization in its various forms (see the section on Water quality). Although it is easy in many parts of the world to take water for granted, in other parts it is a rare commodity. The chemical quality of water can include various types of dissolved and suspended components that can cause problems during cleaning (introduced in Chapter 6, in the section on mixtures, formulations and solutions, summarized in Table 6.2). These vary depending on the water source (reservoir, lake, water table, etc.), any purification steps (e.g. to render it safe for drinking), how it is transported to and within a facility and if any further treatment is done within the facility. It will also vary, depending over time, in particular between seasons. Particular and common problems include hardness (particularly calcium carbonate, $CaCO_3$) that is dissolved in water, but when it is heated becomes insoluble and deposits/sticks on surfaces to form a white or otherwise color precipitate/deposit known as "scale" (Chapter 15, in the section on Water Quality/Purity). Treated tap water usually has various types of chlorine compounds added, used to kill microorganisms (Chapter 6), but when heated can become particularly aggressive on metal surfaces and may cause instrument corrosion. Various other types of chemicals can lead to a variety of damage and changes in color. The impact of water quality on the reprocessing of devices is considered in further detail in Chapter 15, in the section on Water Quality Purity. Overall, it is recommended that water quality, being provided to a site of use for cleaning and reprocessing is periodically tested chemically and, if found to be unacceptable or at a high risk of causing instrument damage, then pre-treatment is considered (Chapter 15, in the section on Water Quality).

• Staff training: staff should be trained in using the cleaning chemistry safely and effectively, as well as in the whole cleaning and decontamination cycle approved by a facility. Staff can provide the greatest variation in cleaning practices, particularly in manual cleaning. But equally, although automated systems (such as ultrasonic baths and washer-disinfectors) can be wonderful provisions, they can do their job only as well as humans allow them. It is also important to remember that these chemical formulations are designed to remove and/or break down patient soil, and will therefore have safety risks to any staff members associated with their use.

An often underestimated principle of correct cleaning is the final step, rinsing. Rinsing should ensure that any cleaning chemicals remaining on the device surface following cleaning are safely removed. Cleaning chemistries are designed to remove and breakdown soil from surfaces, there is no doubt that patient complications can occur if such chemicals remain on the device through any subsequent reprocessing step (e.g. steam sterilization) or even direct use on a patient. Such residues may also lead to damage to the device, particularly if subsequently treated with another chemistry or with heat. Therefore, rinsing is considered an essential step to ensure the device can be safely used/further reprocessed. The most effective and widely used method is by using water. The extent (e.g. number of rinsing cycles and volume of water used) will depend on the cleaning chemistry, and instructions regarding safe rinsing should be provided by the device and cleaning chemistry manufacturer. As pointed out earlier, some high alkaline cleaning chemistries require neutralization with an acid chemistry (to ensure the pH on the device surfaces is returned to neutral, around pH 7) and then rinsing to remove the acid cleaner residues. Note, in these cases, that the amount of acid used to neutralize needs to be carefully controlled, as too much acid can leave the device with a lower (acidic) pH and too little will not adequately neutralize the alkaline, leaving the device with a higher (alkaline/basic) pH.

Following the basic cleaning cycle and depending on any requirement for further reprocessing (disinfection and/or sterilization) the devices may then need to be dried. Drying in this case may be defined as the removal of water or residual moisture. This will be generally true if devices are for immediate patient use and particularly if being prepared for steam or gas sterilization. In other cases drying may not be necessary and it may be sufficient to remove excessive water from and, if applicable, within devices prior to further reprocessing or use. Drying may also be conducted manually, within a washer-disinfector or a separate drying cabinet (that uses hot air and fans to assist drying). In the case of manual drying, care should be taken not to re-soil the devices using dirty towels or cloths that are inappropriate.

Manual cleaning

Manual cleaning may be used as a pre-cleaning step prior to automated cleaning and/or as a full cleaning step when mechanical cleaning facilities are not available or not recommended. For example, many types of delicate or complex instruments that have to be carefully taken apart are often recommended only to be manually cleaned and certain types of devices cannot be submerged in water, such as some electrically operated or air powered drills or certain parts of complex endoscopes.

When cleaning manually (by hand) extreme caution must be exercised by staff in order to reduce hazards.

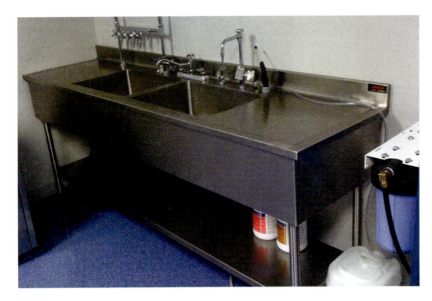

Figure 8.7 A typical double-sink system used for manual cleaning.

These include microbiological (from patient soil), chemical (in particular with the cleaning chemistry) and sharp (device) risks. Personal protective equipment (PPE) is therefore particularly important and should be mandatory in manual cleaning (see the section on receiving and sorting and Figure 8.2).

Recommended PPE for manual cleaning (as discussed in the section on receiving and sorting) will include:
• Face-protection: this can include a full face shield or separate eye and mouth protection.
• Waterproof apron, to protect clothing from splashes and spillages.
• Heavy duty gloves (e.g. nitrile gloves). These are usually longer gloves to cover the wrists and lower arm. Shorter gloves may also be supported by arm guards that go over the elbows.
• Other PPE should also be considered, such as hair/head protection (to protect the operative's hair from aerosols/sprays that may occur in this area when using sprays or during the action of manual cleaning) and special foot protection (e.g. boots and protected footwear, such as steel-toed, to minimize risks from dropping accidents and should be enclosed to protect against spillage accidents).

Manual cleaning is only as good as the person performing it and the tools provided to allow it. The most important consideration to cleaning staff is training, to ensure that they are trained on safe and effective cleaning methods for the variety of devices they may encounter. In the cleaning area, lighting should be good so that the person can visualize the devices for cleaning and to prevent injury. A double-sink set-up is recommended, to allow cleaning in one sink and rinsing in another (Figure 8.7); this can be performed with one sink but particular care should be taken in training on the correct quality of water to use for the final rinsing method to ensure soil/residual chemistry is adequately removed (Chapter 15, in the section on water quality/purity). The sinks are generally recommended to be deep, to minimize splashing during cleaning and should be positioned at the right height for staff to use comfortably. Adequate draining is clearly an important consideration in designing manual cleaning areas. The sink may also be equipped with a spray-hose system, to allow water to be sprayed over devices for pre-cleaning and rinsing; consideration should be given to reducing risks of aerosol generation in such cases. Ready access to compressed air is also common to allow residual water/chemistry to be flushed from devices (particularly lumened devices). It is increasingly common to see sinks being equipped or specifically designed with various equipment that allows the manual cleaning process to be better controlled. Examples include temperature probes (to ensure the optimal use of the cleaning chemistry), dosing systems (that automatically dose in a controlled volume of chemistry, to minimize waste and over/under dosing) and level indicators/sensors (that ensure that the quantity of water used is effective). Sinks are also being designed to allow for adjustable height settings, to improve their safe (ergonomic) use. Specific cleaning accessories are designed for certain types of devices, such as endoscopes to allow for leak-testing and cleaning (flow) of internal channels.

As highlighted earlier in the chapter, a variety of manual aids are often provided to aid in the cleaning process. Examples include various types of soft or specifically designed brushes, syringes (for lumen cleaning/flushing) and sponges. Such cleaning accessories are readily available in most countries. Care should be taken in using these, in particular sponges; they should be routinely replaced on a frequent basis (at least daily if not more), as if they are left wet, bacteria and fungi can multiply in and on them providing an additional risk. It is preferable that such accessories are single-use, disposable items, but if this is not economically viable, re-usable accessories are recommended to be decontaminated (rinsed and heat-disinfected) frequently. Accessories such as scouring pad should not be used, as they can damage device surfaces. If specific types of accessories are required by a device manufacturer to allow cleaning, such as speciality brushes, information regarding brush specifications and how these can be obtained should be provided.

Some cleaning chemistries have been specifically designed and labelled for manual cleaning. Traditionally neutral pH, enzymatic-based chemistries have been used but these are not required; any cleaning chemistry can be used for manual cleaning if instructions are provided by the manufacturer for that purpose. Cleaning chemistries should be used that have been designed for medical/surgical device use. All cleaning chemistries have health risks, but some (such as high alkaline or low acidic chemistries) are often considered of greater risk to staff. For this reason, neutral or mild alkaline chemistries are recommended for routine cleaning, with or without enzymes. Despite this, all chemistries should be handled as being potentially damaging to health and particular care given to review safety data sheets provided with them.

Despite the cleaning chemistry used, the supplied chemistry should be prepared and used according to manufacturer's instructions. Pay particularly attention to the concentration, temperature and recommended exposure times, as well as any requirements for rinsing. Training on the correct use of the cleaning chemistry is essential.

During manual cleaning, care should be taken to minimize any splashing or aerosolization. It is recommended, for this reason, that devices should be cleaned under water (immersion method) and particularly when using brushes or when flushing lumened devices. All surfaces of the instrument/device must be cleaned. To do this, some disassembly may be required (see the section on disassembly and preparation for cleaning). Items that cannot be immersed should be cleaned in a manner that will not produce aerosols/sprays and with particular attention to the instructions provided by the manufacturer. Manual friction is the basis of manual cleaning, with the cleaning chemistry aiding in removal and breakdown of soil from surfaces. The following guidelines are given:

• Appropriate PPE should be worn at all times. Strong gauntlet gloves, a plastic apron, eye protection and mask are recommended to protect staff and reduce the risk of splashes and cuts from sharp items.

• A double sink method is recommended to be used with a dedicated washing and a separate rinsing sink.

• Fill the clean sink with the appropriate measured amount of water and detergent, according to the detergent manufacturer's instructions. The ideal water temperature and concentration should be specified. Water at a temperature of <45°C is preferable for any pre-cleaning (to remove gross soil) as hotter water may coagulate protein materials (found in blood, sputum, etc.) making them very difficult to remove. Water temperatures of greater than >55°C will be too hot for comfortable manual cleaning by staff.

• Medical grade cleaning chemistries that are specific to the type of soil on the instruments/equipment should be used. In most cases these will be neutral or alkaline-based detergents, with or without enzymes; inorganic soil contaminants (such as rust and scale) can be removed using acid-based chemistries (see below). Do not use household or hand soaps as they are not labelled for such use, can be highly foaming, making rinsing difficult and can leave unwanted residues (e.g. fatty acids in the household soap may react with hard water to form a soap "scum" on the instruments).

• Dismantle/disassemble/open all instruments before cleaning, paying special attention to joints, serrations, tips or crevices. A clean soft brush or soft cloth/sponge may be used to clean the surfaces. Do not use abrasive or metal brushers as these will damage the instruments. It is recommended that the number of devices placed and washed in the sink at any time is limited (e.g. no more than six devices). Wash the device using manual friction (e.g. using a brush) below the surface of the water, in order to avoid aerosols and minimize splashing. Pay special attention to grooves, teeth, and joints, etc., when brushing to remove any soil. The brush should be cleaned and rinsed after use and before

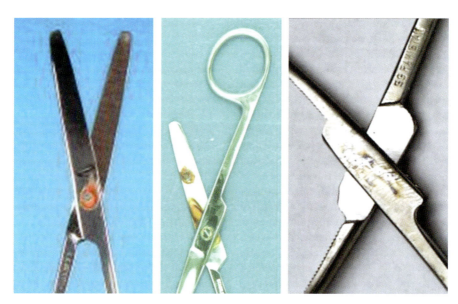

Figure 8.8 Rusting present on a device. Rusting is a sign of damage on a device surface, in particular on stainless steel devices where two metal surfaces interact (e.g. the hinge joints of forceps). Rusting (chemically known as ferric oxide) builds up on the surface when is become visible as a brown stain or deposit.

re-use; any cleaning accessories should be left dried when not in use (or otherwise discarded). Lumened items should be washed externally, but particularly all lumens brushed according to manufacturers' instructions using appropriately designed brushes. Some lumens may require irrigating with a high pressure water-jet spray gun; this should be done below the water surface to prevent aerosolization. Note: manual lumen cleaning is required for two reasons, to remove patient soil and to ensure that lumens are free-flowing (not blocked). Blocked lumens will prevent subsequent disinfection/sterilization and may render the device inoperable. Automated systems (e.g. specifically designed ultrasonic washers, irrigator systems and washer-disinfectors) may be used to replace manual cleaning, but in these cases the system manufacturer's instructions and written claims should be closely inspected and followed to ensure they allow the flow and detect the potential blockage of the range of lumen sizes that can be present in any lumened device (flexible or rigid; Chapter 10, in the section on Rigid endoscopy, Flexible endoscopy).

• Whilst cleaning, visually inspect the item to ensure that all parts are clean. If an instrument is broken, attempt to locate any missing pieces and follow the broken/missing instrument procedure.

• Replace cleaning and/or rinsing water after each set of devices or when the water is obviously soiled/contaminated.

• When rinsing fully immerse cleaned items in a separate sink with clean water in order to rinse off all soil and detergent residues. The number of rinses required may vary depending on the number of devices being cleaned, types of devices and any manufacturer's instructions. Any chemistry or soil left on the items can reduce the effectiveness of further processing and can lead to other patient complications. The quality of water may need to be controlled, if the water quality being provided to a reprocessing area is not considered safe for such purpose (for further guidance on water quality refer to Chapter 15, in the section on Water Quality/Purity).

• If required, instruments should be manually dried before patient use or further reprocessing (particularly when devices are being prepared for packaging and steam or gas sterilization). At a minimum, any large amounts of water remaining on or within a device should be removed.

• Complete any relevant documentation associated with the facility quality and/or tracking/traceability system.

Often brown staining is observed on device surfaces during cleaning. This can be due to rusting (Figure 8.8), dried patient soil or residual iodine (that is sometimes used as a surgical scrub and pre-operative preparation, and can accidentally contaminate device surfaces). It can often be hard to differentiate these, but in general patient soil and iodine should be easily removed during the

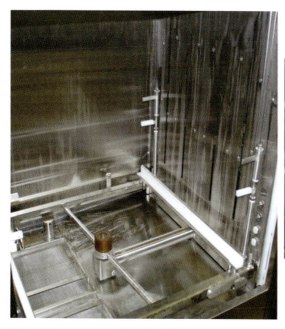 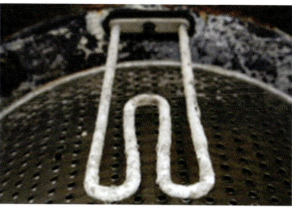

Figure 8.9 An example of "scaling" due to water hardness in a washer-disinfector (left) and on a water heater (right). Note the white precipitate.

cleaning process, but rusting will not. Rusting can be removed by spot treatment with an acid-based, rust-removing cleaning chemistry that is used to dissolve inorganic contaminants such as rust.

A further use of such chemistries is for the routine removal of hardness or "scale" deposits on a surface (generally seen as a white precipitate; Figure 8.9). Note that rusting is a visual sign of device damage, therefore removing the signs of rusting (the build up of rust, specifically the chemical ferric oxide) only removes the visual signs of damage; both the underlying damage and further erosion/rusting of the surface will continue. Excessive use of certain types of acid-based cleaners can itself actually promote rusting, so care should be taken in reading instructions supplied with and using such chemistries.

Automated cleaning

Most modern reprocessing facilities in developed countries use an automated cleaning system resulting in minimal handling of contaminated equipment by staff, enabling process standardization and larger handling capacity of device sets through the reprocessing cycle. Unfortunately this is not always the case in developing countries, which exposes staff and patients to increased

safety risks. At the same time, mechanical washers, like any other tool, will only be effective if designed and used correctly. In comparison to manual cleaning of devices, mechanical cleaning is the method of choice as it removes soil and microorganisms, with minimal risk to staff, through a consistent repeatable automated cleaning and rinsing process, providing higher standards of cleanliness and can be validated (Table 8.2).

Most, but not all, modern instrument washers also incorporate a thermal or chemical disinfection cycle capable of destroying various numbers and types of microorganisms; these are officially known as washer-disinfectors but may also be referred to as "washers", "washer-pasteurizers" and other similar terms (see Figure 8.10). A washer-disinfector is defined as a machine that cleans and disinfects medical devices and other articles used in the context of medical and dental settings (but is equally applicable to other areas such as veterinary and research settings); "clean" in this context is defined as the removal of contamination ("soil") from a surface to the extent necessary for further processing or use. The design and performance requirements for a washer-disinfector, according to international standard requirements, are defined in the ISO 15883 (*Washer-disinfectors*) series of standards (see the section on Cleaning guidelines, standards and testing).

Table 8.2 Manual vs automated cleaning.

Manual cleaning	Automated cleaning
Advantages	**Advantages**
Often recommended for handling delicate, complex devices	Fully automated programmable cycle, including cleaning, rinsing, and (in most cases) disinfection
Required for non-immersible devices	Automated cycles that should expose the device to the same conditions for each cycle, record cycle parameters and can be validated
Often considered cheap	Minimizes instrument handling and safety considerations
Direct and visual inspection during cleaning	Performance easily monitored
Disadvantages	**Disadvantages**
Difficult to ensure reproducibility and to validate that a process is consistent	Often unsuitable for certain types of items, such a non-immersible devices
Cleaning depends on individual performance	Equipment and maintenance can be expensive
Safety issues	Cleaning outcome is design-specific, where inadequate designs can lead to problems
Labour intensive and time consuming	

Essentially, all the cleaning principles described in the section on the basic principles of cleaning are equally applicable to automated cleaning, but in this case the cleaning process is done by a machine rather than a person. This provides many advantages, but it should always be remembered that the machine (and the processes it is programmed to control) will only be as good (safe and effective) as it is designed to be, if used by staff as intended by the manufacturers and maintained in accordance with recommendations. Washers vary considerably in their design, varying from those that are only designed to assist in part of a manual cleaning process to those that provide a fully automated cleaning, and optionally disinfection and drying, process. The same three components for the cleaning process (as outlined in the section on basic principles of cleaning) are still required: water, cleaning chemistry and method of friction. In the case of automated washers, the methods of friction include ultrasonics, flow systems (e.g. through lumened devices), immersion and spray-type mechanisms. One or a number of these mechanisms may be employed within the same washer. As examples, an ultrasonic bath includes immersion and ultrasonics, but may also be equipped with a dedicated flow system; tunnel washers can include immersion/ultrasonics in one chamber and a spray type system in another. In considering the installation and use of an automated washer, important factors will include the required water volumes (and in some cases temperature ranges recommended), water quality/purity requirements, electrical and draining specifications, and even the types of cleaning (or other accessory) chemistries that may or may not be used. All of these requirements, in addition to recommended process cycles, maintenance schedules and instructions for use, should be provided by the washer manufacturer. Examples of such concerns will include the choice and use of cleaning chemistries. As for manual cleaning, certain types of cleaning chemistries are specifically designed for automated cleaning and should be labeled as such. A common concern is the production of excessive foam during the cleaning process (Figure 8.11); foaming is not a bad attribute (in many cases it can be a benefit), but excessive foaming can lead to inadequate cleaning/rinsing as well as damage to the machine's pumping systems (e.g. leading to pump "cavitation", where the presence of air (in the foam) reduces the efficiency of the pump to work and the water pressure being employed for flow or spraying reduces significantly).

Although it will depend on the washer design, the washer should always be capable of providing a consistent process that can include pre-washing, washing and rinsing. Some washers will only be designed for one, two or all of these stages, with most being capable of being specifically programmed to run one or a number of washing cycles to meet the needs of a facility. In all cases, care should be taken to ensure that the cycle settings (that have been designed and preferably tested to meet the facility requirements) are fixed; the ability to change cycle

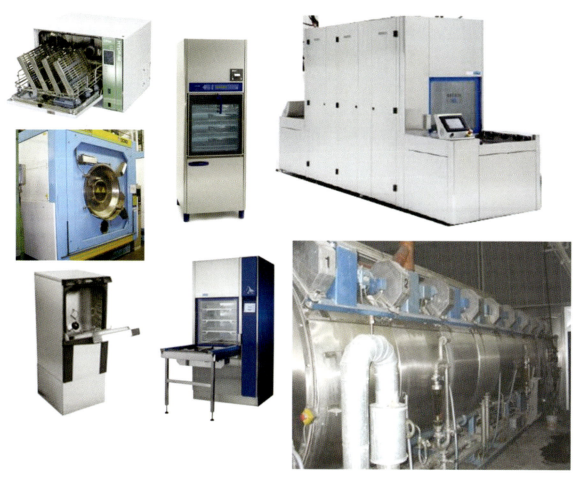

Figure 8.10 Various types of automated washers and washer-disinfectors. These may be used for washing alone (with or without rinsing) or with a chemical or thermal disinfection cycle. They come in various different sizes and types.

parameters (including chemistry dosing volumes, cycle times, etc.) should only be accessed by staff members authorized to do so and who understand the risks and requirements when such parameters are changed. When defined machine cycles are fixed, staff should be trained on the correct use of the machine, including cycle choice, loading/unloading of the washer and alarm resolution.

The main benefits of automated washers should be to reduce handling risks and to provide a consistent, more efficient cleaning process. This, however, may not always be the case, where inappropriate washer design, maintenance or use can lead to problems. Consider some of the following examples that have been reported:
• Open sonication baths can cause aerosolization of microorganisms and chemicals into the reprocessing area and affect the health of those working in this area.

• Washing processes that appear to and have been recorded (documented) as being successfully completed, but in fact have not been (e.g. no cleaning chemistry was dosed into the machine or spray arms/flow ports where blocked, thereby not allowing flow for cleaning).
• National and/or international safety designs have not been adequately considered, despite the obvious risks of mixing electrical components, mechanical parts and water/chemistry within the same machine!
• Devices that have not been loaded into the washer correctly, thereby not allowing the process to have full contact with the various internal or external parts.
• Machine alarms being ignored or even turned off by facility staff, due to lack of servicing/maintenance.
For these reasons, greater attention has been placed in recent years to the adoption and use of washer-disinfector

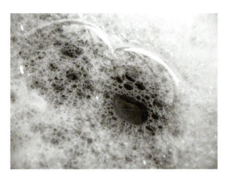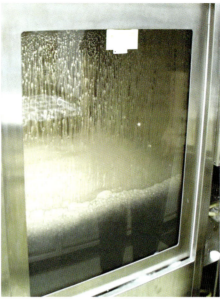

Figure 8.11 Foaming and an example of excessive foaming in a washer-disinfector.

standards (the ISO 15883 series, as international examples) to reduce these risks.

The correct use of the washer will often be dependent on various accessories that are provided to be used with the washer, such as loading tray, racks and flow connectors (Figure 8.12). Instructions on the correct use of such accessories should be provided by the washer manufacturer.

Overall, despite the obvious benefits of automated cleaning, the washing process is always dependent of those using the machine. Therefore, training is important and should, at a minimum, involve:

• Safe and correct use of chemicals (e.g. when changing the chemical provided to the machine or during accidental spillages). In some cases the same cleaning chemistry can be used for manual, ultrasonic/immersion and automated cleaning, thereby minimizing mix-ups and simplifying staff training. In such cases, the cleaning chemistry should be labelled for each specific application.

• Preparation of devices for loading into the washer. Particular attention should be paid to device disassembly (when required), ensuring hinged instruments are open and that device trays are not overloaded (Figure 8.13).

• Loading and unloading of devices in trays/racks into the washer. This can be a manual or assisted by an automated loading/unloading design within the facility. Particular attention should be given to any safety risks in using automated loading/unloading systems as they

include automated moving parts that can cause accidental injury. Manual or automated loading/unloading systems are generally designed to improve ergonomics (preventing or minimizing lifting/pushing/pulling) and to maximize through-put of the available washing machines.

• Correct cycle selection. Washers are often set up with different cycles to be able to handle different types of loads.

• Handling and reporting of any alarms. Alarms can be visual, audible and/or otherwise recorded. For example, most modern washers have independent process monitoring installed (see the section on Cleaning guidelines, standards and testing) and inspection of computer-generated reports or data records may be required to ensure the correct process has been attained. Some washers may alarm, but once a cycle is complete or the alarm has been turned off there is no record, while others will alarm and prevent further use of the machine until the problem is rectified.

• Any subsequent reprocessing steps. For example, ultrasonic and immersion baths may only wash the devices, but may require subsequent manual or automated rinsing. Similarly, devices may require drying following the cleaning/disinfection cycle.

• Routine maintenance. All such machines require routine maintenance and recommendations should be provided by the manufacturer. Failure to follow these guidelines can lead to damage or failure of the washer.

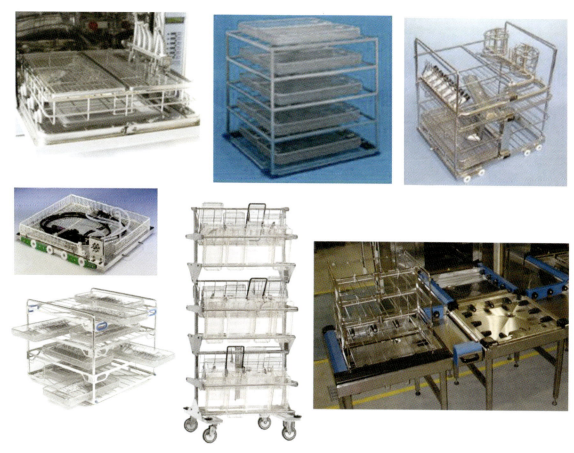

Figure 8.12 Various types of accessories (racks and trays) used with automated washers.

Typical examples of recommended maintenance include inspection of drains (not clogged and free-flowing), spray arms are not moving (not stuck) and jets not blocked, and regular draining and disinfection of immersion baths.

• Routine testing. As mentioned previously, there are international standards now in place (e.g. ISO 15883 series) and users should follow the advice given and carry out the recommended periodic testing. The results of all tests should be logged for each individual machine and retained for future inspection.

As a final note, despite the use of an automated washer, PPE requirements will be similar to those specified for sorting (see the section on Receiving and sorting) and manual cleaning (see the section on the basic principles of cleaning). Although the risks associated with splashing, aerosolization and with sharp instruments may be

less, it is not unusual for staff involved with automated cleaning to be also conducting sorting, disassembly, pre-cleaning and manual cleaning in the same area; therefore PPE consistent with requirements within the area should be considered (Figure 8.14).

Immersion, including ultrasonic baths

Various types of immersion baths can be used for cleaning and provide the benefit of controlling various cleaning variables such as temperature, and friction mechanisms. The most commonly used are ultrasonic baths (Figure 8.15).

Sound (or "sonics"), including the sensation of hearing, is based on a mechanical vibration (or pressure variation); sound, as we perceive it, is essentially a vibration within a certain range (known as a frequency range). "Ultrasonic"

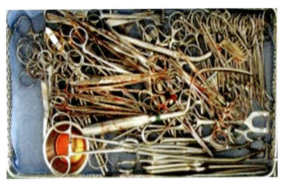
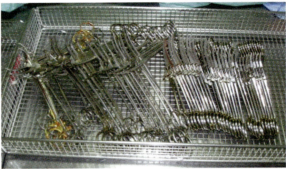

Figure 8.13 Overloading and improper assembly of a device tray (left). A better assembled tray is shown on the right. Note the opened hinged devices on the right.

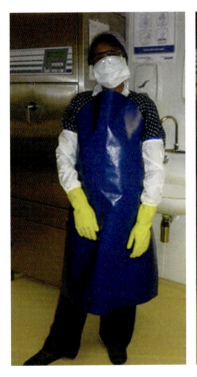
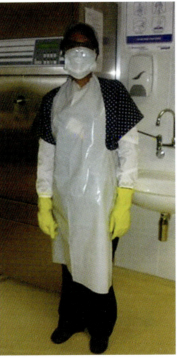

Figure 8.14 Examples of acceptable PPE being used in an automated cleaning area. By all accounts, the recommended PPE is similar, if not identical to that described for manual cleaning (Figure 8.2).

or "ultrasound" refers to sound that is at a higher range than that perceived by the ear (generally >20 kHz).

These mechanical vibrations (at high frequencies) can be used for a variety of medical applications including medical imaging (where very high frequencies are used to visualize various internal organs and structures, such as during pregnancy, known as an "ultrasound" or sonography) and treatments (e.g. high frequencies used to fragment kidney or gall stones into smaller pieces, in a process known as lithotripsy). Lower frequency levels, but still at or higher

Figure 8.15 Ultrasonic baths.

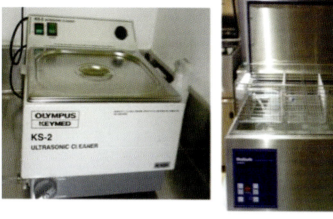

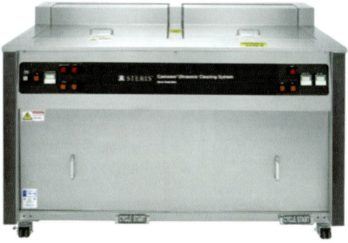

than those that we perceive as sound, are used for cleaning purposes, such as in dental practices (teeth cleaning) and with surgical/medical devices. Cleaning in these cases is assisted by the production of ultrasonics in water/cleaning chemistry. Cleaning is assisted by an effect known as cavitation, where ultrasound production within a liquid causes the production and collapse of small bubbles along the surface of the device that causes soil disruption/removal. A cleaning chemistry should always be present, as well as for assisting in the removal of soil and to prevent soil from re-attaching to the device surface when the ultrasonics are turned off. The cleaning chemistry should be designed for ultrasonic use, or at a minimum not cause any negative effect on ultrasonic production or cleaning effects. Some ultrasonic bath designs allow lumened devices to be attached to a flow system provided in the bath that circulates cleaning chemistry through the device to aid in cleaning.

An ultrasonic washer (also known as a "sonicator" or "sonication bath") can be particularly effective in the presence of a cleaning chemistry to remove soil and hardened debris from instruments. They may be used for pre-cleaning purposes or as part of an automated cleaning process (including cleaning and rinsing). Highly contaminated and difficult to clean instruments (such as those containing tight hinge joints, Chapter 4, see the section on Basic everyday instruments) are often recommended to be pre-cleaned in an ultrasonic bath. For pre-cleaning purposes, the use of an ultrasonic bath is preferred to manual immersion cleaning, as it reduces direct contact with contaminated items, decreases the risk of cuts/puncture wounds to staff and can be an effective cleaning step. It is important to note that some device manufacturers may recommend the use of ultrasonics for cleaning, while others will not (or even recommend against the use of ultrasonics, due to the risks of damage to the device); such recommendations or limitations should be clearly stated in their instructions for reprocessing.

Staff are recommended to always wear personal protective equipment, including heavy duty gloves, masks, protective eyewear, and a gown when handling contaminated instruments and working with the ultrasonic baths. Protective headwear may also be considered. The following general instructions are given, but can vary depending on the ultrasonic bath type and manufacturer:

• Fill the tank with water (typically potable or drinking water) to the manufacturer's designated level (defined volume).

• De-gas the water as recommended by the machine manufacturer. This sonicates the water to remove dissolved gases (Chapter 6, see the section on Mixtures, formulations and solutions) that could interfere with the cleaning process.

• Add the cleaning chemistry to the defined concentration, ensuring the manufacturer's recommendations (of the chemistry and/or ultrasonic bath) are followed. It is advisable to use a suitable neutral or mild alkaline detergent (with or without enzymes) that is effective at lower temperatures (as for manual cleaning, see the section on Manual Cleaning).

• If the tank has a heater, set the temperature control to the set point defined by the cleaning chemistry manufacturer's recommendations.

• When the specified temperature has been reached, place the opened/dismantled instruments into the basket.

• Place the basket of instruments into the tank, ensuring that they are completely immersed in the diluted cleaning chemistry. Never put instruments directly onto the base of an ultrasonic washer as this can short-circuit the ultrasonic transducers and damage the washer. Note that in some designs, lumen devices can be connected directly to flow ports provided within the washer; ensure that these devices are connected correctly (and do not become disconnected during washing) and are also completely immersed.

• Set the timer control to the time specified by the machine or device manufacturer.

• After the washing cycle has been completed, remove the basket from the tank and rinse the items with clean water – unless the machine has an automatic rinse stage, or the load is to be transferred directly into a washer/disinfector for further processing. As for manual cleaning, the quality of water used for rinsing may need to be controlled; potable water may not be sufficient (Chapter 15, see the section on Water Quality).

• Cleaned devices may be further reprocessed, dried and/or clinically used (depending on the Spaulding classification; Chapter 1, see the section on Goals of decontamination and the Spauldings classification).

• Completely drain the bath chamber. If the ultrasonic bath is to be used again, it is to be refilled with fresh water and the steps above repeated. If it is not being used again (e.g. over 2–3 hours), the chamber can be dried (using a non-linted cloth).

• Record the instrument(s) that has been processed, according to facility requirements (such as the method and solutions used and details of the staff member who completed the procedure).

Similar procedures are recommended for other types of immersion (including irrigation) baths.

Automated washers/washer-disinfectors

Most automated washers today are designed for cleaning and disinfection, therefore these processes are introduced here with an emphasis on the automated cleaning phases of the cycle and disinfection specifically discussed in further detail in Chapter 9. Washer-disinfectors are used to clean and disinfect a range of devices and materials that are intended to be re-used. The cleaning and disinfection process is intended to make the items clean but also safe (microbiologically) for staff to handle (as a prerequisite for packaging and sterilization), reducing the load of micro-organisms on device surfaces and also often for direct/indirect use with a patient (in particular non- and semi-critical devices (Chapter 1, see the section on Goals of decontamination and Spauldings classification). Examples of devices that typically go through a cleaning-disinfection process prior to patient use include flexible endoscopes (used for semi-critical procedures, as is generally the case with investigational colonoscopy and gastroscopy: Chapter 15, see the section on Endoscopes and other lumened devices) and miscellaneous non-invasive devices such as trays/carts, wash-bowls and re-usable footwear. Most surgical devices are typically (although not always) passed through a cleaning and/or disinfection process, packaged and then subjected to a sterilization process.

A typical cleaning-disinfection process consists of a number of separate phases to include:

• Cleaning, usually including a prewash with water (<45°C), a washing phase and rinsing; the number of prewashes, washing steps (including type(s) of chemistry used) and rinsing steps can vary depending on the cleaning process.

• Disinfection, using hot water (for such devices that are thermo-resistant) or various chemical disinfectants (in particular for thermo-sensitive devices). In most cases where chemical disinfection is used, the disinfectant is required to be rinsed away at the end of the disinfection phase. Thermal (hot water) disinfection (also known as "pasteurization") is achieved by the action of moist heat maintained on the surface to be disinfected at a particular temperature for a particular time. This time-temperature relationship can vary depending on the types of devices being reprocessed (e.g. non-critical or critical devices) and the design of the washer-disinfector, which is further discussed in Chapter 9, in the section on Physical disinfection). Lubricants (as accessory chemicals) are often added automatically onto device surfaces during the disinfection phase (to ensure that devices, in particular hinged devices are operating optimally), but it is also common for lubricants to be in applied manually onto individual devices following cleaning-disinfection.

• Drying, if and when applicable. Drying is performed using the circulation of dry/heated air within the washer and can be assisted using a chemistry (rinse aid). The rinse aid generally assists in water droplet dispersion, making them easier to evaporate (from liquid to gas) and removed by the drying system. Note: any chemical rinse aid used should be non-toxic, including testing to show that it does not become toxic to patients when sterilized (e.g. by steam).

There are many different sizes and types of washers. They may be single or multi-chamber, single (one) or double (two) door, and varying in size/design. In single-door designs, the devices or materials (referred to as the "load") are introduced and removed from the same door, while double-door designs allow for the introduction and removal through separate doors (pass-through design). The pass-through door washers are preferable as contaminated items can be loaded in the "dirty" area and removed in the "clean". The disadvantage of a single-door washer is that the contaminated and clean items are loaded and unloaded through the same door from the "dirty" side.

The major components of any washer-disinfector will include:

• Washing chamber and draining system, to hold, circulate and remove water/chemistry during the cleaning process.

• Water-pumping system, including pipework, pump(s) and spray/flow systems.

• Dosing system, for the delivery of any chemistries used during the process. Chemistries are normally dosed as liquids using designated pumps and the number of individual dosing pumps can typically vary from 1 to 4. Solid dosing systems are also used, being integrated into the water-pumping system directly or indirectly.

• Air handling system, in particular for use during drying but may also be used during rinsing (to remove large volumes of water/chemistry from the devices and minimizing the use of water).

• Computerized control allowing the cleaning-disinfection process to be automatically controlled, according to defined programmed process conditions; these include process phases (cleaning, rinsing, disinfection, drying), dosing of any associated chemistries, temperature, pressure (used for the control of the flow of water through the system), exposure times and other parameters required for the specific washer design. The control system is therefore linked to a number of sensors that are monitoring the performance of the process (such as temperature sensors). It is typical for the control to include a recording system (either printed out on paper and/or collected by a computer system) to allow for a record of the cleaning-disinfection process to be confirmed/archived.

In addition to the main control system, most modern washer-disinfectors are equipped with an independent monitoring system. This system is separate from the computer system and its associated sensors (e.g. temperature, pressure, etc.), where independent sensors are used to verify that the controlling sensors are operating correctly. As an example, if a dosing system for cleaning chemistry has malfunctioned or the chemistry has been used up (and is now dosing air!) the control system may record that chemistry was delivered to the washer at the right volume/concentration even though it was not. The independent monitoring/sensor would detect that this had occurred. Similar types of systems are often found in modern sterilizers (Chapter 11, see the section on Steam sterilizer design). In some cases the independent monitoring system is integrated into the control system to immediately alarm and inform staff of the problem, preventing the washer-disinfector process from proceeding until the problem is fixed; in other cases, the data collected from an independent monitoring system needs to be manually checked by staff to ensure all the cycle variables were within a given specification (range). Overall, care should be taken to ensure that staff understand how the independent monitoring system operates to ensure its correct use. These systems are designed to reduce the risk of an automated process failing, not to remove the risk.

Washers are also designed to accept single or various types of loading racks that allow devices (directly or within trays) to be placed and introduced into the washer. These are designed to be used as part of the washing process; a common example is that the rack is designed with spray arms, connecting directly with the water flow systems within the washer chamber and allowing water to be sprayed over and/or under the devices for cleaning-disinfection. Typical surgical instrument racks are multi-layered, designed to accommodate a number of wire mesh baskets full of instruments or can be more widely spaced to accept and correctly position large bowls, instrument trays, re-usable rigid containers and similar items. Specific types of racks commonly used include those to accommodate anesthetic equipment and accessories, as well as racks to assist in the washing of minimal invasive surgical and endoscopic (rigid and flexible) devices.

Loading/unloading of automated washers

As introduced above, devices are usually introduced into the washer using a system of baskets and racks. For example, commonly used terms in the capacity of a washer are "DIN" or "ISO" tray/baskets, which refer to the number of standard-sized trays into which devices/device sets are placed into the washer chamber. Typical examples widely used in Europe include 10 and 15 DIN tray racks and washer designs.

Despite the design of the washer and rack system, automated washing will only be effective if the devices/ trays are loaded correctly according to manufacturer's instructions and the cleaning process can contact the various parts of the device. The following are given as a guide to device loading:

• Do not overload trays or racks; if the washer is overloaded, then not all devices may be cleaned effectively, increasing rejection rates (the number of devices that are rejected on visual inspection as not being adequately cleaned and requiring re-cleaning, manual or automated).

• When loading make sure all items are placed into a basket in a manner that will enable them to have direct exposure to the water/detergent (e.g. the spray system). For example, hinged instruments should be placed in the open position.

• Ensure that the correct racks are used for loading the various types of instruments in the load; different types of racks are often designed for specific types of loads/device types.

• Do not place hollow or larger materials (such as bowls/basins) over other instruments as this can cause "shadowing", where the instruments are not in contact with the cleaning process. Hollow items must be turned upside down, otherwise water/cleaning chemistries will collect in them during the process.

• Ensure that spray arms are freely moving within the washer and are not blocked or obstructed from circulating by the load (particularly those integrated into the rack design).

• Ensure that the racks are correctly positioned within the washer chamber to ensure contact with the washer pipework/pumping system (according to the washer manufacturer's instructions).

• Devices and loads should not be left for extended periods of time in the washer, especially if only used for cleaning and not disinfection/drying. Residual moisture can lead to corrosion on some instruments over time.

Smaller washer-disinfector designs will obviously have smaller loading racks and device capacity; these are usually loaded manually in and out of the washer. Similarly, larger washer-disinfectors (e.g. for carts, beds and wheelchairs) are also manually loaded. For larger capacity devices and other material washers (e.g. laundry, see the section on Surgical and medical laundry), the load can be very heavy and difficult to handle for staff without the high risk of back/arm/hand injuries. Ergonomics refers to the design of procedures and equipment to reduce operator fatigue, discomfort and injury. In this case, automated loading-unloading systems are used to minimize such risks of carrying/pushing/pulling and also to improve the operational capacity of the available washers within a department. Automated loading/unloading systems can range from semi-manual types to fully automated systems (Figure 8.16).

In a typical example, the empty racks are placed onto a conveyer belt that is under control of a computer/sensor system. The device-containing trays are then individually loaded onto the rack shelves and once ready can be advanced to an available washer-disinfector. Various levels of complexity and automation design can go into such systems. For example, the conveyor system may assist in moving the rack to and into the washer under control by a person, followed by manual selection and initiation of a washing cycle. In contrast, the loaded racks can be automatically moved along floor, ceiling or wall-mounted conveyor systems and when a washer is detected as being free (or available to take a load) the system automatically moves the rack to the washer, detects the type of devices associated with that rack (e.g. surgical instruments), instructs the washer to automatically open, receive the load, close the door and initiate the defined cycle. Equally, in a typical double-door washer design, similar unloading systems are used on the clean side of the washer to remove the load, which can be manually or automatically moved to an area for packaging and sterilization. Overall, safety considerations are important in the design and use of automated systems, to reduce any risks of accidents.

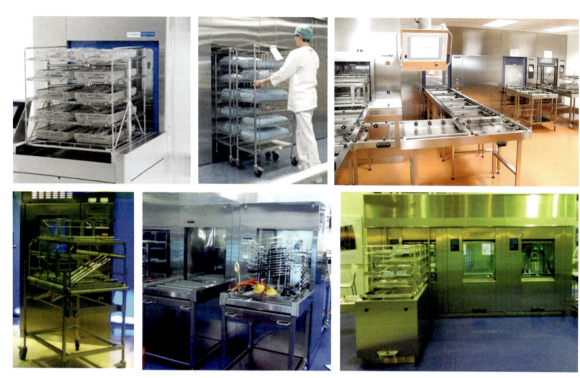

Figure 8.16 Examples of various types of loading/unloading systems. They range from manual, to semi-manual and fully automated (with fully automated examples shown right).

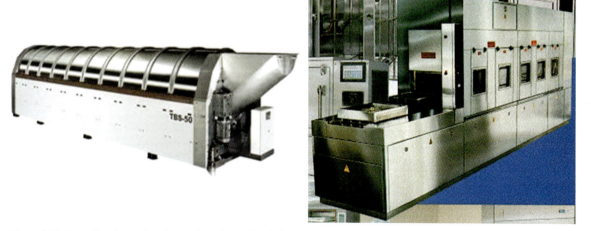

Figure 8.17 Examples of tunnel washers. A laundry washer (left) and an instrument washer (right).

Tunnel (or continuous process) washers

A tunnel washer consists of a series of inter-connected, open chambers (essentially a tunnel) through which the devices are passed through in a continuous process (Figure 8.17); these should not be confused with multi-chamber washer-disinfectors (see the section on automated washers/washer-disinfectors) that consist of separate, distinct chambers with doors separating chambers from each other.

Tunnel washers have been used in the past, with most not designed for cleaning complex or cannulated instruments. These washers typically featured two to five inter-connected open chambers, each with a specific processing task. The instruments move through the pre-rinse, washing (spray, immersion and/or ultrasonic) rinse, and drying cycles on a conveyor belt. Water can typically be sprayed from the top, bottom and sides. For device cleaning, the tunnel washers have largely been replaced by multi-chamber washers, but tunnel washers are still used for certain types of devices and laundry applications.

Multi-chamber washers

A multi-chamber washer is similar to the tunnel washer in that it has two or greater (typically up to four) chambers, but the similarity ends there; these machines have separate chambers with doors at either end and at intermediate positions between chambers (Figure 8.18).

Instead of an open chamber each chamber is separated by an inter-locking door and each chamber has a specific, distinct process associated with its design. During the process, the devices are passed through each chamber sequentially. Only the entry or exit door on each chamber can be open at any given time to prevent cross-contamination between the clean and dirty areas and re-contamination of a chamber containing a processed load. By placing chambers and processes one behind the other, loads can be prepared and passed in sequence through the cleaning-disinfection-drying process (depending on the washer design).

Multi-chamber machines have more than one chamber, where separate stages of the reprocessing cycle are performed in each chamber. The typical phases are cleaning (including a pre-wash for gross debris, cleaning chemistry wash and rinsing), disinfection and generally drying. Additional chambers can include separate pre-cleaning or cleaning chambers (e.g. an ultrasonic bath into which the device rack is lowered for cleaning). Since the load is moved through the machine and separated from phase to phase it is possible to get physical separation between dirty and clean loads. The full range of process stages is only completed when the load is delivered from the final chamber. Typically the chambers will be dedicated to cleaning,

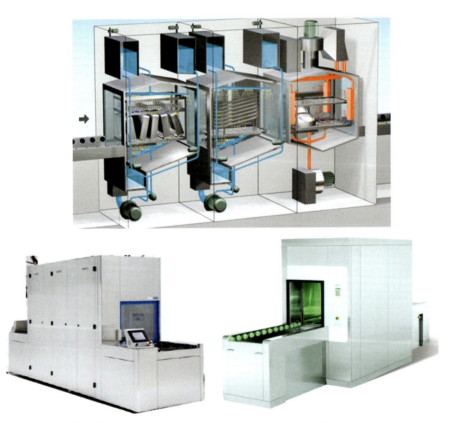

Figure 8.18 Multi-chamber washers-disinfectors. A representation (top) shows three-chambers each with a separate process ongoing (cleaning, disinfection and drying). A three-chamber (left) and two-chamber (right) washer-disinfector is shown below.

disinfecting and drying. Compared with single-chamber machines (where the full washer-disinfector process is included in one chamber), multi-chamber washers have a higher continuous throughput of devices/loads for a similar process, but have a larger footprint requirement (being longer in design they take up greater space within a facility).

Single-chamber washers

Single-chamber washers are widely used for the reprocessing of a variety of devices and other materials. They range in size from smaller table-top washers to large load (such as cart) washers; they may also be single-door or double-door designs. Over time, they are replacing manual cleaning due to their ability to provide a consistent and documented process, to minimize handling risks and to free up staff time from manual cleaning. The entire wash cycle is in one chamber, that is, prewash, main wash, rinsing, and typically disinfection and drying (if applicable). Since all stages of the cycle take place in the same chamber, it is not possible to get physical separation between the dirty and clean stages of the cycle within the washer. Assurance that the load will not be re-contaminated is dependent upon the efficacy of the cleaning and disinfecting stages in decontaminating

the interior of the washer as well as the load. Physical separation with the reprocessing area between a "dirty" and "clean" area is possible with double-door designs, with soiled devices being passed into the washer on one side and removed from the other, typically into a "clean" area (e.g. packaging room). Depending on the design and use of the washer, the machine can include a variety of dosing pumps (with chemistry being applied from outside or inside the washing chamber), pumping/spraying/flowing/immersion systems and an air handling system (particularly when drying is performed).

Three examples of single-chamber washers include:
• Endoscope washer-disinfectors (Figure 8.19). These are specifically designed for the reprocessing of rigid and/or flexible endoscopes. They are generally smaller-sized (including table-top or under-counter washers), but can also be larger, single or double-door design. In one example, the washer is used for a variety of cleaning processes, but specific racks are provided for the handling of rigid or flexible devices and associated accessories. These racks are designed to allow for the support and specific flow of water/cleaning chemistry through the internal device lumens. These are typically used with minimum invasive devices (including

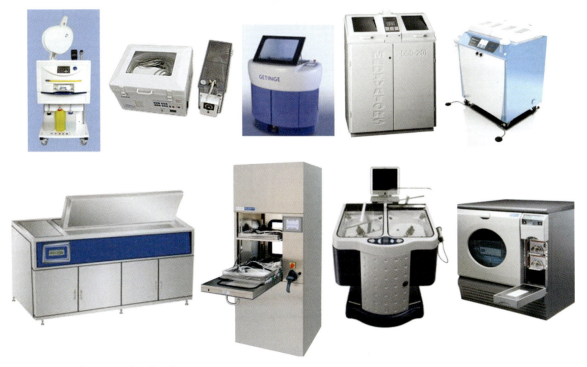

Figure 8.19 Endoscope washer-disinfectors.

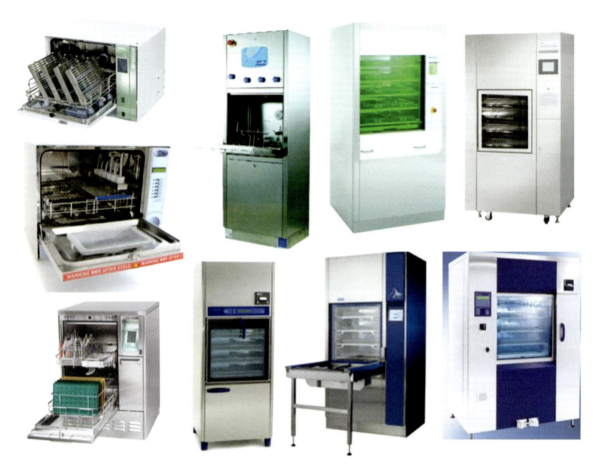

Figure 8.20 Single-chamber surgical and dental device washer-disinfectors.

rigid endoscopes), often referred to as MIS (minimal invasive surgery) racks. Minimal invasive surgery instruments are also automatically washed in some types of immersion/ultrasonic baths that control the various phases of the cleaning cycle (but most ultrasonic baths are semi-manual, see the section on Immersion including ultrasonic baths). In another example, the washer is only designed for use with specific devices, which is typical with flexible endoscope washer-disinfectors. These can include immersion or spray-flow type systems, that allow for cleaning and chemical disinfection outside and within (lumens) of the device. Flexible endoscope washer-disinfectors can be simple or complicated in design; these can be simply immersion baths with or without specific flow connectors for attachment/flow of lumens or more complicated systems that are designed to ensure that the correct number of lumens are connected, flow connectors are checked to ensure that they are not blocked/occluded before, during

or after the cycle. They can include a "leak-test" phase that ensures that the flexible endoscope can be safely immersed in water (in particular that no holes are present on/in the device that would allow water to leak into the internal (fiberoptic) parts of the device. Cleaning and disinfection chemistries can be provided in a variety of ways, and provisions for the correct quality of water (generally, bacteriologically free water) to be used for rinsing of the chemistry following disinfection. Cleaning is historically conducted with neutral, enzymatic cleaning chemistries, but any neutral or mild-alkaline chemistry may be used if labelled as compatible with flexible endoscopes.
• Surgical (including dental) device washer-disinfectors. These can be bench-top, under-counter or larger-chamber washer-disinfectors. They can also be single or double door in design (Figure 8.20).
They are used for reprocessing the variety of surgical/medical instruments, sometimes with multiple, programmed

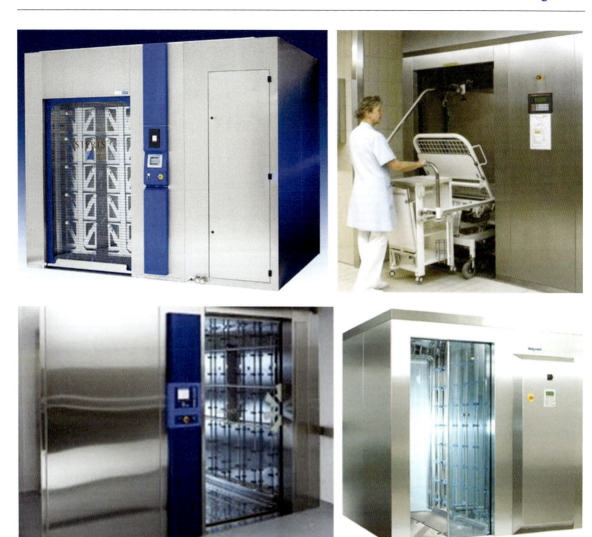

Figure 8.21 Cart or large-chamber washers.

cycles to include critical or non-critical device loads. They commonly have specified cleaning, disinfection and drying phases of reprocessing cycles, where a higher quality of water is generally recommended for use in the thermal disinfection of instruments and potable (drinking water used for cleaning). Such washers most commonly use thermal disinfection. Many larger reprocessing facilities will employ the use of automated material handling systems with multiple single-chamber washers. Such systems position multiple single-chamber washers side by side to reduce the floor space required within a department. The machines are then connected by a oading (and unloading, on the clean side) conveyor belt

positioned at a right angle to the line of washers, with docking stations at each washer. These can be fully or semi-automated and assist the staff in handling and loading of devices for reprocessing.

• "Cart" washers: these are commonly referred to as cart or large chamber washers, but are used for the reprocessing of a variety of non-critical materials such as carts, trays, trolleys, bed-pans and wheelchairs (Figure 8.21). Such devices are placed in the washer in a tilted position to enable water to drain out and prevent restriction of any moving parts within the washer. Due to the volume of water used in such designs and for non-critical items, it is common for water used for various phases to be collected and re-used between cycles; for example, rinse water may be re-used but should be monitored to ensure any soil or chemical load within the rinse water does not accumulate over a safe level that could cause problems. If designed, installed and programmed for such purpose, they can also be used as larger washers for critical surgical/medical devices. In these cases, it is typical for a higher level of disinfection to be programmed. Although chemical disinfection can be used in such washers, they more commonly employ thermal disinfection.

Special cleaning considerations

In this section, consideration is given to cleaning challenges with specific types of devices, due to their design. It is important to remember, as highlighted throughout the rest of this chapter, that every device requiring reprocessing may or may not require specific handling during cleaning. This can include disassembly, limitations on types of cleaning method or chemistries that can be used, and adequate rinsing. Reprocessing instructions should be provided by the device manufacturer, in accordance with various international guidelines and standards (e.g. ISO 17664 *Sterilization of medical devices – information to be provided by the manufacturer for the processing of resterilizable medical devices*). This section only considers some of these devices as examples, but even some devices that appear to be simple may provide similar challenge or considerations.

Microsurgical, including ophthalmological devices

Microsurgical devices are generally small and delicate, often used for surgical procedures using a microscope (see the section on the basic principles of cleaning earlier in this chapter). They are used for a wide range of surgical procedures, including those on the eye (ophthalmology surgery). Reprocessing such instruments can be a challenge as they are delicate and easily damaged by handling or various types of cleaning methods (including chemistries). Cleaning is a challenge due to the size of the devices and difficulty in inspecting such small parts for soil residuals. As highlighted in the section on the basic principles of cleaning, various types of soils or chemicals (from the cleaning process or even from the water used for rinsing) that remain on instrument surfaces can lead to toxicity risks in patients; this is particularly true with microsurgery and can be highlighted with toxicity concerns following ophthalmology procedures. Toxic

anterior segment syndrome (TASS) is a rare and potentially devastating complication of routine intraocular surgery due to a non-infectious toxic agent entering the anterior (front) segment of the eye during the procedure, causing an inflammatory reaction and patient complications. Toxic anterior segment syndrome has been particularly reported in cataract surgery and lens implantation, with complications ranging from partial to complete loss of the eye. The main suspected causes of TASS related to device use include: cleaning chemistry residuals, remaining soil (inadequate cleaning), materials (such as toxins, particularly endotoxins; Chapter 5, see the section on Bacteria) present in water used for reprocessing, and rusting or other chemicals. Equally, TASS may also be caused by particulate contamination, possibly by other materials used during the procedure, such as talc from gloves, topical ophthalmic ointments, lint (from materials), etc. Although not well described, other toxic effects may also be expected from the improper reprocessing and use of other microsurgical devices. To reduce these risks the following guidelines are given:

• Follow the device manufacturer's guidelines regarding handling and reprocessing.
• Ensure cleaning chemistries are correctly prepared and used according to the manufacturer's guidelines. This requires accurate measuring and dilution of the chemistry; do not overdose the chemistry, as it can lead to unexpected problems with rinsing.
• Pay close attention to the quality of water used to rinse the devices post-cleaning (and indeed during any subsequent disinfection and sterilization processes; note that chemical impurities, sometimes at high levels, can actually be transferred in steam onto a device surface). In some countries it is recommended that high purity water (e.g. distilled or reverse osmosis water) is used for rinsing and subsequent reprocessing following cleaning (Chapter 15, see the section on water quality/purity).
• Closely inspect the devices following cleaning (and disinfection, if applicable).
• Ensure that lint-free packaging materials are used following cleaning and powder-free gloves should be used during inspection and packaging following cleaning.

Loan devices and device sets (including orthopedic sets)

It is typical for many healthcare facilities to borrow devices or device sets from a manufacturer, supplier or another facility. Examples include very expensive device sets, when specific devices are needed for patient implantation (e.g. orthopedic screws/pins that are only selected during the

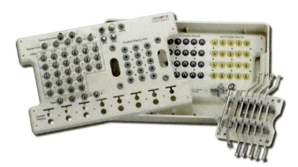

Figure 8.22 An example of a typical, orthopedic loan set. Note the small series of orthopedic screws/pins that are selected for specific use during a procedure; during surgery these can be selected and replaced back into the tray or used on a patient. As such, they can be soiled and contaminated during the procedure, therefore requiring reprocessing.

surgical procedure based on the immediate need of the surgeon; Figure 8.22), using experimental devices or when the required equipment is not routinely available at that facility.

These are commonly referred to as "loan" devices or sets. In some cases, individual devices from such sets are implanted into the patient, while others are returned to the set during the course of the surgical procedure. These sets will therefore become soiled and contaminated, requiring standard reprocessing (cleaning, disinfection and sterilization) prior to use with another patient. In some cases the devices may be returned soiled to a manufacturer or third party reprocessing facility, or are reprocessed within the same facility and provided for a further procedure (at the same or different hospital). It can be seen that the risks associated with such sets/devices should be closely controlled. The following guidelines are given when handling/reprocessing loaned instruments:

• A written procedure should be in place at any facility handling loaned devices/sets, describing how they need to be handled and reprocessed (if applicable). Staff should be trained on the procedure, particularly in any disassembly, cleaning and rinsing instructions. This should be done in advance of receipt of the instrument(s).

• Carefully follow manufacturers' reprocessing instructions. Many loaned sets may provide various types of implantable and non-implantable patient devices, small and large. Reprocessing procedures and particularly cleaning processes should ensure the adequate cleaning, rinsing and subsequent reprocessing of each device. In some cases, the complete set may need to be disassembled from the set tray(s) or multiple trays removed from set-containers to ensure adequate cleaning/rinsing.

• Safe practice dictates that all items entering the reprocessing facility are treated as contaminated, whether open or unopened and whether they appear to be used or not. Loan sets should always be opened, cleaned, inspected, and sterilized before they are issued to an operating room, unless a quality assurance certificate has been received from the previous reprocessor/device manufacturer. Such devices/sets that are not packaged (or if packaging has been compromised) should be considered contaminated and be reprocessed according to documented policies and procedures.

Electrical and robotic systems

Many devices contain various internal electrical components (Chapter 4) and can often be very sensitive to damage. Care should be taken in the handling, but also the cleaning of such devices. For example, it is not usual (although sometimes surprising to find) that a particular device or part of the device cannot be immersed in water. In such cases, close attention to manufacturers' instructions should be given. An example is a part of a device that is inserted into a patient for a particular procedure, while another attached part never touches the patient and is connected to an electrical source; a typical example is with various types of flexible endoscopes, which are further discussed in the next section. In this case, the patient-contacting part of the device may be manually cleaned in a sink, while the other parts of the device are cleaned with a wetted cloth. Protecting this kind of device from patient contamination will assist with the decontamination and can limit the extent of soiling.

Robotic-assisted surgery is a growing area of patient care and can include a variety of associated devices such as flexible/rigid endoscopes, light guide cables, light guide cable adaptors, camera arm sterile adaptors, camera sterile adaptors, instrument sterile adaptor, graspers, scissors, large and small needle drivers, blade instrument arm cannulas (sheath), cannula adaptors, obturators and reducers. All or most of these can contain electronic and microprocessors built into them and it may not always be possible to submerge them in water, which presents a challenge when cleaning. A further consideration is the various parts of the robot itself (Figure 8.23) that may require routine cleaning/disinfection (generally as a non-critical device but within the surgical area around the patient).

Cleaning instructions can vary depending on the specific device/component, to include the process and type of chemistry that can be used. These can include a manual cleaning and disinfection wipe, immersion in a sink or the use of ultrasonic, automated cleaning, etc. In all cases manufacturers' instructions should be closely reviewed.

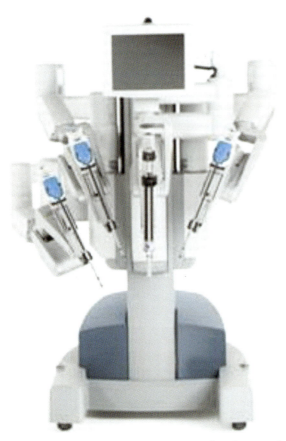

Figure 8.23 An example of a robotic system, where the arms of the root can contain a variety of device types that contact the patient during the surgical procedure.

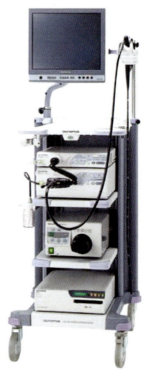

Figure 8.24 An example of an endoscopic system. This is a typical flexible endoscopic system including the endoscope (hanging on the right and connected to the control system), the control system (centre), video screen (top) and water source (middle left).

Endoscopy

Endoscopes are complex viewing instruments (Chapter 4, in the section on instruments for general viewing), being classified as being rigid or flexible in design. They are very delicate devices (particularly due to their internal structure, containing lenses and fiberoptics) and are composed of a variety of parts that are assembled together (often glued together with adhesives). They can range in materials from stainless steel (particularly rigid endoscopes), plastics (flexible endoscopes), glass, etc. In addition, many of these designs include internal channels (or "lumens"), ranging from one to five lumens that can often be interconnected. The endoscope can also have a number of re-usable accessories (Chapter 4, Figure 4.57 and 4.58; Chapter 15, Figure 15.3) that will also need to be considered for cleaning and subsequent disinfection/sterilization. Overall, care needs to be taken in the reprocessing of these devices and particularly during cleaning

to prevent damage; damage may occur during the handling of these devices, and from the various types of chemicals, processes and accessories used for cleaning. Flexible endoscopes are particularly sensitive due to their complex internal structures and use of various types of soft plastics used in their construction. Depending on their use, the levels of soil (including microorganisms) can be very low, but in contrast they can also be very high; consider, for example, the use of a colonoscope for the inspection of and often receiving a sample from the colon (part of the lower intestines).

Endoscopic systems may or may not consist of many parts, such as the endoscope itself (the part that contacts the patient) and a remote power source to which the endoscope is connected (either directly or indirectly; Figure 8.24).

The power source can enable the device to provide light, to view and capture internal pictures of structures within the body (on a video screen) but also to provide a source of water, air (or another gas) and suction that are also used during the procedure. The emphasis for cleaning will be on the endoscope itself (as a critical or semi-critical device, depending on its use), although periodic cleaning (and disinfection) may also be required for the power source. Maintenance may also be required for any utilities (water, gas, etc.) that are provided as part of this equipment.

The following recommendations are given for endoscope cleaning:
• Ensure that staff have been correctly trained on the handling and cleaning of endoscopes and any associated endoscopic equipment. Written procedures may be required and should be considered for individual devices, in particular for flexible endoscopes that contain multiple internal lumens. Remember: following patient use all lumens will be potentially contaminated. One of the most common mistakes made during endoscope reprocessing is not understanding the device design, how many lumens are present and neglecting to clean all lumens.

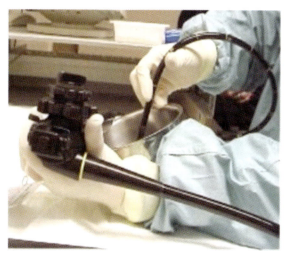

Figure 8.25 Bedside procedure with a flexible endoscope showing the device lumens being rinsed with water/cleaning chemistry (by suctioning) prior to transport for reprocessing.

• Care should be taken in the handling of endoscopes to ensure they are not physically damaged during cleaning. Flexible endoscopes, for example, have a minimum bend radius (how tightly they can be coiled) defined by the manufacturer and sinks or cleaning containers should be provided into which the device can be safely cleaned with adequate room for the process.
• Immediately following a patient procedure with a flexible endoscope, it is normal procedure for the major working lumens of the device to be flushed with water and/or a cleaning chemistry and for the outside of the scope to be quickly wiped down with a cloth. This is often referred to as the "bedside-procedure" as it is usually conducted in the patient room before the endoscope is disconnected from the control system (Figure 8.25). This serves to remove gross soil from the device lumens and surfaces prior to transport for reprocessing.
• Endoscopes should be prepared for immersion in water, prior to cleaning. For example, flexible endoscopes are provided with soaking caps that are placed over the exposed electrical components on their light guide connector ends (Figure 8.26).
• Before cleaning, the device should be inspected for any damage that may restrict how the device should be cleaned. An example is with flexible endoscopes, where the device is recommended to be leak tested before being immersed in water. The internal compartment of the flexible endoscope contains various electrical and fiberoptic components and should not contact patient materials or water; however, in some cases the internal lumens or external parts of the device may become compromised (e.g. through a tear or puncture) and allow materials to enter this compartment. It is therefore important to make sure that these parts do not contact water during cleaning/disinfection. During a leak test the internal compartment of the endoscope is pressurized with air using a leak tester (Figure 8.27) specifically designed for this purpose with the endoscope. The leak tester usually connects to a specific port on the light guide

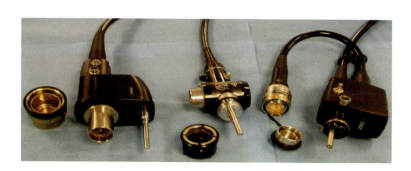

Figure 8.26 Flexible endoscope soaking caps (three different designs shown).

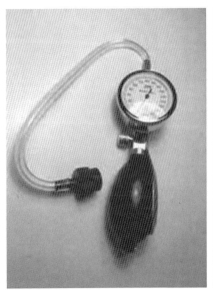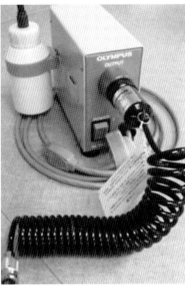

Figure 8.27 Flexible endoscope leak tester. A manual (right) and electrical (left) example.

end of the endoscope. The leak test can be performed manually (with a handheld or electrical leak-tester) and/or in an automated system, essentially using the same types of connectors to the endoscope. During manual leak testing, if a large leak is present, a rapid pressure drop will be observed by the pressure monitoring gauge/system; the test should be repeated and if confirmed as a leak the device should not be immersed in water. For a more sensitive test, the endoscope can be then be completely immersed in clear water to detect small bubbles emerging from the endoscope, particularly while flexing the distal tip of device to check for any leaks around the bending rubber of the device.

• Ensure that the device is disassembled and each re-usable part is cleaned according to instructions. Some parts or accessories may or may not be immersed in water! Other accessories (such as valves or "buttons" used with flexible endoscopes) require special cleaning to ensure that all parts are adequately cleaned (e.g. by actuating, opening and closing, valves in the cleaning solution).

• Recommended cleaning chemistries can range depending on the device or chemistry manufacturer. This can include neutral to mild (or in some cases high) alkaline cleaning chemistries. Neutral chemistries (with or without enzymes) are most commonly used. It is recommended that a fresh solution of cleaner/water is prepared, used for manual cleaning and discarded after each use.

• Manual cleaning is often described by the manufacturer, with or without any subsequent automated cleaning. During manual cleaning, the device should be cleaned on the outside as well as any internal lumens (Figure 8.28). Manual cleaning of internal lumens is performed for two particular reasons: for cleaning purposes (to remove soil) and to ensure that the lumens are free-flowing (not blocked or occluded). Internal lumens can be cleaned by flushing with water – cleaning chemistry and/or the use of specifically designed brushes/sponges (Figure 8.29). This should always be done under water to minimize the risk of aerosol formation during cleaning that could pose a safety risk to staff. Care should be taken to only use the correct brushes/sponges for the size of the lumen; when too small they will not be able to clean the lumen and when too big they can damage the internal structure. Older brushes/sponges should not be used as parts could fall off and get stuck within or otherwise damage the lumen.

• Semi-automated irrigation systems or ultrasonic baths may be used to assist in the cleaning process. It is important to ensure that any lumens are correctly attached to such systems to ensure irrigation (flow of cleaning chemistry/water) through the lumens. Some systems may be capable of detecting a blocked or occluded lumen while others may not. Ultrasonic baths with appropriate cleaning chemistries are often used for cleaning of endoscopes, but it is important to check with the device manufacturer's instructions if the device is compatible or not with ultrasonics. Not all ultrasonic systems are the same (e.g. different ultrasonic power, recommended exposure times, temperature control,

Figure 8.28 Manual cleaning (brushing) with a flexible endoscope. In this case the brush is shown being passed through the biopsy port of the device and being passed down the patient end of the endoscope (suction/biopsy channel). Note the device is brushed while under water to prevent aerosolization.

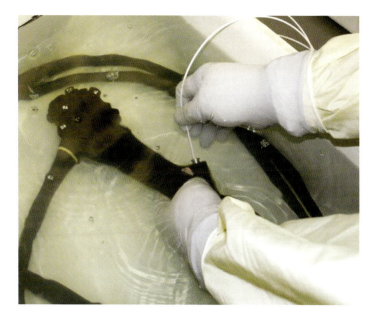

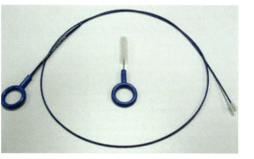 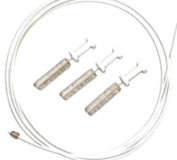

Figure 8.29 Examples of specially designed brushes and sponges used for cleaning of endoscope lumens.

etc.) and some devices may be damaged under certain exposure conditions/limits.

• Ensure that correct rinsing is performed on all external and internal structures. Certain types of enzymatic cleaners may require multiple rinsing cycles with fresh water to ensure that residual enzymes (which are proteins) do not remain on the device prior to disinfection/sterilization.

• There are many different designs of washer-disinfectors that can be used for automated cleaning (see the section on automated washer/washer disinfector and Figure 8.9). They range in complexity, including immersion and/or spray systems for cleaning the outside of the scope and generally irrigation systems for lumen cleaning. Some washers use specifically designed connectors that attach to the endoscope and irrigation/flow system of the machine, while others use a pressurized system at the control head of the scope to provide flow (connector-less washers). They may or may not provide a variety of features such as a leak-test, lumen blockage test, irrigation control, detection of connector attachment/detachment, cleaning process parameter control, rinse-water quality control, etc. Information should be provided by the washer manufacturer regarding the testing and validation of cleaning efficacy, preferably in compliance with local national or international standards/guidelines (see the section on Cleaning guidelines, standards and testing). At a minimum, the washer should be provided with at least one cleaning process that has been shown to be effective for the claimed endoscope application.

Devices known or suspected to be contaminated with prion material

Prions are unusual infectious agents (Chapter 5, in the section on prions and other infectious proteins). They are considered infectious proteins, and are strongly implicated in causing a group of rare diseases known as transmissible spongiform encephalopathies (TSEs), with the most common example being Creutzfeldt-Jakob disease (CJD). They are known to be transmissible through contaminated tissues (particularly brain and other nervous tissues/organs) on items such as re-usable devices, and are considered to have a higher resistance to decontamination methods. In most countries in the world (including older recommendations by the World Health Organization (WHO) published in 1999[1]), additional precautions and handling procedures are recommended in known or suspected cases of prion disease. These are considered in further detail in Chapter 15, in the section on Devices known or suspected to be contaminated with Prion material.

At the time of writing, there are limited studies on the effectiveness of cleaning to reduce the risks of surface prion contamination, but the following conclusions have been made to date:

• As prions are proteins, and cleaning is designed to remove protein, cleaning is considered one of the most important steps in reprocessing device surfaces known or considered at high risk of being contaminated with prion materials.

• Prions are hydrophobic (water-hating) proteins and therefore attach strongly to device surfaces, making them harder to remove and especially with water. The use of surfactants and other cleaning mechanisms can assist this action.

• The highest risk of prion contamination is with the brain and spinal cord tissue. This is not to say that other tissues do not have a risk, but the risk with these tissues is much less. In some cases, with a specific form of the disease known as vCJD, other tissues may provide a higher risk such as lymph nodes, and in certain types of eye procedures. Despite this, standard precautions against prions should be considered if there is a high risk of them being present.

• Drying of prion-contaminated material on a surface has been shown to increase the resistance to subsequent reprocessing, therefore devices should not be allowed to dry prior to decontamination.

---

[1] Report of a WHO consultation, Geneva, Switzerland, 23–26 March 1999. WHO/CDS/CSR/APH/2000/3. http://www.who.int/csr/resources/publications/bse/WHO_CDS_CSR_APH_2000_3/en/

• Cleaning alone can significantly reduce the risk of prion surface contamination by physical removal and even (depending on the cleaning chemistry and process) degrade the prion material. This is, however, not always the case. In some cases cleaning chemistries have been shown to *increase* the resistance of prion material: in others they *decrease* the risk. This appears to be specific to the cleaning chemistry formulation.

• Therefore, at this time, it is recommended that cleaning chemistries should be used only if supported by data that demonstrate directly that an individual cleaning chemistry has been tested and shown to safely reduce the risk of surface prion contamination. It is not sufficient to claim a product to be effective because it is of a certain type (e.g. alkaline or enzymatic). As an example, proteins are generally broken down by enzymes called proteases (Chapter 6, see Table 6.2), but prion proteins are known to be extremely resistant to the effects of most proteases.

• Most cleaning processes alone will not be effective in completely removing the risks associated with prion or indeed microbial contamination. Therefore, cleaning should always to be followed by routine or prion-specific inactivation protocols (Chapter 8, see the section on Devices known or suspected of being infected with Prion material). For these reasons, the following cleaning guidelines are given when handling known or potentially prion-contaminated re-usable devices:

• Ensure that a written facility policy is in place regarding the safe handling and reprocessing of re-usable devises.

• Reduce any risk of devices drying following surgical use and prior to pre-cleaning/cleaning.

• Cleaning chemistries used should be supported with data that shows that such products have been shown to reduce the risks of prion contamination. Cleaning conditions (product concentration, temperature and contact time) should be closely followed, in addition to the normal cleaning guidelines (e.g. manufacturer's instructions regarding disassembly).

• Ensure that devices are correctly rinsed and prepared for subsequent disinfection/sterilization and/or specific prion decontamination recommendations.

Textiles and laundry

Laundering of surgical/medical linens and textiles should follow the same chain of events as the reprocessing of any other surgical/medical devices. This should include the steps of:

• Post-procedure sorting and separation of waste from materials to be reprocessed (Chapter 7, in the section on post-procedure sorting)

• Safe transport to a reprocessing site (Chapter 7, in the section on transportation post-procedure)
• Cleaning
• Disinfection (Chapter 9)
• Sterilization (Chapter 11) if required (e.g. if used directly or contacting critical devices used directly for patient procedures)

Laundry items (linens, textiles, drapes, etc.) are therefore considered as devices in their own right, and in some parts of the world are described as such from a regulatory and legal point of view (e.g. in the European Union as a medical device under the Medical Devices Directive).

All re-usable, soiled textiles should be washed and disinfected/sterilized. While some textiles such as gowns and drapes play a negligible role as sources of infection, they may act as carriers of infectious microorganism and be released into the sterile core environment (Chapter 3, Principles of aseptic (or "sterile") technique). A certain amount of bacterial and fungal contamination can also accumulate in textiles that can offer an even greater risk. Conventional surgical gowns and drapes were often made of cotton; however, cotton materials are not considered a safe barrier against fluids and microorganisms and may also release lint (fluff or fragment) particles. Lint can be released into the environment during procedures and, if introduced into the patient (particularly during surgical procedures) the body may recognize it as a foreign body and it may cause patient complications (e.g. impaired wound healing). Low-linting fabrics with more effective barrier properties are therefore recommended.

The laundry process should begin at the point where they are used (e.g. in the operating theatre) with the proper collection and sorting of textiles into specially provided containers (Chapter 7, see the section on Post-procedure sorting). All items should be correctly sorted to include single-use, disposal items (textiles and devices) for waste disposal and multiple-use, re-usable textiles and devices. Devices should be separated from textiles; a main hazard posed by contaminated linen is negligent waste disposal by staff at the point of use, where instruments such as sharps (needles, razor blades) and surgical instruments are accidentally mixed with the textile. It is for this reason that contaminated textiles are often defined as: *laundry that has been soiled with body fluids or other potentially infectious material or may contain sharps*. Textiles may also be heavily soiled, posing a contamination/infection risk to staff. Therefore the same protection methods (PPE, see the section on Receiving and sorting) should be used in handling soiled linens as described for instruments. Any textiles that may have been exposed to patients, whether used or not, are assumed to be contaminated. Standard or universal precautions are always recommended when handling such items.

The reprocessing process with textiles needs to consider safety (to staff and patients), ensuring cleaning is adequate to remove visible staining, disinfection/sterilization requirements, but also that they are of acceptable quality to ensure patient comfort and textile durability. Surgical laundry, such as gowns, drapes and surgical towels should be separated from general hospital. If textiles are heavily contaminated as much organic material as possible must be rinsed off before placing it into the machine with other washing. The type and cause of stains will affect acceptance or rejection of laundered items. For example, linen with stains from substances, such as lubricants, blood, or body fluids, that cannot be removed, may affect the sterilization process and patient safety and should be rejected. Chemical stains such as methylene blue may appear unsightly but will not necessarily affect the functioning of the textile. A stain protocol should be in place establishing stain acceptance and rejection criteria.

Cleaning and disinfection of textiles (laundering) is usually conducted in specialized washer-disinfectors that can be single-chamber, multi-chamber or, commonly, tunnel washer-disinfectors (Figure 8.30). A typical cycle

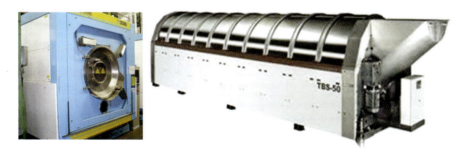

Figure 8.30 Examples of a single-chamber and tunnel washer-disinfectors used for textiles.

will include cold water pre-cleaning, cleaning, rinsing, disinfection and removal of water/drying. Drying may be included in the same machine, or in a separate unit. Depending on the institution the laundry may be an in-house department (separate to or part of a central reprocessing area) or an off-site facility, which often combines general-use and surgical textiles laundry. The textiles may also be owned by either the laundry (therefore on loan) or the medical facility. A variety of cleaning chemistries may be used, similar to those described in the section on Basic principles of cleaning, including neutral, alkaline and enzymatic-based Chemical disinfection Chapter 9 chemistries. Alkaline and enzymatic chemistries are typically used; in both cases adequate rinsing (and in the case of some alkaline chemistries, correct neutralization with an acid) is important to reduce risks of skin irritation on clinical use. ther accessory chemicals may be used for the conditioning the textile loadDisinfection is performed by thermal (>60°C) and/or chemical means (<60°C, e.g. using ozone or peracetic acid under controlled temperature conditions; Chapter 9, in the section on Chemical disinfection).

The following guidelines are given regarding the reprocessing, including cleaning, of linens and textiles:

• Similar to other devices, textile items can be provided as single use or multiple use. "Textiles" are often used to described re-usable items, while "non-wovens" refer to single use. Single-use items are designed to be discarded when used/soiled and are not recommended to be reprocessed.

• Facility staff (including those using, transporting and reprocessing textiles) should work closely together to set standards and allocate responsibilities. A facility has a health and safety responsibility to ensure that there are clear separation and handling procedures for soiled/used materials and clean materials ready for patient use. Decisions should be made regarding what type of laundry equipment and how many systems will be needed to process the anticipated volume, who will be responsible for transporting both soiled and unsoiled items and how they will be transported, who will be responsible for inspecting textiles, who will assemble packs, and whether the laundry or the healthcare facility will store new or uncirculated textiles.

• Re-usable textiles should be separated from instruments and single use items at the point of use. Particular care should be taken to remove any sharp devices, which can be a risk to laundry staff. All masking/autoclave tape should also be removed from the textiles prior to returning them to the laundry.

• Standard/universal safety precautions should be followed when handling contaminated textiles, including the use of personal protective equipment (PPE). Hand washing facilities, including a hygienic sink, soap dispensers and paper towels, must be provided in the soiled-textile laundry. The laundry facility should be designed to have a barrier or functional separation between areas in which soiled textiles are received/reprocessed and areas in which cleaned textiles are handled, stored and or sterilized for distribution to the facility.

• Soiled textiles should be sorted and checked before being loaded into the washer, to prevent damage to machines from other materials (such as paper, sharps and instruments). Some textiles that are heavily soiled may require pre-washing, pre-wetting or the use of a pre-soak chemical to prevent staining.

• Laundry washer-disinfectors are currently excluded from the scope of the international standard for washer-disinfectors (ISO 15883), but many of the requirements included in these standards are equally applicable to laundry applications. These include verifying the correct dosing of chemicals (including cleaning chemistries), verification of temperature control/distribution, correct rinsing, etc.

• As in cleaning of instruments, the way the washers (and dryers) are loaded is also important; if they are not loaded correctly, are overloaded or sometimes under-loaded, it may affect the process. An example is the exposure of all surfaces to the cleaning chemistry: if overloaded there may be insufficient water/chemistry to be effective or lack of sufficient contact for cleaning and if under-loaded, in washers that are calibrated with a given level of chemistry to handle a given load, there may be over-use of chemistry and inadequate rinsing.

• Drying is an important consideration, as the presence of moisture will allow for the growth of microorganisms (bacteria and fungi) on storage of textiles and particularly if these materials are not packaged and sterilized for use. This may be assisted by hot air drying and ironing.

• Inspection of laundered materials should include inspection for cleaning and particularly staining. Textiles can be visually inspected, with the assistance of a light table, for stains, physical defects, foreign debris, labels/tape, against a written quality procedure/standard. Although stained materials may be safe for use, they may be unacceptable to patients/staff. If applicable, the critical zones of gowns, drapes, table covers and sterilization wraps should be particularly inspected. Stains must be removed if possible, holes must be repaired with heat patches, foreign debris (hair, lint) must be removed, labels, etc., removed and tapes on gowns repaired.

• In some cases, materials are separated and packaged for sterilization; these processes should follow the same guidelines as for instruments (Chapters 10 and 11).

• Cleaned/disinfected textiles must be protected from contaminants in the environment, including during transportation and storage to avoid re-contamination. Unwrapped textiles should be placed into transport carts or hampers and covered for transport to a designated area for storage. If the transport cart does not have a solid bottom, it should be lined with heavy plastic before placing clean textiles inside. Barrier packaging may also be used to prevent accidental soiling on transport/storage.

• During storage, unwrapped textiles should be handled as little as possible and be placed preferably in a positive pressure, temperature controlled (68–98°F), properly ventilated area with limited access in order to prevent accumulation of dust and lint. Shelves for clean textiles should be typically 2.5–5 cm (~1–2 inches) from the wall, 15–20 cm (~6–8 inches) from the floor; and 30–46 cm (~12–18 inches) below the ceiling; textiles should never be stored on the floor.

Cleaning guidelines, standards and testing

There are a variety of cleaning guidelines and standards that are used in specific countries and internationally; a number of these are summarized in Table 8.3. Decontamination staff and managers should be familiar with any local, area or country guidelines and standards that apply to their facility; in the absence of specific guidelines, consider the use of international standards and guidance as provided in this and other references.

A particular series of standards apply internationally to washer-disinfectors, being the ISO 15883 series. They define the minimum design, performance and testing requirements for a washer-disinfector. At the time of writing the series includes six parts:

• Part 1: general requirements, definitions and tests. This standard is applicable to all washer-disinfectors and should be used in conjunction with the applicable other standards for specific types of washer.

• Part 2: requirements and tests for washer-disinfectors employing thermal disinfection for surgical instruments, anesthetic equipment, hollow articles, utensils, glassware, etc.

• Part 3: requirements and tests for washer-disinfectors employing thermal disinfection for human waste containers. Examples include bed-pan washers.

• Part 4: requirements and tests for washer-disinfectors employing chemical disinfection for thermo-labile endoscopes. This part considers the reprocessing of flexible endoscopes (that use chemical disinfection).

• Part 5: test soils and methods for demonstrating cleaning efficacy of washer-disinfectors. This is an information document (known as a technical specification) that provides information about various methods used around the world to test cleaning efficacy.

• Part 6: requirements and tests for washer-disinfectors employing thermal disinfection for non-invasive, non-critical medical devices and healthcare equipment. An example would be a cart-washer.

Further parts are under development. Each standard describes the necessary requirements for the design, performance and validation of the washer-disinfector, including cleaning. Design requirements include the mechanical, electrical, safety and control components. Performance requirements include how the washer should perform for cleaning, as well as for disinfection, rinsing and drying (if appropriate). These requirements are tested by the manufacturer and also confirmed (validated) by testing a washer-disinfector when installed into a facility. Further testing is also recommended to be performed routinely or periodically, to ensure that the equipment is operating correctly. Various checks and tests should be determined with the washer manufacturer, but the following are given as a guide:

• Daily tests:
  ○ Check devices are visually clean.
  ○ Check that any nozzles, flow attachments, filters and rotating spray arms (in the machine and on racks) are clean/freeflowing.
  ○ Inspect door seals.
  ○ Confirm that the correct type and volume of chemistry is available for the day.
  ○ Manually clean around the areas, including any carts/conveyors/loading areas are not left soiled.
  ○ Check print-outs (including paper available) and/or associated computers collecting cycle data are working (where relevant).

• Routine tests (these may be quarterly, six monthly, and/or yearly tests):
  ○ Calibration of various washer instruments, such as thermometers, pressure sensors, dosing systems, etc.
  ○ Washing tests, including chemistry dosing and cleaning studies.

Table 8.3 Various internationally used cleaning guidelines and standards. This list is only an example of some of the most widely used documents: it should also be noted that these standards/guidances are periodically updated/revised.

Guideline/standard	Title	Description
ISO 15883 series	*Washer-disinfectors*	A series of standards describing the design, performance and testing of washer-disinfectors, including cleaning requirements. Provided in a series, Part 1 (*General requirements, terms and definitions and tests*) describes the requirements for all washer-disinfectors and subsequent parts provide more details on specific types of machines (e.g. surgical instruments and flexible endoscopes).
ISO 17664	*Sterilization of medical devices – information to be provided by the manufacturer for the processing of resterilizable medical devices*	Specifies information to be provided by the device manufacturer on the reprocessing of re-usable medical devices including preparation at the point of use, preparation and cleaning.
ASTM E2314	*Standard test method for determination of effectiveness of cleaning processes for re-usable medical instruments using a microbiologic method (simulated use test)*	Test for the effectiveness of a cleaning process for re-usable instruments artificially contaminated with mixtures of microorganisms and simulated soil.
ISO 9398 series	*Specifications for industrial laundry machines*	Series of standards on laundry machines, including definitions, testing of capacity and consumption characteristics. For example, Part 3 considers washing tunnels and Part 4 washer-extractors.
ANSI/AAMI ST65 (USA)	*Processing of re-usable surgical textiles for use in healthcare facilities*	Guidelines for the proper handling, reprocessing, and preparation of re-usable surgical textiles, including cleaning. Addresses on-site and off-site recommendations.
AS/NZS 4187	*Cleaning, disinfecting and sterilizing re-usable medical and surgical instruments and equipment, and maintenance of associated environments in healthcare facilities*	Recommendations on the reprocessing of devices, including textiles including sorting, cleaning and safety aspects.
AS/NZS 4815	*Office-based healthcare facilities not involved in complex patient procedures and processes – cleaning, disinfecting and sterilizing re-usable medical and surgical instruments and equipment, and maintenance of the associated environment*	Similar to AZ/NZS 4187 but with an emphasis on office-based (including outpatient) facilities. Includes recommendations on cleaning and associated facilities.
AAMI TIR 30 (USA)	*A compendium of processes, materials, test methods, and acceptance criteria for cleaning re-usable medical devices*	Guideline regarding test protocols, test soils and acceptance criteria to validate cleaning processes for re-usable devices.
AAMI TIR 12 (USA)	*Designing, testing and labeling re-usable medical devices for reprocessing in healthcare facilities: a guide for medical device manufacturers*	Similar to ISO 17664, providing guidance to device manufacturers on developing and testing cleaning processes, including requirements at the point of use, preparation and cleaning.
AORN (USA)		Recommended operating room practices for cleaning and care of surgical instruments and powered equipment.
SGNA (USA)	*Standards for infection control and reprocessing of flexible gastrointestinal endoscopes*	Includes recommendations and guidelines on the care, handling and cleaning of flexible endoscopes.

Table 8.3 (*cont'd*).

Guideline/standard	Title	Description
IAHCSMM (USA)	*Central service technical manual*	A comprehensive guide to reprocessing of re-usable devices, including preparation and cleaning/cleaning processes.
CAN/CSA-Z314.8 (Canada)	*Decontamination of re-usable medical devices*	A Canadian standard describing safe handling, transportation and biological decontamination of contaminated re-usable devices. Biological decontamination includes thorough cleaning and disinfection.
ESGE	*Guidelines on cleaning and disinfection in GI endoscopy*	Includes recommendations and guidelines on the care, handling and cleaning of flexible endoscopes.
HTM 2030 (UK)	*Washer-disinfectors*	Gives guidance on the choice, specification, purchase, installation, validation, periodic testing, operation and maintenance of washer-disinfectors.
HTM 01-05 (UK)	*Decontamination in primary care dental practices*	Recommended decontamination processes, including cleaning in dental practices.
BSG	*Guidelines for decontamination of equipment for gastrointestinal endoscopy, British Society of Gastroenterology*	Includes recommendations and guidelines on the care, handling and cleaning of flexible endoscopes.

○ Thermometric test for thermal disinfection.
○ Water quality tests (note, washers can use up to three different sources of water: cold, hot and treated, e.g. deionized or reverse osmosis water).
○ Check for wear-and-tear on various washer parts (including seals, pumps, racks and other accessories).
○ Security and settings of door safety switches and interlocks.

While such testing is often carried out with washers, little to no testing is conducted with manual cleaning, which can often lead to concerns on the safety of such processes. It is recommended to minimize any risks with manual cleaning by ensuring that written procedures are given, staff are periodically trained, tools are provided to minimize any variables (such as personal protective equipment, automated chemistry dosing and sinks with indicated water volume levels) and regular auditing of manual cleaning practices is conducted.

Cleaning is generally tested by looking at the devices for any signs of soil (visual inspection); this can be often enhanced using a magnifying glass (Figure 8.31). Rigorous inspection of devices is recommended at a minimum to ensure devices are correctly cleaned and fit for further reprocessing or patient use.

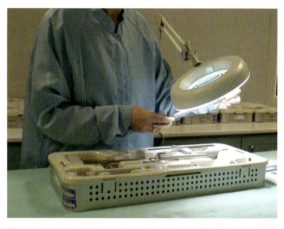

Figure 8.31 Visual inspection of a device set following a cleaning process.

Ensuring a consistent cleaning process provides a further level of security that sufficient cleaning has been performed. For manual cleaning, this can be encouraged by having written protocols, well-trained staff and periodic audit. Greater assurance can be provided with washers and washer-disinfectors by monitoring various process parameters (including temperature, pressure, chemical

Table 8.4 Various types of test soils used for testing cleaning efficacy[1].

Test soil/country	Components	Uses
German test soil (Germany)	Test pieces (screws and tubes) contaminated with blood, semolina pudding or egg yolk test soils and *Enterococcus faecium*	General surgical instruments, glassware and anesthesia equipment
Austrian test soil (Austria)	Heparinized blood test soil	General surgical instruments
KMNE test soil (Austria)	Nigrosine, plain flour, eggs, instant potato flakes	Bed-pan washers
French test method (France)	Tubing contaminated with a *Pseudomonas aeruginosa* biofilm	Flexible endoscope washers
Swedish test method (Sweden)	Citrated blood with $CaCl_2$	Surgical instruments, wash bowls, bed-pans, urine bottles, anesthesia equipment, baby bottles and suction bottles
Edinburgh test soil (UK)	Egg yolk, defibrinated blood, dehydrated hog mucin	Surgical instruments, surgical instrument trays, bowls, dishes and receivers
Hucker's test soil (UK)	Glycerol, horse serum, dehydrated hog mucin, unbleached plain, safranine	Flexible endoscopes
ASTM E2314	Mixtures of microorganisms (including and with an emphasis on bacterial spores) and simulated organic soil; soils types are not specified	Re-usable instruments, with an emphasis on lumened devices (such as flexible endoscopes)

[1] Based on Washer-disinfectors – Part 5: test soils and methods for demonstrating cleaning efficacy of washer-disinfectors.

dosing, etc.); however, these do not replace the need for correct staff training, audits and device inspections.

An area of increased discussion internationally is the need for standardized methods to define cleaning endpoints. As mentioned at the beginning of this chapter, visually clean is the only consistent endpoint currently used, but others that have been used include biochemical, chemical or even microbiological endpoints. It should be noted that most of these methods of assessing the efficacy of cleaning are laboratory based and are generally not considered to be routinely used in healthcare facilities. Examples include the detection of protein, carbon or microorganisms on surfaces following a cleaning process. These are primarily used by manufacturers (or devices, materials, washers and cleaning chemistries) to assess cleaning on or with their various products. Despite this, some tools and methods are being recommended and used to assess cleaning in healthcare facilities; these include:

• Defined types of cleaning soils that are used to soil devices and then tested for being clean after a cleaning process. ISO

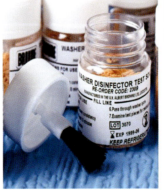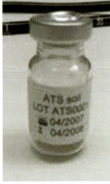

Figure 8.32 Two types of commercially available test soils.

15883-5, in its current form, describes the various types of soils that are used around the world for testing cleaning. Examples include Edinburgh, Hucker's, Blood and Austrian test soils (Table 8.4). Most of these are made up from given recipes, but a few are available commercially (Figure 8.32).

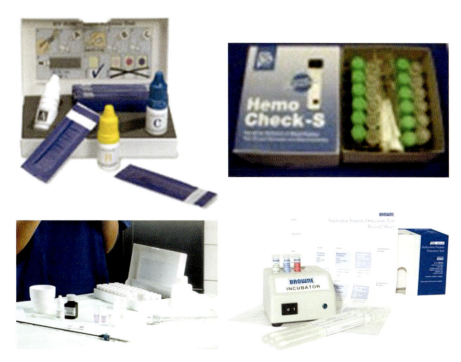

Figure 8.33 Various types of soil detection kits.

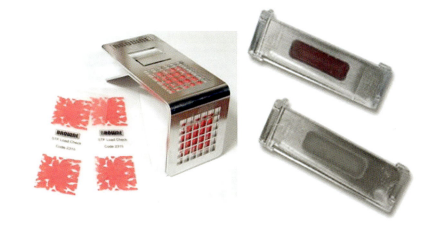

Figure 8.34 Various types of cleaning indicators used to test cleaning performance.

• Detection kits are used for the specific identification of certain components of soils, such as protein, blood and ATP (a molecule found in most living cell-based materials). An example is the use of a chemical called ninhydrin that reacts with protein and when heated gives a purple color. These often give lower detection levels than are visually observed (Figure 8.33).

• Cleaning indicators (Figure 8.34). These are defined surfaces (e.g. stainless steel or plastics) that have a known amount of soil applied and dried. They are used to test the efficacy of cleaning in washer or washer-disinfectors. It should be noted, as for all types of indicators, that they can be used to ensure that a cleaning process has taken place, but cannot ensure that the devices in the process are clean.

Troubleshooting cleaning problems

Inadequate cleaning is a common problem in the reprocessing of devices/materials. This may be observed directly by the presence of visual soil or by using other more sensitive soil detection methods (e.g. protein detection). This is usually detected on inspection following cleaning disinfection, but may also unfortunately be detected at the point of use. In both cases the device or devices will be rejected for further reprocessing or use; this is often monitored by the reprocessing facility as a rejection rate (the number of devices rejected compared to the number reprocessed). Rejection rates should be minimized and rejected items investigated for potential causes. Any rejected devices will need to be re-cleaned and subjected to further reprocessing before clinical use, which in some cases can lead to patient procedure delays and even cancellations. The most common causes of inadequate cleaning with automated washers are:

• Overloaded baskets/trays allowing some items to shadow others from spray jets (e.g. a bowl placed over instruments).

• Devices not disassembled according to instructions or not placed in the optimum position for cleaning. A typical example is with hinged instruments that are not opened prior to washing, thereby not allowing cleaning to occur within the joint. If certain hinged instrument designs are constantly being rejected, despite being placed in the open position, these devices may require specific manual pre-cleaning or disassembly.

• Inadequate maintenance of immersion/ultrasonic bath, including build-up of soil in the bath that is carried over on the device to a subsequent reprocessing stage.

• Blocked spray jets and/or spray arms that are not free to rotate. These should be periodically checked. A common problem is that the washer racks are not correctly aligned/attached to the water flow system within the washer.

• No cleaning chemistry used (e.g. dosing system is broken or chemistry has run out). This may or may not be detected by the washer-disinfector.

• Blocked strainer in the chamber base, leading to inadequate draining from the chamber and spray patterns for cleaning.

• Soiled instruments that have been stored for prolonged periods with no pre-cleaning or pre-treatment. Blood, protein and other materials can become fixed and coagulated when dried, making soil difficult to remove.

• Inadequate cleaning cycle design: this can include many variables such as pre-cleaning, subjecting devices to high temperatures (45°C) prior to cleaning (allowing soil to be fixed onto the device), cleaning chemistry (type, concentration, temperature and exposure time) and inadequate rinsing.

• The water quality being used (for cleaning and rinsing): the formulation of the cleaning chemistry should be able to work under good or bad water qualities, but this is formulation-specific. Water hardness (scale) is a particular concern and is often detected by the presence of "spotting" or a white, grainy deposit on device surfaces. It can only be removed by treatment with an acid or acidic-based chemistry (Chapter 6, see the section on Non enzyme based cleaners).

• Soils can be from the patient, various chemicals used during or following the procedure on the device or even from the reprocessing cycle itself. Care should be taken to inspect for the presence of patient soil compared to other materials that may be present. The methods used to remove the problem can be different. In the case of patient soil or chemical such as iodine, these should be removed by repeating the normal cleaning process. Other soils will not remove by repeating the normal cleaning process, with examples being the development of rust, water hardness and presence of cement. The first two are generally water quality concerns, although rusting can be promoted by aggressive cleaning or other chemicals used on the device (in particular low quality stainless steel devices). Rusting may often be mistaken as being dried blood, as they can have the same brown appearance; a simple test for rusting (and hardness deposits) is to place a small amount of an acid cleaner onto the material and it should quickly dissolve, while patient soil will not. Both can be removed using an acid-based chemistry, but this only hides the problem and will persist unless the water quality is improved and/or better cleaning chemistries are used. Cement is a particular concern with orthopedic devices, as when it dries it becomes very hard on a surface; it is recommended that cement deposits should be removed at the site of a patient procedure, as when it sets it may only be removed by chipping off the surface (also assisted by an acid cleaner) that may damage the device. Overall, in many cases inadequate cleaning rates can be reduced by staff training for both manual and automated cleaning procedures. This may not only include the correct handling and inspection of the device but also any of the tools used for cleaning (chemistries, machines, loading systems, etc.). Other problems, such as persistently high rejection rates, appearance of chemical deposits and device damage may require more detailed analysis of the cleaning process in place and the variables associated with that process.

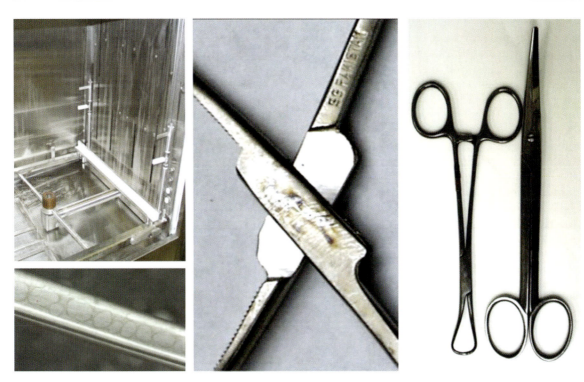

Figure 8.35 Examples of various types of surface changes commonly observed following cleaning, disinfection and sterilization processes. They include water hardness deposition (far left, seen as white precipitate in a washer-disinfector and "spotting" on a device surface), rusting (centre) and staining (black staining on stainless steel devices, on the right).

In addition to inadequate cleaning, various surface changes can be observed following a cleaning process (Figure 8.35).

Note, that many of these problems will be seen following cleaning, disinfection and/or sterilization. A simple process of elimination can be used to investigate such problems. For example, if rusting is not observed following cleaning and disinfection (on inspection prior to packaging), but appears to be present on a device presented to a theatre this potentially highlights a problem with a steam sterilization process. Another example is the sudden occurrence of a problem, when the cleaning and other reprocessing steps have remained unchanged; this often highlights a problem with variable water quality that can actually change from day to day with a facility. These surface changes include:

• Milky white to grey, grainy deposits or films. This is typically an indication of high hardness levels in water being used for cleaning or rinsing. Hardness (or scale) refers to the concentration of calcium and magnesium ions in water (measured chemically as parts per million (ppm) or milligrams per litre (mg/L) $CaCO_3$). Water can have high concentrations of hardness (e.g. over 400 ppm) without being seen, but such high concentrations will precipitate out when heated. It may also be otherwise colored (e.g. appearing more green or brown due to the presence of other metals such as copper in the water that precipitate with the hardness). At lower concentrations, hardness may appear as "spotting" or brown rings on a dried device surface. To reduce these effects, hardness levels in water of ≤150 mg/L $CaCO_3$ are recommended for cleaning. In some countries ≤10 mg/L is recommended for water used for disinfection/final rinsing.

• Reddish brown, partial discolorations, crater-shaped or pinhole-type impressions on the device surrounded by brown or multi-colored, edges. These are the hallmarks of corrosion or rusting; rusting is a visual sign of surface damage and particularly on stainless steel devices. The main cause of rusting is the presence of chlorine (but also other halogens such as iodine and bromine) that can be present in patient soil (e.g. in blood), water and other solutions (such as iodophors used in theaters and physiological saline which is sodium chloride, NaCl). High levels of chlorine in water are a common concern, particularly when heated. Typical recommended chlorine levels for cleaning should be ≤120 mg/L. Chloride concentrations greater that 240 mg/l chlorine can be very damaging to stainless steel and plastic surfaces, with higher temperatures being more aggressive at even lower concentrations (in the 10–120 mg/L range). Other causes can be due to wear-and-tear (e.g. in hinge mechanisms) and aggressive cleaning chemistries (especially acid chemistries).

• Multicolored stain (often seen as a rainbow effect including yellow, brownish, blue and violet) covering large areas or drop-shaped or irregular, insular shapes are usually due to increased content of silicates in water, particularly final rinse water. This can also be seen on stainless steel devices on exposure to excessive (often dry) heat.

• Whitish grey corrosion or deposits on surface of carbon steel and naturally anodized aluminium. This is usually due to incorrect chemical (e.g. strong acid or alkaline chemistries) being used on such devices that are incompatible with such metals. In these cases, cleaning products that are labeled as being "aluminum-safe" should be used, such as neutral and mild alkaline cleaners (depending on the formulation and specific manufacturers' claims).

• Orange-brown staining: often due to high levels of phosphates in the water or even sometimes associated with the cleaning chemistry.

• Black staining: typically due to levels of acid remaining on device surfaces (e.g. when used for neutralization of an alkaline cleaner or for removing of rust in manual cleaning).

• Other types of deposits, including white or otherwise colored grainy films observed on drying. These may be simply due to residual chemistries remaining on the device because of inadequate rinsing; when dried the chemistry remains. Close attention should be paid to rinsing post-cleaning. In contrast to hardness deposits, these should be easily dissolved/removed with water alone. In some cases, white spots can be due to high levels of silicates or sulphites in water used for reprocessing.

Although these are the most common problem associated with cleaning, other staining can be observed after steam sterilization, such as any of the above associated with water (used to make steam) or purple/black stains (due to overdosing of amines often used to prevent corrosion of steam lines) and gold-tinting (from chlorine and other chemicals present in water treatments systems).

As many of these problems are associated with water, the quality of water used for the various stages of reprocessing is an important consideration and is further discussed in Chapter 15, in the section on water quality/purity.

9   Disinfection

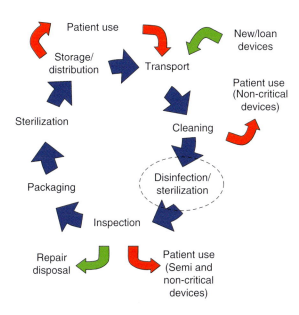

Introduction

Disinfection is defined as the antimicrobial reduction of microorganisms on a surface to a level determined to be appropriate for its intended further handling or use. A disinfectant is a product or/process used for this effect. In this chapter, disinfection of re-usable devices is addressed. During the decontamination cycle, devices may be subjected to cleaning, disinfection and/or sterilization prior to patient use (Chapter 1, see the section on the decontamination process). Some consideration is also given to the various types of disinfectants used for other, general surface applications. Microorganisms remaining on devices can lead to patient infections. Antimicrobial products and or processes such as disinfection are

designed to reduce these risks when using devices or materials with patients, as well as to protect staff handling these devices. As introduced in Chapter 1, re-usable devices can provide different levels of risks to a patient and therefore various levels of disinfection or even sterilization are recommended to reduce these risks (as summarized in Figure 9.1).

In the reprocessing cycle, disinfection should follow cleaning (Chapter 8). Cleaning itself can significantly reduce the number of microorganisms on a re-usable device, but can only be considered as the sole treatment for non-critical devices (those that may contact intact skin). Even in these cases, low or intermediate-level disinfectants are also often used (as part of or as a separate step to cleaning). A "high level" of disinfection is the recommended minimum requirement for semi-critical devices that can directly contact patient mucous membranes. The different levels of disinfection are considered further below. Disinfection is also used as a common step in the reprocessing of critical devices, for example in a washer-disinfector process with surgical devices to render the devices safe for handling during packaging. Other terms such as pasteurization (use of moist-heat disinfection) and antisepsis are forms of disinfection; other definitions such as sanitization may have local, specific definitions and care should be taken to understand the data provided to support any disinfectant product claims and local requirements (for further discussion see Chapter 6, in the section on disinfectants, including preservatives).

As introduced in Chapter 5, microorganisms consist of a wide range of viruses, bacteria, fungi, protozoa and helminths; they range in their resistance levels to disinfection, as summarized in Figure 9.2 (also introduced in Chapter 1 and Chapter 6, in the section on disinfectants, including preservatives). Different levels of disinfection

A Practical Guide to Decontamination in Healthcare, First Edition. Gerald McDonnell and Denise Sheard.
© 2012 Gerald McDonnell and Denise Sheard. Published 2012 by Blackwell Publishing Ltd.

Patient contact	Examples	Device classification	Minimum inactivation level
Intact skin	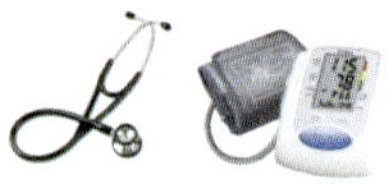	Non-critical	Cleaning and/or low/intermediate level disinfection
Mucous membranes or non-intact skin	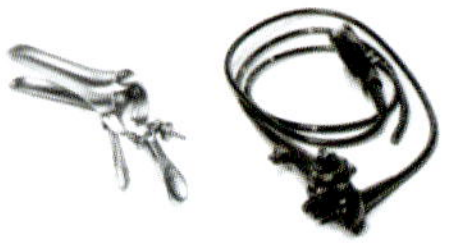	Semi-critical	High-level disinfection
Sterile areas of the body, including blood contact	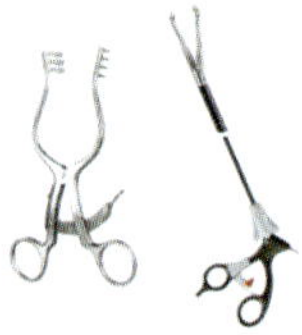	Critical	Sterilization

Figure 9.1 A summary of the Spaulding classification system, recommending various levels of disinfection or sterilization for the reprocessing of devices based on their potential risk to patients.

are traditionally defined based on their ability to inactivate such microorganisms. A common classification includes the designation of high, medium or low-level disinfection, being dependent on the types of microorganisms that they kill. Specific definitions of disinfection levels can vary from country to country, with a widely used example given in Table 9.1.

Sterilization is therefore the highest level of microbial inactivation; sterilization is more than the demonstration of a product to be effective to kill all types of microorganisms. It is the recommended minimum practice during the reprocessing of critical devices and the various thermal/chemical methods used in healthcare facilities are described in further detail in Chapter 11. According to this classification scheme, high-level disinfection is considered effective against the range of microorganisms, including mycobacteria and even has some activity against bacterial spores. Examples include disinfectants based on glutaraldehyde or peracetic acid, as well as moist heat processes at greater than or equal to ($\geq$) 90°C for one minute. A further term used is "chemical sterilant", describing a high-level disinfectant

that is effective against bacterial spores, but might require extended contact time for such activity; it can only be effective as a sterilant under those specific conditions that are recommended by the manufacturer. Intermediate-level disinfection includes activity against enveloped viruses, most fungi and non-enveloped viruses, and bacteria, but not necessarily mycobacteria. Due to their unusual structure, mycobacteria are highly resistant to disinfection in comparison to other types of bacteria (Chapter 5). Finally, low-level disinfection is also considered effective against enveloped viruses and most bacteria, but might only be practically active against some types of fungi and not more highly resistant forms such as non-enveloped viruses and mycobacteria.

These defined levels of microbial inactivation, and the types of microorganisms that a product is effective against, are (or should be) confirmed by identified test methods, such as those defined by the Association of Analytical Chemists (AOAC), the American Society for Testing and Materials (ASTM), the Comité Européen de Normalisation (CEN, French; translated as the European

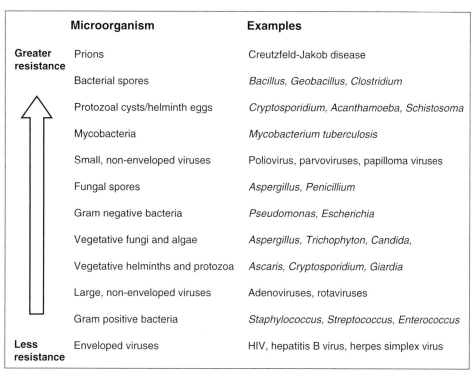

Microorganism	Examples
Greater resistance Prions	Creutzfeld-Jakob disease
Bacterial spores	*Bacillus, Geobacillus, Clostridium*
Protozoal cysts/helminth eggs	*Cryptosporidium, Acanthamoeba, Schistosoma*
Mycobacteria	*Mycobacterium tuberculosis*
Small, non-enveloped viruses	Poliovirus, parvoviruses, papilloma viruses
Fungal spores	*Aspergillus, Penicillium*
Gram negative bacteria	*Pseudomonas, Escherichia*
Vegetative fungi and algae	*Aspergillus, Trichophyton, Candida,*
Vegetative helminths and protozoa	*Ascaris, Cryptosporidium, Giardia*
Large, non-enveloped viruses	Adenoviruses, rotaviruses
Gram positive bacteria	*Staphylococcus, Streptococcus, Enterococcus*
Less resistance Enveloped viruses	HIV, hepatitis B virus, herpes simplex virus

Figure 9.2 The resistance of microorganisms to inactivation. Microorganisms are listed as being of lower (bottom) to higher resistance (top) to inactivation. This list is given as a guide only, as the actual level of resistance can vary depending on the disinfection/sterilization method used. For example, the designation of prions as showing the highest resistance is generally accepted, but is not always the case. Also, bacterial spores are often considered the most resistant to disinfection/sterilization, but in some special cases other types of microorganisms are equally or even more resistant. Certain types of microorganisms are not as well studied from a disinfection/sterilization point-of-view, but this list gives an estimate of what is known.

Table 9.1 A commonly used classification system for disinfectants, describing their different levels of efficacy against various forms of microorganisms. The definition of the specific disinfection levels and their requirements for efficacy can vary from country to country.

Microorganism	Sterilization	Disinfection		
		High	Intermediate	Low
Bacterial spores				
Mycobacteria				
Small, non-enveloped viruses				
Fungi				
Bacteria				
Enveloped viruses				

Committee for Standardization) and the Organization for Economic Cooperation and Development (OECD). In many countries such disinfectant claims are regulated by national agencies such as the US-FDA (for medical devices) and US-EPA (for environmental surfaces) in the United States and Therapeutic Goods Administration (TGA) in Australia; this is, however, not always the case. As different countries/regions can have different requirements, care should be taken to ensure that any disinfection/sterilization claims are substantiated and, if necessary, approved for use in that region/country. In addition to statements of effectiveness against specific microorganisms (e.g. "effective against HIV") or levels of disinfection, other commonly used terms with disinfectants include:

• –static, implying the ability of a product to inhibit the growth of a specific microorganism, for example "bacteriostatic", sporistatic or fungistatic.

• –cidal, implying the ability to kill a specific microorganism, for example "bactericidal".

• Bactericidal: ability to kill bacteria. This may often be misleading. It is clearly not possible to test all types of bacteria and so surrogates are generally selected. In the USA, a bactericidal claim is based on testing against three types of bacteria: *Staphylococcus aureus*, *Pseudomonas aeruginosa,* and *Salmonella enterica*. This is also specifically referred to as a "germicidal" claim. It does not, however, include mycobacteria.

• Mycobactericidal: ability to inactivate mycobacteria. In some regions this is different to specific tuberculocidal claims, referring specifically to a test method to confirm activity against *Mycobacterium tuberculosis*.

• Sporicidal: activity against bacterial spores. As bacterial spores (or more correctly "endospores") are generally considered as some of the more resistant microorganisms, this will generally imply activity against other dormant forms, in particular fungal spores. The test methods to verify sporicidal activity can range considerably from region to region.

• Virucidal: ability to inactivate viruses. There are two major types of viruses based on their resistance to disinfection (Chapter 5, in the section on viruses), enveloped (being relatively sensitive) and non-enveloped (demonstrating higher resistance). Non-enveloped viruses can be further sub-classified into large and small forms, based on their resistance profiles (Figure 5.2). Therefore, specific virucidal claims can vary, ranging from an individual virus tested (which may be enveloped but demonstrating low resistance) to a range of viruses (e.g. one test virus from each type/group).

• Fungicidal: ability to kill fungi.

• Other, less used, terms may include cysticidal (effective against specific types of protozoan cysts) and even priocidal (referring to reducing the risk of prion contamination).

Disinfection can be considered as physical or chemical in nature, though both can be employed together. The main types of antimicrobial methods are summarized with examples in Table 9.2. The most common physical methods are various forms of heat, including the use of hot water (also known as pasteurization). Other physical methods can include radioactive or light sources (e.g. UV-light); these are considered only briefly as they are rarely (if ever) used for the reprocessing or re-usable devices. Chemicals (chemical disinfectants) are widely

Table 9.2 Examples of disinfection and sterilization methods. These are given as examples only. Note that the formulation/use of a chemical disinfectant can have a dramatic effect on the activity of an antimicrobial chemical (biocide). Exposure time is also a critical variable and the manufacturer's written instructions (see product labels) must be followed.

Inactivation method	Examples
Sterilization	Physical: steam (e.g. at 121°C for 15 minutes or 134°C for 3 minutes)
	Chemical: ethylene oxide or hydrogen peroxide gas
High-level disinfection	Physical: moist/wet heat (e.g. hot water at 90°C for 1 minute), UV light
	Chemical: glutaraldehyde, peracetic acid, ortho-phathalaldehyde (OPA), sodium hypochlorite (chlorine), hydrogen peroxide
Intermediate-level disinfection	Physical: moist/wet heat (e.g. hot water at 80°C for 1 minute), UV light,
	Chemical: phenolics, sodium hypochlorite (bleach) (chlorine), iodophor, alcohols
Low-level disinfection	Chemical: quaternary ammonium compounds (also known as QACs/QUATs), alcohols

used for environmental surfaces (including many non-critical device surfaces) and device disinfection; they are also used as part of controlled processes for sterilization (Chapter 11). Chemical disinfectants are designed for use under specific conditions, which may include the correct control of various physical factors (such as temperature; the combination of a chemical/thermal process can be referred to a *chemo-thermal*).

Disinfectant and disinfection products are also provided or conducted in a variety of forms, such as:
• Boiling water baths.
• Washer-disinfectors, where disinfection can be achieved by chemical, thermal or thermo-chemical means.
• Concentrates that require dilution and/or suspension in water prior to use.
• Ready-to-use products that require no dilution prior to use.
• Wipe or cloth-impregnated disinfectants.
• Two (or more) component or activated disinfectants, requiring two or more parts to be mixed together to prepare the disinfectant (some products will require a certain "activation" time to allow the disinfectant chemistry to be generated prior to use).
• Electrochemically generated systems that generate the disinfectant from water/chemical mixtures.
In addition, as is typical with many high to low-level disinfectants, they can be designed for single or multiple use, depending on the product design and labeling. These terms are used to differentiate the use of a disinfectant for a particular application once (e.g. for the disinfection of a semi-critical device) and it is then discarded as in the case of single use, while multiple-use disinfectants are prepared (if applicable) and used for many applications and even over multiple days (as in the case of low, intermediate and high-level disinfectants).

Basic principles of disinfection

Disinfection products and processes are designed to reduce the level of microbial contamination on surfaces (but also in the air or water). Device disinfection is used to prepare a device for direct patient use or staff handling, and also as an intermediate step in the reprocessing cycle (e.g. prior to packaging and sterilization). This can range from the use of low or intermediate-level disinfectants to wipe down various types of equipment used medically with the patient such as blood pressure machines, monitors, etc., to high-level disinfectants and high temperature processes used to treat more critical

devices. The choice of disinfectant will depend on two major considerations:
• Efficacy or how effective a product is. As described in the introductory section in this chapter, this depends on the designation of the device as being critical, semi-critical and non-critical, and the ability of a disinfectant to inactivate various types of microorganisms. While low-level disinfectants have limited effectiveness to include enveloped viruses and most bacteria, high-level disinfectants or processes are expected to practically inactivate all forms of microorganisms with the exceptions of high numbers of bacterial spores (and unconventional agents such as prions).
• Safety, including primarily safety of the patient and protection of functionality of the device. An example of a patient safety consideration is in the use of a chemical disinfectant, where residuals of the chemical or its by-products remain on or within the device; these can lead to toxic problems in patients. Device safety is often referred to as compatibility, being the ability of a disinfectant to be used on the device but without damaging it. Compatibility (or indeed incompatibility) can be obvious following treatment or may only be observed over time. For this reason, it is highly recommended that any disinfectant being used on a device, particularly semi-critical and critical devices, is demonstrated to be safe for use on that device. A typical example is the description of a device being "thermo-sensitive" or "thermo-resistant"; thermo-sensitive devices are designed with components/materials that cannot tolerate high temperatures (generally greater than 60°C) that are required for thermal disinfection/sterilization. Such devices can only be reprocessed in low temperature disinfection/sterilization processes; common examples include flexible endoscopes (Chapter 15). Thermo-resistant devices are less restrictive, in particular they are able to withstand higher temperatures. Equally, many devices cannot tolerate certain types of chemicals or formulations due to negative effects on their materials of construction; examples can include the chemical compatibility of various types of adhesives (glues) that are used to bond materials together. Other safety considerations include any risks to those using the disinfectant (with close attention given to material safety data sheets (MSDSs), that should always be provided with the chemistry) and any environmental concerns (which is a growing issue in many parts of the world).
Efficacy and safety are the major considerations, but there are others. These include:
• Product design and practical considerations. Formulation plays a major role in the efficacy of a chemical

disinfectant (Chapter 6, Mixtures, formulations and solutions). Therefore, close attention should be paid to the product labeling (including any associated documentation provided by the manufacturer) to ensure that the product can be safely used for a given application. First, is the product designed for a particular application? Many disinfectants are to be used only on general, environmental surfaces and are not designed for device use. Second, how is it to be used: diluted, directly, activated and, particularly, for what exposure time? The product might be effective against a particular organism but may take an impractically long time to be effective. The concentration of the active chemicals (or biocide) in the product is important to ensure efficacy and safety, but so are other variables such as recommended exposure times, concentrations, temperatures, etc. Close attention should be given to the types of test methods that have been used to prove that the disinfectant is effective against various types of microorganisms; in some countries these claims are tightly controlled while in others they are not. Instructions on how the product is used are important; these should be provided by the manufacturer and closely followed by the user. Some products may only be designed for manual use, while others for automated disinfection. In manual type applications care should be taken to ensure that all surfaces of the devices (particularly internal surfaces) are fully exposed to the disinfectant for the required exposure time/conditions. As with other chemistries, the choice of a disinfectant or process may also depend on its esthetic qualities (e.g. smell is often a concern in manual disinfection).

• Regulatory approvals: is the product/process approved for use in a general country/region. Note that because a product is available for sale it does not mean that it meets the legal requirements of the country/area!

• Product efficacy variables: these include the concentration, temperature, mode of preparation/use, exposure time, etc., that can all significantly influence the effectiveness. Low temperatures can decrease product efficacy, depending on the design; temperature control is essential in the case of thermal washer-disinfectors. Equally, low concentrations of chemical disinfectants can be ineffective but may also allow bacteria/fungi to grow within the formulation; this can be a particular concern in multiple-use disinfectants, where, particularly for semi-critical applications, indicators are available to check that the product is capable of disinfection.

• Water quality: water quality can affect the outcome of physical and chemical disinfection. Some chemical disinfectants can essentially lose their activity if the water quality is inadequate; this should always be clearly stated in the instructions for use/labeling of a disinfectant.

Thermo-chemical disinfection can also cause some concerns, for example the presence of high levels of chlorine when heated can cause significant damage (pitting/corrosion) to stainless steel surfaces and damage other types of materials. The impact of water quality is considered in further detail in Chapter 15.

• Staff training: disinfectants, physical and chemical, are designed to kill microorganisms and can therefore have immediate or even long-term effects to staff on exposure. Essentially there is no such thing as a "safe" disinfectant and all products/processes should be treated with caution. Staff should be trained in using the disinfectant safely and effectively. This will include, where applicable, the preparation, handling, use (or re-use), rinsing, checking and disposal of the product. Care should be taken so that the correct PPE and environment is provided to ensure staff safety; examples can include ventilation, safety cabinets, accidental spill procedures, access to water, etc. This is particularly important in manual disinfection. As highlighted previously, automated processes can provide greater assurance, but staff need to be trained on their use and equipment needs to be maintained and serviced according to manufacturers' guidelines.

It should be noted that all of these considerations apply not only to disinfection, but are also important for cleaning or sterilization processes. It is clear that close attention should be paid to reading and understanding the instructions for use, labeling and associated materials provided with a product and/or process used for disinfection.

Disinfectants can be classified in many ways, with the most common including:

• The type of antimicrobial agent, usually classified as being physical or chemical. This classification is considered in further detail in the following sections of this chapter.

• Sterilization or various levels of disinfection for critical, semi-critical and non-critical devices; the use of a disinfectant/sterilant for these applications has been considered in the introduction to this chapter. Note: the use of a disinfectant for these applications will depend on its associated labeling; if the product is not described for use for particular medical applications then it should not be used for that purpose. A common example is the use of antiseptics (disinfectants designs for use on the skin/mucous membranes) being mistakenly used to disinfectant devices used on patients because they are considered medical-grade. If the product is not labeled for purpose it is not fit for purpose!

• Manual or automated disinfection. Examples of manual disinfection include the use of disinfectant impregnated wipes and soaks, while automated are most commonly washer-disinfectors.

Physical disinfection

Physical methods of disinfection include heat (thermal disinfection), radiation and filtration. Heat can include dry (hot air) heating and moist/wet heat (essentially hot water). Wet heat methods are the most commonly used and reliable methods of disinfection, for example in thermal washer-disinfectors or boiling water baths. All other physical methods, including dry heat, radiation methods and filtration are less used for device disinfection but may often be used as part of another process; these are discussed later in this chapter.

Moist/wet heat disinfection

Hot water is a very effective and simple disinfection method. Most microorganisms, with the exclusion of heat-resistant bacterial spores are inactivated at temperatures in excess of 65°C; however, the intrinsic resistance of various types of microorganisms can vary depending on the temperature. Most bacteria and fungi, in their vegetative form, are unable to grow at temperatures greater that 45°C (113°F) and are inactivated at ~60–65°C (140–149°F). This is essentially the basis of pasteurization methods that are widely used to treat liquid foods, including milk (e.g. 65°C for 30 minutes). Most viruses are inactivated at this range but some have been shown to be more resistant (e.g. requiring 70–80°C (158–176°F) to be inactivated). These direct high temperature effects cause the coagulation and loss of structure/function of the various parts that make up microorganisms (Chapter 5).

It is widely accepted that heat disinfection is based on a time-temperature relationship: essentially as the temperature increases, less time is required for disinfection. Therefore, examples of thermal disinfection conditions used for the reprocessing of surgical devices will include:

80°C (176°F) for 10 minutes
90°C (194°F) for 1 minute
100°C (212°F) for 0.1 minute

Such time-temperature relationships are used to define the disinfection conditions for immersion disinfection and washer-disinfectors. An example is the A_0 concept described in the ISO 15883 series of standards for washer-disinfectors. The A_0 is defined as the equivalent time (in seconds) at a temperature of 80°C (176°F) for disinfection; this definition is with reference to microorganisms with a z value of 10°C (the z value is a concept further discussed in steam sterilization, which is also based on time-temperature relationships; Chapter 11, Steam (moist heat) sterilization). It is mathematically given as:

$$A_0 = \sum 10^{[(T-80)/z]} \times \Delta t$$

where
A_0 is the A value when z is 10°C;
t is the chosen time interval, in seconds;
T is the temperature in the load, in degrees Celsius.
A minimum temperature of 65°C (149°F) is required under this concept. From this concept, recommended levels of disinfection are given in various parts of ISO 15883 and times/temperatures can then be applied in order to provide these levels (Table 9.3). Essentially, as the exposure temperature increases, the time for disinfection decrease (Table 9.3). It should be noted that where temperatures are over 65°C within such disinfection processes that reaching the defined minimum temperature and also cooling down below 65°C after the defined exposure time will contribute to the overall disinfection efficacy (a summary of this is shown in graph form in Figure 9.3).

In defining such a disinfection process, it is important to consider that the water temperature alone is not sufficient to confirm a thermal disinfection process; the temperature distribution in the exposure chamber and particularly the load to be disinfected need to be within the required temperature ranges during a disinfection process.

Thermal disinfection of devices is usually conducted by a water immersion or spray method (Figure 9.4). Water immersion, where devices are immersed into hot water for a given period of time, was a common method but is less used today. It is still an effective method, but

Table 9.3 Examples of A_0 values and their practical application in disinfection processes.

Device types	Disinfection level	A_0[1]	Examples
Non-critical, e.g. bedpans, wash bowls, carts	Low or intermediate	60	80°C (176°F) × 1 minute 90°C (194°F) × 6 seconds
Semi-critical or critical, e.g. surgical instruments	High	600	80°C (176°F) × 10 minutes 90°C (194°F) × 1 minute 100°C (212°F) × 6 seconds

[1] The minimum recommended A_0 is in accordance to ISO 15883.

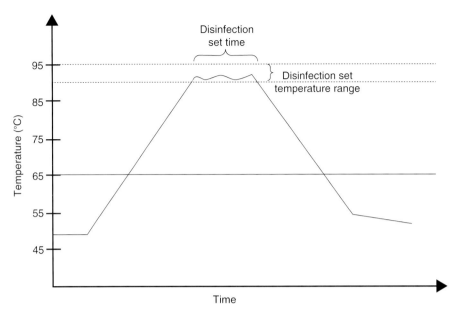

Figure 9.3 An example of a thermal disinfection process in a washer-disinfector. Thermal disinfection is based on a time-temperature relationship; the graph shows this relationship with the time on the X (horizontal) axis and temperature on the Y (vertical) axis. The temperature over time is plotted during the disinfection cycle. In this example, a minimum disinfection time and temperature is set (at 90°C, but in a range of 90–95°C; dotted lines). Under these conditions, the minimal A_0 is based on the time at the set temperature of 90°C, but the actual A_0 can be determined based on the amount of time at each temperature above 65°C (solid line across the graph).

care should be taken to ensure that the water temperature and exposure time are controlled and that air bubbles do not collect at the device surface. The safe handling of devices during or following disinfection is important, to ensure that staff are not burned during the process of placing and removing devices in the bath and that devices are not re-contaminated following the process (particularly if being prepared directly for patient use). Spray-type methods are used in many types of washer-disinfectors for thermal disinfection (Figure 9.4). Washer-disinfectors are defined as machines intended to clean and disinfect devices and other articles. They are widely used in medical, dental, pharmaceutical and veterinary practice. They have already been introduced and discussed in detail in Chapter 8 for automated cleaning. They are provided in a variety of sizes and designs, ranging from smaller bench-top or under counter disinfectors, to larger free-standing machines (Figure 9.4). With emphasis on thermal disinfection in washer-disinfectors, water is generally introduced into the load chamber, circulated by a pump system including a spray system) and heated to the programmed disinfection temperature. The load is then held at a given range of temperature (e.g. between 0 and +5°C of a set temperature, which at 90°C is 90–95°C) for the required

disinfection time and then drained. This is commonly achieved by spraying the load using the same mechanism as during the cleaning cycle (Chapter 8). The load may then be cooled (with or without drying) prior to removing from the chamber (to reduce any risks of burns). Different types of chemicals can be applied during the disinfection phase to include lubricants and drying/rinsing aids (Chapter 6, Classification of cleaning chemistries). Lubricants are applied as an alternative to manual application to ensure that devices, in particular hinged devices are in good working order. Rinse aids assist in water droplet dispersion, making them easier to remove during drying. In both cases, these chemicals should be proven to be non-toxic to a patient, either if used alone or if subsequently sterilized.

In addition direct heating of large volume of water for thermal disinfection (in immersion or spray-type systems), steam-exposure chambers may also be used, where steam is provided or generated within a chamber under atmospheric pressure and allowed to contact the device load for the desired temperature/time. Although the mechanism of heating is different, these types of disinfectors follow the same principles of time/temperature as immersion/spray based disinfectors; in all cases, the

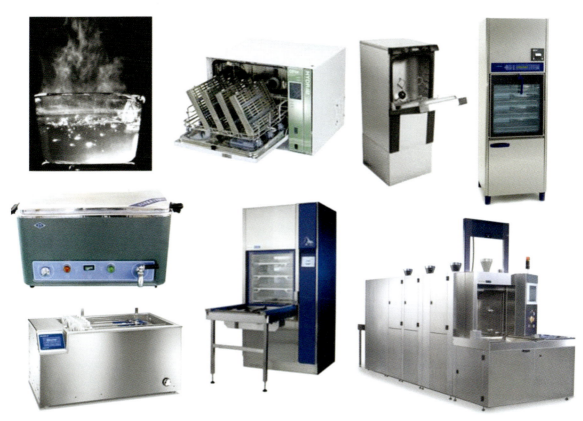

Figure 9.4 Examples of thermal disinfection methods. On the far left are various types of immersion methods, including a simple pan of boiling water (top) to specially designed immersion disinfectors. On the right are various types of washer-disinfectors using thermal disinfection, including bench-top, single chamber and multi-chamber washers. The design of various types of washer-disinfectors is discussed in further detail in Chapter 8 (in the section on automated washers/washer-disinfectors).

distribution of the correct temperature within the load is important to ensure a correct disinfection process.

Dry heat

Dry heat disinfection follows the same principle as wet/moist heat but in the absence of moisture/water. Many types of bacteria, enveloped viruses and vegetative fungi are inactivated by drying alone and this can be enhanced at higher temperatures; however, it is important to note that the mechanisms of action and efficacy of dry heat are different to those with wet/moist heat. In general much higher temperatures and exposure times are required for dry heat to be as effective as moist heat, and for these reasons dry heat methods are not widely used for disinfection. Dry heat disinfection/sterilization can be achieved in specific machines, also referred to as ovens or convection ovens (Figure 9.5). Convection refers to the method of heat transfer through a liquid (water) or gas (air), in this case through hot air; conduction is another term used that refers to a method of heat transfer from one surface or material to another. Dry heat disinfection is effective by the transfer of heat by conduction and convection. Note that if a device is placed wet into a dry heat disinfection process, then the water will be heated and the presence of this moisture actually increases the effectiveness of the process by moist-heat mechanisms.

Dry heat may be considered as a reasonable method for low or intermediate-level disinfection (even at temperatures of 70–80°C (158–176°F) over time to ensure treated surfaces are dried); higher temperatures may be used to achieve higher levels of disinfection (such as up to 140°C (284°F) for one hour). Even higher temperatures and extended exposure times (over many hours) are used

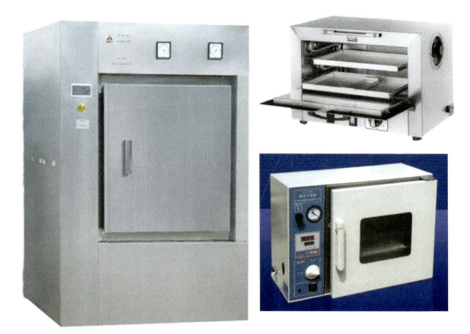

Figure 9.5 Dry heat disinfection ovens.

for some limited sterilization methods (Chapter 11). Types of devices/materials that are disinfected with dry heat can include oils/powders, needles, glass syringes and some clothing; many devices are restricted from dry heat disinfection due to risks of damage.

Radiation

Radiation and various forms of light (in particular high energy sources such as γ radiation) can have disinfection and sterilization properties; they are, however, not widely used for re-usable device reprocessing and are not covered in detail. The various different forms of radiation were identified in Chapter 6 (in the section on light, radiation and the electromagnetic spectrum). High energy radiation sources and generators are more widely used for the disinfection and sterilization of single-use materials within healthcare facilities such as bandages and types of single-use devices. There are three forms that are sometimes used routinely, either on their own right or as part of a particular system. These are:

• Ultraviolet (UV) light: light is much greater than what we see, which is known as "visible" or white light. In technical terms, light refers to the electromagnetic spectrum (Chapter 6, Figure 6.9). Ultraviolet light refers to wavelengths of light that have a higher energy level just above visible light (specifically in the 10–400 nm wavelength range). Ultraviolet light is generated from specifically designed types of lamps; the most effective range of UV against microorganisms is considered to be in the 200–280 nm wavelength range. Ultraviolet light is primarily used for exposure to general environmental surfaces (including various types of equipment/devices that may be present in a given area), the air and liquids (e.g. in water treatment). Ultraviolet light is not very penetrating and therefore will only be effective on those surfaces that directly make contact with the light. It is used for both preservation and disinfection, but rarely for direct disinfection of devices. The specific efficacy of different types of UV-disinfection systems can range considerably, therefore close attention should be paid to the claims and support evidence provided by suppliers.

• Infrared (IR) light: both IR light and microwaves are on the opposite end of the visible light wavelength range, being lower in energy (longer in wavelength). IR light is in the 0.7–1000 μm wavelength range; at this range they are considered to have low to no direct antimicrobial properties, but are used as a method of applying dry heat (see the section on dry heat).

• Microwaves are commonly used for heating purposes (for foods/liquids); they have an even lower energy level than IR and, similarly, have little to no direct antimicrobial activity. Microwaves are used as a heating mechanism

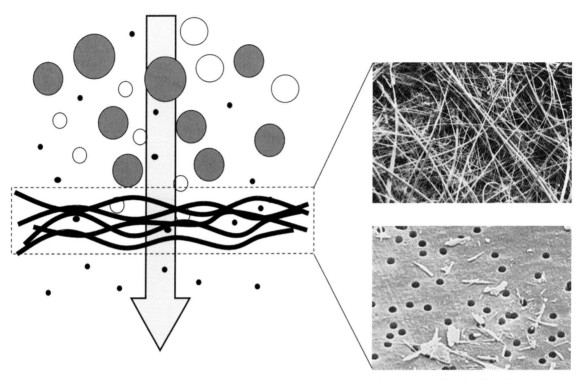

Figure 9.6 Mechanisms of physical removal of microorganisms by filtration. On the left is an example of a liquid/gas containing particles at various sizes being passed through a filter (center); only the smallest particles will pass through the filter (this is often called the "filtrate"), while the others are retained on the dirty side of the filter. Examples of the microscopic structure of two types of filters are shown on the right.

for water, thereby acting as a moist heat disinfection method (see the section on physical disinfection below).

Filtration

Filtration is commonly used as a physical mechanism of disinfection (and even sterilization), especially with air, gases and liquids (including water). It is distinct from the other methods of disinfection discussed in this chapter in that the method of disinfection is by physical removal of microorganisms rather than inactivation of them. The theory of filtration is presented in Figure 9.6. Filters are used to remove various microorganisms due to their size. The filter itself (also known as a membrane) is essentially a mesh of fibrous material, or contains holes of specific sizes as defined by the manufacturer; if the gas/liquid, microorganism, chemical or any other substance is too large it will be trapped on one side of the filter while those that are smaller can pass through.

Filters can be designed from a variety of types of materials and in a variety of forms, depending on their application. Typical examples include HEPA (high efficiency particle air) filters used for filtering air and water filters (Figure 9.7).

Filters are generally classified based on their size exclusion characteristics (or the size of particles, microorganisms, etc., that they can prevent the passage of). Examples of various types of filters and their size exclusion capabilities are shown in Figure 9.8.

In addition to being designed for size exclusion, some filters are made to specifically remove various contaminants by attachment to the filter material; examples include carbon filters and HEPA filters. Carbon (also known as charcoal or granular activated carbon) filters are composed of activated (positively-charged) carbon and are used for water treatment; they can, depending on their design, remove particles down to ~1 μm (therefore including some bacteria), but actively bind chlorine that can be present in the water. They are often used for pre-treatment of water prior to further purification (e.g. by reverse osmosis).

High efficiency particle air (HEPA) filters are used to filter air, but are designed to have a variety of retentive abilities (often designated by letters/numbers such as

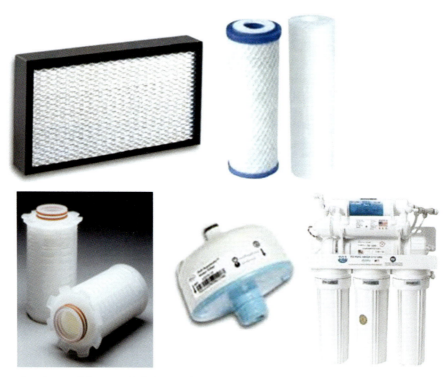

Figure 9.7 Examples of types of filters. On the left are air filters, with a HEPA filter (top) and sterile air filters (bottom). On the right are water filters of various types (upper), a tap filter (lower left) and an under-counter reverse osmosis (RO) filter system.

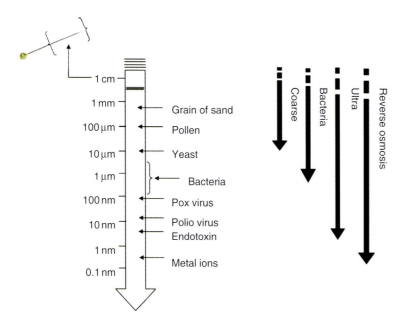

Figure 9.8 The various sizes of microorganisms, particles and chemicals and types of filtration methods. The head of a pin is shown for perspective (note: there are 10 mm in a cm). Filters can therefore be referred to as coarse (or gross), bacterial-retentive, ultrafilters, etc. The specific retentive abilities of an individual filter will depend on its sign and can vary considerably, even within these estimated ranges.

E10, H13 and U17). Typically these filters have the capacity to retain particles down to a 0.3–1 μm range (thereby removing most bacteria), but this will depend on their specific design. They can also cause removal of smaller materials due to attachment to the filter material. High efficiency particle air filters are used for treating air in a defined clean area (such as in surgical theatres and in some "clean", packaging area of decontamination facilities), as well as treating air that is used in various washer-disinfectors (for drying) or sterilizers (for releasing vacuums during sterilization cycles).

Reverse osmosis (RO) filters, known as a semi-permeable membranes, are specifically designed for generating purified water in that they can remove most microorganisms and chemicals. The RO process is not just the use of the membranes but includes a designed pressurized system and constant water flow/movement; the water moves along the surface of the membrane and contaminants are constantly swept away while the pure water passes across the membrane.

It is important to note that while the various types of filters can theoretically exclude various sizes or remove materials, the successful use of filtration is dependent on how filters are used. An example is that mechanical or chemical damage to the filter may not be detected and can compromise the filter allowing contaminants to pass through. If filter based systems are not designed and maintained correctly, they can easily become compromised. There are test systems available to ensure the correct installation and maintenance of filters; these include filter integrity (air or water) and leak tests. Filters can also become blocked, thereby not allowing air/water to pass through; in the case of water, this is typically detected by reduced flow over time. Another example is that while most bacteria are retained by a 0.2 μm micro-filter some bacteria can "grow-through" the filter over time and contaminate the clean side of the filter. Overall, as with any disinfectant, filters should be used and maintained according to manufacturers' instructions to ensure their correct use.

Chemical disinfection

There are many types of chemicals and chemical processes used for disinfection (Figure 9.9). These have been introduced briefly in Chapter 6 (in the section on disinfectants, including preservatives) and are discussed in further detail in this section. In many publications and guidelines the various types of biocides used for disinfection are often classified as being capable of killing certain types of

microorganisms and therefore being capable of low, intermediate or high-level disinfection. For example, non-critical devices/surfaces may be treated with a wide range of disinfectants, including those based on surfactants, oxidizers, alcohols, phenols and aldehydes; a much more limited selection of biocides are used for semi-critical/critical applications such as the peroxygens and aldehydes. This approach can be useful (as shown in Figure 9.1) but often misleading. The ability of a disinfectant or chemical disinfection process to be effective can vary significantly depending on how the biocide is formulated and how it is used. This section discusses some of the major types of biocides used and gives some general guidance on their advantages/disadvantages. It should, however, be remembered that specific efficacy claims, methods of preparation/use and any safety considerations should be provided by the disinfectant manufacturer and should always be closely reviewed.

Alcohols

There are three types of alcohols used as disinfectants: ethanol ("alcohol" or the major component in "methylated spirits"), isopropanol (also known as "rubbing" or isopropyl alcohol) and n-propanol. Alcohol solutions are used directly at specified dilutions or as formulated products typically within the optimal 60–80% range (note that although higher concentrations are available they are often *less* effective). Alcohols are widely used as antiseptics, known as hand rubs or hand disinfectants; they have been particularly highlighted for routine use in hospitals and healthcare facilities due to their ease of use, good antimicrobial activity on the skin and because they do not require rinsing in water. The formulation of the alcohol can be important to maximize the efficacy of the alcohol, particularly on the skin, but also to ensure that it does not irritate the skin. An example is the use of lower concentration of alcohol (in the 60–65% range) with other chemical ingredients that help to prevent drying effects on the skin; these extend the contact time of the alcohol on the skin and leave the skin feeling smooth after use. Some alcohol-based disinfectants can contain other biocides, in particular chlorhexidine (see the section on other biocides), that remain on the skin following use to continue to provide antimicrobial activity (this is known as residual activity or persistence). Alcohols are not generally used as device disinfectants, but can be used to wipe down various surfaces. They have a benefit of evaporating (drying) very quickly and are therefore often used to aid in the drying of devices, in particular lumened devices such as flexible endoscopes.

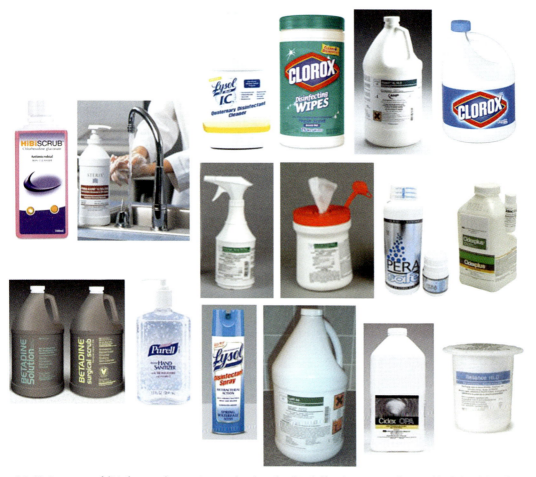

Figure 9.9 Various types of disinfectants, from antiseptics (used on the skin; left) to low, intermediate and high-level disinfectants (from left to right). They include concentrates, ready-to-use and wipe-type products, also one and two-component chemistries.

Alcohols are generally considered as intermediate to high-level disinfectants. They have rapid bactericidal activity (including against mycobacteria), are somewhat slower but effective against fungi and viruses (with the exception of most non-enveloped viruses) and have little to no activity against bacterial spores.

Alcohols have the advantages of being easy and rapid to use as disinfectants, with little odor, residues and toxicity. Disadvantages include no sporicidal activity (and limited activity against some non-enveloped viruses), they are flammable (at high concentrations), and can damage/irritate surfaces (by drying).

Aldehydes
The main types of aldehydes used as disinfectants are glutaraldehyde, orthophthaldehyde (OPA) and formaldehyde.

Glutaraldehyde and OPA are widely used as high-level disinfectants for temperature-sensitive devices, in particular flexible endoscopes. They are available as single or multi-use types of disinfectants. They are also used for low/intermediate-level disinfection for other types of devices, and in the case of some glutaraldehyde-containing products for environmental surfaces in some jurisdictions.

Glutaraldehyde has been traditionally used as a high-level disinfectant for over 40 years, but its use has been decreasing over recent years due to safety and efficacy concerns. It is typically used for disinfection in the 1.5–3% range and supplied as one or two-component chemistries. The one-component (usually stabilized acidic formulated) chemistries do not require any pre-activation and can immediately be used (either directly or by dilution in water); two-component formulations require activation (mixing and contact time) before they are used for disinfection. They are generally provided in two parts: an acidic solution containing the aldehyde to which a smaller activator is added to make the solution neutral or alkaline for use. Once prepared the product is ready for use, within the defined shelf-life of the activated solution (e.g. 14 days or as defined by the manufacturer). Remember, in these cases the product is *not* effective as a disinfectant unless it is activated correctly! As with any activated and/or multiple use formulation, care should be taken to follow manufacturers' instructions and in particular those relating to any means provided to ensure the disinfectant can be safely used; an example of such a means is the use of a chemical indicator that is specifically developed for use with the disinfectant to show that it is correctly activated/fit for use (Figure 9.10). Glutaraldehyde-containing formulations may also include high concentrations of other antimicrobials that work together with the aldehyde to provide the disinfection efficacy; examples include various types of surfactants, alcohols and phenols (Table 9.4).

Orthophthaldehyde formulations are normally provided as concentrates or ready-for-use solutions (not requiring activation), and are typically used at ~0.4–0.6% range for disinfection at room temperature (18–25°C). With both OPA and glutaraldehyde, the efficacy of disinfection increases at higher temperatures (e.g. within a heated bath or washer-disinfector); in these conditions low concentrations may be used (by dilution in water) in accordance with any label claims (Table 9.4).

As high-level disinfectants, the biocidal properties of glutaldehyde and OPA have been well described as being effective against most bacteria (including mycobacteria), viruses and fungi. Glutaraldehyde is also effective, in particular over extended exposure times (e.g. as chemical sterilants in the USA), against bacterial spores; OPA is considerably less effective against spores and this activity may be enhanced at increased temperatures. Both aldehydes are considered effective against protozoal vegetative forms, but not always the dormant (encysted) forms, in particular *Cryptosporidium* oocysts and *Acanthameoba* cysts. Some types of mycobacteria, other bacteria and fungi have demonstrated the ability to develop high-level resistance to aldehydes (in particular with glutaraldehyde).

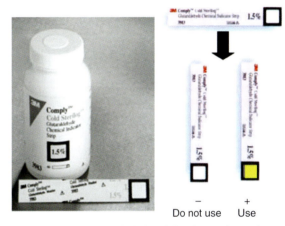

Figure 9.10 A glutaraldehyde-based disinfectant chemical indicator, used to confirm that the disinfectant is activated/safe to use. In this case, a white to yellow color change indicates that active glutaraldehyde is present.

Table 9.4 Examples of label claims on glutaraldehyde and OPA-based high-level disinfectants. Note: due to county or region-specific regulatory requirements, the recommended disinfection time may vary on the same product. These are typical claims on US-FDA registered products.

High-level disinfectant	Recommended exposure conditions
2.5% glutaraldehyde with surfactants	35°C for 5 minutes; 28 day re-use. One component
3.4% glutaraldehyde with 26% isopropanol	20°C for 10 minutes; 14 day re-use. Two component (activated)
1.12% glutaraldehyde with 1.93% phenol	25°C for 20 minutes; 14 day re-use. Two component (activated)
2.5% glutaraldehyde with surfactants	25°C for 90 minutes; 28 day re-use. Two component (activated)
2.4% glutaraldehyde	25°C for 45 minutes; 14 day re-use. Two component (activated)
0.55% OPA	20°C for 12 minutes; 14 day re-use. 25°C for 5 minutes; 14 day re-use. One component

Both glutaraldehyde and OPA are well recognized as high-level disinfectants for flexible endoscope and other device (e.g. dialysis machine) disinfection. Formulations generally show good material compatibility and are low cost. Orthophthaldehyde is also considered less irritating than glutaraldehyde, due to its lower vapor pressure (essentially it evaporates into the air less), but does cause staining of materials in the presence of protein. Aldehydes are cross-linking agents, therefore (as is the case for all disinfectants) devices should be well cleaned prior to aldehdye disinfection as any remaining materials can become fixed onto device surfaces and can lead to complications over time. Particular care should be taken to follow manufacturers' instructions regarding activation (for two-component disinfectants), handling, use (in particular re-use to ensure the disinfectant remains active) and disposal of aldehyde-based disinfectants. An example of bad practice often observed in the use of aldehyde disinfectants is referred to as "topping-up". This is where the re-usable disinfectant is used for a certain time and then a smaller amount of a freshly prepared solution is added to the disinfectant so that it can be used for longer. Such practices are not safe and are unlikely to be recommended by the disinfectant manufacturer (if they are this should be verified in writing). Glutaraldehyde and OPA can be irritating to the skin, mucous membranes and respiratory tract; in addition to short-term effects, long-term exposure to either biocide can have other consequences. Glutaraldehyde has been reported to lead to dermatitis and asthma, with some debate regarding the biocide being classified as a carcinogen (an agent that can cause cancer). Orthophthaldehyde is also known to be a potent sensitizer, but overall is less studied to date than glutaraldehyde. In both cases, risks can be reduced with the proper design of a facility using the biocides for disinfection; this particularly includes the use of closed baths (preferably enclosed washer-disinfectors) and for correct ventilation (e.g. 10–15 air changes/hour in the room or the use of a chemical fume hood). Some facilities recommend the use of respirators for all staff handling or using aldehdye-containing baths. The use of adequate PPE is important, including use of safety glasses, face shields and nitrile/rubber gloves when handling solutions. In certain countries, it is recommended that the levels of glutaraldehyde exposure to staff is closely monitored, with a typical "safe" level being considered at or below 0.05 ppm; at the time of writing no such level had been set for OPA. Glutaraldehyde-monitors including personal or area monitors and periodic or constant sensors are available for such purposes. High levels of

glutaraldehyde and OPA remaining on device surfaces following disinfection is also a concern, in particular in reports of colitis (irritation of the colon) and complications following eye surgery. Care should be taken to ensure that any high-level disinfected devices are correctly rinsed, according to manufacturers' instructions prior to patient use; this may include up to 4–6 individual fresh water rinses, ensuring that all surfaces (internal and external) are correctly immersed in water for each rinse. Finally, specific instructions are usually provided on the safe disposal of aldehyde disinfectants due to environmental concerns; in certain regions/countries there is a requirement for the neutralization of glutaraldehyde-based disinfectants (e.g. by mixing with other chemistries such as glycine or sodium bisulfite) prior to disposal down a public drain. Such instructions will be provided by the manufacturer or by local agencies.

Formaldehyde is considered separately, as today it is not widely used for healthcare facility disinfection. It is, however, more widely used for gas sterilization applications and this is considered further in Chapter 11 (see the section on Formaldehyde gas); this will include humidified formaldehyde gas and chemical vapor (formaldehyde with alcohol) sterilizers used in certain parts of the world. Formaldehyde is particularly used in pathology laboratories as a disinfectant/preservative for tissue; it is primarily used as "formalin", a 37% solution of formaldehyde in water/methanol. Older liquid disinfection applications used dilutions at 4–8% in water and/or alcohol, but these are no longer recommended due to material compatibility and toxicity concerns. Such formulations were considered to provide intermediate to high-level disinfection, but at recommended long contact times (e.g. 4% formaldehyde at 24 hours); although liquid formaldehyde is effective against most bacteria, viruses and fungi, efficacy concerns were observed with some types of bacteria (with resistance mechanisms), non-enveloped viruses and bacterial spores requiring higher concentrations and/or extended contact times. Of particular concern are the safety aspects of using formaldehyde, as it is associated with irritating fumes; it is a known carcinogen, but also with known short and long-term toxic effects (such as dermatitis and asthma-like complications). The recommended safety level is in the range of 0.75 ppm. In addition to liquid use, gas-based formaldehyde was traditionally used for laboratory and even hospital area disinfection (also known as fumigation). In these processes, the gas is produced by heating paraformaldehyde (a dry form of formaldehyde) or formalin solutions in the presence of high humidity (>80%) and holding this in a room/area for many hours (e.g. seven hours); the room is then aerated (typically over 12–24 hours) to remove the gas. Overall, long cycle times and safety concerns have limited the use of liquid or gas formaldehyde for healthcare disinfection applications.

Halogens

"Halogens" describe a group of similar chemicals (Chapter 6) and some of which are widely used as disinfectants, particularly chlorine and iodine. Both have been used as disinfectants for many years and in a variety of applications.

Iodine (specifically in water, the biocidal molecules I_2 and HOI) is used for both antiseptic and general surface disinfectant (low, intermediate or high) applications; it is not generally recommended for re-usable medical device reprocessing. Iodine is traditionally provided in two forms: tinctures (for use on skin/wounds, e.g. iodine dissolved in ethanol) or iodophors (iodine-releasing agents, e.g. PVPI). A common example is the Betadine® range of iodophor-containing hand washes and surgical scrubs (Chapter 6, Antiseptics). Iodine, depending on the biocidal concentration and contact time, can provide high level disinfection including bactericidal, fungicidal, virucidal and even sporicidal activity. Antiseptic products are generally used as lower biocidal concentrations to minimize damage to the skin and at higher, sporicidal concentrations for general surface disinfection. Note: these products should not be used for device disinfection unless labeled for such use. At higher concentrations iodine can be staining (browning), irritating and damaging to some surfaces, but the alternative use of iodophors has reduced these negative effects.

It is hard not to come across the use of chlorine on a daily basis, as one of the most widely used chemicals for disinfection. Chlorine is widely used as a general surface, water and in some cases device/equipment disinfectant. When chlorine is dissolved in water, the main active molecules are Cl_2, HOCl and OCl⁻; they are provided by directly dissolving chlorine or chlorine-containing chemicals, with common examples being sodium hypochlorite (NaOCl; typical household "bleach" solutions contain 5% NaOCl in water), calcium hypochloride (solids or tablets) and chloramines (e.g. monochloramine or T-chloramine). Chlorine should not be confused with chlorine dioxide (ClO_2, which is a peroxygen-based chemistry and is considered separately on associated safety and efficacy). Similar to iodine, the antimicrobial activity of chlorine is dependent on its available active concentration over time. It is widely respected and tested as being effective against

all microorganisms, with higher concentrations or contact times being required for dormant forms (spores and cysts). High concentrations/exposure times (e.g. 2.5% sodium hypochlorite for one hour) have also been particularly shown to be effective against prions (Chapter 15). Note that many chlorine-containing products do not have associated disinfectant claims, such as household bleach, while others are registered disinfectants with specific recommended dilutions/preparation methods and claims. Despite this, chlorine solutions such as those based on household bleach are widely used for environmental disinfection applications. For example, many guidelines recommend the use of a "10% household bleach solution", which can be misleading. Inspection of household bleach products will show that they range in concentration. Typical concentrations are in the 5–6% range of sodium hypochlorite and other ingredients may also be present (e.g. surfactants); 5–6% sodium hypochlorite is approximately equal to 50,000–60,000 ppm of available chlorine (depending on the product formulation and its age/storage conditions). As a guideline, freshly prepared bleach dilutions at ~500 ppm available chlorine (a 1:100 dilution of a 5% sodium hypochlorite solution in water) are considered effective low-level disinfectants at contact times of ~1–2 minutes. However, bleach solutions are readily neutralized by many materials and the "10% household bleach solution" or about 5000 ppm available chlorine is more reliable as an intermediate to high-level disinfectant; mycobacteria might be inactivated in ~5 minutes whereas 10 minutes or more might be needed for many types of bacterial/fungal spores. Further important variables include the quality of water that chlorine-based products are diluted into, which may also affect the actual available activate chlorine concentration and the types of surfaces that it will be used on. The presence of soil, as for most disinfectants, can dramatically affect the antimicrobial activity, as available chlorine reacts with the soil and may therefore not be available for inactivation of microorganisms present.

For device or equipment disinfection application, staff should ensure that chlorine will not damage the surfaces (in particular referring to manufacturers' instructions); one of the leading causes of rusting on stainless steel devices is chlorine (particularly in water when heated as part of cleaning, disinfection or sterilization applications). Other material compatibility concerns will include the "bleaching" (loss) of colored materials, hardening of plastic surfaces, degradation of some types of rubber materials such as o-rings; premature wearing of devices/general surfaces and degradation of anodized aluminum.

Chlorine is widely used as a water disinfectant, where a low level of chlorine is often present to maintain the microbial content in the water at a low and safe level for drinking. Levels of chlorine can range from season to season and even from day to day. In addition, chlorine is often used at high levels as a disinfection method for equipment and facility pipework/water handling systems. An example in hospitals is the treatment of facility water pipework systems to reduce the levels of certain infectious microorganisms such as *Legionella* (the causative bacteria in Legionnaires' disease). As highlighted above, chlorine can be a leading cause of device damage (e.g. rusting) when present in water used for reprocessing and particularly when heated. Therefore, it is important to monitor and potentially control the levels of chlorine in water used for reprocessing of devices (Chapter 15, Water Quality/Purity). Typical recommended levels of chlorine in water used for cleaning and disinfection is less than 120 mg/L available chlorine, with even lower levels being recommended when heated to higher temperature (such as for steam sterilization (less than 10–120 mg/L; note, in this case chemically 1 mg/L is ~1 ppm).

Chlorine-based products are widely used and inexpensive disinfectants, with good broad spectrum antimicrobial efficacy (depending on the available chlorine concentration and including sporicidal activity), are fast acting and have generally low associated toxicity. The "chlorine" smell is commonly associated with cleaning/disinfection. Higher concentrations of chlorine can be irritating and sensitizing, depending on the concentration and the individual. Chlorine can also damage surfaces (metals and plastics), ranging from loss of color (bleaching) to more serious damage such as pitting and rusting. Chlorine products should never be mixed with acid chemistries (e.g. descalers), as the reaction can lead to the release of chlorine gas that is poisonous. Chlorine chemistry is very pH dependent; when stored as an alkaline solution (household bleach) it is quite stable but on dilution with water the pH drops and the solution is more rapidly active but less stable. Diluted chlorine-based products can be unstable (in particular in the presence of poor water quality and soil), therefore they are not recommended to be stored for extended periods of time and should be prepared fresh for use (unless otherwise described by the product manufacturer).

Chlorine-generation systems are also used for device, general surface and even wound disinfection applications. These are often referred to as "activated", "electrolyzed" or "super-oxidized" water applications (Figure 9.11). Most of these system work on a process known as electrolysis, where an electric current (or other form or energy) is applied to water with a low concentration of salt (typically NaCl, sodium chloride). The salt solution has little to no antimicrobial activity, but when the electric current is applied active chlorine species (primarily HOCl but also Cl_2 and OCl^-) are formed and can be concentrated in the design of the generator. Other antimicrobial molecules can also be formed during this process that adds to the disinfection activity (such as ozone). These preparations have powerful antimicrobial activity (based on its oxidation potential) for use when diluted into water for device disinfection (e.g. with flexible endoscopes and other semi-critical devices) and water disinfection (including low concentrations added into water to be used for disinfectant rinsing). The preparations are, however, not stable; therefore activated water is not stored but freshly made at or close to the time of use (although this may vary depending on the exact generator type, e.g. stored for up to 24 hours). The concentrated antimicrobial solution prepared is at a very low pH and this may be modified by the generator (in concentration and pH) for particular applications depending on the specific antimicrobial process designed and tested. Overall, depending on the concentration and pH used, it can provide low to high-level disinfection (and has even been used as a sterilant, due to powerful sporicidal activity). Antimicrobial activity is generally very rapid, with typical intermediate to high-level disinfection (at 100–250 mg/L available chlorine) for 2 minutes and 5–10 minutes for sporicidal efficacy. Similar to chlorine solutions (discussed above), the quality of water used and presence of soil (in water or on the device/surface being disinfected) can affect the antimicrobial activity (depending on the dose). In addition to providing powerful antimicrobial activity, these systems are easy and generally safe to use. Activated water does not have the strong odor/irritation associated with high-level hypochlorite solutions and, after the initial purchase of the generator, the overall running costs are considered low. Disadvantages have been reported to include device damage (e.g. with flexible endoscopes protective coatings are often recommended to prevent damage to the external surfaces of these devices) and the importance of controlling water quality used for generation (that can lead to other negative effects in the generator and surfaces treated with the activated water produced, such as strong odor and device damage).

Figure 9.11 Examples of super-oxidized or activated water generators.

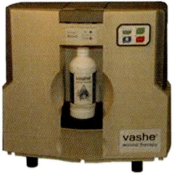

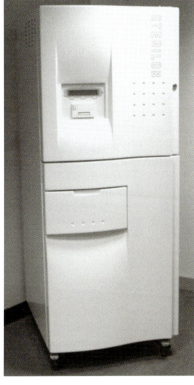

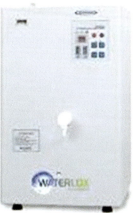

Peroxygens

Peroxygens are a group of chemicals widely used for disinfection; they include hydrogen peroxide (H_2O_2), peracetic acid (CH_3COOOH and often called PAA) and chlorine dioxide (ClO_2). In addition, ozone (O_3) is also considered in this section. Depending on how they are used, all are potentially effective disinfectants and sterilants (including sterilization applications that are further discussed in Chapter 11).

Hydrogen peroxide is widely used in liquid and gas form. Simple liquid solutions of peroxide in water (such as 3–6%) have been traditionally used on wounds or in laboratories for wiping surfaces, being considered as low to high-level disinfectants depending on the concentration and exposure time. However, these have now been largely supplanted by hydrogen-peroxide containing formulations that have been developed to enhance the antimicrobial activity of peroxide and minimize negative effects on device compatibility, thus allowing the use of lower concentrations of peroxide to achieve the same effects that would not be possible with the unformulated chemical alone. These formulations are specifically developed for certain applications (environmental surface or device disinfection) and may or may not contain other biocides (e.g. peracetic acid-containing products always contain a certain, low concentration of hydrogen peroxide, and some products that are primarily hydrogen peroxide might contain some additional peroxygen compounds, including PAA). Hydrogen peroxide concentrations are used in formulation range from <1 to 10%; an example is a series of "accelerated" peroxide formulations used for low to high level disinfection within 5–10 minutes; at higher concentrations this includes high-level disinfection of re-usable devices. The material compatibility of these peroxide-containing preparations can vary significantly; therefore care should be taken to examine any evidence provided of compatibility with metals and other materials sensitive to oxidation damage. Antimicrobial activity also depends on the specific formulation, but they typically provide high-level disinfection, with some activity against bacterial spores. Other liquid formulations mix 6–8% peroxide with silver (as an antimicrobial metal), claiming a combined benefit in antimicrobial activity; these are used for environmental surface applications and in particular in the generation of peroxide/silver containing droplets/gas mixtures that are released into the air for the purpose of air/surface disinfection within a room/area. Hydrogen peroxide gas is also a very powerful antimicrobial, being much more effective than liquid preparations at lower concentrations (e.g. 0.00001–0.001% in gas form is typically used). Depending on the concentration and contact time, peroxide gas is a rapid bactericide (including against mycobacteria), fungicide, cysticide, virucide and sporicide; it has also been shown to be effective under certain conditions against prions and to penetrate over time through organic soils (including blood) that may be associated with microbial contamination. The gas is easy to make (usually from liquid preparations ranging from 6 to 55% peroxide in water) by heating/aerosolization and can also degrade naturally into water and oxygen, therefore having a good safety (including environmental) profile. In addition to being an effective antimicrobial the gas, when correctly controlled, is safe for use on most materials, including electricals and electronics. For these reasons, peroxide gas is used for a variety of disinfection and sterilization applications. For disinfection, its major use is for room/area and equipment fumigation; fumigation refers to the use of disinfectant indirectly within an area (as opposed to manually applying a liquid disinfectant). These include routine or high-risk (e.g. isolation wards) areas within a facility. With the use of gaseous peroxide, equipment may also remain in or specifically be taken into an area during the fumigation process as a method of disinfection (such as hospital beds, stands and other non-critical items). A variety of peroxide gas generators are used for this purpose and vary in their particular application, generation methods and safety/efficacy.

Some systems are used to generate gas (also known as vapor) phase peroxide only, while others make a mixture of gas and liquid peroxide or even just liquid alone. They can vary in the type and concentration of peroxide used as part of the process. Some generators are designed to make peroxide gas and then safely remove it (to allow staff to re-enter the room) and others just generate a peroxide liquid aerosol, leaving it in the room to naturally degrade. Peroxide gas can be noxious at low concentrations (e.g. 5–10 ppm), and a recommended safety level within an area is typically defined at 1 ppm. Overall, the safety and efficacy data associated with any system should be closely inspected prior to use as they can vary significantly. Sterilization applications with peroxide gas are considered in Chapter 11.

Overall, hydrogen peroxide in liquid or gas form can be a powerful disinfectant; liquid products can vary depending on their formulation and gas/aerosol products depending on their concentration and process control. Gaseous peroxide is a particularly effective antimicrobial, including sporicidal activity, but its use is constrained to areas not under active occupation. Peroxide has a relatively good safety profile and has become a popular alternative to other biocides with greater safety (staff, patient or environmental). Although liquid concentrations at 3–6% can be safely handled, even at these lower concentrations they should be respected as potent chemicals (use of PPE, including gloves and safety glasses); higher concentrations (e.g. 35% solutions used to generate gas peroxide) can have serious effects, such as skin burns, on contact. Low concentrations of the gas can be irritating (especially to the eyes) and at higher concentrations (e.g. at 75 ppm) can do significant damage to various tissues, including the lungs, with potentially serious complications. Depending on the application/product, peroxide can lead to loss of color (bleaching). It also degrades on contacting certain types of materials (e.g. paper, wood and brass/copper, thereby losing disinfectant activity) and can damage some surfaces. These side effects can vary significantly depending on the formulation and/or process used for disinfection.

Peracetic acid (PAA) is primarily used in liquid form for disinfection; it has not been successfully used to date in gaseous form. Solutions of PAA always contain a certain level of hydrogen peroxide and acetic acid, with the acetic acid being responsible for the typical pungent odor associated such products. It is also widely used as a general surface disinfectant in industry, but in healthcare facilities its most important function is as a high-level disinfectant/sterilant for semi-critical and critical devices. Sterilization applications with PAA are considered in Chapter 11 (Chemical sterilization). It is also used for equipment, in particular water-handling equipment (e.g. RO water generation and storage systems) disinfection. Peracetic acid is provided for disinfection applications in many ways (Figure 9.12): single components (ready for use or diluted in water), two components (requiring mixing to provide the disinfectant or allowing the component to generate PAA), activated or not. Dry (solid) or liquid formulations are also available as single or multi-use products for manual application/immersion or as part of a defined washer-disinfector or disinfector/sterilizer processor.

Peracetic acid disinfectants can be used in open trays for manual immersion, but the strong odors associated with such applications can be undesirable and minimized by the use of chemical hoods or appropriate ventilation

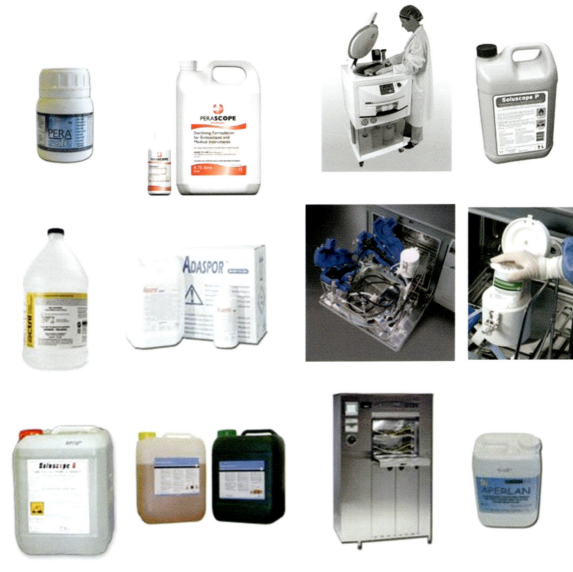

Figure 9.12 Various types of peracetic acid-containing disinfectants and disinfection/sterilization systems. Various types of one or two component formulations are shown on the left (the top, far left, is an example of a solid product that is diluted in water to generate the PAA). Washer-disinfectors and their associated PAA-containing disinfectants for flexible endoscopes are shown on the right; some designs are restricted to one type of disinfectant and others are not.

(frequent air exchanges) within the reprocessing area. Peracetic acid is also used as a common disinfectant in many types of washer-disinfectors for flexible endoscope disinfection (Figure 9.12). These systems not only control the exposure to the disinfectant (in particular for delivery through device lumens and under controlled temperature conditions) but minimize any handling (staff safety) risks and should also ensure that disinfectant residuals are adequately removed prior to patient use.

Peracetic acid-containing formulations are very effective high-level disinfectants/sterilants against all types of microorganisms including bacterial spores; relatively low concentrations (e.g. 0.1–0.2%) are required for such activity and can be particularly enhanced by controlling the temperature of the disinfection process (if labeled for such applications). Temperature-controlled processes have been shown to have cysticidal activity, but overall this can be product-specific. Some formulations will also have cleaning and biofilm removal effects, but this strictly depends on the product formulation. It is considered an effective biocide at low concentrations, even in the presence of organic/inorganic soils. Similar to other per-oxygens, it also degrades naturally into safe, non-toxic by-products such as water and a low concentration of acetic acid. There are, however, some disadvantages. Some formulations can have strong, irritating odors that are undesirable when being used or stored. Peracetic acid can cause skin burns at low concentrations, with the eyes being particularly at risk from accidental splashing. Material and device compatibility is a frequent complaint with PAA formulations, and this can vary significantly from product to product; as for any disinfectant, compatibility claims should be supported by documentation from the manufacturer and not contra-indicated by the device manufacturer.

Chlorine dioxide-based disinfectants are popular in many parts of the world, for both non-critical device/general surface disinfection and for high-level device disinfection applications. Similar to PAA, it is also used for equipment disinfection, such as water handling systems, and for water disinfection itself (as an alternative to chlorine). The efficacy and safety of chlorine dioxide should not be confused with chlorine (see the section on halogens), as they are separate and distinct biocides. Its primary use to date is as a liquid-based disinfectant and it is rarely, if ever, used at this time in gas phase. As it is a very unstable biocide, it is always provided as a one or two-component generating system where the chlorine dioxide is generated by mixing two components together or by dissolving similar components in dry tablet form into water. A variety of delivery systems have been developed to accommodate the biocide generation. These include two-component liquid systems (to generate a concentrated chlorine dioxide solution that is then diluted in water at the indicated concentration), ready-to-use pump systems (two components are mixed on spraying out onto a surface), tablets (that activate when mixed with water) and wipe-systems that are activated prior to use using the indicated mixing method and time. These are used for manual application/device immersion or in automated washer-disinfector systems. The antimicrobial effects of chlorine dioxide depend on its concentration, formulation and contact time/temperature; with these considerations it can be similar if not more superior to

chlorine formulations. Typical bactericidal/virucidal concentrations have been reported in the 0.2–1 mg/L, with high level disinfection requiring higher concentrations (1–2 mg/L) at which it is also effective against spores and some types of cysts. It also maintains efficacy in the presence of soil, but this is concentration-dependent. Unlike chlorine, chlorine dioxide disinfectants are not associated with strong odors (although they may have a slight "chlorine" odor) or other negative effects observed with chlorine. It is considered non-toxic and safe for the environment, as it degrades naturally. As such disinfectants require generation, care should be taken to ensure that they are activated correctly according to manufacturers' instructions at the time of use and should, preferably, be confirmed using a type of chemical indicator specific for chlorine dioxide. High, generally sporicidal, concentrations are often considered damaging to certain types of materials (including stainless steel and plastics) but these effects are formulation-specific; loss of color is frequently observed over time. Release of chlorine dioxide gas from disinfectants can be a safety concern, with relatively low levels (over 0.1 ppm) considered to be toxic.

Ozone is not widely used for disinfection purposes in healthcare facilities today and is only briefly described here; specific sterilization processes using ozone are considered in more detail in Chapter 11. The main applications for ozone include laundry, for water or waste disinfection and less commonly for area (environmental) and air disinfection. It is generated in air or water from available oxygen (including water, H_2O, as a source of oxygen) at the point of use (e.g. from an ozone generator or within a washer-disinfector). In a typical ozone-water system, the ozone is generated from air (or from an oxygen gas source) by application of an electrical charge and then, as a gas, bubbled into the water (e.g. using an injector/mixing system; Figure 9.13); the ozonated water is then used in a disinfection process. Ozone has become a popular low-temperature chemical alternative for healthcare laundry applications (typically at 30–35°C), in that it can provide an intermediate to high level of disinfection but also is a deodorizer and degrades naturally to give safe by-products (oxygen), therefore minimizing water consumption. As a gas, it is generated and used directly in the air (for air and surface disinfection), but requires high humidity levels (75–95%) for optimal activity.

Ozone is a particularly powerful biocide and, like other peroxygen biocides, disinfectant activity will depend on the ozone concentration and process control. For example, in air disinfection and device sterilization

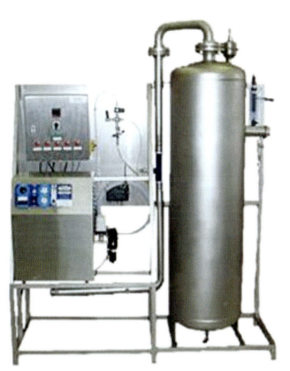

Figure 9.13 An ozonated-water generator system. In this system the ozone is generated as a gas from the oxygen in air by application of an electrical current and then added into the water by bubbling. The ozonated water is then used for disinfection applications.

(Chapter 11) applications, in addition to ozone concentration, the temperature, contact time and humidity control are important; humidity (usually over 80%) is particularly important to ensure that ozone can be effective and at higher temperatures there can be a benefit of increased activity, but a negative effect degrading the available ozone concentration. Disinfectant activity can therefore range from low to high level, and can even be used for sterilization purposes as part of a controlled process. As a highly reactive disinfectant, it reacts with all microorganisms and, with sufficient activity, will render them non-viable. Typical conditions of bactericidal and viricidal activity are in the 0.2–0.5 mg/L range, with higher concentrations generally required to inactivate fungal and bacterial spores, as well as protozoal cysts. Overall, the advantages of ozone are its wide antimicrobial activity, ease of generation and being environmentally friendly. Ozone is also used to neutralize various types of chemicals that are associated with foul odors (such as aldehydes and some phenols) and other unwanted molecules. Disadvantages are: its rapid

neutralization by surface and soil contact, it can be toxic at low levels (with a typical safety limit being 0.1 ppm), and it may damage surfaces (including stainless steel and plastics, depending on the concentration and disinfection process).

Phenols

"Phenol" is a specific chemical and is not routinely used as a disinfectant; "phenols" or "phenolics" refer to biocides used for disinfection that are based derivatives of phenol or have similar chemical structure. Examples include cresols, 2-phenylphenol, chlorocresol, chloroxylenol (commonly known as PCMX) and triclosan. They are used as low to intermediate-level disinfectants for environmental surfaces, but are generally not considered safe and effective for device reprocessing. They are available as concentrated or ready-to-use disinfectants for general housekeeping (floors, walls, general contact surfaces, etc.), but are often not recommended in certain applications (e.g. in nurseries and particularly incubators) due to strong odors or toxicity (in some cases). Depending on the formulation (including types of specific phenols), concentration and application time, phenols can provide rapid bactericidal, fungicidal, and virucidal (enveloped) activity, with some formulations having practical activity also against mycobacteria and some non-enveloped viruses. Phenols have little to no activity against bacterial spores. Overall, phenolic disinfectants retain good activity in the presence of soils (used for cleaning/disinfectant activity), are often associated with the "hospital" smell (generally sweet, aromatic type) and some are readily biodegradable (but equally some are not). Formulation plays an important role in the activity of these disinfectants and as with many other disinfectants they are usually combined with surfactants to aid in cleaning-disinfection applications. They are, however, often associated with a strong odor (particular when used at high concentrations), should not be used if particular applications where toxic residues could be a concern (e.g. neonatal and food contact surfaces) and (again depending on the formulation) can damage certain types of plastics and rubbers.

Two particular phenols, triclosan and PCMX (or chloroxylenol) are widely used as antiseptics, including for routine (antiseptic) hand washing and surgical scrubbing (Chapter 6). Other examples of phenol-derived antiseptic type biocides include hexachlorophene and salicylic acid. These are all considered separately from the hard surface disinfectants above as they are distinct in safety and efficacy considerations. Triclosan is one of the most widely used biocides in antiseptics and is often integrated into surfaces that have antimicrobial claims. In formulation, concentrations typically range from 0.1–2%. Its antimicrobial activity is very good against Gram positive bacteria but poorer against Gram negative bacteria; formulation is essential to optimize the activity of triclosan for use in antiseptics. Such antiseptics are considered as low-level disinfectants and for use only for hand washing (or in combination with alcohol, for hand rubbing). Chloroxylenol (in the 0.5–4% range) is essentially very similar, but is less used than triclosan. Antiseptics using either biocide often claim activity against fungi (yeast and molds) and non-enveloped viruses. Both can also remain on the skin following washing to give a sustained (persistent, bacteriostatic) antimicrobial activity. Triclosan and chloroxylenol have been popular in antiseptics due to their low irritation profiles and mildness to the skin. They do, however, have limited antimicrobial (low level) activity and are often a concern due to persistence in the environment.

Quaternary ammonium compounds

Quaternary ammonium compounds belong to a group of chemicals called surfactants ("surface active agents"). These are unique chemicals that can hold dirt (including fats and oils) in water; for this reason they are widely used in cleaning and disinfection chemistries (Chapter 6). Many types of surfactants also have antimicrobial activity and particularly a group known as quaternary ammonium compounds (or QACs, QUATs for short). These are usually associated with rather long chemical names such as hexadecylpyridinium chloride and hexadecyltrimethylammonium bromide (commonly known as "cetrimide"). Other types of surfactants used for their disinfection activity are known as the "amphoteric" surfactants (e.g. alkyldimethyl oxide). Quaternary ammonium compounds are used in disinfectants, particularly low level for combined cleaning and disinfection. They are also widely used with surfactants in a range of other cleaning and disinfectant formulations due to their soil removing and capturing activity. They are typically provided as concentrates, ready-to-use and wipe-impregnated disinfectant products for general environment and non-critical device applications. They are generally known to have a pleasant, clean odor that can also be used for deodorization in general ward use. Similar to the phenols (see the section on phenols), the QACs range dramatically in activity depending on the chemicals used (they are often used in mixtures of two or three QAC types) and their formulation. In general, QAC-based products provide good bactericidal and viricidal (enveloped) activity, but can

range in activity to include fungi and even (rarely) mycobacteria and therefore might have claims as intermediate-level disinfectants. They have important advantages in being used as both cleaning and disinfectant agents, and are considered non-corrosive and safe for use. They are limited in antimicrobial activity and can be irritating or damaging to some surface materials (e.g. copper, depending on their formulation).

Other biocides

There are many other types of biocides that can be used for disinfection purposes, in addition to the main types discussed above. It is difficult to consider all of these in detail and, even then, individual products and applications can range considerably. In all cases of existing and new biocides, consideration should be given to the claims made with the product, with particular emphasis on safety and efficacy (in the section on basic principles of disinfection). A few additional biocide types are discussed briefly below.

Glucoprotamine (or glucoprotamin) is a relatively new biocide used for low to high-level disinfection of environmental surfaces and device reprocessing (including semi-critical devices, depending on the disinfection product). Formulations have claimed bactericidal (including mycobactericidal activity at defined contact times/conditions), fungicidal and viricidal (particular enveloped viruses) activity. There is little to no activity with certain types of non-enveloped viruses and bacterial spores. Typical concentrations used are in the range of 0.25–0.5% in formulation; formulation effects include optimizing antimicrobial activity and surfactants to aid in cleaning activity. Such disinfectants are generally considered to have good material compatibility, but are also irritating to the skin/mucous membranes.

Strong acids and bases (low or high pH respectively; Chapter 6, in the section on the pH scale: defining acids and bases) are sometimes used for their antimicrobial activity, especially in product formulations. Examples may include low pH (acidic) and high pH (alkaline) based formulations. Cleaning solutions may also have some antimicrobial claims (used for cleaning and low-level disinfection), with particular emphasis on bactericidal and viricidal (enveloped) activity. Strong alkaline solutions have also been recommended to be effective against prions (such as 1–2 N sodium hydroxide for one hour on surgical devices), but these are not generally recommended for routine use for device reprocessing. Although they may provide some antimicrobial activity, care should be taken in their use from a personal safety and device compatibility point of view (in particular as strong acids and bases can be damaging to device materials). pH also plays an important role in the activity of other chemical disinfectants (as discussed above), as an important part of a disinfectant formulation (Chapter 6, in the section on mixtures, formulations and solutions).

Chlorhexidine (commonly known as CHG for "chlorhexidine gluconate") is a widely used biocide in antiseptics (hand washes and hand rubs), for general hand washing, pre-operative patient bathing, pre-operative skin preparation and as a surgical scrub. It is an example of a group of biocides known "biguanides". Other examples, although much less used in this group, are alexidine and octenidine in antiseptics and the polyhexamethylbi-guanides (PHMBs) for general surface/water disinfection. Chlorhexidine-based antiseptics generally provide bacteri-cidal and virucidal (non-enveloped) activity, with some activity against fungi (depending on the product). Some products provide a combined effect of chlorhexidine and alcohol (in hand rubs), as well as other formulation effects to increase the overall antimicrobial activity of the product. Typical concentrations range from 0.5% to 4%, but overall activity is based on specific formulation effects. As antiseptics they are considered gentle on the hands but effective against many of the transient bacteria/viruses found on the skin. In addition to its immediate activity during the wash/application, chlorhexidine can remain bound to the skin and provide a persistent antimicrobial activity over time. This is often a benefit during long surgical procedures to prevent the growth of bacteria (in particular under gloves). Despite these benefits, the over-all antimicrobial activity is limited (low-level disinfection) and some formulations can be irritating to those using them; residual activity can be neutralized by certain types of skin creams and hand washes (e.g. those containing non-ionic surfactants). The PHMBs are not widely used as disinfectants and then only for general, environmental surfaces as low-level disinfectants (with specific claims dependent on the disinfectant formulation).

Certain types of metals are used for disinfection purposes in healthcare; these particularly include silver and copper. Copper has become more widely used as a naturally occurring antimicrobial integrated into sur-faces; these surfaces usually consist of a certain amount of copper mixed with other metals (these are known as "alloys", e.g. brass is an alloy of copper and zinc). Copper-containing surfaces are used to provide a low-level (specifically bactericidal or bacteriostatic) disinfection on surfaces if contacted. Typical applications include light switches, tray tables, etc. Silver is also used for antimicrobial purposes, but rarely for surface/device

disinfection and more commonly for certain antiseptic-types applications (e.g. wound dressings). Copper-silver ionization systems (where an electric current provided to copper/silver plates releases a low level of both biocides into water) are used for water-treatment (e.g. to reduce lev-els of certain types of bacteria such as *Legionella* that can be a concern in water-handling systems). The activity of these types of antimicrobial metals can range considerably and close attention should be given to any label claims that can include bactericidal/bacteriostatic, fungicidal/fungi-static activity over time. Like all metals, they can be toxic to humans if exposed at higher concentrations.

Disinfection guidelines and standards

As highlighted in introductory section, disinfection claims may or may not be regulated in different countries/regions, with some countries closely controlling the use of disinfectants and others not. Examples include:
• USA: the FDA CDRH (Food & Drug Administration Center for Devices and Radiological Health) regulates the disinfection and sterilization of devices, including thermal and chemical processes, as well as antiseptics (as they contact the skin/mucous membranes). The EPA (Environmental Protection Agency) regulates the use of chemical disinfectants for general environmental sur-faces. Products are registered and approved for use based on scientific evidence of safety and efficacy. Some states may also have specific requirements regarding the use of disinfectants, including restrictions on disposal of chemi-cals through public drains.
• European Union: in Europe, if a disinfectant or disin-fection process is used for reprocessing a device for patient use they are also considered "devices" and are therefore regulated under the Medical Devices Directive (93/42/EEC). There are various classes of devices, depending on the risk to the patient, ranging from the lowest risk (class 1) to the highest risk (class 3). Device disinfectants and disinfection processes are currently considered as class 2b devices. The general (essential) safety requirements for these products are described in the directive itself and specific require-ments are also outlined in applicable EN and/or ISO standards (note: under the Vienna Agreement 1991, there is technical cooperation between ISO and CEN to make such standards compatible or even identical). An example is for washer-disinfectors as defined in the EN ISO 15883 (washer-disinfector) series of standards. Further considerations for washer-disinfectors and

disinfection machines include the Machinery Directive (2006/42/EC, if moving parts are used as part of the process) and electrical safety requirements. There is also a series of EN standards under development regarding the demonstration of the antimicrobial activities of antiseptics and disinfectants. These range from simple suspension tests (phase 1), laboratory antimicrobial tests that simulate the practical use of the disinfectant (e.g. on the hands or a hard surface; phase 2) and "field" tests where the disinfectant is tested as used in practice (phase 3). In addition to these tests, other country-specific tests or requirements may be specified in certain countries (e.g. French AFNOR, British BSI and German DIN tests). Chemical disinfectants used for other purposes (environmental or water disinfection) are also affected by other European Directives. These include the Biocidal Products Directive (BPD, 98/8/EC) that regulates chemicals used for antimicrobial purposes, with a particular emphasis on environmental concerns. Others with a similar remit that affect disinfectants (or the use of other chemicals in disinfectant formulations) include the EC Detergent Regulation (648/2004) and the REACh Regulation (Registration Evaluation and Authorisation of Chemicals EC 1907/2006). As a note, a further exception is that antiseptics are regulated as medicines under the EU Medicinal Products Directives 2001/83/EC and 2004/27/EC.

• Australia: disinfectants are regulated by the Therapeutic Goods Administration (TGA) under the Therapeutic Goods Order (TGO) No. 54. This applies to antiseptics and disinfectants. A range of international and national standards and test methods are recognized to establish disinfection efficacy.

• Canada: disinfectants, including antiseptics, are regulated under Health Canada's Therapeutic Products Directorate (TPD). Products are registered and approved for use based on scientific evidence of safety and efficacy. Antimicrobial hand soaps must also have a Drug Identification Number (DIN) that is displayed on the product label.

• Brazil: disinfectants to be registered with the National Health Surveillance Agency (ANVISA), including safety and efficacy (e.g. with standard test methods).

• Korea: disinfectants are registered with the Korean Food and Drug Administration (KFDA) including safety and efficacy (e.g. with standard test methods).

• International: examples of international requirements include the ISO standards (e.g. EN ISO 15883 for washer-disinfectors) and antimicrobial test methods described by the Organization for Economic Cooperation and Development (OECD). In the case of ISO standards, although these are internationally harmonized, many countries may specifically decide to modify the text for publication as a local standard and others will adopt them without modification.

In addition to these country-specific requirements, a variety of country or organization-specific guidelines have been developed and are frequently updated. They generally provide guidance regarding antisepsis and disinfection, including types of disinfectants and local or device-specific considerations regarding safe and effective use. Guidelines are not a replacement for country/region-specific regulations, but they are often used together to establish best practices in facilities. A summary of some types of guidance on disinfection is given in Table 9.5.

Particular consideration has already been given to the various parts of the ISO washer-disinfector standards, the ISO 15883 series (Chapter 8, in the section on cleaning guidelines, standards and testing). Thermal disinfection is specified as the minimum temperature and contact time necessary to provide an A_0 applicable to the type of washer-disinfector; for example surgical devices are required, in compliance to ISO 15883 Parts 1 and 2, to be disinfected at a minimum A_0 of 600 (e.g. 90°C (194°F) for one minute; Table 9.5). The temperature distribution within the washer-disinfector is verified using temperature sensors (e.g. thermocouples) and associated recording systems (Figure 9.14); these are placed at various locations within the chamber, load and load carrier (rack, tray, etc.). The measurement system should have a specified accuracy, precision, etc., and be periodically calibrated to ensure it is functioning correctly. For ISO 15883 compliance, the disinfection temperature should be between −0°C and +5°C (32–41°F) of the set temperature; an upper limit is also set to prevent the washer-disinfector from accidentally overheating the load, which could lead to damage.

Testing and confirming temperature distribution may be conducted during the design, installation and periodically (e.g. yearly) during clinical use. It should be pointed out, however, that the A_0 concept is not accepted in all countries as being enough to make a thermal disinfection claim and thermal disinfection cycles may need to be further verified by antimicrobial test methods (discussed further in this section and summarized in Table 9.6). These test methods and pass/fail criteria will be defined by local government regulatory agencies. Although there are tight controls and testing requirements defined in ISO 15883 for automated washer-disinfectors, there are little such controls on manual thermal disinfection; despite this the same concepts can be applied. The temperature of the water used for disinfection should be verified, exposure conditions should ensure that the device is fully immersed for disinfection and the contact time should be controlled.

Table 9.5 Examples of disinfection guidance documents.

Publisher	Title	Description
US-CDC HICPAC[1] Guideline for Disinfection and Sterilization in Healthcare Facilities	*Guideline for disinfection and sterilization in healthcare facilities*	Recommendations on methods for cleaning, disinfection and sterilization of patient-care devices and the healthcare environment
Canadian General Standards Board (CGSB)	*CAN/CGSB-2.161-97 assessment of efficacy of antimicrobial agents for use on environmental surfaces and medical devices*	Guidance on the registration of disinfectants, including safety and efficacy requirements
British Society of Gastroenterology (BSG)	*BSG guidelines for decontamination of equipment for gastrointestinal endoscopy*	Guidelines on cleaning and disinfection of flexible endoscopes
World Gastroenterology Society (WGO)	*WGO/OMED practice guideline endoscope disinfection*	Guidelines on cleaning and disinfection of flexible endoscopes
Association for the Advancement of Medical Instrumentation (AAMI)	*AAMI/ANSI ST58 chemical sterilization and high-level disinfection in healthcare facilities*	Guidelines for the selection and use of high-level disinfectants (and chemical sterilants) approved in the USA
Society of Gastroenterology Nurses and Associates (SGNA)	*Guideline for use of high-level disinfectants and sterilants for reprocessing flexible gastrointestinal endoscopes*	A guide to the types and use of disinfectants/sterilants for endoscope reprocessing
American Professionals in Infection Control (APIC)	*Guideline for hand washing and hand antisepsis in healthcare settings*	Guidelines on the type and use of various antiseptics in healthcare applications
World Health Organization (WHO)	*Infection control guidelines for transmissible spongiform encephalopathies*	Guidelines for infection control practices against prion diseases, including decontamination[2]

[1] Center for Disease Control (CDC) Healthcare Infection Control Practices Advisory Committee (HICPAC).
[2] These where initially published in 1999 and are now considered outdated.

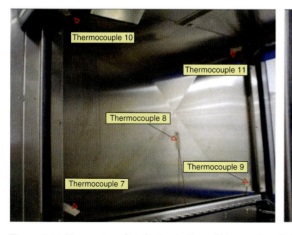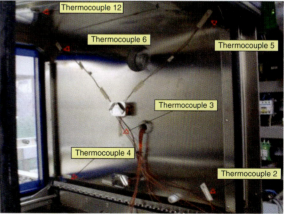

Figure 9.14 Temperature distribution testing within a washer-disinfector chamber. Note the use of various temperature sensors (thermocouples) located at various places in the chamber.

Table 9.6 Examples of published and widely used disinfection test methods.

Test method	Title	Description
EN 1500	*Hygienic hand rub – test method and requirements (phase 2/step 2)*	Volunteer hands are artificially contaminated with a controlled number of test organisms. The number of test organisms before and after application of the hand rub are tested.
EN 14347	*Basic sporicidal activity: test method and requirements (phase 1)*	Bacterial spore (*Bacillus* species) suspensions added directly to the disinfectant to test sporicidal ability.
EN 13727	*Quantitative suspension test for the evaluation of bacterial activity of chemical disinfectants for instruments used in the medical area: test method and requirements (phase 2, step 1)*	Vegetative bacteria (Gram positive and negative) suspensions added directly to the disinfectant in the presence of interfering substances.
AOAC	*965.12 Tuberculocidal activity of disinfectants*	*Mycobacterium bovis* (or test modified using *M. terrae*) inoculated onto small cylinders, dried and exposed to the disinfectant.
AOAC	*966.04 Sporicidal activity of disinfectants*	Two types of spore-forming bacteria (*Bacillus* and *Clostridium*) in the presence of soil inoculated onto two types of carriers, dried and exposed to the disinfectant.
EN ISO 15883:1	*Washer-disinfectors – part 1: general requirements, terms and definitions and tests*	Describes the A_o concept for thermal disinfection and testing of temperature distribution in a washer-disinfector.
EN ISO 15883:4.	*Washer-disinfectors – part 4: requirements and tests for washer-disinfectors employing chemical disinfection for thermolabile endoscopes*	Microbiological testing of a range of microorganisms (including bacteria, viruses, fungi and spores) inoculated into surrogate lumen devices and tested for microbial inactivation (log reductions) following the disinfection process.
American Society for Testing and Materials (ASTM) E1837	*Standard test method to determine efficacy of disinfection processes for re-usable medical Devices*	Simulated use testing for disinfection of re-usable medical devices using bacteria, viruses and/or fungi.
ASTM E1174	*Standard test method for evaluation of healthcare personnel hand wash formulations*	Activity of an antiseptic on the hands using an artifical inoculum of *Serratia marcescens*.
ASTM E1838	*Standard test method for determining the virus-eliminating effectiveness of hygienic hand wash and hand rub agents using the finger pads of adults*	Activity of an antiseptic on the fingerpads contaminated with different viruses.
ASTM E-2197[1]	*Standard quantitative disk carrier test method for determining the bactericidal, virucidal, fungicidal, mycobactericidal and sporicidal activities of liquid chemical germicides*	Method tests the ability of disinfectants to inactivate microorganisms in the presence of a soil load on disk carriers, representing environmental surfaces and devices.
ASTM E2111	*Standard quantitative carrier test method to evaluate the bactericidal, fungicidal, mycobactericidal and sporicidal potencies of liquid chemical germicides*	Known quantity of microorganisms are inoculated onto carriers and exposed to a disinfectant to determine a given reduction.

[1] This test method, at the time of writing, is being proposed for adoption by the Organisation for Economic Cooperation and Development (OECD) as a recommended international series of test methods for various types of microorganisms.

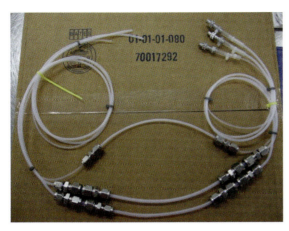

Figure 9.15 Example of a surrogate test device for demonstration of disinfection efficacy in a washer-disinfector.

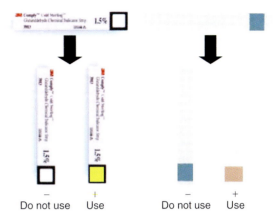

Figure 9.16 Examples of two different types of chemical indicators and their typical color change on exposure to a chemical disinfectant.

Chemical disinfection can be achieved by a chemical disinfectant alone (usually at room temperature, either manually or in a disinfector machine) or by a chemical-thermal process (where the temperature is also controlled during the disinfection process). A wide range of test methods may be used to show that a product is effective as a disinfectant and/or antiseptic. Examples of such tests are given in Table 9.6. It is important to note that these tests are designed to show that a product is effective when tested in a laboratory under a particular set of conditions and that the disinfectant can be effective when used in accordance with labeled directions.

Some of these tests are specifically designed to demonstrate the effectiveness of a chemical disinfection process in a washer-disinfector; an example is in ISO 15883 Part 4, describing tests for washer-disinfectors employing chemical disinfection for thermolabile endoscopes. As an example, in the recommended testing a range of microorganisms may be tested to include bacteria, mycobacteria, viruses, fungi and bacterial spores. Preparations of each are inoculated into plastic (specifically PFTE) tubes of 2 mm or 1 mm diameter x 150 mm in length and placed at various positions along an overall length of tubing at 1.5 meters; two of the 2 mm sizes and one of the 1 mm sizes are then used for testing in the washer-disinfector (during the disinfection process; Figure 9.15). Bacterial spores are used to test for physical removal during the process and the other microorganisms to demonstrate antimicrobial efficacy, where a given level of microbial reduction is expected to be demonstrated. Such tests can demonstrate a combination of physical removal and disinfection.

Other test methods, given in Table 9.6, are used to show that the chemical disinfectant is effective under laboratory conditions and/or within a washer-disinfector. They are used to establish and register a chemical disinfectant as being effective; in certain countries specific test methods are defined and reviewed, while in others they are not. A further series of tests may be required for a chemical washer-disinfector regarding "self-disinfection". A self-disinfection cycle is described as a programmed cycle for use without any load in the washer-disinfector that is used to periodically disinfect all liquid transport systems including piping, chamber(s), tanks and all other components that may come into contact with the water and/or solutions used for cleaning, disinfecting and rinsing the load. This is a periodic disinfection cycle designed to reduce the risk of the development of biofilm formation (Chapter 5, in the section on Bacteria), where a different type of chemical or preferably thermal disinfection process is provided within the disinfector to reduce biofilm. This is particularly important in water rinsing or a storage system provided within the washer-disinfector that may or may not be routinely disinfected.

A further consideration in the use of chemical disinfectants is chemical indicators. Chemical indicators (or CIs) are defined as test systems (usually in the form of test strips) that reveal a change in one or more pre-defined process variables, based on a chemical and/or physical change resulting from exposure to a process. They are generally provided as color-change indicators (Figure 9.16) that are used to verify that a chemical or physical disinfectant or disinfection process (or indeed cleaning or sterilization process) is fit for use or has been conducted.

Table 9.7 The classification of chemical indicators[1].

Class	Indicator type	Description
Class 1	Process indicator	These are simple indicators to demonstrate exposure to a process and also to distinguish between processed/unprocessed units. A pass result may not mean the process has been achieved.
Class 2	Indicators for use in specific tests	Used to indicate a specific type of test, generally established in another standard.
Class 3	Single variable indicators	Designed to respond to only one critical process variable (e.g. concentration of a biocide).
Class 4	Multi-variable indicators	Designed to respond to two or more of the critical variables (e.g. temperature, time and concentration of a biocide).
Class 5	Integrating indicators	Designed to respond to all critical variables of the process, in particular to be equivalent to a biological indicator (e.g. indicators containing bacterial spores used to test sterilization processes); Chapter 11.
Class 6	Emulating indicators	Designed to react to all critical variables for a full specified cycle (that may be over and above that matching a biological indicator).

[1] Defined based on ISO 11140 *Sterilization of healthcare products – chemical indicators*.

They are often used with re-usable disinfectants (in particular, high level disinfectants), where the disinfectant is verified to be under the right conditions (e.g. presence of sufficient biocide) to be effective according to the manufacturer's claims. In the case of re-usable disinfectants, this is important as they may become watered down over time with use, be incorrectly prepared/maintained, or be used in a manner that may have exhausted the presence of the biocide. A typical term used is the minimum effective concentration (MEC), where the indicator is designed to show that a minimum amount of the disinfectant is present. They are also used for single-use disinfectants/sterilants, for example to ensure that they have been delivered correctly at the right concentration or generated/mixed correctly (in cases where the biocide is made or activated by mixing two chemicals together). In addition to chemical disinfection, they are also widely used to verify thermal and chemical sterilization processes (Chapter 11). Chemical indicators, according to the ISO 11140 series of standards titled *Sterilization of healthcare products – chemical indicators*, are defined into six different classes depending on monitoring abilities and information they may (or may not) provide about the process being monitored (Table 9.7); although this series of standards relate to sterilization process, they are introduced at this stage in reference to the use of chemical indicators for disinfection. At the time of writing there are no standards defining the requirement for CIs used for disinfection. But overall, most indicators used with chemical disinfectants are generally similar to class 1, 3 or 4 types.

As the various regulatory requirements can periodically change, it is important to understand any local requirements and to review any disinfectant product claims closely. This is particularly important in countries where no specific product registration (including technical review) is required and independently reviewed. Do not hesitate to get an expert microbiological review of any test data to ensure that the disinfectant or disinfection process is fit for purpose.

Special considerations

Many of the special considerations previously outlined in Chapter 8 on cleaning of various device types equally apply to disinfection. These include close attention to any manufacturers' guidelines on disinfection practices (e.g. restrictions on temperature, preparation, chemical compatibility, etc.) and/or local guidelines, requirements or legal rules. For example, many biocides or chemicals used in disinfectant preparations may or may not be used in certain geographical regions or will especially require local registration with an authorized regulatory authority prior to use in healthcare facilities. These may include various efficacy and even safety requirements (e.g. environmental safety is a growing concern worldwide). Care should therefore be taken to understand any local requirements and to ensure that any changes or updates are considered in the use of chemical or even thermal disinfection products/processes. The particular concerns related to microsurgical devices, ophthalmological instruments, loan devices/sets, devices with integrated electrical components, robotics, endoscopes and textiles should be considered as outlined in Chapter 8 in the section on special cleaning considerations.

Thermal and chemical disinfection can be particularly affected by the quality of water provided. In some cases, chemical contaminants such as high chlorine and water hardness levels can lead to device damage (rusting) or the deposition of chemical deposits (scaling) on surfaces. In both cases these can lead to patient complications. Further, the chemical quality of water can affect the ability of a chemical disinfectant to be effective (in particular the presence of water hardness and even heavy metals that can significantly affect the disinfection activity of these products, depending on their formulation). The microbial water quality can also be important. High levels of microorganisms in water used as part of a chemical disinfection may affect the overall efficacy of the product. This is particularly a concern in water used to rinse a device following disinfection, where the disinfection may be successful but then the water used for rinsing can re-contaminate the device and lead to patient infections; this has been particularly highlighted in the inadequate reprocessing of flexible endoscopes and even due to the inadequate design or maintenance of washer-disinfectors used to reprocess such devices. But equally, high levels of certain types of bacteria (in particular Gram negative Bacteria) may be inactivated but can release toxins (with Gram negative bacteria endotoxins; Chapter 5, see the section on bacteria) that can lead to subsequent patient complications; note that endotoxins are known to be very resistant to thermal disinfection and even sterilization processes in particular.

Flexible endoscopes

Various considerations in the cleaning and reprocessing of flexible endoscopes have been outlined in Chapter 8 in the section on endoscopy. These equally apply to disinfection. Remember that the use of a flexible endoscope can contain various components, including the endoscope, its accessories and the control system (with its own accessories). The control system is a non-critical device, but may require routine cleaning/disinfection of various surfaces using low to intermediate-level disinfectants (e.g. daily or after each use); various parts may become soiled or otherwise contaminated during procedures (in particular due to staff handling). Some systems provide a source of water for use with the endoscope

during the procedure (e.g. for cleaning lenses at the distal tip of the scope or for irrigation of internal tissues during the procedure); such water bottles are usually provided with sterile water, but also should be routinely cleaned and disinfected/sterilized. A typical example is to rinse the water bottle with water, assist drying with 70% alcohol and follow by steam sterilization. Specific device manufacturers' instructions should be considered regarding the disinfection of the control system and associated water bottles.

Flexible endoscopes are generally temperature sensitive, being restricted to cleaning and disinfection processes below 60°C and are therefore commonly reprocessed using chemical disinfectants and sterilization processes. These can be conducted under manual immersion methods or as part of disinfection (washer-disinfection) processes (Figure 9.17).

It is important to ensure, in both cases, that all parts of the device are adequately immersed in (or contacted with) the disinfectant to ensure antimicrobial activity, this includes ensuring that all bubbles are removed from the device lumens during manual immersion (e.g. by immersion and flushing of the lumens under the disinfectant) and by correct attachment of all lumens to an automated irrigation system. Further, it is important to also consider any accessories that are used as part of the device or during the device procedure (Chapter 15, Figure 15.3); this particularly includes the control valves ("buttons") used with the device. Remember that these valves may be single use or be required to be cleaned and disinfected/sterilized as an important component of the device; due to their design, they may require to be correctly opened (or actuated, by opening and closing) to ensure that all parts of the valve are correctly exposed.

The different steps in reprocessing of a flexible endoscope include:
- Manual pre-cleaning (bedside procedure).
- Automated and/or manual cleaning and rinsing.
- Manual or automated disinfection.
- Rinsing (if applicable). Note, in rare cases rinsing may not be required in certain types of washer-disinfectors; if claimed by the manufacturer, this should be verified and documented by the facility.
- Drying, if applicable.

Further consideration is given to the disinfection and drying stages below.

The most widely used biocides for the disinfection of flexible endoscopes include the aldehydes (glutaraldehyde and OPA), oxidizing agents (particularly peracetic acid and hydrogen peroxide, but to a less extent chlorine

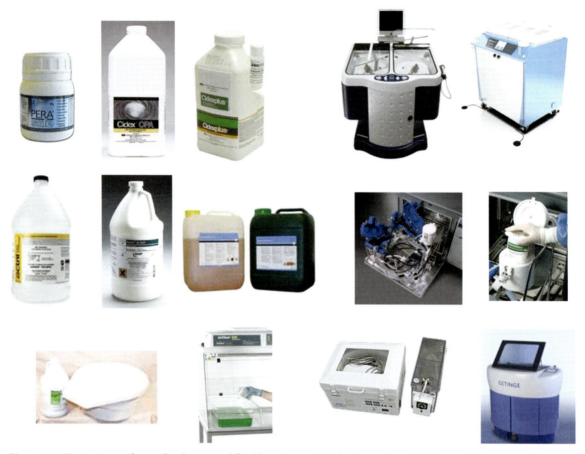

Figure 9.17 Various types of manual and automated flexible endoscope disinfection products/disinfectors. Various types of disinfectants (single and two-component; top left), manual immersion baths (bottom left) and automated disinfectors (right).

dioxide and super-oxidized water methods) and other miscellaneous biocides or mixtures of biocides such as quaternary ammonium compounds and glucoprotamine. All of these are used in formulation and individual formulations will vary on required exposure conditions and antimicrobial claims; it is not sufficient to consider the concentration of the biocide alone as this can be misleading. Remember that each formulation will vary, depending on safety, efficacy, device compatibility, preparation method, shelf-life (when being used or stored), temperature, monitoring systems (e.g. use of chemical indicators to confirm the MEC; see the section on disinfection guidelines and standards), number and method of rinsing, etc. In all cases, care should be taken to read and understand the label claims and instructions provided with the disinfectant. In some countries, specific soaking times may be recommended in independent guidelines that are different to product label claims; in these cases, this is a facility decision, and should be specified and approved in a written protocol to prevent staff confusion. Due to differences in country/region testing and registration requirements, it is not unusual for the same disinfectant to have different label claims in different countries; it is therefore important to understand any local requirement or restrictions in the use of disinfectants (e.g. certain biocides may not be recommended for use in a given region or may have specific handling/disposal requirements). Some formulations are only designed for use in automated systems under temperature control, while others are designed for manual and/or automated reprocessing. In manual immersion systems, care should be taken to ensure that all surfaces of the device are adequately immersed/covered in the disinfectant, including the internal lumens. The presence of

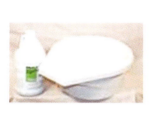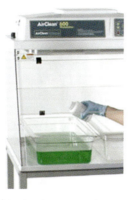

Figure 9.18 Manual immersion safety, showing a covered soaking bath (left) and use of the disinfectant in a chemical safety cabinet.

air bubbles, for example, on immersed surfaces can limit disinfection efficacy. Automated systems generally provide various types of irrigation or flow type systems that are designed to flow the chemistry through the internal channels; they may also use spray and/or immersion type methods to disinfect the outside surfaces of the endoscope.

In addition to ensuring disinfectant/disinfection efficacy, consideration should be given to the safe handling of the chemical disinfectant. Safety considerations include risks to staff, devices, patients and the environment. All disinfectants are potentially hazardous to health; therefore contact with the disinfectant should be minimized. This can be done manually using a well ventilated area, chemical extraction hoods (Figure 9.18) and covering open disinfection baths; automated systems are often preferred as they should limit access/exposure to the disinfectant. Safety has been particularly highlighted with the use of aldehyde-based disinfectants due to occupational hazardous (e.g. irritation to the skin, mucous membranes and respiratory tract; see the section on aldehydes), but may be equally true in the handling of other types of disinfectants. Exposure risks should be specified in the material safety data sheets provided with the disinfectant; if these are not provided the disinfectant should not be used. Information regarding the compatibility with the device and device materials should be provided by the disinfectant manufacturer; it is preferable that the disinfectant is approved for use by the device manufacturer, but failing this a written statement of compatibility should be provided by the disinfectant manufacturer. In general aldehyde-based disinfectants are widely compatible with flexible endoscopes, while

oxidizing agent and other biocide-disinfectants can vary considerably.

Rinsing is an important consideration following chemical disinfection, to minimize any patient safety risks. The endoscope should be rinsed, manually or in a programmed/validated automated system according to the disinfectant manufacturer's instructions to ensure that no chemical toxic residual remain on the device. In some cases, up to five or six rinses in fresh water may be required to ensure that all external and internal surface residuals are correctly removed prior to patient use. Disinfectant residual can lead to patient complications. A typical example is with the use of glutaraldehyde and OPA; both types of disinfectants can be difficult to rinse away from surfaces and have been associated with complications such as colitis (irritation of the colon) following colonoscopy procedures. Toxicity may not only be related to the biocide, but also to the other components of the disinfectant formulation. There is a further consideration with rinsing: contamination of the rinse water being used. Water can include a variety of chemical and microbial contaminants, even if it has been previously treated to reduce such risks (Chapter 15 in the section on Water Quality). Therefore, the control of water quality is an important consideration to ensure that the device is not re-contaminated prior to patient use. National and regional guidelines can vary considerably on this point to include:
• Rinsing with tap water, followed by flushing internal lumens with alcohol to aid in drying
• Rinsing in filtered water (generally using a "sterile" or bacterial retentive filter)
• Rinsing with water previously sterilized by steam or provided sterile
• Rinsing with highly purified water, such as deionized, distilled or reverse osmosis water
All of these methods may be considered safe depending on the quality (chemical and microbial) of the water being used and the subsequent use of the endoscope. For example, the quality of tap water can vary widely, even from day to day, including microbial and chemical contamination. But equally, treated water (by filtration or purification) can become re-contaminated on storage or transfer to the point of use for rinsing. For low-risk endoscopy procedures (e.g. an investigational colonoscopy), reprocessing of the endoscope followed by a rinse with tap water can be used to remove disinfectant residuals and bacterial contaminants present in the tap water can be reduced by alcohol flushing and drying; however, tap water and even 70% alcohol (remembering that alcohol is not an effective disinfectant for certain types of

microorganisms, particularly bacterial spores) can often be contaminated. Therefore it is always optimal for the microbial quality of the water to be maintained at a low or essentially no contamination level. For microbial contamination, an example that is used on the routine monitoring of bacterial contamination is:

- <1 cfu/mL: satisfactory
- <1–9 cfu/mL on a regular basis: acceptable, indicates that bacterial numbers are under reasonable control
- 10–100 cfu/mL: unsatisfactory, investigate the potential problem and/or repeat testing
- >100 cfu/mL: unacceptable, out of service until quality is improved

These levels may or may not be acceptable depending on the use of the endoscope (procedure, blood contact, etc.). Any system providing, treating or holding water for rinsing should be correctly maintained to ensure it does not become contaminated; for example, biofilms (e.g. with bacteria such as *Pseudomonas* and *Mycobacterium* species) can easily form within these systems, leading to cross-contamination of endoscopes during rinsing. Maintenance may include routine disinfection (by heat and/or chemical) of water storage/handling lines or self-disinfection cycles of the washer-disinfector/separate

water treatment equipment. Equally, certain types of chemical contaminants may cause problems, such as high levels of chlorine, leading to device damage over time (see the section on troubleshooting disinfection problems below). Overall, local guidelines should be considered and regularly monitored in providing staff with facility-approved instructions. In some cases this needs to be validated by the washer-disinfector manufacturer and in other cases to be routinely monitored by the facility.

Drying of the endoscope is a further consideration, particularly when the device has been disinfected and is to be stored for some time. This will particularly prevent the growth of bacteria/fungi in the device lumens during storage. Guidelines are equally variable on this topic, but include:

- Purging of water from the device lumens using air and wiping down the external surfaces with a clean cloth
- The use of alcohol (typically 70%) to assist in lumen drying, following and during air purging as described above
- Purging of any large volumes of water from internal lumens and placing the device into a specifically designed flexible endoscope storage cabinet that allows HEPA-filtered air to pass through the lumens to dry and/or maintain during storage (an example is shown in Figure 9.19)

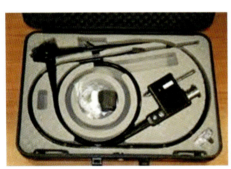 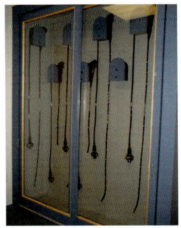 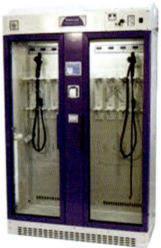

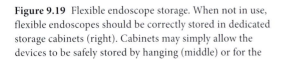

Figure 9.19 Flexible endoscope storage. When not in use, flexible endoscopes should be correctly stored in dedicated storage cabinets (right). Cabinets may simply allow the devices to be safely stored by hanging (middle) or for the device lumens to be connected to a HEPA-filtered air source to allow for and/or maintain drying (far right). Flexible endoscopes should *not* be stored in their transport cases (left).

Drying may therefore be done as a manual or automated method. In some washer-disinfectors, this may be by the use of air to purge the majority of water from the lumens (or external device surfaces) and/or providing a 70% alcohol rinse. Drying with the use of 70% alcohol is sometimes recommended after each and every reprocessing cycle, particularly where tap water is used for rinsing, or more commonly at the end of the day/patient list prior to device storage; equally, the 70% alcohol may not be required or may even be recommended against. As a minimum, flexible endoscopes that have been high-level disinfected and are not in use should be stored under dry conditions (including the lumens) in a dedicated area/cabinet to prevent damage (Figure 9.19). It is recommended that they are hung vertically, not over-coiled, and protected from accidental breakage. Specially designed storage cabinets are used for this purpose that provide HEPA-filtered air to pass through the device lumens (when correctly connected) to assist in drying. In most cases, it is recommended that the device is re-disinfected immediately prior to patient use following storage; however, if the device has been correctly dried and maintained dry during storage (e.g. according to instructions provided by storage cabinet manufacturers) this may not be necessary. Local guidelines should be reviewed in considering safe and acceptable practices for a facility.

Following disinfection (and drying, if applicable), chemicals may be used for the maintenance of the device (such as lubricants). These should be used safely under the guidance given by the manufacturer.

A variety of automated systems may be used for the reprocessing of flexible endoscopes, such as disinfectors or washer-disinfectors (Figure 9.17). These can vary in complexity and include immersion and/or spray systems for disinfecting the outside of the scope and irrigation (flow) systems for lumen cleaning. Some washers use specifically designed connectors that attach to the endoscope and irrigation/flow system of the machine, while others use a pressurized system at the control head of the scope to provide flow (connector-less washers). They may or may not provide a variety of features such as lumen blockage test, irrigation control, detection of connector attachment/detachment, disinfection process parameter control, rinse-water quality control, fault alarm systems, etc. Remember that a machine is only as good as how it is used and maintained. A common problem is that a lumen connector has not been attached (or is not attached correctly) or has become detached during the cycle. A further problem is in the maintenance of the system, where bacteria biofilms may develop in the system (or particularly the rinse water system/lines) can

cause re-contamination of the device during the automated process; the disinfector manufacturer should provide an assurance that these risks are minimized in the machine design. Information should also be provided by the manufacturer regarding the testing and validation of disinfection efficacy, preferably in compliance with local national or international standards/guidelines. At a minimum, the disinfector should be provided with at least one disinfection process that has been shown to be effective for endoscope disinfection/rinsing. The disinfector may be designed for use with one or many types of disinfectants. Useful standard to consider are ISO 15883 Part 1 and 4, Part 4 being specific.

One of the prevalent causes of failure in flexible endoscope reprocessing is human error. Examples include:
- Failure to clean/disinfect the whole device, including the accessories
- Failure to detect and ensure that all lumens are cleaned/disinfected
- Failure to use the disinfectant or disinfection machine according to manufacturers' instructions
- Recontamination due to inadequate water quality
- Inadequate endoscope storage

These risks should be minimized by correct and frequent training of staff; this is particularly important where a department has a high turnover of staff. Flexible endoscope reprocessing can be a difficult task and is often performed in departments that have little time to ensure it is performed correctly. Training should highlight the structure and safe handling of flexible endoscopes, manual cleaning, how to use and troubleshoot automated reprocessing systems, manual or automated washing-disinfection, rinsing requirements (manual or automated), maintenance of the endoscopes and reprocessing equipment, and safety. Health risks should be specifically highlighted, to include the risks associated with manual cleaning (including brush), use/disposal of chemicals and personal protective equipment (PPE).

All facilities should have a written policy on the safe reprocessing of flexible endoscopes. Various international and regional endoscopy organizations provide and periodically update guidelines on the safe reprocessing of flexible endoscopes. Due to differences from country to country, these may vary and even contradict each other in some cases; therefore it is important to ensure the correct local requirements are considered in establishing and maintaining written facility instructions. These organizations include:
- USA:
  ○ SGNA: Society for Gastroenterology Nurses and Associates

○ ASGE: American Society for Gastrointestinal Endoscopy

○ APIC: Association of Professionals in Infection Control and Epidemiology

• Europe:
  ○ ESGE: European Society of Gastrointestinal Endoscopy
  ○ ESGENA: European Society of Gastrointestinal Endoscopy Nurses and Associates
  ○ BSG: British Society of Gastroenterology

• Australia:
  ○ GESA: Gastroenterology Society of Australia
  ○ GENCA: Gastroenterological Nurses College of Australia

Laundry

Textile reprocessing (preparation, cleaning and disinfection) has already been considered in some detail in Chapter 8 in the section on textiles and laundry. Textiles may often become heavily contaminated (in particular with soils, such as blood and feces and microorganisms), but are generally considered as being at low risk of transmission to staff/patients, particularly when cleaned and disinfected. Despite this, standard safety precautions (including PPE) should be taken in handling contaminated or patient-used materials (Chapter 8, section on textiles and laundry). Disinfection of textiles provides some unique challenges given the types of materials being treated. Healthcare laundry disinfection is usually conducted in a washer-disinfector design (Chapter 8, Figure 8.30) and some materials may also require further packaging and sterilization. Disinfection is performed by thermal (>60°C) and/or chemical means (<60°C, e.g. using chlorine, ozone or peracetic acid under controlled temperature conditions). The cleaning and disinfection process may be conducted as part of the same stage or separate stages of the reprocessing cycle. Other chemicals are used as part of the process, including for cleaning, specific stain removal and load conditioning.

Thermal disinfection is conducted in the same manner as for instrument disinfection, in a time-temperature dependent manner. A typical recommended condition is at a minimum temperature of 71°C (160°F) for 25 minutes. Temperature distribution is an important consideration and should be confirmed for a specific weight or load of textiles; remember, under or over loading the washer may lead to negative effects. Following moist heat disinfection, hot air drying and ironing are also considered effective to reduce microbial loads in textiles. Lower temperatures can be used in combination with chemical biocides.

Chlorine (specifically the addition of bleach/sodium hypochlorite at ~50–150 ppm) and the use of alkaline detergents (at high pH, >10) at temperatures ranging from 20–50°C are traditional examples; it is important to note that high alkaline applications need to be adequately neutralized (to a neutral pH) if used for cleaning (prior to disinfection with another biocide) or on completion of the cleaning-disinfection cycle during rinsing. Other types of chemical disinfectants that have become popular in recent years, due to cleaning/disinfection effects or reducing the consumption of water/energy, include direct application of peracetic acid or ozone. Peracetic acid (PAA) is added as a liquid or solid-generation type of disinfectant and then rinsed to remove any residuals (and odors, as PAA has a strong associated vinegar smell). Ozone (O_3) is a popular alternative, being produced in a generator (e.g. based on passing dried air or oxygen source through a corona discharge or UV light, and directly injected into the washer water (e.g. by bubbling/diffusion) for the desired concentration/contact time. In general, chemical applications are used at lower temperatures to reduce energy costs and for optimal antimicrobial activity.

Antiseptics

Antiseptics are disinfectants that are used on the skin and mucous membranes. They include hand washes/hand rubs, surgical scrubs, pre-operative preparations and various other types of preventative and therapeutic products (e.g. mouth rinses, biocide-containing creams, etc.; Figure 9.20). They are generally low-level disinfectants, being specifically designed to remove/inactivate microorganisms (particularly bacteria) but also not to irritate the skin. The most widely used antimicrobials are alcohols, iodine, chlorhexidine and triclosan. The role of antiseptics in infection prevention and control is discussed in Chapter 5 and further consideration is given to their use in Chapter 6, in the section on antiseptics.

Environmental disinfection

Environmental disinfectants are specifically used for the disinfection of a variety of hard surfaces such countertops, beds and bedrails, wheelchairs, floors, toilets, phones, computers keyboards and various types of non-critical devices such as non-invasive monitors and other general medical equipment. These surfaces can be a source of unseen contamination, particularly within a healthcare facility, for the transfer of microorganisms to patients (Chapter 5 in the section on infection control and prevention strategies). This can be expected to occur

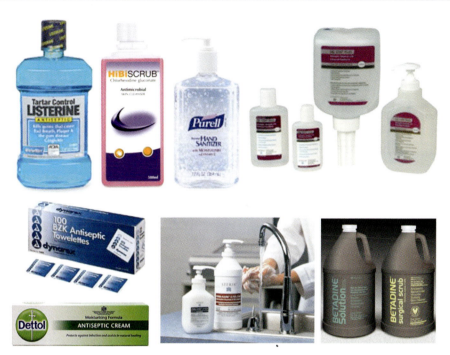

Figure 9.20 Examples of various types of antiseptics.

directly by the patient themselves (by touching contaminated surfaces and cross-contaminating themselves, such as by eating, accidentally contaminating a wound, etc.), or by contact with medical/surgical staff and visitors (contaminating their hands/gloves and transferring the microorganisms to a patient). Examples of commonly used surface disinfectants are formulations that include phenolics, quaternary ammonium compounds, alcohols, chlorine-based solutions (such as "bleach", being preparations of sodium hypochlorite that release chlorine), iodophors (that release iodine), hydrogen peroxide, chlorine dioxide and peracetic acid. They can also be provided in a variety of forms such as in concentrates (requiring dilution in water for use), ready-to-use preparations, two-component chemistries requiring mixing (activation) prior to use, disinfectant-integrated wipes and even fumigation systems (where gas or liquid-based disinfectants are automatically distributed around an area/room).

Overall, environmental disinfectants will be similarly labeled for use as that described for device disinfectants, but with specific consideration to their recommended environmental use. It is important to note that it is extremely rare that a disinfectant is labeled for use as a device and environmental disinfectant. In fact they are most often considered different products and, as a rule,

should *only* be used according to their specified label claims. Environmental disinfectants are also often classified as low, medium or high-level disinfectants, but more often will have specific antimicrobial claims provided with their recommended conditions of use. These include claims such as being bactericidal, viricidal, germicidal and sporicidal. Care should be taken to closely inspect any such label claims and how they have been verified (as highlighted previously in the first two sections in this chapter). For example, in the USA the term "germicidal" only refers to antimicrobial activity against certain types of bacteria, specifically, *Staphylococcus aureus, Salmonella enteric* and *Pseudomonas aeruginosa* in a standardized test method (noting that this excludes other bacteria with higher resistance to inactivation such as *Mycobacterium tuberculosis*). Label claims (regulated and unregulated) can vary significantly from country to country, based on various test methods and exposure conditions (such as exposure time, presence/absence of interfering soils, etc.).

Environmental disinfectants are often not used correctly to ensure that they are safe and effective. A typical use pattern will be applying the disinfectant to a surface and wiping it off immediately. The disinfectant may not have even contacted all required surfaces or have had any time to be effective against target microorganisms.

The presence of soil will also significantly affect the ability of the disinfectant to provide the desired antimicrobial activity. As highlighted for other disinfectants, the disinfection efficacy will only be as good as how the disinfectant is used (see the first two sections of this chapter). Most importantly, the disinfectant needs to be prepared (if applicable) and used in accordance with the manufacturer's instructions. An important consideration is the contact time for disinfection. Typical test conditions can range from five minutes to three hours for certain types of standardized test methods and associated disinfection claims! Overall, disinfectant label claims should be closely inspected and manufacturers' instructions for use should be followed to ensure the optimal use of environmental disinfectants.

It is not necessary for all surfaces in a healthcare environment to be regularly disinfected. In many cases (such as floors and ceilings) cleaning (or the physical removal of microorganisms and visual soiling) is considered sufficient and will adequately reduce patient safety risks. But care should be taken to ensure that many high-touch or high-risk surfaces are routinely and adequately disinfected. This includes high-risk surfaces around the patient such as bedrails, emergency call buttons and potential food contact surfaces, as well as surfaces that are routinely used by healthcare workers such as computer keyboards, touch surfaces on patient monitoring equipment and even door handles. In certain microbial outbreak situations, where there is a sudden increase in the numbers of cases of an infection, putting other patients/staff in the vicinity at risk, more detailed consideration of environmental disinfection is often considered necessary (Chapter 5, in the section on the role of infection prevention and control). Within a device reprocessing area, routine environmental surface disinfection should be particularly considered in any manual cleaning or soiled device handling areas (e.g. as described in Chapters 7 and 8), where the risks of microbial contamination and accidental transmission to staff can be a concern.

Prion disinfection

Prion disinfection has been the subject of recent research. Traditionally prion disinfection (and/or sterilization) methods have included the use of chemicals. Examples of these, as recommended by the WHO (1999[1]) include:

---

[1] Report of a WHO consultation, Geneva, Switzerland, 23–26 March 1999. WHO/CDS/CSR/APH/2000/3. http://www.who.int/csr/resources/publications/bse/WHO_CDS_CSR_APH_2000_3/en/

- Immersion in 1–2 M NaOH (sodium hydroxide, a strong alkali; Chapter 15) for one hour at 20°C. Equally effective was immersion in 1 M NaOH and subjecting to extended steam sterilization cycle (e.g. gravity displacement cycle at 121°C for one hour) or disinfection temperatures (e.g. boiling for ten minutes). "Steam sterilization" in this case refers to a mechanism of heating only, as these experiments consisted of prion material immersed in NaOH solutions and did not consider what exact temperature was achieved, air removal, etc., that are required for steam sterilization processes (Chapter 11 in the section on Physical sterilization). It is noted that recent experiments have shown that lower concentrations of NaOH may be effective at higher temperatures.
- Immersion in ≥20,000 ppm, (~2%) NaOCl (sodium hypochlorite, the major component of household "bleach") for one hour at room temperature (~20°C).

Some of these methods are not only considered to be effective against prions, but will also have significant activity against bacteria, fungi and viruses; however, in both cases, significant damage may occur on device surfaces with the use of such chemical procedures and they are generally not recommended by device manufacturers. These aspects are considered in further detail in Chapter 15 in the section on Devices known or suspected to be contaminated with prion material. More recently, alkaline cleaning and disinfection processes have also been shown to be effective (depending on their formulation and process conditions, such as concentration, exposure time and temperature). Similarly, some other chemical formulations and process conditions have been described as being effective against prions, including gaseous hydrogen peroxide, some phenolic disinfectant formulations and other formulation mixtures. Any claims associated with such products should be carefully inspected and understood.

To date, the typical conditions of thermal disinfection have been shown to have little to no effect on prion decontamination. In general, much higher temperatures are considered to be required and even then at longer exposure times than those typically used for sterilization (e.g. 121°C for one hour or 134°C for 18 minutes; Chapter 15). Chemical disinfectants or disinfection processes may or may not have some effect. Some types of biocides are not recommended due to their known mechanisms of action. Examples include aldehydes and alcohols in that they may even increase the risks of transmission due to their cross-linking or protein fixation effects. Others, such as the oxidizing agents, including chlorine, peracetic acid and hydrogen peroxide (particularly in gas form) may have some benefit, but this will depend on the product formulation or process conditions. It is incorrect to conclude that oxidizing agents can reduce the risk due to any potential claims of protein degradation or removal from a surface. Overall, chemical disinfectants should not be considered to have any beneficial effect to reduce the risk of prion contamination, unless specific testing is completed to demonstrate that the product is safe for such use (Chapter 15, in the section on Devices known or suspected to be contaminated with prion material). This may or may not be predicted based on the type of chemical biocide.

Troubleshooting disinfection problems

Many of the considerations discussed in the section on troubleshooting problems with cleaning (in Chapter 8) are also applicable to disinfection. Unlike cleaning, where a visual examination of the device may be acceptable to say the device has been cleaned or not, the evaluation of the success/failure of disinfection is difficult to ensure. Microorganisms may be present, but will not be seen! The greatest risk for device disinfection is with manual disinfection (thermal and/or chemical); therefore it is recommended that any variables of the disinfection process are monitored and, if possible documented. These include exposure times, temperatures, preparation methods for the disinfectant, chemical indicators for use with chemical disinfectants (to verify the MEC), etc. Thermal disinfection will not be achieved unless all parts of the device are contacted for the minimum specified temperature and contact time; equally, chemical disinfection requires the correct formulation/biocide concentration, contact time and exposure to all parts of the device, but may also depend on temperature, pH, etc. The same concept applies to any risks of residual toxicity remaining on the device in the use of chemical disinfectants, for example number and times of rinses, etc. These risks can be reduced but not eliminated with automated washer-disinfector or disinfector designs. These machines need to be correctly designed, used and maintained to ensure a reproducible and adequate disinfection process. Modern washer-disinfectors, in particular those compliant to ISO 15883, are provided with the means to verify that important variables of the process have been achieved. In such cases, known as independent monitoring, variables such as temperature, pressure, dosing volumes and contact times are controlled by the machine, but independently verified by a separate set of monitoring sensors. The data collected from these sensors may be checked directly by the machine and compared to the control sensors, providing an instantaneous

alarm if detected to be incorrect; in other systems the data may need to be downloaded from the washer-disinfector (e.g. onto a computer or printed out) and manually checked to ensure that the process is correct. In addition to these sensors (known as "parametric" sensors), chemical indicators are also used in automated systems to ensure that the disinfectant has been present during the process (although it is important to note that these will not confirm that the disinfectant has actually contacted all surfaces of the device/load). Although these automated systems can reduce the risks of inadequate disinfection they should be used (loaded) and maintained correctly, as highlighted in Chapter 8 in the section on troubleshooting problems with cleaning. Overall, in both manual and automated systems, human error can be an important variable; the best way to reduce this risk is by having written procedures and routine training of staff.

Disinfection, both by heat and particularly with chemical disinfectants, can be compromised by the presence of patient soils (blood, lipids, fats, proteins, etc.) that have not been adequately cleaned from device surfaces. This is due to the protection of microorganisms within these soils and the effect of the disinfectant and the reaction of the biocide with the soil preventing contact with the microorganisms. Aldehydes, for example, can potentially fix soils onto device surfaces, thereby protecting any internal microorganisms from disinfection, and oxidizing agents can be rapidly inactivated (depending on their concentration) by the presence of organic soils. Further negative effects can be due to the presence of cleaning chemistry residuals (e.g. enzymes used in cleaning formulations are proteins and can remain on inadequately rinsed devices following cleaning) and with poor water quality (e.g. where the presence of water hardness or chemicals such as heavy metals can compromise the activity of the disinfectant formulation). In conclusion, if the device is not cleaned it cannot be assumed to be disinfected (or even sterilized; Chapter 11).

A limited but increasing number of devices cannot withstand the typical thermal disinfection conditions, such as flexible endoscopes (see the section on flexible endoscopes); it is obvious that these devices should not be heated to over 60°C, to prevent damage. Heat tolerances are usually described by the device manufacturer in their instructions for use or reprocessing guidelines. Device compatibility is often an important consideration in the use of chemical disinfectants. As highlighted in section on flexible endoscopes earlier in this chapter, aldehydes often provide better device compatibility with such devices/ materials but are difficult to rinse away, while oxidizing agents can range considerably based on their use and formulation. Therefore, in consideration of chemical disinfectants, it is optimal for the device manufacturer to provide a statement of compatibility with a given product (not type of biocide); but as this is not always practical a written assurance of compatibility should at least be provided by the disinfectant/washer-disinfector manufacturer.

Water quality can also play a role with both thermal and chemical disinfection techniques (as previously highlighted in Chapter 8 in the section on troubleshooting problems with cleaning). These include:
• Interference with the activity of chemical disinfectants (e.g. high levels of water hardness and "heavy" metals such as copper, chromium and lead).

• Filter damage, leading to break-through of bacteria and other microorganisms over time (e.g. with high levels of chlorine).
• Device damage and rusting (due to chlorine and other chemicals, particularly when heated).
• The build-up of various deposits and color changes on devices and equipment surfaces (these have previously been highlighted in Chapter 8 in the section on troubleshooting problems with cleaning). Examples include water hardness (white, grainy deposits), phosphates (orange-brown staining) and acids (black staining).

The importance of water quality and troubleshooting problems associated with it are discussed in further detail in Chapter 15, in the section on Water Quality.

10 Inspection, packaging and loading for sterilization

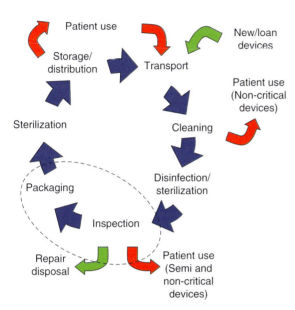

Note: re-usable instruments can be subjected to cleaning and disinfection and/or sterilization. Inspection and/or disposal may be conducted at any or at many step(s) during the cycle. In some cases devices are packaged for sterilization and storage prior to a patient procedure.

Introduction

This chapter considers the inspection of instruments prior to direct patient use or for subsequent packaging and presentation to a sterilization process. As discussed in Chapter 1 (in the section on The decontamination process), instrument reprocessing can include a number of steps such as cleaning, disinfection and, if applicable, sterilization. Following cleaning and disinfection (or even flash sterilization; Chapter 11), for non-critical and semi-

critical, or even in some situations critical devices, many instruments will be immediately used on a patient or subsequently prepared for and subjected to sterilization.

Inspection and packaging area design considerations

As discussed in Chapter 1 (in the section on The design of a decontamination area), reprocessing facilities should be designed to prevent the inadvertent mixture of contaminated/soiled instruments with decontaminate/clean instruments. Following cleaning and disinfection (if applicable), instruments should be held in a designated "clean" area, where decontaminated instruments are checked for cleanliness and functionality. Following this the instrument(s) can be correctly assembled (if required), transferred to a patient area for use in a procedure or prepared for further sterilization. Thousands of instruments may pass through these areas daily, and each instrument has the potential to significantly influence a patient outcome. Instruments that are not correctly cleaned can pose a serious risk of infection or other patient adverse effects (e.g. toxicity). Likewise, if instruments are not disinfected correctly, microorganisms or other contaminants may be transferred to a patient with significant health consequences.

Area design

The design of "clean" areas can range from a designated part of a room to a physically separated area of a facility design that includes a dedicated air handling system.

In most cases, instruments may be cleaned alone (e.g. non-critical devices) and/or disinfected (non-critical or semi-critical devices). They should be handled in a designated 'clean way' but are generally not handled in a specifically designed air-handling room; however, with

A Practical Guide to Decontamination in Healthcare, First Edition. Gerald McDonnell and Denise Sheard.
© 2012 Gerald McDonnell and Denise Sheard. Published 2012 by Blackwell Publishing Ltd.

the increasing concerns regarding the use of certain semi-critical devices (such as flexible endoscopes that may often be used for semi-critical or critical procedures) such designated facilities are often considered necessary. For critical devices, which need to be prepared for subsequent sterilization, a designated assembly and packing area should be considered. Such areas are designated as "controlled environments" (note: a controlled environment is defined as a zone in which sources of contamination are controlled by specified means. It is distinct from a "clean room" that may require a higher level of environmental control that may not be necessary for sterile reprocessing areas). Such areas are controlled to prevent cross-contamination with air contaminants that may come from "dirty" areas (e.g. cleaning areas), other hospital or external areas and even from staff and materials that are present in the clean area. Cleaning/ "dirty" areas are designed to keep contamination within a given risk area, whilst, clean areas should be designed to keep contamination out. Ideally these designated areas are maintained at a differential, positive pressure (e.g. at a 10 Pa pressure difference to the cleaning or external areas), and are physically separated from the cleaning area, with restricted access. Specific air handling systems can be employed to maintain these conditions and to circulate the air in such a way as to maintain the particle count low in the area. In such designs, the circulation of air can be controlled, but also the quality of the air can be maintained by passing the air continually through designated filter (HEPA filter) systems that will remove contaminants above a certain size. Examples of air contaminants that may cause concern include bacteria, fungi, hair, skin cells, dust particles, lint and other materials. Regular air particle counts are recommended in this area and staff should wear non-lint clothing to ensure that specifications are met.

In summary, design criteria for designated "clean room" areas should include:
• Separation of "clean and dirty" (preferably physical or a separate room)
• Controlled limited access
• The clean area must meet specific temperature, humidity and air exchange controls
• Controlled monitored air quality and environment, ten air exchanges per hour
• Positive pressure to control airborne microorganisms (e.g. 10 Pa with respect to external areas)
• Comfortable working environmental temperature (18–2°C or 66–73°F)

• Comfortable air humidity levels (e.g. 40–70%)
• Adequate space for handling and packaging of surgical trays
• Adequate availability of materials for packaging, sterilization and process monitoring

Maintenance

The effective management of microorganisms and the quality of air in these areas is solely dependent on the people who work there following facility guidelines. Guidelines should be in place to protect both the workers and patient and to maintain the "clean" environment. Routine cleaning/disinfection of all work area surfaces and equipment will assist in controlling the spread of microorganisms. A maintenance schedule must be in place to ensure that the temperature, humidity and air control is kept constant, as well as the routine maintenance of the air handling system (e.g. periodic changes in HEPA filters). On installation and periodically, the air handling system may be checked for the adequate flow of air through the system/room (e.g. using air flow visualization tests such as smoke tests) and even the air microbiological or particle counts (e.g. using air particle sampling systems) to ensure they are correctly maintained.

Personal attire and other material consideration

As discussed in the chapter on cleaning, personal attire (including personal protective equipment, PPE) is designed to protect staff from various microbiological and chemical risks encountered during receiving, sorting and cleaning of devices/materials (Chapter 8). In the clean area, personal attire and materials should be used to prevent any microbiological or chemical risks from being transferring from the technician to the patient. The following should be considered:
• Wear and use non-linting materials; linting materials, such as cotton, can lead to complications if introduced into a patient during a surgical procedure.
• Defined clothing only to be used within the clean area (e.g. surgical scrubs). Staff and visitors should wear these on entering the room and remove them on leaving, usually in a designated ante-room.
• Hair covering should be worn.
• Closed shoes should be worn and shoe covers may be considered (to reduce transfer of floor contamination from outside into the area).
• Gloves may or may not be worn; if they are used, it is recommended that they are powder-free.

Further guidance

It is important to understand and employ the best practices when inspecting, assembling and packaging instruments, to ensure the instruments are maintained safely for patient use. Inspection, assembly, packaging and labeling policies and procedures should be established within a facility. These procedures should define the facility practices regarding the handling of instruments within these areas and the monitoring of care and use of instruments and equipment. Guidelines and standards regarding facility design can vary from region to region. Examples of such guidelines include:

• ISO 14698 is a series of standards on clean rooms and associated controlled environments; these and similar standards/guidelines will be published by local organization such as the Association for the Advancement of Medical Instrumentation (AAMI) in the USA.
• Health Building Notice (HBN) 13 on *Sterile services departments*, Department of Health, England.
• AAMI ST79 is a comprehensive guide to steam sterilization and sterility assurance in healthcare facilities.

Inspection

Cleanliness

The objective of cleaning is to remove or significantly reduce the presence of contaminants, including microorganisms (bioburden) and other contaminants (protein, lipids, etc.) from an item to an acceptable level. Cleaning is regarded as having been effective if the item is free of these contaminants. An acceptable level is defined as the reduction of contamination so that a surface (e.g. non-critical device) so that it can be used safely or safely disinfected or sterilized, as soiling can inhibit the effectiveness of physical or chemical microbial inactivation methods. Inadequate cleaning may result in damage to the device (such as corrosion, rusting, and pitting of an instrument) and the transfer of toxic residues to a patient. These will not be removed or neutralized by subsequent sterilization. Cannulated or lumened instruments may become obstructed due to dried organic or inorganic materials. Where possible the inspection and functional testing of surgical instruments should be carried out independently. All non-conforming products, for example those that are dirty or stained, should be rejected and returned to the wash area for re-cleaning and/or disinfection, before being used directly on a patient or packaged and sterilized.

There are many different types of methods that can be used to determine that a device has been adequately cleaned, including visual assessment, determination of the levels of bacteria/fungi (microbiological methods) and chemical or biochemical detection methods. The microbiological and biochemical test methods are generally restricted to investigational or laboratory-based studies (e.g. by device manufacturers to study the cleaning efficacy of a process, including compliance to some cleaning standards such as the test methods described in ISO TS 15883-5 *Test soils and methods for demonstrating cleaning efficacy* (Chapter 8, in the section on Cleaning guidelines, standards and testing). For most hospital-based applications, the assessment of cleanliness is done by visually inspecting the devices and, in some cases, by using simple biochemical tests. Routine tests to evaluate cleaning efficacy within a washer-disinfector have already been considered in Chapter 8, in the section on Cleaning guidelines, standards and testing; this section discusses typical methods used to evaluate cleaning efficacy on device surfaces on a routine basis within a reprocessing facility.

Visual inspection

Visual inspection is the most common method used to provide evidence of cleaning and proper functioning of most instruments (Chapter 8, in the section on Introduction). Inspection using the naked eye alone may not always be effective as it relies on the individual's eyesight and ability to detect residual soil. Further, visual inspection is not practical with any device that has internal components, such as cannulated (lumened) instruments, or where parts of the device cannot be seen. The original condition of the item before cleaning will have a significant effect on how adequately it can be cleaned. Instruments that are subjected to prior rough handling (either on surgical/medical procedures, reprocessing or transport) will develop scratches and roughened surfaces that can harbor materials that are difficult to detect. Damaged surfaces will allow dirt and microorganisms to collect, and also be potentially dangerous for both staff and patients. Therefore, visual inspection is not limited to inspecting the device for cleanliness but also to ensuring that it is not damaged and is fit for use (see the section on functionality testing below).

Optical aids are available to assist with the inspection of instruments, for example lighted magnifying glasses are ideal (Figure 10.1). However, some body fluids that contain no obvious color are transparent and create more of a challenge as they cannot be seen easily with the naked eye. Even if a device looks clean to the naked eye, there

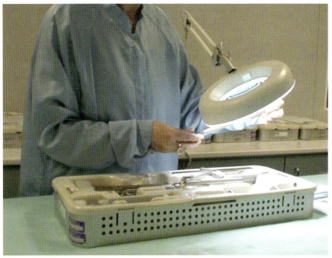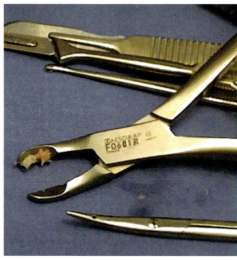

Figure 10.1 Use of an optical aid (magnifying glass and light source) to inspect devices for cleanliness and damage. An example of a soiled device is shown on the right (note the jaws on the bone nibbler).

may still be microscopic particles of dirt and bacteria present that cannot be seen. For this reason, many guidelines will also recommend the use of additional, biochemical tests to be able to provide a more sensitive method of evaluating cleaning.

Biochemical tests

Biochemical or chemical tests are often used as they are more sensitive and less subjective than visual assessment; however, this is not always the case. Consider, for example, how the device is tested: is the whole surface sampled or only part? Is the method of testing effective to remove what may or may not be present on the device? What is the detection method specifically detecting? All these should be considered (in particular they should be defined by the manufacturer of the method or kit being used to detect soil), but it is important to highlight that as for any indicator it may be useful to ensure that a cleaning processes has been conducted but may not ensure that the device(s) has been cleaned. These tests are not a replacement for visual inspection, but may provide a more sensitive method for the detection of soil and if a device is clean. At the time of writing, as discussed in Chapter 8 (see introductory section), visual cleanliness is considered adequate to indicate that cleaning has been effective, but in some parts of the world more sensitive methods are recommended.

The most common biochemical marker used is protein (Chapter 8, Table 8.4). Proteins are one of the four major types of molecules that make up cellular structure and function (including human and microbial cells), and are therefore a key component of soils found on devices. Laboratory studies that have investigated the various different soil components which are found on devices after patient use have highlighted the presence of protein; it is not only a major component of soiling on a device but is also considered a sensitive marker as to whether a device has been cleaned or not. Protein detection methods can be very detailed, generally requiring a biochemical laboratory to evaluate; however, various types of test kits have been developed for routine healthcare facility use. These are generally swab-based tests, where the swab is used to wipe the surface (note: without touching the hands or other surfaces that can themselves contain high levels of protein), and then exposed to a chemical that detects the presence/absence of protein at a certain level. These may range from simple color-change reactions to more sophisticated light-emitting type of assays (where the level of light equates to the level of protein). Example of various types of protein test kits are shown in Figure 10.2. These kits can vary in the methods used for protein recovery and detection, guidelines on how they should be used/controlled and protein detection levels. These test kits are based on the use of chemicals for protein detection, such as ninhydrin and the Biuret reaction. As a general guide, a level of protein that may be considered as "clean" has been suggested to be about 6–7 µg/cm^2 levels of protein on a device, but such levels are not currently universally accepted.

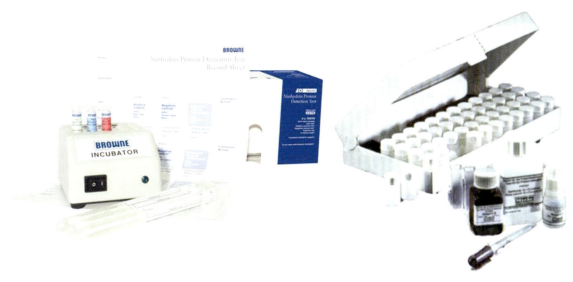

Figure 10.2 Various types of protein detection test kits.

Other types of biochemical tests are used to aid in soil detection. These include:
• Adenosine triphosphate detection kits: ATP is a molecule that is present in most living cells, including human and bacterial cells. Therefore the detection of ATP can be an indirect indicator of the presence of contamination (including bacteria/fungi and patient soil) on a surface. Adenosine triphosphate test kits are available, based on the swabbing of surface and detection of ATP within a monitoring device or simple color-change types of indicators.
• Blood/hemoglobin detection can be achieved using hydrogen peroxide; various different types of enzymes that found in blood cells break down the peroxide to release oxygen, shown as bubbling. Kits are available for the sensitive detection of blood contamination, such as swab-based tests that give a color change in the presence of low levels of blood.

Functionality testing

As well as checking that devices have been properly cleaned, all items should be subject to functionality testing to ensure that they will perform the tasks for which they are designed. It is also the duty of the reprocessing area to manage the inventory of instruments, this involves knowing how to care for instruments, which individual parts must be tested and when instruments should be repaired, refurbished, or even replaced. Instruments that are not cared for and handled correctly have a shorter lifespan, which leads to increased repairs, replacements and costs. It is the responsibility of reprocessing staff to ensure that instruments are functional, available and assembled in the right sets to meet the demands of the theatres and wards. For patient safety it is crucial that all instruments are maintained in optimal working condition. Damaged instruments can cause clinical delays or cancellations, and, if undetected, can even cause patient injury.

Only trained staff familiar with the manufacturer's instructions and/or local policy should carry out inspections, which include checking for damage and ensuring that the medical device is functioning. To ensure staff safety and reliable functioning, it is recommended that instruments are only tested for function once cleaned. If any problems are noted during the inspection process, the item may need to be sent for repair depending on the problem observed.

Manufacturers' guidelines

Follow the manufacturer's instructions at all times when handling and inspecting instruments. Disregarding the manufacturer's recommendations may damage or shorten an instrument's life. Device manufacturers should supply guidelines on the use, safety considerations, care and maintenance of their products (Chapter 1, in the section on where to start). Such written instructions and any other technical documentation should be provided by the manufacturer on delivery, to ensure that the device will be used in a safe and effective manner, and to minimize the risk of harm to either the user or patient. Legally, this document absolves the manufacturer of liability in the event that the guidelines are not followed, which is why it is important that all reprocessing staff are aware of the instructions and trained in the appropriate use and care of the device. If these guidelines are not adhered to then the manufacturer's warranty will generally become null and void. The appropriate manufacturer's guidelines should be directly accessible to all staff working in the reprocessing area at any time. If these documents are lost or unavailable, a new set needs to be obtained from the manufacturer.

The manufacturer's guidelines or instructions for use should include the following important information on the proper use and care of the device:
• Definition of the intended use of the device.
• Provision and explanation of safety-related information regarding proper handling, use and operation of the device.
• What may constitute misuse, including any particular warnings.
• Functional and safety tests.
• Cleaning, disinfection and/or sterilization instructions (where applicable). It is recommended that at least one method of manual and automated reprocessing instructions have been validated by the device manufacturer.
• Types of physical or chemical processes/products that may or may not be used during device reprocessing or maintenance.
• Lists of accessories and consumables that may be used with the device.
• Requirements for safety inspection of the device/equipment.
• Requirements for planned maintenance (e.g. lubrication, repair, etc.).
Ignoring, not fully recognizing or not understanding the manufacturer's instructions may result in decreased efficiency of the device, deterioration of the equipment or harm to the user or patient. It is essential that appropriate staff training is given and that the training program is documented, and regularly reviewed for new equipment and/or new employees. In many cases, as with complex devices, training should preferably be given by the manufacturer with regular refresher courses.

General guidelines on device inspection

Each instrument should be individually examined and inspected for cleanliness, proper functioning and alignment, defects, sharpness of cutting edges, looseness of pins and chipping of plated surfaces.

The following general guidelines are given for the inspection of devices:
• Ensure that instruments with serrations or inserts on the jaws are free from any visible materials.
• Check instruments for corrosion (rusting, surface damage) that may lead to further damage or device breakage. While visible stains and rust can be removed using commercial stain removers (acid cleaners, see the section on Classification of cleaning chemistries and Non enzyme cleaners), the underlying instrument damage is already present and will likely continue to be further damaged at this site, leading to permanent damage.
• Open and close ratchets using one hand and feel if it moves easily. Stiffness in the joint is an indication of debris in the joint; if not cleaned, over time the joint will fail.
• Check that the tension is being maintained on instruments with box locks or ratchets.
• Check hinged instruments such as clamps and forceps for stiffness.
• Test instruments that grip or clamp for holding strength.
• Check instruments with cutting edges such as scissors, rongeurs, curettes, etc., for sharpness. There should be no dull spots, chips, or dents. Red and yellow Therab and can be used for checking the sharpness of scissors and rongeurs (Figure 10.3).
• Check that moving parts (such as hinges and box-locks) move smoothly throughout the intended range of motion. Lubricate hinges, threads and other moving parts with a commercial, water-based, surgical grade, instrument lubricant (such as instrument milk) to reduce friction and wear. Follow any specific manufacturer's guidelines regarding lubrication.
• Check that tips are properly aligned, jaws meet perfectly and joints move easily.
• Run your fingers down the shaft to feel for dents. Check for bends and dents in instruments with lumens, that is, trocars.
• Check that where individual parts form part of a larger device assembly that all parts are present, matching and can be assembled.
• Check the condition of instrument marking systems, for example instruments with marking tape or instruments that have coating rings. If either of these methods is used to identify sets, they must be routinely replaced if they are chipped, torn and rough, or if the edges of the tape start to curl or come off, or if there is an excess of glue residue at the edge of the tape.
• Check insulated instruments carefully, ensuring that there is no breach in the insulation.

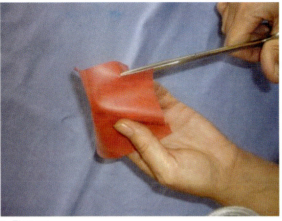
1. First cut.

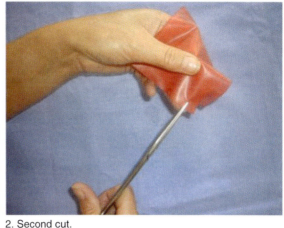
2. Second cut.

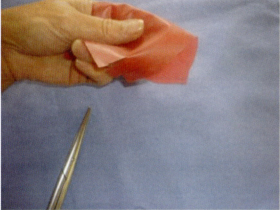

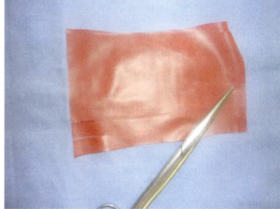

3. Two cuts in theraband.

Figure 10.3 Sharpness testing with red Theraband.

Examples of specific device inspections
Scissors

Scissors are designed to cut tissue and suture materials and should not be tested on any paper, types of tubing, etc. All scissors are designed to be re-sharpened, with the exception of those with serrated edges, which are replaced when found to be blunt. Scissors dull first at the distal tip, where most of the cutting occurs. Inspection may include:

• Check the scissors' cutting action by opening and closing the scissors to assure a smooth glide that is not too loose, too tight, grinding or jumping. The cutting blades should glide smoothly past each other.

• When testing scissors for sharpness use a Theraband red test material for scissors larger than 4.5 inches, and yellow test material for scissors smaller than 4.5 inches

(Figure 10.3). Make at least two cuts in the test material. The scissors should cut all the way through to the top of the blade. Check for catching or snagging and ensure that the scissors cut all the way through to the tip.

• Check that both tips are present and not damaged. Device tips are rounded and should not have burrs, which could cause puncturing and tearing.

• Check the distal ends (surgeon handling end) for bent blades or damage.

• Inspect for chips or burrs on cutting surfaces.

• Inspect tungsten carbide inserts for cracks, and check for pitting where the tungsten carbide meets the stainless steel. Tungsten carbide blades cannot be repaired and should be discarded if damaged.

• Don't over sharpen scissors; if the carbide coating is ground off then the scissors will no longer be useful.

• Inspect both sides of the hinge for cracking, staining or bioburden trapped inside the screw or screw head.
• Inspect the finger rings for cracks which could cause the handles to break.
• Inspect the jaws for blood or bioburden.
• Check that the jaws are in alignment and fit together, not overlapping.
• If box-joints are present check for soil and cracks on both sides of the hinged area (in particular the closed sides).

Tissue and dressing forceps

Forceps inspection should include:
• The tips (jaws) to see if they are even and undamaged.
• Check that there is no overlap and that tips meet evenly.
• Check that teeth are not broken and inter-fit smoothly.
• Check distal serrations for blood or baked on-debris.
• Check proximal ends (handle, spring and forceps link) for cracks.

Hemostatic forceps

These are used primarily to occlude vessels and control blood flow. Hemostats are designed to clamp blood vessels and should not be tested on any type of tubing, etc. Typical inspections include:
• Check that tips are rounded and do not have burrs, which could cause puncturing and tearing.
• Check that both tips are present.
• Check distal ends for bending or damage.
• Check that the forceps do not stick abnormally.
• Inspect for chips or burrs on tissue holding surfaces.
• Check tips of serrated hemostat forceps, that is, Crile/Kelly, etc., for alignment; they should meet equally, with no overlap.
• Check that the teeth of hemostat tissue forceps, that is, Allis/Kocher, etc., are intact, straight and that jaws inter-fit. Check the space between the teeth for tissue.
• Inspect teeth and any serrations for soil.
• If box-joints are present check for soil and cracks on both sides of the hinged area.
• Test the ratchets by opening and closing, the action should be smooth and the ratchet should hold on each engagement (click). The tips should meet just before the ratchets engage as the ratchets engage the entire jaw should mesh, clamping closed.
• To test the spring, set the clamp on the first ratchet and gently tap the instrument on a flat surface, if the instrument is "sprung" the ratchet will pop open.
• Check the spring area for cracks and soil.

Needleholders

These are used for holding suture needles and should not be tested on any type of tubing, etc.:
• Check that tips are rounded and do not have burrs, which could cause puncturing and tearing.
• Check that both tips are present.
• Inspect for worn or chipped edges.
• Check the tread for wear on the tips.
• Check that cardiovascular needleholders are demagnetized by holding a needle against the tips; if the needle is drawn to the trip the holder must be demagnetized.
• Check smooth jaws for wear and tear by holding them up to light, if light is seen it is worn and will not hold a needle.
• Check that shanks are not bent or mis-shaped.
• Check for cracked/missing inserts.
• Inspect the neck for cracks, the larger the crack, the longer it has been there.
• Inspect tungsten carbide inserts for cracks, and check for pitting where the tungsten carbide meets the stainless steel; tungsten carbide blades cannot be repaired.
• Inspect both sides of the hinge for cracking, staining or soil trapped inside the screw or screw head.
• Inspect the finger rings for cracks which could cause the handles to break.
• Inspect the jaws for blood or other soils.
• Jaws of needleholders must be able to hold a suture needle. Check that the jaws are in alignment and fit together, not overlapping.
• If box-joints are present check for soil and cracks on both sides of the hinged area.
• Test the ratchets by opening and closing, the action should be smooth and the ratchet should hold on each engagement (click). The tips should meet just before the ratchets engage as the ratchets engage the entire jaw should mesh, clamping closed.
• Check the spring area for cracks and soil.
• To test the spring, set the clamp on the first ratchet and gently tap the instrument on a flat surface, if the instrument is "sprung" the ratchet will pop open.

Suction nozzles

These are used to extract fluids from a surgical site or area of the body:
• Inspect for sharp or abraded edges, dents.
• Inspect the holes/cannula for blockages and trapped debris.
• Inspect the shaft for bending or dents, visually and by running your finger down the shaft to feel for dents.
• Check the suction control is unblocked and working.

• Check any soldered areas of the device for cracks and soil.
• Check that the stylet can be inserted at the proximal end of the device.

Hooks and spatulas

These are used for retracting skin in various procedures:
• Inspect the entire area, in particular the edges for cracks and chips.
• Check for any buckling or bending on the device.

Self-retaining retractors

These retractors are used to open up the working space and improve visualization of the operative site for the surgeon. Tissue damage may result from mismatched retractor blades or points, causing tissue healing problems. Inspections should include:
• Check that flexible retractors are in their original shape and flat.
• Check that any small accessories with the device (e.g. washers, screws) are present – these systems cannot be used if such parts are missing.
• Inspect all parts to ensure that they are completely clean.
• Check that all parts are in proper working order.
• Particularly inspect any screws and springs for cracks/soiling.
• Check that all parts are moving freely – lubricate according to manufacturer guidelines using an approved lubricant that is compatible with the device and any subsequent reprocessing stages (e.g. sterilization).
• Inspect distal ends for bent blades and prongs.
• Check release lever – when the release lever is "flicked" it should spring back into place.
• Retractors should open and close smoothly.
• Check that the ratchets hold in the open position by opening the retractor and simultaneously applying pressure to both shanks, the ratchet should unlock with minimal pressure.

Microsurgical instrumentation

Various types of microsurgical instruments have been previously considered in Chapter 4. They are used for particularly delicate surgical/medical procedures (Figure 10.4). Because of the high risk of damage, such devices should be handled with care. The tips of delicate and sharp medical devices should be protected at all times to avoid unnecessary damage. These instruments are extremely fragile and must be inspected before and after every endoscopic procedure. Some eye micro-instruments can be unhinged to ensure proper cleaning (confirm with manufacturer). Ensure that all instruments are reassembled correctly after cleaning. Very delicate or sharp instruments may have their tips covered with instrument caps.

Rigid endoscopes and accessories (such as trocars)

It is recommended that after cleaning, endoscopes are visually inspected for defects such as rough surfaces, sharp edges or prominent parts as these defects could harm the end user or patient. Endoscopes should also be inspected for any soil residues, but this is not easy, depending on the design of the endoscopes (e.g. for those black in color and visually inspecting internal lumens is virtually impossible). The following guidelines are given:
• Inspect the telescopes for scratches, dents, protrusions, distal tip burrs or other surface irregularities by running your fingers down the length of the endoscope.
• Pay attention to dents or defects due to high frequency or laser surgery instruments as well as cracks at the ocular (patient) end of the endoscope.
• Check that the surfaces of the light inlets and outlets are smooth and clean. If the surfaces show deposit layers, or rough fibers can be felt this could lead to decreased illumination. If the endoscope is used or prepared in this condition, it may be continuously damaged over time.
• Test any moving components to ensure they are functional.
• If present, check the eyepiece and its seal on the device for visible signs of damage. Inspect and detach the eyepiece of the lens if it is detachable.
• Do not touch the telescope's ocular or the objective lenses to avoid fingerprints and debris that will impair the view and possibly cause scratches.
• Endoscopes with damaged glass surfaces (e.g. cracks), impaired image quality or noticeable surface damages or distortions should not be used. In some cases they may be checked by directly viewing through the endoscope (with or without a light source).
• Check any proximal or distal glass surfaces of the endoscope surface. The glass surfaces must be clean and free from deposit layers.
• Check the image through the scope it should be sharp and clear. This can be done by looking at a piece of nonglare white paper with printing. Start with the scope's distal tip about three inches from the paper and move the tip until it is about one-quarter inch from the paper. The printing should appear crisp and clear, with minimal distortion. Discolored or unclear print could be due to improper cleaning, disinfectant residue, a cracked or

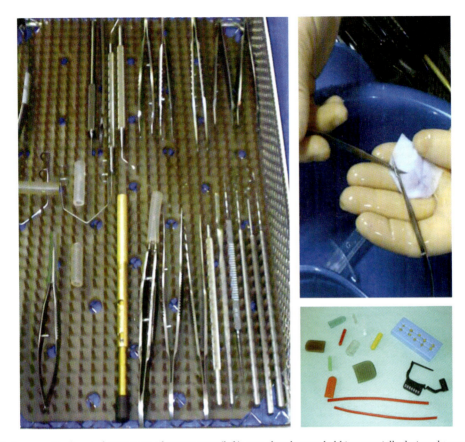

Figure 10.4 An example of a set of microsurgical instruments (left); note that they are held in a specially designed transport tray to prevent damage to the devices. These devices should be closely inspected (e.g. tip inspection, top right) and tips or various other parts of the device may need to be protected using device caps (bottom right).

broken lens, moisture within the shaft, or external shaft damage which has broken some fibres.

• Check the light transmission through the fibres by holding the light guide connector against a light (not a cold light source). If numerous black spots appear on the distal end, the light output is insufficient. The black spots are broken fibres and the scope should be sent for repair (Figure 10.5).

• On inspection of the proximal and distal lenses, they may be further cleaned with a lint-free cloth/swab saturated with 70% alcohol; repeat the inspection process. If the view through either lens remains cloudy or distorted after cleaning, the scope is damaged and should be sent for repair.

• Before re-assembling, any stopcocks provided with the device may need to be treated (on their sliding surfaces) with a small amount of silicone grease/lubricant according to the manufacturer's instructions.

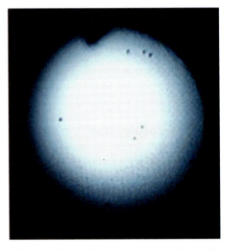

Figure 10.5 Checking endoscope light transmission. Broken light fibers are shown by black spots within the field of view.

• Re-assemble the scope according to instructions.
• Check and disconnect any associated light cables. These may be reprocessed separately from the other parts of the device.

Flexible endoscopes

Flexible endoscopes are also very delicate instruments with unique complexity. Close attention should be paid to the inspection of such devices prior to patient use or further processing. These include:

• Inspect for any extraneous materials or cracks at the working end of the scope (scope tip), including any moving mechanisms. A particular example is with the distal tip of a duodenoscope (Chapter 4, Figure 4.57) that contains an elevator mechanism; this area of the scope is particularly difficult to clean and soil can get trapped within the moving mechanism.
• Check the seals around the various parts of the distal tip lenses and other components. These are generally held in place by adhesives and may become loose or detached over time.
• Visually inspect the entire shaft of the instrument for nicks and cuts, as well as kinks or other irregularities along the length of the device.
• Physically check the instrument for any obvious damage and functionality. Ensure that all moving parts are moving freely.
• Ensure that all detachable buttons, valves or caps are free of soiling and move freely. These parts will need to be re-assembled with the device for patient use.
• Inspect any electrode and light cables for damage.
• Inspect the connection post for the light source.
• Lightly pull back on the insulation; if you can slide it (or it becomes detached), the insulation needs to be replaced.
• If possible, inspect that all channels are clear (e.g. by passing sterile or medical grade air down each lumen). Such inspections are normally conducted during cleaning/disinfection and are also checked on setting the device up for a patient procedure.

Electrical equipment considerations

Electrical equipment should be handled with care and tested according to manufacturer guidelines. Failure to adequately inspect these instruments can be dangerous for both the patient and staff.

• The re-usable appliances should be disconnected from any mains current before cleaning and inspecting.
• Check for corrosion – electrical equipment (and indeed any device/equipment) should never be cleaned with saline as this causes corrosion.

• Move and check that any control switches are operating.
• All insulated instruments should be visually inspected for breaks in the integrity of the insulation each time the instruments are processed to avoid possible injury to the patient and/or surgical/medical team. Instruments that have an outer insulation coating, for example diathermy forceps, require close inspection to ensure that the insulation remains intact. Check that the insulating material and electric cables are not damaged in any way and look for cracks and splits for damage or wear.
• Check the battery pack if the equipment is battery driven.
• Lubricate all powered equipment and attachments according to manufacturers' written instructions.
• Check that attachments fit firmly – improperly fitting attachments can be thrown from powered equipment, resulting in injury to patients and personnel.
• Check that any trigger handles are in the safety position to prevent accidental activation of powered equipment, causing injury to patients or personnel.

Maintenance, repairs and replacements

All devices should be accompanied by instructions on routine and periodic maintenance and repair in order to maintain their safe and effective use. These instructions should give information on the type and frequency of maintenance, safety and calibration check requirements and should be directly accessible to the reprocessing staff as well as the persons in charge of the maintenance. It is recommended that a maintenance plan is put into place and that all maintenance or repairs performed are recorded; some of these may be performed by in-house staff (e.g. by trained biomedical engineers), an external third party group and/or the device manufacturer.

Instruments are often damaged during their intended use or suffer from general wear and tear for a number of reasons, but are more often damaged due to inappropriate use, poor handling or contact with corrosive chemicals/processes. Instruments may be physically damaged due to being dropped on the floor or rough handling, or as a result of contact with agents during surgical/medical use, for example iodine or saline solutions. Damage typically seen with the naked eye can include rusting, pitting or general surface corrosion (Figure 10.6).

If during inspection and function testing items are found to be faulty or damaged, or if a fault is identified by surgical/medical staff, they should be taken out of use and either repaired or replaced. A written procedure

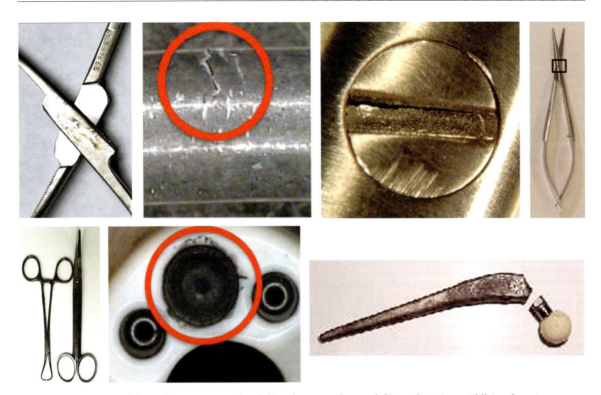

Figure 10.6 Examples of device damage. Rusting (top left) and staining (bottom left), cracking (top middle) and erosion of adhesives on flexible endoscopes, and stress cracking on devices (left). Some of these effects may be very obvious while others are not.

should be in place describing which procedure to follow when an instrument is found to be damaged. The procedure should be agreed by both the reprocessing staff and user. It should include details about who should be notified, how it will be recorded, how replacements can be obtained, who should be notified if a replacement is not immediately available, and whether the set can be packaged and sterilized without the missing item and, finally, if an incomplete set is approved for sterilization, how it will be labeled so that the user is made aware of the missing instrument before the surgical procedure begins.

Instruments identified as needing repair should be placed in a dedicated tray in the preparation room following the wash/decontamination procedure and recorded in a "damages" or "repairs" file. A decision must be taken whether it is viable to repair the instrument or whether it needs to be disposed of and replaced. Instruments for repair must be clearly marked, then cleaned and autoclaved before being sent for repair, in order to protect the engineers. Instruments for repair should be returned to a trained biomedical engineer/maintenance department, the manufacturer or a reputable repair company.

Items sent for repair should be identified on the checklist (see the next section on device and tray assembling) and the set to which they belong or in the case of individual instruments (for example endoscopes) the particular instrument noted. If only parts of an instrument are sent for repair the instrument should be held in a quarantine area until the repair has been completed and the device reassembled/prepared for re-use.

Instruments that cannot be repaired should be removed from use and if a replacement is not available a note should be made on the instrument checklist to alert users. Where instruments, which are part of instrument "sets", are taken out of use the set should ideally be removed from use until the instrument has been repaired/replaced and returned to the set. This should be agreed with the surgical/medical personnel concerned.

If the manufacturer has limited the number of times that a re-usable medical device can be reprocessed, then accurate records must be retained in order to achieve compliance. The device must be discarded once that usage limit has been reached and the item replaced.

Device and tray assembling

Medical and surgical devices are used for a variety of procedures in healthcare facilities (Chapter 3). These procedures can range from the use of a single device to a whole complicated set of devices (e.g. as is the case with most surgical procedures).

In all cases, ensuring that the proper types of devices (and any accessories) for a given procedure are ready and available is important, and particularly in endoscopic and surgical procedures. It is therefore an important role of the decontamination staff to ensure that devices/sets are correctly prepared for patient use. For non-critical and semi-critical devices this is most often a direct or combined role of staff available within designated departments/facilities; but with critical (and sometimes semi-critical) devices that are reprocessed by centralized departments, the devices are organized into sets for particular procedures according to the surgical/medical needs, packaged and sterilized prior to distribution/use within a facility.

General considerations

Surgical instruments are organized into trays, and then into sets if applicable, to meet specific requirements for specific procedures. Each set will contain those instruments required to perform a specific procedure. Sets may also contain basins, bowls, receivers, drills, implants and other items that may be needed for that particular procedure. Therefore trays/sets can range in complexity and on the number of instruments that are needed for different procedures. This section provides guidance on how these trays/sets are assembled for sterilization and then subsequent patient use.

Given the range of instruments that can be used for a given surgical procedure, the weight of device trays should be controlled. Consider, for example, an orthopedic set that may contain particularly heavy instruments such as mallets. By limiting the weight of devices in a tray, this can reduce the risk of damage to devices and also reduce any staff injury risks (as an ergonomic precaution). Note: ergonomics is the design of procedures, work areas and equipment to reduce operator fatigue, discomfort and injury. In this case, heavy trays can lead to back or arm strains and even more serious injury. The guideline weight for an object being carried using extended arms is 7 kg for a female and 10 kg for a male. As part of best practice and safety of staff, these weights should form a basis for how heavy trays should be in assembly.

When assembling instrument trays/sets it is critical that staff understand what the instruments are used for, that they are functioning correctly and that each set is assembled in the proper manner for any given procedure. Training of staff is therefore important and can be assisted by the use of assembly aids, such as "pick list" or "tray checklist" (Figure 10.7). Tray or set checklists provide a list of instruments that should be in the tray/set and can include pictures, device identification codes/numbers, item description, quantity of devices, etc. These may be paper or computer-based systems that assist staff to assemble the tray/sets correctly and in a standard manner. In computer-based systems, the device may be scanned (to read a unique identification code) and confirmed as being in the applicable set (including, for example, particular checks, assembly, maintenance, etc., that need to be made on the device at that stage).

These checklists can form the basis of a tracking and traceability system for devices within a facility. Therefore, the set when verified in a central reprocessing/assembly area will be signed by staff responsible for checking/packing, maintained with the set/tray during sterilization and transport/storage, and then further verified by staff receiving, opening and preparing the devices for surgical/medical use. Further, the same tray/set checklist should be used to verify that all devices are accounted for following a procedure and on transfer to a reprocessing area. It is recommended in these cases that each responsible person in this cycle should indicate and sign that the quantities are correct and that nothing is missing. This allows instruments to be traced back to a specific person and located if applicable. It is not uncommon for devices and accessories to go missing, to include removal of instruments from one set to replace in another set (instead of introducing a new device to the incomplete set), accidental loss by mixing with linens or waste following a procedure in an operating room or, in extreme though unfortunate cases, where a device is accidentally left within a patient following a procedure. Ultimately, such checklists can be archived, depending on whether it is used as a patient safety document or for inventory control; this may include staying with the instrument set throughout (from processing to procedure and back to reprocessing) or to be filed with the patient's records post-procedure.

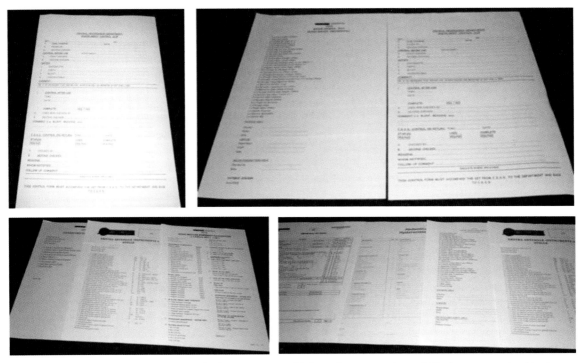

Figure 10.7 Examples of device tray and set checklists. A variety of different formats may be used. The lists are completed by the member of staff assembling the tray/set and are usually signed on completion.

Operating theatres use the greatest number and variety of instruments and are by far the largest users of reprocessed and particularly sterile items in a healthcare facility; accuracy is thus vital when assembling instrument sets. The contents of instrument sets are usually decided by the surgical team. The assembly of a tray should be agreed by both the reprocessing area and theatre managers, as best fits the clinical need. However, it should be remembered that the assembly of a tray may have some safety (e.g. weight) restrictions and may also be crucial for effective sterilization. For example, the overloading or inappropriate placement of certain items in trays can affect the outcome of a sterilization process. Overloaded and heavy trays/sets may not be adequately conditioned/sterilized by pre-programmed steam sterilization cycles (Chapter 11) and may in some cases remain wet; this can lead to residual moisture (water) remaining in or on the pack ("wet-pack", Chapter 11, in the section on Troubleshooting steam sterilization problems), which can be subsequently rejected when presented in an operating room for use. Instruments that are distributed evenly within a tray will enhance the drying process.

Trays are usually packed in the order that instruments are used. When the scrub sister sets up for a case in the operating room (Chapter 3, in the section on Operating room set up) the following may be typically prepared:
• The sterile trolley/surfaces to work from (e.g. including a Mayo trolley if it is an abdominal case). Drapes and trolley covers will be needed to cover these surfaces.
• Instruments are then laid out onto the surface in the order of use. Depending on the types of surgery the following are most commonly used first: BP handle and scalpel blade (for cutting), diathermy (bleeding control), scissors (cutting/dissecting), retractor/dilators and forceps.
• A cleaning/disinfecting solution is placed into a bowl and often with an instrument to clean with (e.g. a swab holder), if applicable.
• The patient is cleaned and draped (towel clips and drapes are needed, unless self-adhesive disposable drapes are used).
• All are assembled on and around the operating table to establish the sterile core. Sterile light handles will be

applied, suction, diathermy, drills/camera light sources, etc., will be attached by operating room staff.

These steps should be considered in the preparation of sets/trays with the operating room staff to aid in an efficient process.

Overall, it is important that the following points are taken into consideration when choosing a tray/set and packaging method:

- The type of pack
- The size and weight of items to be packed
- The number of times the pack will be handled before use
- The number and training of personnel who may handle the pack
- The distances that packs will be transported
- Whether the storage system is open or closed
- The condition of the storage area (cleanliness, temperature, humidity)
- If secondary packaging (e.g. Asepto bags or dust covers) will be used or are necessary
- The method of sealing packs

Once the tray and/or packaging system has been chosen the following factors need to be taken into consideration when assembling the instrument trays (examples are given in the section on assembling a tray below).

- The correct type of carrier tray must be used (see the section on instrument trays and pouches). When choosing trays, allowances should be made for extra length, ungainly, heavy or delicate design, all of which are more susceptible to damage than "regular" shaped instruments.
- Trays should be perforated to allow penetration of the sterilizing agent and efficient drying.
- The assembly should allow a subsequent user (e.g. an operating room scrub nurse) to remove the items aseptically without causing contamination.
- The weight of packs must be taken into consideration when assembling trays. Consider, for example, that a guideline weight for an object being carried using extended arms is 7 kg (~15.5 lbs) for a female and 10 kg (~22 lbs) for a male. Some standards and guidelines may also provide recommendations, such as ANSI/AAMI ST77 (*Containment devices for re-usable medical device sterilization*) and ANSI/AAMI ST79 (*Comprehensive guide to steam sterilization and sterility assurance in healthcare facilities*) recommend a maximum weight limit of 25 lbs (~11.5 kg) for instrument trays, which includes the packaging system.
- Instrument trays must be assembled to maximize instrument exposure to the sterilant, as well as sterilant (e.g. water) removal.

- In order to allow the sterilant to touch all surfaces of the instrument; instruments with ratchets or hinges should be held in an open and unlocked position, sliding/ extended/complex multiple-part instruments should be disassembled or sufficiently loosened to permit the sterilizing agent to come into contact with all parts of the instrument.
- Instruments should be left slightly open to allow for sterilant penetration, rings should be slightly separated.
- Unusually dense instruments/trays or design characteristics that may create moisture problems (i.e. wet packs) should have absorbent tray liners. Items that could hold water during steam sterilization must be placed in a way that allows easy drainage.
- Heavy instruments should be placed at the bottom of the tray as the weight of heavy instruments or retractors lying on top or over other instruments can cause the instruments at the bottom to bend and become misaligned.
- The variety of angles and curvatures pose a challenge when assembling trays. It is difficult to organize "unusually shaped instruments which can become damaged when they are "forced" to fit into trays. If trays are over packed and instruments do not lie flat the tips of instruments can become entangled and easily damaged.
- Placing the instruments in a single layer will provide more protection to the instruments.
- Taller rigid containers will permit segregation of delicate instruments.
- The relative size of different instruments must be the same, for example when using a 7"/17.5 cm pair of scissors, a 7"/17.5 cm needleholder and 7"/17.5 cm forceps will also be used.
- Tips of instruments should all be facing the same direction.
- Due to fragile nature of distal tips, the use of tip protectors is often advised by the manufacturer. These should have been tested to ensure they are compatible and safe to use for the designated sterilization process.
- Always make sure that all parts of the instruments are present and trays are not overloaded. The inclusion of a tray checklist/instrument set count sheet is part of quality management and/or inventory control and is an essential communication strategy between reprocessing staff and end users.
- In-pack, chemical process indicators should be placed in the most challenging part of the tray (Chapter 14, in the section on Monitoring sterilization). It is recommended that the indicator is placed in the densest part of the tray. This is also an important part of quality control,

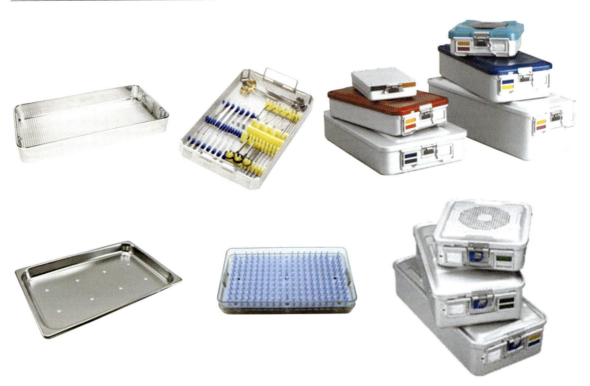

Figure 10.8 Various types of instrument trays and containers. On the left, a wire-mesh tray (upper) and a semi-solid (perforated; upper) tray, in the middle are example of specific types of set-trays for holding delicate instruments and on the right are a variety of rigid containers.

as the in-pack indicator should be checked for the correct indicator change (e.g. change in color) by the theatre staff when opening the pack immediately prior to use.

Instrument trays and pouches (supplementary devices)

Choose a tray to suit the dimensions of the instruments and type of sterilization technique to be used. The various types of trays available should be specifically developed and tested to be compatible with the specified sterilization process (e.g. Figure 10.8). These trays may be provided by the device/instrument set manufacturer, the sterilization process manufacturer or a third party supplier. They may be open in design (therefore loaded with devices and wrapped with packaging materials for sterilization) or provided with rigid containers with lids that are locked/sealed in preparation for sterilization. They can be constructed from a variety of materials, such as stainless steel, anodized aluminium and plastics. The ideal tray will have a perforated base and sides that will allow for even distribution of the sterilant; a solid base or sides may impede distribution of the sterilant. Too much metal from solid or semi-solid trays may also result in negative effects (e.g. in steam sterilization, leading to wet packs due to increased condensation). Edges should be smooth to prevent damage to packaging materials due to sharp edges that could have cut or punctured the package.

In addition to trays/containers, some individual devices or smaller sets are also prepared with medical grade packaging pouches or wraps (Figure 10.9), which are also designed for particular types of sterilization processes. These may also be made of a variety of materials such as paper and various types of plastics (e.g. a common material is Tyvek®, a trade name for a strong type of material made of polyethylene fibers. Further consideration is given to the various types of packaging materials in the section on Medical grade packaging systems.

Assembling a tray

To assemble instruments for surgical trays the following steps should be performed:

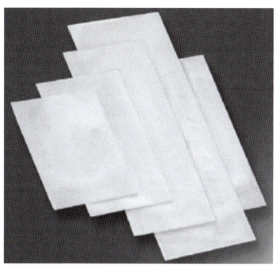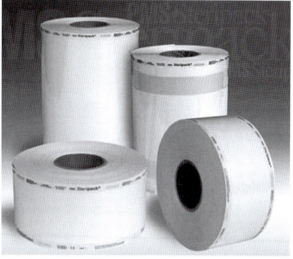

Figure 10.9 Various types of pouches and wraps used as sterilization barrier (packaging) systems.

• Make sure that all instruments are dry and have been opened or disassembled to allow sterilant penetration.
• Place all hollow items face down.
• Place a tray-liner in the bottom of the tray to assist with absorption of moisture (if applicable).
• Count instruments and place them into the tray according to the tray checklist.
• Place large instruments such as retractors at the bottom and more delicate instruments on top to prevent damaging the instruments.
• Do not substitute instruments.
• Place ring-handled instruments on pins or stringers according to type to facilitate counting.
• Do not band flat instruments together with rubber bands or in steripeel.
• Cover sharp or delicate tips in order to protect them.
• When packing single instruments make sure that the handles are at the end which is opened.
• Separate different metals, for example stainless steel and brass BP handles as they may become discolored due to oxidation.
• Place cannulated instruments such as suction nozzles at a slight angle (e.g. to allow for drainage of moisture during a steam sterilization process).
• Arrange the instruments according to the checklist, usually in a pattern that will evenly distribute the weight, protect sharp edges and facilitate their removal in the OR. The various steps in assembling a typical tray are summarized in Figure 10.10.

It is important to remember not to overload the tray (Figure 10.11). If too many devices are required for a particular procedure, they should be redistributed into a number of trays that are then provided as a set for surgical/medical use.

Examples of different procedure device sets and prepared trays

Figure 10.12 is given as an example of various different types of device sets and prepared trays.

Medical grade packaging systems

To create ideal packaging conditions, where the sterility of the packaged and sterilized device/material is maintained until it is used, is one of the day-to-day challenges that healthcare facilities need to consider. The purpose of a sterilization packaging system is to provide a safe and effective method of protecting sterile supplies and equipment while handling, transporting and storing, as well as allowing for aseptic presentation. The question of how many layers of wraps should be used, and whether this has been validated in the performance qualification of the sterilizers should be asked when choosing a wrapping system. Most countries routinely use a minimum of two layers of wrap, the outer being the transport wrap and the inner the sterile field (allowing the tray to be opened and placed on a Mayo table/trolley perhaps).

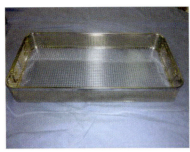

1. Select the appropriate tray.

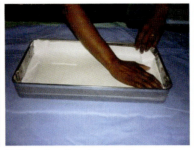

2. Place tray liner in the bottom of the tray.

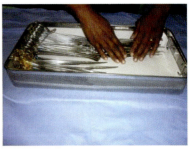

3. Inspect and pack instruments according to tray layout.

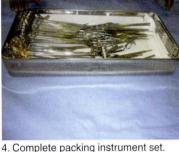

4. Complete packing instrument set.

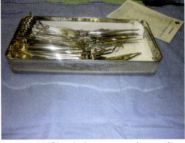
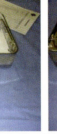

5. Check the type and quantity of instruments against a check list.

Figure 10.10 A general guide in assembling a tray. Note: not all steps are required, depending on the tray load and sterilization process in use (e.g. may not be necessary or advisable to use a tray liner).

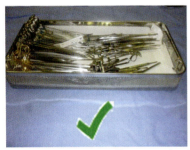
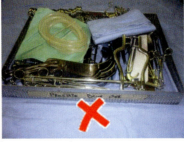

Do not overload instrument sets!

Figure 10.11 Do not overload device trays/sets.

Traditionally, sterile wrapping of individual items or trays consists of two separate layers of various different types of wrap materials, linens, see-through packaging or a combination of different packaging materials. A variation on the same theme may be a container with or without an inner wrapping. In strict terms, a single barrier layer should be sufficient but is not ideal as, if the wrap is exposed to contaminants during its transport to the point of use, often through corridors of hospitals and theaters, etc., where the pack could be heavily exposed to all sorts of bioburden, there is no additional layer protecting the tray/instruments. The use of two layers of wraps reinforces the strength of the packaging, affording greater protection during handling, transport and storage prior to its use in a surgical/medical situation. Folding the two wraps separately, one after the other makes the pack more secure, as the greater the number of folds the more tortuous the path becomes for micro-organisms to penetrate into the packaging. The double wrap with two sequential folds also affords a two-step unwrapping process which assists in aseptic presentation and creation of a sterile field for users in the operating theatre; the outer wrap is

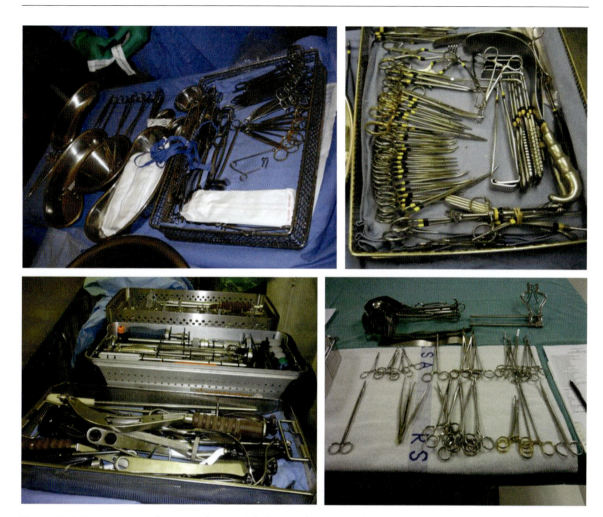

Figure 10.12 Device set examples. A complete Trendelenburg set for removal of varicose veins (top left), general surgical tray for appendix/hernia procedures (top right), an orthopedic set (can have up to 33 trays, bottom left) and a set for devices for an abdominal hysterectomy.

removed before entering the operating room or by an assistant.

Inappropriate handling will cause contamination of the outer packaging. In the case of a single layer this means that the entire barrier has been contaminated; in the case of a double layer, the inner pack remains sterile even on its outside until it is removed. In the case of a single layer, there is also a risk that sterile goods can become contaminated, during opening, by micro-organisms which cover the outside of the pack while the pack is opened. Therefore, whenever aseptic handling is necessary, especially in theatres, double layers are recommended in order to guarantee contamination free removal, particularly after longer storage times.

Practically packaged materials will not become compromised due to natural degradation of the packaging material but due to a specific event (e.g. damage to the packaging material such as ripping, wetting, etc.). It is therefore recommended (unless otherwise recommended by the packaging material manufacturer) that sterile packaged materials are not issued with a specific expiration time ("time-related shelf-life"), but that the shelf-life is based on any event that may recontaminate the device/set ("event-related shelf-life"). In this case, where no adverse event has occurred, the device/set may be used at any time in the future. Storage times are limited because of any risk of recontamination, such as during the handling, storage, transport or opening the package. These concepts may often be challenged when new packaging materials or concepts are introduced; any such claims should be based on sound principles and scientific verification. The choice of packaging and how it is used within a facility should be based on their own risk analysis. Healthcare facilities have traditionally used more than one packaging material/method, as all materials/methods have advantages and disadvantages. It is up to the facility to make an informed choice from the extensive range available, bearing in mind that the choice of packaging is extremely important as it must meet the primary aim to guarantee the sterility and integrity of the contents until the time of use.

Following the preparation and assembly of devices into trays/sets, the next step is to package the sets for sterilization and subsequent sterile storage. The term "sterility" implies that the devices have been subjected to a validated sterilization process *and* that the microbial barrier has not been compromised and the packaging is intact when being inspected for use. Therefore, sterilization packaging materials/containers have two main functions:

• To keep instruments together in sets before, during and after sterilization.
• To maintain the sterility of the instruments/sets during storage/transport until the time of use.

There are many different types of packaging materials and equipment available, with most healthcare facilities using a variety of these types. Items classified as critical devices should be packaged for sterilization (with the exception of flash sterilization methods; Chapter 11), transport and storage. Developing a packaging and labeling system that meets patient safety and user requirements can be complicated, especially when issues such as cost, distribution and storage facilities are taken into account. The packaging system chosen should be appropriate for the items being sterilized and compatible with the specific methods of sterilization being used. Packaging material used in steam sterilization, as an example, must be able to withstand high temperatures, allow for adequate air removal, be flexible in considering changes in pressure during the process, permit steam penetration to the pack's contents and allow for adequate drying. Similarly, packaging materials used with low temperature sterilization processes (e.g. ethylene oxide and gaseous hydrogen peroxide processes) must have similar properties, particularly being compatible with the sterilization chemicals, moisture, pressure changes and temperature ranges. During and following such processes, heat or chemical based, the sterilization packaging systems should provide an effective barrier to microbes, particulates and liquids, whilst maintaining sterility of the contents until used. All these requirements should be supported by testing and validation by the packaging materials/container manufacturers, particularly to meet international and national standards and guidelines.

Choosing the correct packaging is therefore a critical component of sterility assurance and critical device reprocessing, with each different type of packaging having advantages and limitations that must be understood by staff. High quality sterilization packaging systems can optimize infection control and patient safety. Only validated products that protect the contents and provide a reliable barrier system against microbial penetration, during handling and storage, should be considered for use.

Selection of packaging materials

When choosing a packaging system, turnover, ease of use, material compatibility and storage space need to be balanced with patient, and staff safety and instrument protection and cost. The correct selection, care, use and performance of sterilization packaging systems is critical if sterilization of the contents is to be achieved and maintained until the package is opened for use.

When choosing a sterile packaging system the following ideal properties may be taken into consideration:
• Provide an adequate barrier to microorganisms, particulates, and fluids.
• Compatibility with the sterilization process.
• Strong enough to withstand sterilization and subsequent handling.
• Medical grade packaging that will not cause any harm, that is, be non-reactive, stable, free of toxic ingredients and non-fast dyes, and non-odorous, ensuring product integrity and patient safety. Examples of non-medical grade packaging are cardboard boxes, which are not recommended!
• Permit adequate air removal.
• Allow the chosen sterilant (or sterilization process components) to penetrate and come into direct contact with the all surfaces of the contents.
• Allow for removal of the sterilant, especially toxic biocides or their by-products.
• Securely and completely protect and enclose the contents.
• Provide adequate seal integrity and be tamper-proof.
• Be able to maintain sterility during handling, transport and storage until use.
• Be easy to use.
• Be puncture and tearing resistant.

- Be easily disposed of/or recyclable.
- Be available in various sizes.
- Low-lint content.
- Allow for easy identification of contents.
- Provided manufacturers' instructions for use.
- Facilitate aseptic opening and allow for removal of the contents without re-contamination. When removing sterile items from the packaging, it should not be possible to accidentally touch the un-sterile outer side of the packaging. Here, factors such as the ease of peeling for opening such packaging materials without tearing are important.

Types of packaging

Traditionally, re-usable packaging systems such as sterilizing drums and textiles were the only packaging choice available in most healthcare facilities. Due to a better understanding of packaging systems and advancements in technology this is no longer the case, and a wide range of packaging systems are now available, including disposable and re-usable packaging materials (summarized in Figure 10.13).

The choice of packaging will generally depend on the sterilization method being used. In general, packaging

Type	Properties	Examples
Re-usable woven textile	Textiles are supplied in sheets of woven materials and in a range of different fabrics.	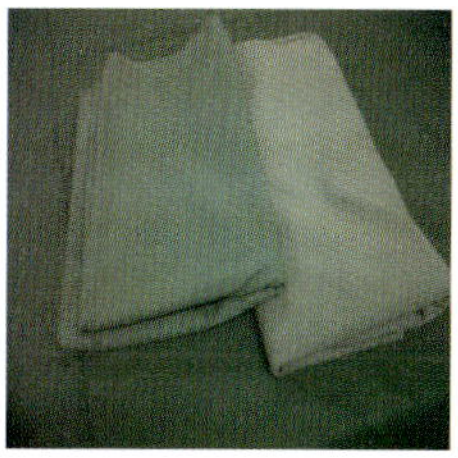
Non-woven	Non-wovens consist of a bonded web made of textile and/or non-textile fibers. They are usually supplied in sheets.	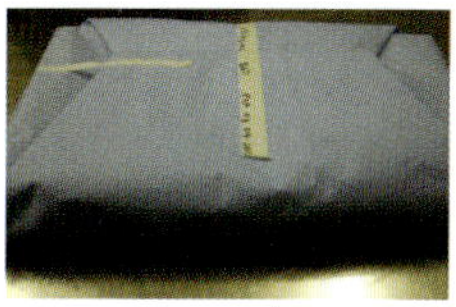
Paper	Paper wrapping materials come in several forms, including sheets of plain or crêpe paper and bags.	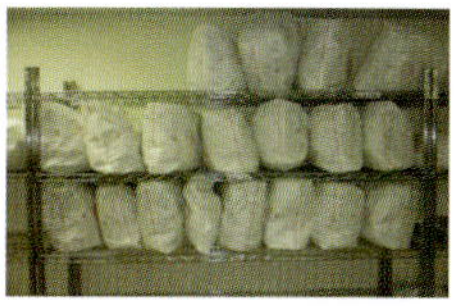
Paper-plastic	This combination is usually heat sealed together along the lengthwise edges to form peel-open packaging. It is supplied as pouches or reels that can be cut to size.	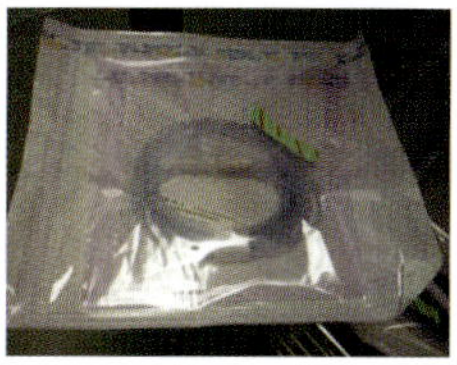
Rigid containers	Rigid containers are usually made of aluminum or plastic and are often used for large or heavy items that require a robust form of packaging.	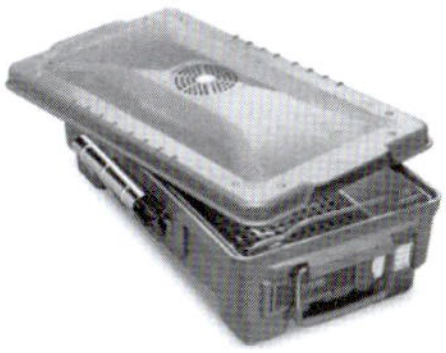

Figure 10.13 Summary of the various types of packaging materials/system.

materials should only be used that have been tested to be compatible and safe for each sterilization purpose. This is true for both high and low temperature sterilization. It is important to note that packaging materials are generally only tested to be effective under claimed conditions and using them outside these claims may compromise the sterilization efficacy of the load, cause damage to the materials used (compromising storage) and other disadvantages.

Re-usable woven textile wraps

Woven textiles were used almost exclusively for sterile packaging until the 1980s, when non-wovens that provided a more effective barrier against microbial contamination were introduced. Traditional woven textiles had a thread count of 140 which provided an ineffective microbial barrier, potentially allowing most microorganisms to pass through. Such woven textiles are still used to form sterile barrier systems in certain countries, but they are generally not optimal for this purpose and should be actively discouraged. Modern woven textiles have, however, now been developed and as long as they comply with international or national sterilization packaging standards (see the section on Standards and guidelines for sterilization packaging systems), they are suitable to be used as wrappers for this purpose.

The advantages of woven textiles are that they are soft, re-usable, inexpensive and drapeable (has little or no "memory" and falls flat when opened). Re-usable woven textile fabrics may be woven from cotton, linen or blends of cotton and synthetic materials, such as polyester. Due to the nature of woven threads the textiles will degenerate over time the more often they are processed. The manufacturer should provide information about the number of laundering and sterilization cycles that the material can withstand.

Before use, such textiles should be laundered, delinted and inspected, preferably over light boxes, for holes, worn spots, tears and stains (for guidance on general laundering, see the sections on Chapter 15, Surgical and medical laundering and Chapter 8, Textiles and laundry). Any tears should be repaired on both sides with a vulcanized patch applied using heat. It is important to launder any previously sterilized textiles as prior to reprocessing woven textile will need to be rehydrated. Textiles should be thoroughly rinsed to ensure that they are free of detergents, bleaches or other chemicals that may react with the sterilant and cause discoloration and/or adversely affect the contents of the pack. A laundering mark-off system should be used to monitor the number of times that the wrap has been used.

Single-use, non-woven wraps

Various non-woven, single-use disposable products are available, for example spun-bonded olefin, fibre-reinforced tissue, spun-bonded polyethylene and spun-laced, wood, pulp-polyester materials. Non-woven fabrics are designed as single-use disposable products and *should not* be re-used. Non-woven fabrics are not woven, they are made up of fibres that have been pressure bonded together to form sheets of fabric. Special non-wovens have been developed, for sterilization, to meet the requirements for primary packaging of sterile goods specified in standards.

Non-wovens are suitable for steam, steam-formaldehyde and low temperature sterilization processes, such as ethylene oxide, vaporized hydrogen peroxide and gas plasma; they are considered to provide excellent bacterial barrier properties. However, not all non-wovens may be compatible for all types of sterilization methods as they contain varying amounts of synthetic material. For example, packaging that contains cellulose cannot be used in hydrogen peroxide or ozone sterilization. Non-wovens are virtually lint free and due to the very small spaces between the fibers are generally resistant to dust penetration. Plastic polymers, such as polyolefins provide excellent water vapor (steam) transmission, but some may resist liquid penetration altogether. Non-wovens generally repel liquids; they are hydrophobic ("water-hating"). Although these fabrics have the flexibility and handling qualities of woven materials, when wrapping they can be torn or punctured by sharp edges of devices and/or instrument trays. Non-wovens are available in a range of weights and a wide variety of sizes.

Papers

Paper is essentially a non-woven material intended for single use. Special papers have been developed to meet the requirements for primary packaging of sterile goods specified in various standards (see the section on Standards and guidelines for sterilization packaging systems). There are many types and grades of paper that include:
• "Kraft"-type papers are generally smooth-surfaced and are used in the manufacture of bags and peel-open pouches.
• Crepe-type paper wrap has been specially treated to allow it to stretch and adapt to the types and sizes of items that it is used to wrap. It also makes the paper softer and easier to handle. This type of paper has "memory", which means that it tends to revert back to the way it was folded and not lie flat when opened to form an adequate sterile field.
Prior to use, paper must be inspected for pinholes, tears, creases or other flaws that would compromise the integrity of packaged items. Crepe-type papers are easily penetrated by steam, ethylene oxide, low-temperature

steam/formaldehyde and are suitable for these sterilization processes. They are not suitable for hydrogen peroxide gas or ozone processes, because of their cellulose content.

Disposable peel-open pouches and reels

Disposable peel-open pouches and reels are composed of paper/plastic combinations. They are designed to contain lightweight or small items and are available in various sizes, for single use only. Peel-open packaging should not be used for heavy or bulky items because the seals can become stressed and rupture. Pouches may be self-sealing or sealed by heat-sealing the open end (see the section on sealing of pouches and reels). Pouches are available in many sizes. The open end of the pouch is closed with a sealing device. It is essential that the heat sealer is functioning effectively in order to get an adequate seal. Both ready-made pouches and reels are available flat or with side gussets for packing bulkier objects. The user can cut reels to any size needed, in which case both sides of the pack will need to be sealed by the user.

Peel-open packaging is useful when visibility of the contents is important. When packaging items, care must be taken to leave a minimum of 1 inch (2.5 cm) of space between the end of the item and the seal of the pouch or reel in order to facilitate aseptic opening. To label, use a felt-tip, indelible, non-toxic ink marker on the clear plastic side of the pouch. Peel-open pouches should be placed upright in a grid basket or container during sterilization. Also they should not be too tightly packed together, such that a hand can slide in between them.

Double peel-open packaging is not routinely required, but if items are double pouched, they must be packaged paper against paper, plastic against plastic in order to enable sterilant penetration. The inner pouch should be at least a size smaller than the outer pouch to prevent folding, which may entrap air and inhibit the sterilization process.

Paper/plastic peel-open packaging materials are suitable for steam, steam formaldehyde and low temperature sterilization processes such as ethylene oxide. It is not suitable for use in hydrogen peroxide gas and ozone sterilizers, again due to the paper (cellulose) content. The plastic front cannot be penetrated by steam or air, so removal of air and penetration of steam or gas is through the paper backing only.

Re-usable rigid container systems

Sterilization containers are a durable sterilization packaging system constructed of a rigid material such as metal, or plastic. They are re-usable, easy to use, cost-effective and versatile. They provide excellent protection as they are rigid and cannot be easily crushed. A variety of sizes can accommodate a wide range of instrument sets. Containers are a box-like structure comprised of a lid and base, carrying handles and a latch or locking mechanism that secures the lid to the base (Figure 10.14). A gasket is used to seal the lid to the base. Inner baskets, trays and various inserts organize and protect the instruments within the container. Nameplates or tags identify the sets and disposable items such as filters, tamper evident seals/locks and load cards/external chemical indicators complete the system.

As such containers are manufactured from non-porous rigid materials they create a barrier to the sterilization process as well as microorganisms; therefore they need to have a means by which the sterilant can enter the container. This is achieved by either a filter or through a valve in the lid, which opens and closes with the varying pressure in a sterilizer (e.g. in steam sterilization process). Filters can be single use or re-usable.

Containers need to be disassembled and cleaned after each use, following the reprocessing instructions supplied by the container manufacturer. Remember: such containers are classified as devices themselves and as such should be reprocessed after each use, not just wiped down. Containers must be cleaned in the same way as any other re-usable device. Following reprocessing they should be checked to include:

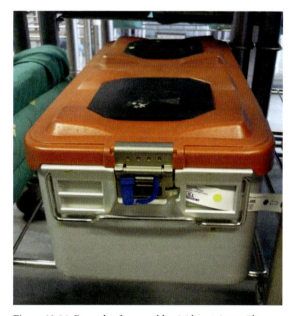

Figure 10.14 Example of a re-usable, rigid container with tamper proof lock (blue, shown in the center).

• Checks of gaskets for fraying, cuts, missing pieces, bubbling or compression.
• Cleaning re-usable filters and inspecting them for cracks or chips. The number of uses also needs to be logged and the manufacturer's recommendations not exceeded.

Choose cleaning products according to manufacturer guidelines, that is, neutral pH or aluminum-safe alkaline detergents are required in order to prevent damaging the fabric of the container, for example color changes.

Wrapping and sealing methods

Training should be provided on the correct methods of using the various different types of sterile packaging systems. In all cases, particular attention should be given to any instructions provided by the sterilization packaging system manufacturer. Three issues are highlighted in this section: standardization of tray wrapping methods, securing of packs and the sealing of pouches/reels.

Wrapping of trays for sterilization

The delivery of sterile products depends not only on the effectiveness of the sterilization process but also on effective packaging of the tray. The wrapping procedure should be precise and performed reproducibly. Wrapping the surgical instruments incorrectly or using the incorrect type of wrap can lead to instrument re-contamination. There are a number of wrapping options, but the facility should agree on their own methods and guidelines that best suits their needs. An example is shown in Figure 10.15. The wrapping sequence should be done in such a manner as to avoid "tenting" or "gapping", which will allow the ingress of dust and microorganisms. Double layers remain common practice due to the rigors of handling within the facility, even though the barrier efficacy of a single sheet of wrap has improved over the years. A sequential wrapping process uses two sheets of sterilization wrap, one wrapped after the other, creating a package within a package, thereby decreasing the risk of contamination. The non-sequential process uses two sheets wrapped at the same time so that the wrapping needs to be performed only once, but the risk of contamination in this case may be higher. Once the tray is wrapped it must be effectively sealed to prevent re-contamination. Likewise, if the package is packed too tightly the seal may loosen during sterilization, transport or storage, leading to a re-contamination event. The final step in the wrapping process is to seal and label the package.

Securing of packs

Various types of masking tapes can be used, including specifically designed process indicator (e.g. autoclave) tape designed to change color on exposure to the sterilization process. Packs and packets should be secured with a medical grade masking tape and/or a process indicator tape (Figure 10.16).

Process indicator tapes are useful to be able to verify whether a pack has been subjected to sterilization. Such process indicators are generally classified as being class 1 chemical indicators (Chapter 14, see the section on Process Indicators), in that they are simple indicators designed to demonstrate exposure to a process and/or to distinguish between processed/unprocessed units. If the tape is designed as a process indicator, it should show a clear color change when exposed to a sterilization process.

The ideal tape should:
• Have good adhesive qualities
• Be easy to remove
• Not leave any glue or ink residues

Sealing of pouches/reels

Some pouches are provided with self-adhesive sealing tabs, where the instruments are placed into the pouch and sealed for sterilization. Other pouches and reels are designed to be heat-sealed as the final step before the packaged devices are loaded for sterilization. Examples of heat-sealing machines are shown in Figure 10.17.

It is essential that the sealing apparatus (and settings of temperature, time, etc.) is used in when sealing pouches and reels. The heat sealer must be set to the packaging manufacturer's specifications, that is, the correct:
• Pressure
• Temperature
• Sealing/hold time

The various steps in the packaging and sealing of a set of devices are shown in Figure 10.18.

The strength and integrity of the seal depends on the appropriate application methods, as well as the correct temperature and pressure being applied for the correct length of time. Heavy instruments are often recommended to be packed with two layers of peel-open packaging, due to the risks of tearing. Instrument protector caps can be used to prevent sharp instruments damaging the pack. In some facilities, the contents of the package may be written on the external surface of the pack for identification purposes.

Note: it is common for devices in peel-open pouches to be placed into wrapped sets or containers. This is not necessary and in some cases may create problems for sterilization

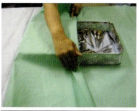

1. Select correct wrap size. Lay two layers of wrap on a flat surface (shown as green and blue) and place the instrument tray in centre. Fold one side to the centre, folding back to create a cuff.

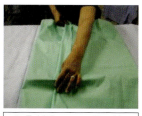

2. Fold the opposite side to the centre and fold back to create a cuff.

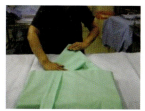

3. Fold both ends of the wrap to create a V-shape.

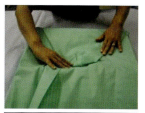

4. Fold the V to the centre of the set, making sure the two ends overlap. Do not pull the wrap too tight.

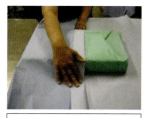

5. Fold the first side of the outer layer to the centre, folding back to create a cuff. Fold the opposite side to the centre, again forming a cuff.

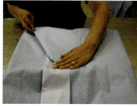

6. Fold both ends of the wrap to create a V and fold to the centre of the set, making sure the two ends overlap.

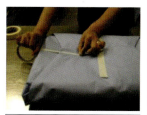

7. Secure the wrap with a length of tape (medical grade and/or autoclave tape).

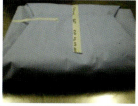

8. Label pack according to hospital policy.

Figure 10.15 An example of a two-layer wrapping process for an open tray set.

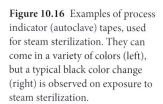

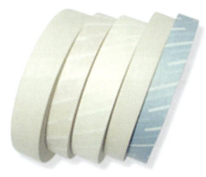

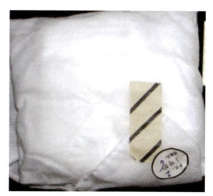

Figure 10.16 Examples of process indicator (autoclave) tapes, used for steam sterilization. They can come in a variety of colors (left), but a typical black color change (right) is observed on exposure to steam sterilization.

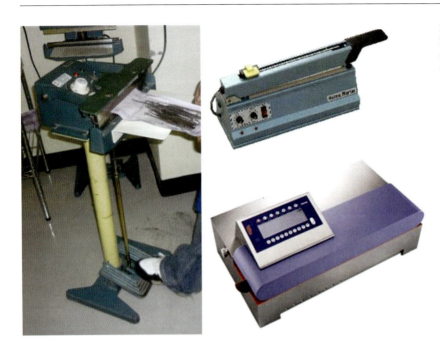

Figure 10.17 Examples of heat-sealing apparatus, with upright (left) and bench-top (right) designs shown.

1. Preparation

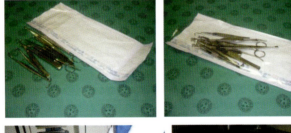

2. Sealing

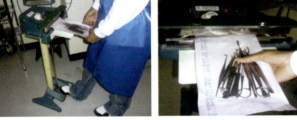

3. Ready for sterilization

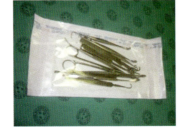

Figure 10.18 The steps in packaging and sealing a set of instruments into a sterile packaging pouch.

(e.g. adequate air removal, sterilant contact and drying, if applicable). Such devices should either be placed directly into the tray (unwrapped) or sterilized as a separate pack.

Standards and guidelines for sterilization packaging systems

Device packaging systems are regulated as an essential part of the process of maintaining sterility of devices/materials through storage, distribution and to a final site of use. The harmonized international standard for packaging is ISO 11607 *Packaging for terminally sterilized medical devices* – Parts 1 and 2. This standard has been adopted by many countries throughout the world and in this case the country adopting the standard will rename it to reflect this as follows:

- BS EN ISO 11607-1 (United Kingdom)
- ANSI/AAMI/ISO 11607-1 (USA)
- SANS ISO 11607-1 (South Africa)

ISO 11607 has two parts: Part 1 focuses on materials and packaging structures and Part 2 covers validation requirements and provides detailed guidance to healthcare facilities on the requirements for material qualification, package system design and testing, and packaging process validation. Guidance of the use of these standards is defined in ISO/TS 17665 *Packaging for terminally sterilized medical devices – guidance on the application of ISO 11607-1 and ISO 11607-2.*

Further regional standards and guidelines may also be used, such as EN 868 series of standards that specify particular requirements for a range of commonly used packaging materials. A summary packaging standards and guidance documents is given in Table 10.1.

Label identification of packaged devices

It is good practice for reprocessing facilities to implement appropriate systems to allow for the tracking of re-usable devices throughout the decontamination process and from patient to patient (Chapter 14, in the section on materials management). Examples of manual methods include the use of checklists (see Figure 10.7) and appropriate labeling of packaged devices/device sets. Labels can be applied to the external packaging, prior to sterilization to allow ease of identification. This is not only important in the loading and unloading of the sterilizer, but also in the subsequent transport and storage and to also correctly identify the contents of a package before it is opened for medical/surgical use. Proper labeling is also important for quality assurance, inventory control and stock-rotation purposes.

In reprocessing areas packaging should be labeled prior to sterilization in a way that does not compromise the integrity of the pack. In some cases this may be by writing directly on the pack, but in many cases this is not recommended by the packaging material manufacturer (due to damage to the material or leaking of ink through the barrier and onto the device); in such cases, information may be written on the indicator tape or an attached label. Labeling should not damage the packaging material; never use a ballpoint pen on any packaging material as it can create holes in the material. Recommended labeling methods include the use of:

- Soft-tipped, alcohol-based, felt marking pens
- Pre-printed tapes
- Pre-printed bags
- Stamping systems
- Pre-printed labels
- Dedicated or automated labeling systems may also be used

If using a manual system (Figure 10.19), the required labeling information must be written down on a sheet identifying the operator, the cycle printout and any other monitoring devices linked to the particular load. An electronic system allows the items to be scanned by a handheld scanner with the information downloaded to produce a batch report. Labels may be pre-printed directly onto packaging materials, or packaging materials can be printed in-line. Often a combination is used, with generic information pre-printed and lot and date-specific information printed at the time of packaging. Alternatively, labels can be directly written and affixed to the packaging system. Automated systems can also be used (Figure 10.20). A common method involves the use of bar codes used to identify packs (these are further considered in Chapter 14, in the section on materials management) and device locations by a scanning process. More sophisticated systems scan digital photos into the system to provide visual assistance in tracking and identification.

It is recommended that packaging systems should be labeled with the description of the package contents, identification (e.g. initials) of the person assembling the package and a lot control number. Further, the label may include other information such as:

- The date of sterilization
- Sterilizer and cycle number
- Any expiration date/shelf-life statement applicable to the facility policy (Chapter 12)
- The procedure and department where the package is to be sent after sterilization

Table 10.1 Examples of packaging standards and guidance documents.

Organization	Title	Description
ISO	ISO 11607-1:2006, Packaging for terminally sterilized medical devices – part 1	Sets the requirements and test methods for materials, sterile barrier systems and packaging systems.
ISO	ISO 11607-2:2006, Packaging for terminally sterilized medical devices – part 2	Specifies the requirements for development and validation of processes for packaging medical devices that are terminally sterilized.
EN	EN 868 Parts 2–10	Specifies particular requirements for a range of commonly used packaging materials.
Association for the Advancement of Medical Instrumentation (AAMI)	TIR 22:2007/A1:2008	Interpretive guidance for the applications of ANSI/AAMI/ISO 11607-1:2009, Packaging for terminally sterilized medical devices Part 1: requirements for materials, sterile barrier systems and packaging.
Australian Standards (AS)	AS 3789.2-1991	Textiles for healthcare facilities and institutions – theatre linen and pre-packs.
	AS 3789.8-1997	Textiles for healthcare facilities and institutions – recyclable barrier fabrics.
	AS 1079.1-1993	Packaging of items (sterile) for patient care – selection of packaging materials for goods undergoing sterilization.
	AS 1079.2-1994	Packaging of items (sterile) for patient care – non-re-usable papers – for the wrapping of goods undergoing sterilization in healthcare facilities.
	AS 1079.3-1994	Packaging of items (sterile) for patient care – paper bags – for single use in healthcare facilities.
	AS 1079.5-2003	Packaging of items (sterile) for patient care – single-use, non-woven wrapping materials – for goods undergoing sterilization in healthcare facilities.
AORN	Recommended practices for selection and use of packaging systems for sterilization	Guidelines for the evaluation, selection and use of packaging systems for items to be sterilized.

Labels must be able to withstand exposure to the sterilization process, storage and transport. Labeling must not:
- Affect the sterility or integrity of the pack
- Become illegible
- Transfer to pack contents
- React with packaging
- Interfere with the decontamination process
- Become detached in sterilization or subsequent storage

Loading and unloading sterilizers

An important part of reprocessing that it is often underestimated is the correct loading and unloading of a sterilizer. It is important to understand when loading a sterilizer that, in order to achieve sterility, all surfaces of the item must have direct contact with the sterilizing agent for the prescribed amount of time. In order to achieve this, all items should be placed in a manner that

Figure 10.19 Examples of manual labeling systems.

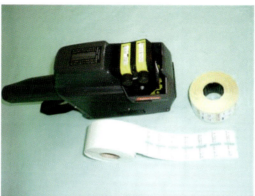
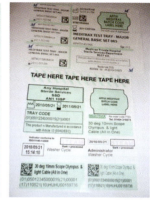

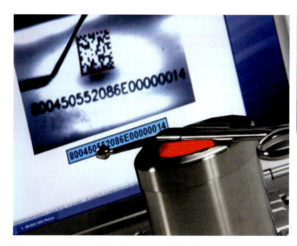
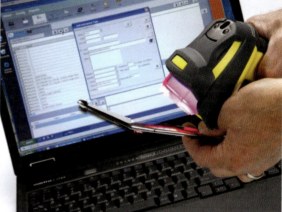

Figure 10.20 Examples of automated labeling systems.

will allow contact of the sterilant to all surfaces. Specific guidelines and recommendation may be provided by the sterilizer manufacturer that should also be considered. Only trained skilled reprocessing personnel should be responsible for the loading/unloading and operation of sterilizers. Sterilization itself is dependent on many parts of the decontamination process and associated procedures being undertaken correctly (Chapter 11). These include:

• Adequate cleaning, packaging and handling of items
• Use of a defined, validated and correctly installed sterilizer
• Correct loading and operating of the sterilizer
• Correct unloading the sterilizer
• Routine maintenance of the sterilizer and re-validation and any associated accessories

Loading the sterilizer

Recommended personal protective equipment (PPE) must be used when loading the sterilizer. An important example is with steam sterilizers (autoclaves), where the internal walls can be very hot to touch; therefore special heat-protecting gloves or gauntlets may be needed in loading such sterilizers (Figure 10.21). In addition, safety glasses are also important if there are various risks of steam or chemical exposure in the area.

Whatever method of sterilization is being used, low or high temperature, the basic rule to consider in loading the sterilizer chamber is that all items need to be properly prepared and arranged in a way that will allow the process to be effective (e.g. present the least possible resistance to the extraction of air and the passage of the sterilant throughout the load). Always follow

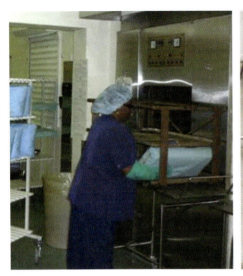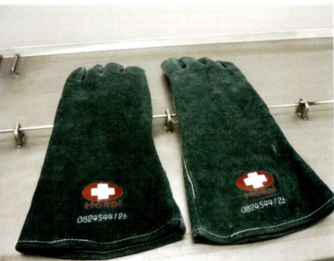

Figure 10.21 Loading of a steam sterilizer (left) using heatproof gauntlets/gloves (shown right).

manufacturers' recommendations when loading the sterilizer. For example, most sterilization processes (sufch as steam, ethylene oxide and hydrogen peroxide gas systems) recommend that devices are dry prior to sterilization, as they are not generally designed to remove excess moisture. Sterilizers should never be overloaded; there should be sufficient space between items to allow for the sterilant to permeate around the package and packages must not touch the top, bottom or sides of the sterilizer. Overloading in both high temperature and low temperature sterilization processes can compromise the effectiveness of the process, as designed for use. The correct load for a sterilizer is determined by the size of the sterilizer chamber and number of items to be sterilized, their characteristics, and how they are prepared and positioned within the sterilizer. These requirements should be specified by the sterilizer manufacturer and may include material/device, positioning and weight restrictions. A single large item, for example, may be the maximum load for the type of sterilizer being used. Large and small items can be included in the same load, but only if applicable. The sterilization process will be effective if items are properly prepared and positioned, so they get adequate contact with the sterilization process for the correct amount of time.

The are a number of considerations when loading a sterilizer (see Figure 10.22):
• Verify integrity of packaging before loading.
• Load according to manufacturers' recommendations.

• Place peel pouches on their edge so they can expand and contact during the cycle. These can expand considerably during a steam/gas based process. Arrange so that the plastic of one pouch touches paper side of the next for penetration and aeration. Consider specific recommendations, for example placing pouches plastic side down can increase the risk of moisture remaining in the pouch during a steam sterilization cycle.
• Use only perforated or wire mesh bottom instrument trays, wire baskets or specially designed pouch baskets. Do not use plastic coated baskets unless designed and validated for sterilization and aeration.
• Load items in a loose fashion to facilitate air removal, humidification (if applicable), circulation and penetration of all surfaces, and removal during aeration.
• Load baskets and carts so hands won't touch packs if you need to transfer them to an aeration cabinet.
• If using approved rigid containers, follow the manufacturer's validated loading instructions.
• Packages must not touch the walls, floor or ceiling of the chamber, otherwise package damage from heat, moisture or other effects may occur.
• Never place items directly on the floor of the sterilizer chamber as this could block the discharge of air from the sterilizer, or allow air and sterilants to be trapped in pockets, resulting in sterilization failure and "wet packs" in the case of steam sterilization. Packs touching the chamber walls can be scorched or contents damaged due to excessive heat of the metal walls or become wet due to excessive moisture on the walls, in the case of steam

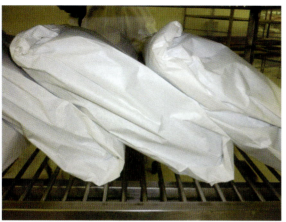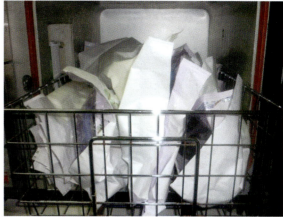

Items should be loaded loosely.

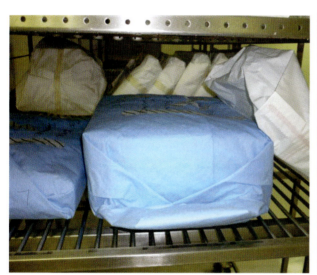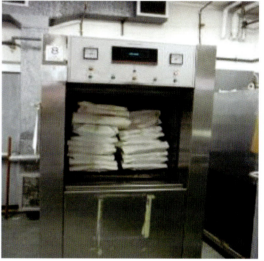

Leave space between packs. Do not layer packs, or touch walls or base of the sterilizer.

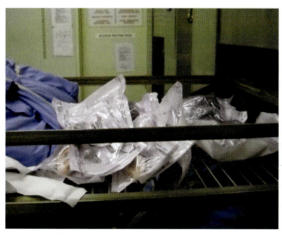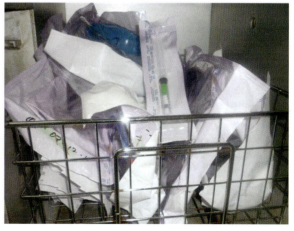

Place small packs in holders.

Do not overload.

Figure 10.22 Guidelines for loading a sterilizer, the basic principles apply irrespective of the type of sterilizer. Note: Many bad examples are shown!

sterilization. Always allow 7–8 cm (3 inches) of space between top-most package and top of chamber. This allows displacement of air and free flow of the sterilant.

• Loading racks or holding trays will help establish package separation. In combination loads of soft packs and instruments trays, place soft packs on top shelves and trays on lower shelves. In the case of steam sterilization this prevents condensation forming when the steam initially comes into contact with the cool metals, from dripping onto soft packs below.

• Soft packs (linen, gauze) should be placed on their sides/edges with folds perpendicular to shelf, this makes it easier for the sterilant to penetrate by flowing down through the folds than through flat compressed surfaces. Never place packages directly on top of each other; this will compress the packages, preventing air removal and sterilant penetration.

• Place solid utensils (basins/bowels) on their sides. Instrument trays should be placed flat on the shelves. Nested packs should be positioned in the same direction to help prevent air pockets, so condensation can drain and steam can circulate freely. Slatted trays, mesh baskets or a loading cart must be used to ensure proper loading.

• Liquids (for steam sterilization) must be sterilized by themselves in a separate dedicated cycle according to manufacturers' instructions. The length of the sterilization cycle will be determined by the amount of liquid in the bottle. Use only heat-resistant glass (Pyrex®) and automatic self-sealing caps for closure as there is always a possibility that solutions will explode.

• Place all empty bottles and empty rigid containers on their sides with lids held loosely in place. This will allow air to drain out and sterilant to take its place.

• If instruments have been assembled in a solid tray or Mayo tray, the tray should be placed on the side and tilted slightly forward. This will prevent the instruments from falling into a "clump" and allow for the run off of moisture in the case of steam and facilitate drying. Rigid containers should be spaced about one inch apart from each other. Stacking should not be performed unless the container manufacturer gives specific information on this process. Peel packs should be placed on their edge in a peel pack separator or basket to stop them moving around during sterilization.

• Always place the heaviest trays on the lowest shelf of the carriage.

Unloading a sterilizer

Recommended personal protective equipment must be used when unloading the sterilizer. For heat-based processes, the processed load and inner sterilizer/rack surfaces may be hot at the completion of the cycle and could result in serious burns. In the case of high temperature sterilizers the load should be allowed to cool before safely removing.

Sterilized packs should be handled gently and as little as possible to avoid re-contamination. All sterilizers should be unloaded in such a manner as to maintain the sterility of the items that have been processed. Remove the loading cart/tray/individual packs from the sterilizer and place them in a dedicated area, where there are no open windows/fans in close proximity as there may be residual humidity in the packages, and dust and dirt could be forced through the wrappers, contaminating the contents. If a pack is dropped, tears or comes in contact with moisture, it must be considered re-contaminated. If there are water droplets or visible moisture on the outside of the wrapper or package, or on the tape used to secure it, the package may also require further drying prior to transport/storage. When unloading, packs should be checked that they are not incorrectly wrapped, that seals are intact, that the process indicator on the outside of the pack has changed, that a tracking date/label is present and that the package is in a good condition.

The use of carrying trays or baskets when loading the sterilizer will reduce the amount of handling when unloading. Hot packs should not be placed on cold metal surfaces, as condensation will occur, resulting in an unsterile or rejected pack. The actual time for cooling should be based on professional judgment, experience and the environmental conditions of the area. Only handle packs once they have reached room temperature. The most important rule to follow is to allow the packs to cool and dry completely before handling.

11 Sterilization

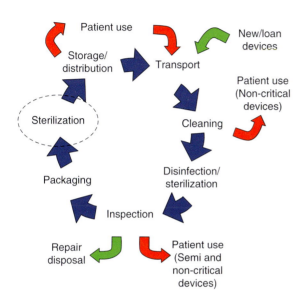

Patient use

Storage/distribution

New/loan devices

Transport

Patient use (Non-critical devices)

Cleaning

Sterilization

Disinfection/sterilization

Packaging

Inspection

Repair disposal

Patient use (Semi and non-critical devices)

Introduction

Sterilization is defined as a process used to render a surface or product free from viable organisms, including bacterial spores. Disinfection and sterilization products/processes are both antimicrobial, but while disinfection may only provide a reduction in microorganisms (Chapter 9) sterilization processes are designed to completely destroy all viable microbial life that may be present (i.e. "sterile" or has been "sterilized"). As previously defined in Chapter 1, re-usable devices can provide various different levels of risks to a patient and therefore various levels of disinfection/sterilization are recommended to reduce these risks. In the Spaulding classification, disinfection (ranging from low, intermediate to high levels) is widely used for the safe reprocessing of non-critical and semi-critical devices (Chapter 9 and

Table 11.1); however, critical devices that penetrate skin or mucous membranes or enter a sterile body cavity, including blood contact, have the highest risk to patient safety and should be sterilized.

How can sterilization assurance be provided and confirmed? Although the term "sterilization" may be commonly used, it is a condition that can be difficult to achieve and hard to guarantee. In fact, sterilization is only the result of a well-defined, repeatable and measurable process in a well-organized and well-operated reprocessing department. This process must at a minimum be shown to be effective against all types of microorganisms, including bacterial spores that are considered highly resistant to inactivation (Table 11.1). The only exception to this requirement is for efficacy against prions, which is considered separately and may or may not be shown for individual sterilization processes (see the section on Prion sterilization). But the demonstration of antimicrobial effects against all representative types of microorganism is in itself not sufficient. Consider, for example, that many of the disinfection products/processes described in Chapter 9 may also be effective against the same range of microorganisms (in particular certain types of high-level disinfectants), but they are not used for sterilization. It is important to remember that "sporicidal" or even "sterilant" refers to a biocidal product/process that is effective against spores, but this is not the same as sterilization. Further, it cannot be assumed that a product is sterile merely because it has passed through a sterilization technique; the process may only be effective if designed for that application, installed/maintained according to instructions, correctly used by staff and even verified to have taken place. These aspects will be further considered in this chapter.

Given the wide range of antimicrobial chemicals/processes available (Chapter 6), only a limited number of technologies have been widely used in sterilization processes. Similar to disinfection, these may also be

A Practical Guide to Decontamination in Healthcare, First Edition. Gerald McDonnell and Denise Sheard.
© 2012 Gerald McDonnell and Denise Sheard. Published 2012 by Blackwell Publishing Ltd.

Table 11.1 A commonly used classification system for disinfection and sterilization, based on the antimicrobial activity of the product/process. The different types of microorganisms are shown on the left (from those that are considered the least resistant to inactivation at the bottom and most resistant at the top), with the expected levels of activity shown for each product/process on the right. In the case of sterilization processes, the minimum criterion is that they are effective against bacterial spores, but the ability to be able to effective against all microorganisms (including bacterial spores) is only the beginning of defining a sterilization process.

classified as being physical or chemical in their main mechanisms of antimicrobial activity. The most widely used physical method is based on moist heat (steam sterilization), which is also the most commonly used method of sterilization worldwide for reprocessing of re-usable devices. Other methods such as dry heat, radiation and filtration have limited applications in healthcare facilities today and are only discussed briefly in this chapter. Chemical sterilization methods have traditionally been used only as low temperature alternatives to steam for the reprocessing of devices that are temperature-sensitive or otherwise not compatible or practical to be used with steam processes. These technologies are based on chemicals such as ethylene oxide gas, formaldehyde gas, hydrogen peroxide gas (that may or may not employ plasma generation), liquid peracetic acid and ozone gas. These are all based on particularly effective antimicrobials, but are used in well-defined processes to ensure their safe and effective use for sterilization. Most large healthcare facilities will employ at least two or more types of sterilization systems to allow for the reprocessing of different types of devices. Staff training is therefore always important to ensure that such processes are used correctly, according to manufacturers' instructions and in compliance with

any written facility policies (concerning loading, unloading, process monitoring, safety, maintenance, etc.). The choice of process can be inappropriate for a particular device, causing damage to the item and possibly even compromising sterility, both with patient complication and increased costs to facilities.

As discussed for disinfection (Chapter 9), assurance of sterilization occurs even before the sterilization process itself. Any effective decontamination process is dependent on effective cleaning as the higher the level of soil and microbial load that may be present on a device or load the lower the probability of reaching sterility can be. The effective cleaning of a re-usable item that is to be sterilized is of critical importance, with failure to clean potentially resulting in failed sterilization (the survival of microorganisms) and other significant patient risks (Chapter 8). Cleaning and disinfection can both play a role in reducing the amount of microorganisms present; this may be important even though the sterilization process is actually designed to provide a significant "overkill" of microorganisms (see the next section on basic principles of sterilization). Further sterilization may be achieved, but the item may not be maintained sterile by the time it is used on a patient (e.g. packaging compromised or device accidentally re-contaminated).

Therefore, sterilization and the provision of a sterile device for a patient procedure is dependent on the whole cycle of decontamination, including cleaning, packaging, sterilization, storage/transport and even to the point of preparing and using the device on a patient. Remember, if you cannot clean a device you cannot sterilize it.

Basic principles of sterilization

As for disinfection (Chapter 9), any sterilization processes needs to be effective against microorganisms and safely applied to devices. Efficacy and safety are the minimum requirements, but to this other considerations may be added, such as practical issues (installation and maintenance issues, ease of use, sterilization time, etc.), regulatory approvals, water quality/purity (water is an important part of the process), staff training and even environmental concerns (such as energy costs, water consumption, chemical safety, etc.). The choice of a sterilization process for a particular application will depend on the needs (today and in the future) of any facility. An ideal sterilization process will include:
• Demonstrated broad spectrum antimicrobial efficacy
• Demonstration as a sterilization process (e.g. sterility assurance level or alternative in compliance to international/national standards or guidelines)
• Compatibility with a range of devices and materials (not damaging)
• Capability of penetrating a range of loads, packaging materials and device complexity
• Safe for staff to use with minimal risks
• Leave no toxic residues that could present a risk to staff or patients
• Rapid cycle time (and not requiring additional holding times before use)
• Allowing for sterile storage, if required following sterilization
• Having a good environmental profile
• Being available in a range of sizes to accommodate various types of loads
• Economic to acquire, use and maintain
• Easy to install
• Methods available to monitor and confirm that the sterilization process has been adequately applied to a load
• Compliant to international and any national standards or requirements (including registrations)
This is not an exhaustive list, but it is clear that no such ideal process exists. This list highlights that there are strengths and weaknesses to all true sterilization processes,

which is why it is important to understand the needs of the facility when defining sterilization needs, but also in understanding any limitations of the various types of sterilization processes that may be available for use.

Further consideration is given to defining the minimum criteria for any sterilization process and in particular efficacy. It is important to note that a first requisite when designing a sterilization process is that the process is capable of demonstrating effectiveness against all types of microorganisms (Chapter 9, Introduction). This will include at least a representative number of bacteria (Gram negative and Gram positive bacteria), viruses (enveloped and non-enveloped forms), fungi (molds and yeasts, vegetative forms), protozoa, mycobacteria and bacterial spores (Chapter 5). A variety of test methods, including those used to establish and register disinfection claims (Chapter 9, see the section on Disinfection guidelines and standards) are often used to verify the effectiveness of such processes. Bacterial spores are particularly highlighted as they generally represent those microorganisms with the greatest resistance to inactivation due to their structure (Chapter 5, see the section on bacteria). But the particular strain (or type) of bacterial spores that are considered the "most-resistant organism" (commonly referred to as the "MRO") can be different depending on the sterilization process (Table 11.2). For example, *Geobacillus stearothermophilus* spores are considered the most resistant to steam and hydrogen peroxide gas (including gas plasma) processes, while *Bacillus atropheus* is considered the most resistant to ethylene oxide sterilization methods.

On successful completion of these tests, the proposed sterilization process has been established as demonstrating broad spectrum antimicrobial activity. The next step is to ensure that the process can provide a defined level of assurance of sterility. International standards, such as ISO 14937 *Sterilization of healthcare products – general requirements for characterization of a sterilizing agent and the development, validation and routine control of a sterilization process for medical devices*, provide guidance on how this can be achieved. One approach, primarily used industrially, is based on knowing the types and numbers of microorganisms that are present on the device or load to be sterilized; given the range of surgical and medical procedures, this is not currently considered a practical method for defining a sterilization process for re-usable devices. A more common method, typically used for defining sterilization processes for re-usable devices, is by studying the inactivation of the most resistant organism to the sterilizing agent (steam, a chemical, etc.) and developing a process that provides an "overkill"

Table 11.2 A list of different sterilization methods and their most resistant organisms. Note, other microorganisms may show unusually high level resistance to the sterilization method, but this may be due to other factors such as presence of soils, etc., rather than a true resistance to the sterilizing agent. These microorganisms are widely accepted and used for the testing of their respective sterilization method.

Sterilization method	Most resistant organism
Steam under pressure	*Geobacillus stearothermophilus* spores
Humidified ethylene oxide	*Bacillus atropheus*[1] spores
Hydrogen peroxide gas (with or without plasma)	*Geobacillus stearothermophilus* spores
Humidified formaldehyde	*Geobacillus stearothermophilus* spores
Liquid peracetic acid	*Geobacillus stearothermophilus* spores
Dry heat	*Bacillus atropheus*[1] spores
γ (gamma) radiation	*Bacillus pumilus*

[1] Previously known a *Bacillus subtilus*.

Table 11.3 An example of results from studying the antimicrobial activity of a sterilizing agent/process over time. The number of microorganisms (usually bacterial spores) remaining on a test surface is determined over exposure time to the sterilizing agent. The number of spores remaining can be given as the actual number counted or, for the purpose of mathematical analysis, converted into a "$\log_{10}$" scale. This mathematical scale expresses the actual number in a scale of 10; as an example, 10 spores would be a $\log_{10}$ of 1 (or 1×10^1), 100 is $\log_{10}$ 2 (or 1×10^2), 1000 is $\log_{10}$ 3, etc. Therefore 300 is 3×10^2 or about $\log_{10}$ 2.5.

Exposure time (minutes)	Number of microorgansims remaining	
	Number of spores	$\log_{10}$ number of spores
0	1,000,000	6
5	500,000	5.7
10	100,000	5
15	10,000	4
20	1,000	3
25	200	2.3
30	30	1.5
35	5	0.7
40	0	0

of this organism. When this is studied by microbiological methods and analyzed by mathematical techniques, the survival of a microorganism can be expressed in terms of probability of a single viable microorganism surviving after sterilization or a "sterility assurance level" (SAL). The most commonly used SAL in healthcare applications is called an SAL of 10^{-6}, defined as the probability of survival following a sterilization process of one in a million. Any SAL can theoretically be used (e.g. 10^{-1}, 10^{-3} or 10^{-6}), as they can all give a minimal assurance of sterility when the relationship between the exposure to a sterilization process and how it kills the most resistant organism to that process is understood. Note that a 10^{-6} SAL is considered a *higher* level of SAL than 10^{-3}, for example where 10^{-3} is a 1 in 1000 probability of a survival, a 10^{-6} is a 1 in 1,000,000 probability of survival. Why is 10^{-6} so widely used? This is traditional and has been widely used since the concept was first proposed. The use of such sterility assurance levels provides a level of "overkill" to ensure that following the sterilization process the items can be considered "sterile".

The correct definition of a sterility assurance level (SAL) is *the probability of a single viable microorganism occurring on an item after sterilization*. We will investigate a typical method used to demonstrate such a SAL of 10^{-6}, to understand the level of safety that is associated with such processes. Consider a surface with a known population of bacterial spores at 10^6 or one million (1,000,000) spores. This can be exposed to a sterilizing agent (under the conditions proposed as the minimum for its use in a sterilization process) over time and the level of microorganisms remaining at different times shown by microbiological techniques. An example of this data is shown in Table 11.3.

These results can also be shown in graph form (Figure 11.1). It can be seen that the sterilization process provides a rapid reduction in the number of spores, but it is the structure of the graph showing the results in log form that we are particularly interested in as it shows a "straight-line" or, to the mathematician, a "linear" response. The graph shows a 6-$\log_{10}$ reduction of the test spores in about 40 minutes, but because the rate of kill is linear (shows a straight line response over time), this allows us to predict the time for an additional theoretical 6-$\log_{10}$ reduction (Figure 11.2).

Therefore, in this example, when starting with a population of the most resistant organism of one million (10^6, 6 $\log_{10}$) and testing under the minimum process conditions for the sterilizing agent, a 6 $\log_{10}$ reduction is shown

Figure 11.1 The spore reduction results in Table 11.3 shown in graph form, with the number of spores surviving (Y or vertical axis) at various exposure times (X or horizontal axis. At the top is a graph showing the actual number of spores surviving and at the bottom with $\log_{10}$ (number of spores surviving).

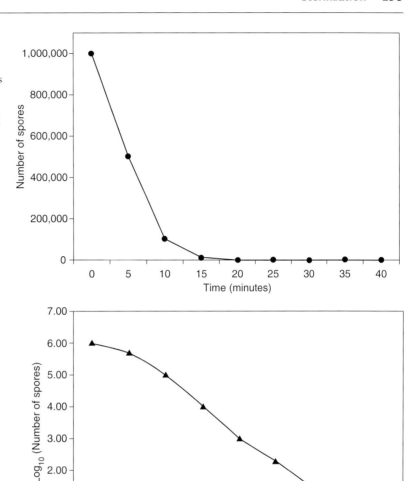

in about 40 minutes and a 12 $\log_{10}$ reduction is predicted mathematically to be within 80 minutes. Therefore, for a SAL of 10^{-6} the process time would be at least 80 minutes; equally a SAL or 10^{-3} would be about 60 minutes. Remember, that in most cases with critical devices, following use on a patient the device is cleaned (Chapter 8) and usually disinfected (Chapter 9) prior to sterilization. These processes remove and inactivate most of the microorganisms that may or may not be present; therefore the level of microorganisms on a device is generally considered to be very low when placed into a sterilizer. With this in mind, the level of "overkill" and therefore safety level to ensure that the device is sterile following such a sterilization process is considered exceptionally high.

Further analysis of the data, as presented in Figure 11.2, is often done in defining a sterilization process. An example is determining the D-value. The D-valve may be defined as the average time (in seconds, minutes, etc.) to give a 1 $\log_{10}$ reduction of a test organism. In the example shown in Figure 11.2, the D-value for the test organism in the sterilization process would be approximately 6.7 minutes. Further experiments can look at other relationships, such the effect of the D-value on the temperature or the concentration of a chemical sterilizing agent. The temperature relationship is particularly well described for steam sterilization; for example a Z-value (defined at the average temperature change required for a 1 $\log_{10}$ change in the D-value) is often

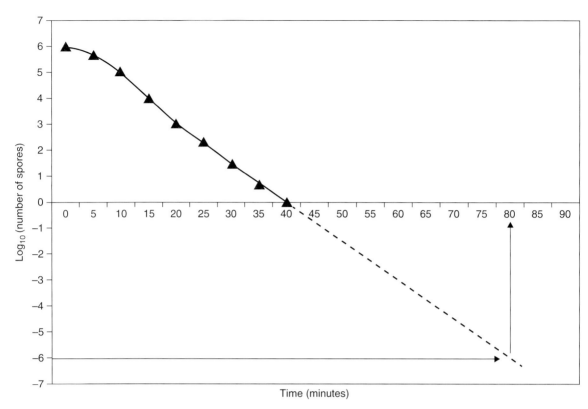

Figure 11.2 Demonstration of a sterility assurance level (SAL) of 10^{-6}. In this case, an SAL of 10^{-6} (or a predicted 12 $\log_{10}$ reduction from a starting population of 6 $\log_{10}$) would be defined for this sterilizing agent, under the process conditions tested, at about 80 minutes. Equally, a SAL of 10^{-1} would be about 47 minutes and 10^{-3} at about 60 minutes.

used to describe the relationship between the temperature and the average D-value. A typical Z-value for steam is 10°C. A further term used in steam sterilization is the D-reference at 121°C ($D_{121°C}$), being the D-value of a population of spores when exposed to steam under pressure at 121°C. When the $D_{121°C}$ and the Z-value is known for a population of spores, the D-value at any temperature of steam under pressure can be estimated and therefore the minimum time for sterilization under those conditions (i.e. for a SAL of 10^{-6}, this is the D-value at the sterilization temperature × 12). For example, at 131°C a typical D-value would be six seconds, therefore a minimum sterilization time would be 72 seconds (just over one minute). In general, most sterilization times are well overstated to give even greater overkill (e.g. 134°C for three or four minutes is typical).

In such a way, the minimum process conditions (e.g. temperature, time, concentration of chemical, humidity, etc.) are defined to provide a minimum SAL of 10^{-6}. During this analysis, these process variables and their effects may also be studied and further understood. When this is complete, the sterilization process itself needs to be developed that allows these minimum process conditions for sterilization to be achieved in the various types of loads ("product") that the process will be used to sterilize. This will define the type of equipment necessary to be able to apply and control the sterilization process. The number, type, design and packaging of different types of devices can provide different challenges to any process. An example is with air removal from the load, as air can prevent the penetration of the sterilizing agent(s) to all areas of the load. Devices that have internal lumens ("cannula" or cannulated devices) are examples of instruments that are considered difficult to remove air from and/or allow a sterilizing agent to fully penetrate. Other variables, depending on the sterilizing agent, may include temperature, the antimicrobial chemical and humidity distribution within the load. It is therefore important that examples of such loads are tested and conform to be sterilized by the chosen process. In addition to the anti-microbial efficacy, the process is also tested for any material effects on the devices to be sterilized ("compatibility"), including the various different types of materials used to make devices as well as the devices themselves, and for safety aspects. The process should not damage the devices or may be restricted from being used on certain types of materials or device types. Safety aspects will include staff safety when using or working in the same area as the sterilizer; patient safety should be ensured by making sure that there are no toxic residues present after the process, from the sterilizing agent and any associated by-products as well as safety of the environment. All of these aspects should be considered and verified through testing in the design of the final sterilization process and associated equipment.

A typical sterilization process will include three stages:
• Conditioning, ensuring that the load is correctly prepared to be sterilized under defined conditions. This can include air removal, adequate temperature distribution, drying, chemical agent distribution (under the conditions required for it to be effective as a sterilizing agent), etc. The specific requirements that need to be verified during conditioning will depend on the sterilization process.
• Sterilization, where the minimal SAL of 10^{-6} is ensured.
• The safe release of the load. This can include removal of toxic chemicals (aeration or ventilation), which is typical of chemical sterilization processes, and drying/cooling (as required following steam sterilization). In some cases, such as certain designs of ethylene oxide and formaldehyde gas sterilizers, additional and often extended acration may be required in a separate equipment design to ensure that the load does not contain high levels of these actives or their by-products.

As a final note, consideration needs to be given to ensuring that the proper instructions and tests are provided to enable the equipment to be installed, operating and performing correctly at a healthcare facility, including requirements for routine monitoring of the process and maintenance of any associated equipment (see the section on Maintenance and quality control). There are many standards and guidelines that may need to be considered during the design, testing and routine monitoring of sterilization processes. These may be specific to the mechanism of sterilization (e.g. steam under pressure or humidified ethylene oxide) or general, in considering any newer sterilization method.

Further consideration is given here to some of the methods used for routinely monitoring sterilization processes to ensure that they have been conducted within expectation. There are four main methods used to routinely monitor sterilization processes. They include:
• Parametric release (or control). This refers to the monitoring of the important conditions (parameters) that have been specified as being required for sterilization to be achieved. Steam is a useful example, as its successful application for sterilization is dependent on reaching the correct temperature (that can only be achieved by steam under pressure; see the section on Steam (moist heat) sterilization). Therefore, the physical monitoring of the temperature and time of the process, are good indicators that the process has been correctly applied. Others may include various types of air detector systems, as effective air removal is an important consideration for steam sterilization. Steam is, however, somewhat more complicated than this (see the section on Steam (moist heat) sterilization). For a chemical sterilization process, this may include the concentration (directly or indirectly) of the sterilizing agent, humidity levels, temperature, pressure and other process variables, depending on the sterilization process. Overall, these various types of sensors can be used for monitoring the effectiveness of the process and can provide this information immediately for inspection/control. There are, however, limitations and they are often complemented by the chemical and or biological indicators discussed below.
• Biological indicators (BIs): these are defined as test systems containing viable microorganisms providing a defined resistance to a specified sterilization process. Various examples are shown in Figure 11.3(a). For sterilization processes, BIs usually contain a known population of bacterial spores (e.g. 10^5 or 10^6) placed onto a carrier material (e.g. paper or a stainless steel disc). The bacteria spore type is usually the defined most resistant organism for the process, such as *Geobacillus stearothermophilus* spores for steam sterilization and *Bacillus atropheus* spores for ethylene oxide (Table 11.2). A BI is designed to be able to show growth or no growth following incubation of the BI on exposure to a sterilization process. Growth would be a failed result and no growth a pass result. This can take time, with the incubation time ranging from one day (24 hours) to seven days before the result is known. Some BI designs (known as "rapid-read") include an indirect, chemical indicator of this final result, such as a color change (based on a change in pH in the growth media) or the presence of enzyme activity (indicated by the production of light), both suggesting that spore growth is occurring; in both cases, these early indications are considered preliminary and require verification of growth/no growth for

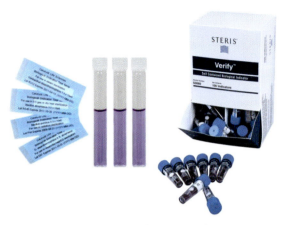

Figure 11.3 (a) Various types of biological indicators (BIs). They may be provided separately (left), where the BI is exposed to the sterilization process, placed into growth media (shown as blue media in glass vials) and then incubated at the defined temperature/time to show growth or no growth. In other more commonly used examples, known as self-contained BIs (SCBI) the indicator is contained in an all-in-one pack that is exposed to the sterilization process and mixed directly afterwards, with little handling by the operator.

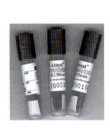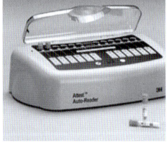

Figure 11.3 (b) An example of a widely used, self-contained and rapid read-out biological indicator (the 3M™ Attest 1292) used to monitor steam sterilization. Indicators (left) and indicator incubator (right).

the final result, and must be verified at a later stage according to manufacturer guidelines. An example of a widely used rapid-read BI is shown is Figure 11.3(b). Biological indicators may also be included in specially designed challenge packs (known as process challenge devices, see below) as a further challenge to a sterilization process. Biological indicators are discussed in further detail in the section on Monitoring sterilization in Chapter 14.

• Chemical indicators (CIs): these have already been briefly introduced in Chapter 9, in the section on disinfec-

tion guidelines and standards, and will be discussed in more detail in Chapter 14, in the section on Monitoring sterilization. They are defined as test systems (usually in the form of test strips) that reveal a change in one or more pre-defined process variables based on a chemical and/or physical change resulting from exposure to a process. They are generally provided as color-change indicators and are widely used in monitoring sterilization processes. They are classified as defined by ISO 11140 *Sterilization of healthcare products – chemical indicators* into six classes (Table 11.4). For sterilization monitoring, class 1 indicators are widely used to indicate on the outside of a pack that it has been exposed to a sterilization process; they are usually applied during packaging (Chapter 10) and provide a visual color change to differentiate sterilized from non-sterilized packs. A typical class 2 indicator is a Bowie-Dick test that is specifically used to monitor air removal from and steam penetration into a "porous load" in a vacuum-assisted steam sterilizer (see the section on steam (moist heat) sterilization); the test simulates a towel pack that can be difficult to remove air from, with a chemical indicator in the centre of the pack to detect that air removal/steam penetration has been effective. Types 3, 4, 5 and 6 indicators may also be used; they are usually placed inside packs to be sterilized and can be checked on opening just prior to use in a surgical/medical procedure. The most widely used internationally (in particular for steam sterilization) are class 5 and 6 indicators. Class 5 indicators simulate the response to a biological indicator (but without the need for incubation) and class 6 are designed to indicate that all critical parameters of the sterilization process have been met, including the full exposure time for the process. Class indicators have the advantage over BIs in that they give an immediate result, and are sometimes used in combination with BIs as dual indicators.

• Process challenge device: a process challenge device (or PCD) is designed to be able to provide a specific challenge (e.g. penetration challenge) for a sterilization process, being used as a more robust method to monitor the performance of that process. Examples are shown in Figure 11.4. They are usually combined with a CI, BI or even both as the indication system(s), but provide a defined additional challenge unique to a sterilization process.

Overall, the specific methods used to routinely monitor sterilization processes can vary significantly internationally and are based on the individual preferences/needs of a healthcare facility. Each facility should have a written policy regarding how and when these various methods and indicators are used, as well as describing the action items to be taken in the event of a fail result being detected.

Table 11.4 The classification of chemical indicators[1].

Class	Indicator type	Description
Class 1	Process indicator	These are simple indicators to demonstrate exposure to a process and also to distinguish between processed/unprocessed units. A pass result may not mean the process has been achieved.
Class 2	Indicators for use in specific tests	Used to indicate a specific type of test, generally established in another standard.
Class 3	Single variable indicators	Designed to respond to only one critical process variable (e.g. concentration of a biocide).
Class 4	Multi-variable indicators	Designed to respond to two or more of the critical variables (e.g. temperature, time and concentration of a biocide).
Class 5	Integrating indicators	Designed to respond to all critical variables of the process, in particular to be equivalent to a biological indicator (e.g. indicators containing bacterial spores used to test sterilization processes).
Class 6	Emulating indicators	Designed to react to all critical variables for a full specified cycle (that may be over and above that matching a biological indicator).

[1] Defined based on ISO 11140 *Sterilization of healthcare products – chemical indicators*.

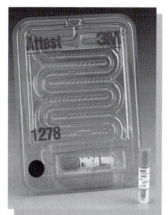
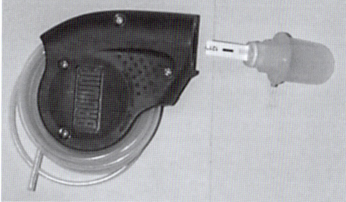
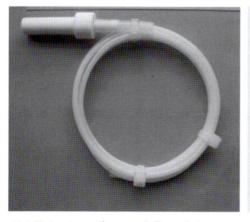
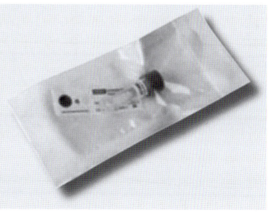

Figure 11.4 Various types of process challenge devices.

Physical sterilization

The most widely used method of sterilization in health-care facilities today is steam (or specifically steam under pressure). Other physical methods are less commonly used and are briefly considered in this section, including dry heat, radiation and filtration.

Steam (moist heat) sterilization
Principles of steam sterilization

High temperature steam (steam under pressure or commonly known as moist heat) is the most widely used and studied method of sterilization. As introduced in Chapter 6, in the section on solids, liquids, gas and plasma, water can be present as a solid (ice), liquid (water) or gas (steam) depending on the energy (e.g. temperature) provided to it. Under atmospheric pressure conditions, under which we all live, water forms steam at 100°C (212°F). We can see this by boiling water to produce steam. As a gas, steam follows the gas laws, therefore if you have a fixed amount of steam in a fixed volume (such as a sealed sterilization chamber), there is a direct relationship between the temperature and the pressure as the pressure increases the temperature of the steam increases (Figure 11.5).

Therefore, higher temperatures of steam can be achieved by increasing the pressure of the steam in a dedicated chamber (steam sterilizer or "autoclave"). This is achieved during the steam sterilization process by the introduction of steam into the chamber, but controlling the amount of steam that is released to cause an increase in pressure, and continuing to provide heat to a defined point. The point at which steam forms under controlled conditions of pressure and temperature is considered the most efficient for sterilization (referred to as being "saturated"). Typical sterilization times, pressures and temperatures are summarized in Table 11.5.

When steam at these high temperatures comes into contact with cooler surface (such as a load of devices to be sterilized) it immediately condenses (goes from being a gas to a liquid) as water on the surface. Condensation has two powerful effects:
• It releases the thermal energy of the steam with a tremendous antimicrobial effect on any microorganisms present as well as heating the surface.
• It causes an enormous reduction in the volume of steam present as it changes into water, causing further steam to be drawn towards the items being sterilized.
Under such conditions, saturated steam is extremely efficient, with an enormous heating and penetrating capacity. This direct application of energy/heat destroys microorganisms, but this destruction is hastened by the addition of moisture as steam is a much more efficient carrier of thermal energy or heat than air. Steam can have many direct effects on the structure and function of microorganisms that culminate in their death or loss of viability. One of the major mechanisms of action is the destructions of proteins, which are essential to the structure and function of microorganism; heat causes proteins to denaturize ("unfold") and coagulate. Steam will also have negative effects on all the other molecules that make up these structures, such as lipids and nucleic acids.

If the steam contains too much water, it is considered too "wet" and if it contains less water it is considered too "dry", also known as "superheated". Wet steam already has a lot of condensed water present, so will be less efficient

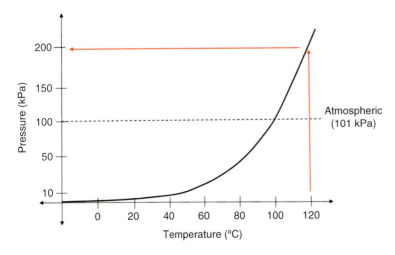

Figure 11.5 The relationship between the temperature and pressure of water according to the gas laws. The line in the graph represents the point at which steam is formed from water at a given temperature and pressure. Atmospheric pressure (101 kPa) is shown by a dashed line. As the pressure is increased the temperature at which steam is formed also increases, giving it more energy. Therefore, as an example, steam at 120°C can be made at a pressure of 200 kPa.

Table 11.5 Typical steam sterilization conditions. The related temperatures and pressures are shown, with the estimated minimum time for sterilization (providing a SAL of 10^{-6} with a population of bacterial spores at a $D_{121°C}$ of 1 and a Z-value of 10°C) and typical examples of exposure times used.

Temperature[1]		Pressure[2]			Minimum exposure time (mins)[3]	Actual exposure times used (mins)[4]
°C	°F	kPa	Bar	psi		
121	249.8	205	2.05	29.7	12	15–30
125	257	232	2.32	33.7	6	10–15
132	269.6	287	2.87	41.6	1	3–5
134	273.2	304	3.04	44.1	0.6	3–4
138	280.4	341	3.41	49.5	0.2	1–18[5]

[1] To convert from °C to°F, use the following formula:

$$°F = (1.8 \times °C) + 32$$
$$°C = (°F - 32) \times 0.5555$$

[2] 1 kPa is equivalent to 0.01 bar, 7.5 mmHg, 7.5 Torr, 0.145 psi.

[3] Estimated to provide an SAL of 10^{-6} with a population of bacterial spores at a $D_{121°C}$ of 1 and a Z-value of 10°C.

[4] Note that these exposure times generally provide a significant overkill, in excess of the minimal requirement of a SAL of 10^{-6}; they are given only as traditional times used.

[5] 134°C for 18 minutes are often used as specific steam sterilization cycles to reduce the risk of prion contamination (Chapter 15, see the section on Devices known or suspected to be contaminated with prion material).

at transferring its antimicrobial effect to a surface. Superheated steam may be formed by temperatures higher than those required to generate steam at a specified pressure, therefore it has less water available to condense and essentially acts like dry heat (which is known to be a much less efficient sterilization method). Therefore, although the concept of steam sterilization at defined temperatures and pressures is straightforward, the control of such processes is important to ensure that it is optimal for sterilization. In fact, the essential process conditions for adequate steam sterilization are:

• The absence of air (or specifically non-condensable gases that can interfere with the process). Note that air may be present in the sterilization chamber, the load to be sterilized and even in the water used to make the steam. As introduced in Chapter 6 (in the section on mixtures, formulations and solutions), air is a mixture of gases, consisting of about 78% nitrogen, 21% oxygen and a range of other gases at much lower amounts (e.g. carbon dioxide, CO_2, and water vapor). Water can also contain an amount of air and therefore types of gases, particularly carbon dioxide and oxygen, but also others such as nitrogen, hydrogen, helium, chlorine, sulfur oxide, etc. Water likes to be a liquid at room temperature and atmospheric pressure, and when in gas (steam) form it is known as a "condensable" gas, being defined as condensing to its liquid form (water) under the typical conditions of pressure/ temperature used during steam sterilization. The gases present in steam (and in the air) have different requirements and are therefore known as "non-condensable" gases under these steam sterilization conditions; they therefore remain in gas form and can impede the penetration of steam to or within the load. Therefore, it is important not only to remove air from the chamber/load but also to reduce to a minimum any non-condensable gases present in the water used to make steam for the process.

• The presence of saturated steam, as the defined temperature and pressure. Remember, saturated steam is at the midpoint between condensation and evaporation of water (Chapter 6, in the section on solids, liquids, gas and plasma).

• The attainment of the minimum specified temperature in the load for the specified sterilization time.

Steam sterilization processes are therefore designed to ensure that these conditions are met for particular types of loads. A typical steam sterilization cycle will therefore include a number of stages:

• Conditioning: air removal and pre-heating to the desired sterilization temperature. There are many different ways to remove air from the load (see the next section on types of steam sterilization processes, based on air removal), most often assisted by the use of steam itself (known as "displacement") that is used to heat the load to the desired sterilization temperature under pressure.

• Steam sterilization: the steam temperature and pressure is maintained at a "constant" level for the desired sterilization time.

• Cooling and drying (optional). Cooling is essential to ensure that the materials can be safely unloaded and transported for storage/use. Drying is also important, as if water remains in the pack it may be suspected of being compromised when opened for a patient procedure (referred to as a "wet-pack"). Excessive water present within a pack can be due to excessive wetness in the steam and the product may not have been sterilized correctly (see the section on Troubleshooting steam sterilization problems).

Steam sterilization processes are developed and tested by the manufacturer for a variety of different applications, including:

• Wrapped devices/instruments (generally referred to as non-porous cycles).

• Textile packs (known as "porous" loads). Porous refers to the ability to trap air/liquid within the structure of such materials due to their structure. Examples of porous materials include textiles, fabrics, paper and even some types of plastics. These are often some of the more difficult materials/loads to sterilize with steam.

• Lumened or hollow devices (e.g. rigid endoscopes and dental hand-pieces, sometimes these require special cycle conditions).

• Utensils and glassware.

• Mixtures of porous and non-porous loads.

• Liquids and solutions: in general, such items are infrequently sterilized in healthcare facilities, being supplied pre-sterilized by manufacturers (e.g. sterile water or saline). Note: specific cycle conditions are required to ensure the correct sterilization of such materials.

• "Flash" (or 'immediate use') sterilization, refers to the sterilization of items for immediate use with a patient (not being stored sterile). Specific flash steam sterilization cycles may be designed for certain types of loads (e.g. porous or non-porous materials) and are usually for quick treatment of materials (e.g. in the case of a dropped instrument during a surgical procedure that is required and there is not a replacement available). Items are usually unwrapped, although they may be wrapped or included in specifically designed rigid containers which have been specifically designed and tested for such a purpose. Despite being wrapped or unwrapped, flash sterilization is designed for immediate use of the device and items should not be stored prior to use, but aseptically transferred to the patient for use. Immediate use steriliza-

tion is further considered as a special consideration (see the section on Flash or immediate use sterilization).

Overall, specific cycles will be defined and tested by the manufacturer, not only to include the types of materials, but also recommended loads and loading practices. Care should be taken to ensure that the right cycles are available/selected for the various types of loads to be sterilized, as well as ensuring that the sterilizer chamber is correctly loaded so that the defined process is effective (Chapter 10, in the section on loading and unloading sterilizers).

Steam sterilization processes are performed in specific sterilizers deemed to be capable of handling the pressures and temperatures during the steam process; these are referred to as steam sterilizers, "autoclaves" or pressure vessels. They are designed in a variety of ways to provide the required steam process, including ensuring that the air can be efficiently removed from the load being sterilized. Steam sterilizers can be classified based on the methods used for air removal, such as upward displacement, downward displacement, pressure pulsing and vacuum assisted. These are discussed in further detail in the next section, on types of steam sterilization processes, based on air removal. In many cases, in particular large steam sterilizers, multiple steam sterilization processes including different methods of air removal (e.g. pre-vacuum and gravity displacement cycles) are provided in the same sterilizer design in order to accommodate the variety of different types of materials to be sterilized.

Overall, steam sterilization has many advantages, being a simple process (with two key variables: time and temperature), well described, easy to monitor, rapidly effective against all types of microorganisms (including prions, but generally recommended at longer contact times) and with a variety of sterilizers (sizes, types, etc.) available. Once installed, these sterilizers are economical, providing a low cost per cycle and relatively short sterilization times (with the longest times of a typical process taken up by conditioning and cooling/drying). Despite these advantages, steam sterilization is not appropriate for temperature or moisture-sensitive materials/devices and may not be applicable for certain types of pressure-sensitive items. Successful steam sterilization is dependent on an adequate supply of water, with water "quality" and "purity" being an important consideration to reduce any negative effects (see the section on water purity and steam quality).

Types of steam sterilization processes, based on air removal

The removal of air is important to ensure an efficient steam sterilization process. Air can prevent the penetration of steam into a load coming into contact with all surfaces. While hot air can have some antimicrobial effects, it is a much more inefficient sterilizing agent than saturated steam. Due to the physics and thermodynamics of steam, air and water mixtures, each method can be used in certain circumstances but has its own deficiencies. Further, while the general types of air removal cycles are discussed, the specific cycle conditions can vary in air removal/steam penetration efficiency and care should be taken to review all manufacturer instructions regarding their use.

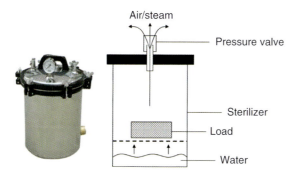

Figure 11.6 An example and the basic design of an upward displacement steam sterilizer. Water is placed at the bottom and heated, to produce steam that rises to push the air out from the top of the vessel.

Upward displacement

These are simple, yet older designs of steam sterilizers based on the concepts used in pressure cooking. They are usually smaller type sterilizers and recommended for smaller, non-porous loads. In these designs (shown in Figure 11.6), water is placed at the bottom of the sterilizer design and heated; as steam is generated it rises to push the air/steam out of the top of the chamber (therefore the air is displaced by upward displacement). Once air has been removed for the desired length of time, a pressure valve can be manually placed at the point of steam/air exit (or controlled automatically); this will allow the steam pressure to build up to the desired pressure/temperature for sterilization. Such designs are often used for simple devices, in particular for flash sterilizations, but overall have poor air removal capabilities. They are not widely used by healthcare facilities.

Downward displacement

Downward (or gravity, non-vacuum) displacement sterilizer designs and steam sterilization cycles work on the opposite principle to upward displacement but have the benefit that steam is lighter than air (Figure 11.7). During a typical cycle, the steam is introduced slowly into the top of the sterilizer and as more steam enters the chamber it will begin to push the air down (due to the weight or mass of steam present). As more steam is introduced the air is continually displaced downwards and out through the bottom of the vessel. When the air removal phase is complete and the correct steam/pressure is

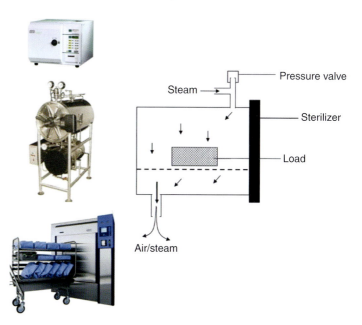

Figure 11.7 Examples and the basic design of a downward displacement steam sterilizer. The steam sterilizer shown at the bottom offers downward displacement and a vacuum assisted steam sterilization cycle option. Steam enters at the top of the vessel that falls by gravity ("gravity displacement") to force the air out from the bottom of the vessel.

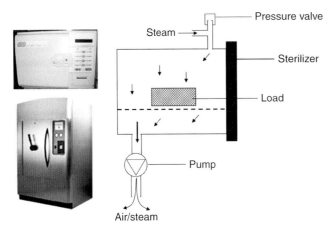

Pressure valve

Steam

Sterilizer

Load

Pump

Air/steam

Figure 11.8 Examples and the basic design of vacuum-assisted steam sterilizers. The steam sterilizer shown at the bottom offers downward displacement and vacuum assisted steam sterilization cycle options. Air is removed by pulling a vacuum (low pressure) within the chamber. Steam then enters at the top of the vessel to replace the increases to the desired pressure for sterilization.

achieved the load is held for the desired sterilization time. Downward displacement sterilizers, when designed and operated correctly, are more efficient at air removal than upward displacement designs, but are generally less efficient at air removal from porous loads and lumened devices. Note: steam sterilization processes based on gravity displacement air removal cycles can be designed for non-porous, lumened devices and porous load, depending on the manufacturer's cycle and testing conditions.

Vacuum assisted

Vacuum-assisted air removal cycle and sterilizer designs are examples of dynamic air removal processes, using a vacuum pump to extract the air prior to introduction of steam (Figure 11.8). In its simplest form, the air is forcibly removed by pulling a vacuum (a low pressure) within the vessel and then steam is introduced to replace the air. When the correct temperature and pressurized conditions are met, the steam sterilization process proceeds. Such cycles are particularly effective at removing air from porous loads (such as fabrics and towels) and lumened devices. Some types of loads/devices may be restricted from such cycles due to being pressure (vacuum) restricted by the manufacturer. Note that many sterilizer designs will be programmed with both downward displacement and vacuum-assisted types of conditioning cycles to meet the needs of the variety of load/device types that may need to be sterilized. The vacuum levels, number of vacuum pulses, etc., can vary from manufacturer to manufacturer and design to design (e.g. as shown in Figure 11.8), therefore care should be taken to closely inspect the instructions regarding the load configuration/restrictions for each type of defined cycle.

In general, the lower the pressure/vacuum the more air is removed from the load, but this may also be compensated for by various vacuum/steam-pulsing cycles. Vacuum-assisted cycles are also the basis for many different other types of dynamic air-removal cycle conditions (see the next section on variations of pressure and/or vacuum pulsing). In addition to conditioning advantages, vacuum conditions may also be useful in assisting with drying and cooling following the steam sterilization cycle.

Variations of pressure and/or vacuum pulsing

The role of steam sterilization conditioning cycles is to remove air *and* preheat the load to the desired temperature for sterilization. Over the years, many different types of efficient conditioning cycles have been described and used for these purposes, in order to minimize the overall sterilization process time, optimize air removal for various types of loads (even complex) and to reduce sterilizer costs. Examples of such steam sterilization processes are shown in Figure 11.9. They can include various pulsing conditions of high pressure and low pressure (vacuum) to various extents in order to optimize air removal. As in the other cases, care should be taken to understand any instructions, restrictions or limitations of such defined cycles in order to ensure that they are used correctly; even such efficient conditioning cycles may be compromised if not used according to manufacturers' instructions.

Steam sterilizer design

Although steam sterilizers can vary in size, shape and complexity, they can all be described as having the same essential design features. This section should not be considered as an exhaustive introduction to the various design criteria and sterilizer types that are available, but

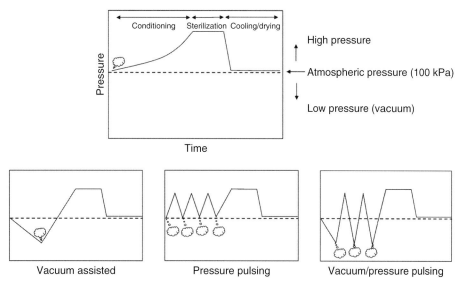

Figure 11.9 Simplified examples of different types of steam conditioning cycles, as part of the overall sterilization process. A typical steam sterilization process will include conditioning, sterilization and cooling/drying phases. The upper cycle shows these phases, in a typical gravity displacement cycle (with steam introduced at the start of the cycle); the dashed line indicates atmospheric pressure. Examples of vacuum-assisted, pressure-pulsing and vacuum-pressure pulsing cycles are shown below, with steam introduction times shown during the cycle. Note that the cycle times are not drawn to scale, but in general gravity displacement cycles are the longest, followed by vacuum-assisted cycles and then the various types of pressure/vacuum dynamic cycles. Such cycles and their efficiencies will vary from manufacturer to manufacturer.

does provide a description of some of the basic components of a steam sterilizer.

A simplified drawing of the basic design of a steam sterilizer is shown in Figure 11.10. The major components include:

• The sterilization chamber, also known as the pressure vessel. The chamber is commonly constructed of a high grade of stainless steel and needs to be designed (and verified) to meet various different safety codes as a pressure vessel (as a chamber designed to withstand high pressures). There may be one or two entry doors into the chamber, in single or double-door designs respectively. In single-door designs the load is placed into and removed from the chamber through the same door, while in double-door designs the load is placed into the chamber on one side and removed following sterilization from the other (allowing for physical separation of unsterilized and sterilized packs). In addition, the chamber may be designed with an external "jacket", that allows the walls of the sterilizer to be heated (e.g. with steam) during the process. Jacketed sterilizer designs have advantages over non-jacketed, such as improved cycle time (as the heat up time for the load and even the drying times may be quicker) and preventing excessive condensation during the cycle (which can lead to "wet" packs or loads that require extended drying in order to ensure there is no residual moisture remaining during storage/transport).

• A steam supply: steam can be injected into the chamber via an internal steam source within or close to the sterilizer (such as an integral steam generator) and/or it can be supplied separately, usually from a main facility supply. In both cases, the volume of water provided is controlled within a steam generator or boiler. With main hospital steam supplies, the steam is produced in large boilers and piped to the autoclave "plant room"; pressures in these systems can be very high (e.g. 1000 kPa), much higher than the actual pressure required by the autoclave (e.g. ~260 kPa) and is therefore reduced using a pressure reducing valve. An isolating steam valve is used to shut off the steam to the autoclaves for maintenance. In other designs, or as a back-up to facility supplier, a steam generator may be built into the design of the sterilizer or closely associated with it. In other designs, water is introduced directly into the base of the autoclave chamber and heaters are provided that heat the water until it boils and produces steam directly within the chamber. Most steam sterilizers are designed with a system that will decrease

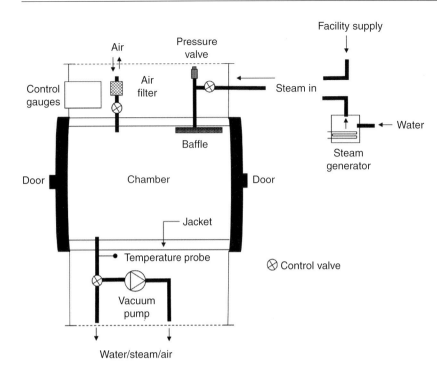

Figure 11.10 The major components of a typical, larger steam sterilizer (in this case showing a double-door, jacketed sterilizer, with a vacuum pump and optional steam generator).

the amount of condensed water present in the steam and direct only saturated steam into the chamber. An example is a baffle plate, located on the entrance of steam into the chamber. Another example is the use of a "steam separator" or "steam trap" to remove condensate from the steam pipework. Remember, increased water content in the steam means excessive water and may result in wet loads; wet packs are a sign of an inefficient sterilization process for the type of load being sterilized and increases the risk of being cross-contaminated during storage/transport (see the section on Process failures).

• Piping systems to aid in conditioning, sterilization and drying/cooling may be made from high-grade stainless steel or other metals (such as copper). These pipes transfer steam/air in and out of the chamber by a system of control (including pressure) valves, generally under an automated control system. In vacuum-assisted sterilizers this may also include a vacuum pump that assists during the conditioning and drying phases of the cycle, as well as various different temperature or other monitoring systems. Sterilizers are often designed to conserve the use of water and energy, for example by re-using water and using heat-recovery systems.

• Air venting system: this allows air to be vented into the chamber at various times during the cycle, where the air is passed through a microbial (bacteria-fungi) retentive filter.

• Control system and gauges: the control system automatically controls the pre-programmed cycle when selected by the user and may be associated with various sensors and gauges (for variables such as temperature and pressure) that aid in controlling and/or monitoring the process. In addition to controlling temperature/ pressure, safety limits are also set to avoid over-temperature or over-pressurization. An example is a "jacket over pressure switch" that is used to shut off the steam supply to the jacket should the temperature probe fail and the pressure goes too high in the jacket; if such a switch failed there is often a further safety valve that will release if the maximum safe working pressure is exceeded. In such extreme cases, where a sterilizer safety valve blows, the machine must be turned off and the steam supply isolating valve shut off immediately. Steam sterilizers are often provided with a printer, to provide a simple or detailed description of the cycle and associated conditions; this may be part of the sterilizer design or connected separately to a computer/recording system. In some designs an independent monitoring system may be provided, which independently monitors the various different cycle parameters (e.g. temperature, time, pressures) in parallel with the control system to ensure that the process is performing within specified limits.

Maintenance and quality control

Regular maintenance and quality control testing is essential to ensure that the sterilizer is functioning adequately. This can include daily, weekly, monthly, quarterly and annual tests, and should be carried out according to department policy and the manufacturer's guidelines.

Maintenance refers to the routine care of equipment in order to reduce malfunction of critical components that could cause sterilization failure and downtime. Manufacturers should provide clear written care and maintenance schedules and instructions which must be adhered to by the user, as only a properly maintained sterilizer will consistently provide sterile packs. Maintenance may be routine or preventive, being performed by in-house or outsourced staff. Maintenance instructions are usually recommended by the manufacturer in their instruction manual, but as examples they should include:

• Wiping and checking the door sealing gasket (seal)
• Removing debris or foreign bodies from the chamber, trays/rack and drains as these may block filters or damage sterilizer parts (e.g. vacuum pump and door gasket)
• Regularly inspecting, cleaning and/or replacing filters, such as water, air and drain filters
• Regularly confirming the calibration of the sterilizer sensors (e.g. temperature and pressure sensors)
• Checking and, if applicable, replacing pressure relief valves
• Performing vacuum leak tests and steam penetration tests (such as, Bowie-Dick or Helix tests).

Regularly scheduled preventive maintenance is required for safe and reliable operation of steam sterilizers. When doing maintenance appropriate safety procedures must be followed at all times. Before commencing maintenance work always follow lockout/tagout and electrical safe work practice standards, by disconnecting all utilities to the sterilizer before commencing work. Any recommended, routine cleaning should only be performed by trained staff and maintenance, repairs and adjustments should only be performed by fully qualified service personnel. It is important that the sterilizer chamber and accessories are allowed to cool to room temperature before performing any cleaning or maintenance procedures. Maintenance and cleaning performed by inexperienced or unqualified staff could result in personal injury or costly equipment damage.

A standard cleaning procedure for the steam sterilizer chamber should be in place in the decontamination facility. Remember to make sure that the chamber is not hot before cleaning. Not only is it easier to remove stains when the machine is cold, but it also ensures that accidental burns do not occur. Manufacturers' recommendations should be followed when choosing any types of cleaning detergents, brushes and equipment. The frequency of cleaning can vary depending on the use and water purity used in the sterilizer. This can range from daily, weekly, monthly and even yearly. The inside of the chamber should be cleaned with a mild detergent-containing cleaning solution, using equipment (e.g. a mop or brush) that is kept especially for the purpose. Strong abrasives or steel wool should never be used on the chamber walls as they may scratch the surface and allow corrosion (rusting) to develop. It is recommended to wipe the door gasket clean daily with a lint-free cloth. While doing so, it is important to check for any defects or signs of wear and tear, especially if the sterilizer utilizes vacuum as part of its sterilization cycles. Any associated carts and loading baskets should also be frequently washed with a mild detergent and any castors and rollers cleaned, checked and lubricated when necessary. The drain strainer at the bottom of the chamber should be removed daily and cleaned thoroughly; this may be done by cleaning under running water using a brush and mild detergent. If debris has been allowed to build up, it may be necessary to soak the strainer (e.g. in an acid cleaner) before further cleaning.

The sterilizer should also undergo periodic maintenance inspections, as recommended by the manufacturer, where the correct functioning of all valves is checked, filters are replaced and the temperature/pressure sensors are calibrated. This should be conducted by trained service engineers (from the healthcare facility, the manufacturer or an applicable third party). It is also recommended that in order to trace any vacuum leaks, the sterilizer has a maintenance plan and is checked to make sure that it is leak-proof. This is typically done using a pre-programmed sterilizer vacuum leak test.

Whereas maintenance deals with routine cleaning and care of equipment in order to reduce malfunction of critical parts, quality control deals with process monitoring (Chapter 14, see the section on Monitoring sterilization and as introduced in section on the basic principles of sterilization, at the beginning of this chapter). The sterilization process is monitored through a combination of parametric, chemical and biological indication methods that are intended to evaluate the sterilizing conditions and the process effectiveness. Steam sterilization generally relies on the integration of parametric, biological and chemical indicators for process monitoring. These include:

• Parametric monitoring of the cycle time (including the sterilization exposure phase), temperature and pressure during the process. These conditions must be monitored as part of the process and, if included, independently monitored by a parallel set of sensor/gauges. In some cases of independent monitoring the sterilizer control system will compare these sensor readings to ensure an effective process (e.g. if two temperature sensors give significantly different results, one or both sensor will require re-calibration); in other cases the data is collected but needs to be manually inspected for accuracy. Other parametric monitors may also be included in the steam sterilizer design, such as a mechanical air detector.

• Biological indicators (BIs), using the most resistant microorganism for steam (i.e. a known population of bacterial spores of *Geobacillus stearothermophilus*). Biological indicators are often used for individual load monitoring as well as for routine (e.g. weekly) monitoring. They can include traditional growth-no growth indicators or, more oftenly used, rapid read-out indicators (see the section on the basic principles of sterilization, at the beginning of this chapter). Biological indicators are more widely used in some geographic locations than others depending on local or regional guidelines.

• Chemical indicators are also widely used for monitoring steam sterilization processes, both internal and external to individual packs. These can range in classification from class 1 (e.g. autoclave tape) to class 5 or 6 (see the section on the basic principles of sterilization, at the beginning of this chapter, and Table 11.5). In some cases class 5 or particularly class 6 indicators are used as replacements for BIs.

• Process challenge devices (PCD) are used in steam sterilization to test for steam penetration and air removal capability in a steam sterilizer. Air removal and steam penetration tests are recommended to be conducted daily within the steam sterilizer. Chemical indicator test systems are available for this purpose. The most common example is the Bowie Dick (B-D) test, which is classified as a class 2 chemical indicator (Figure 11.11). This test simulates a load containing porous materials, consisting of a pile of cotton towel within the middle of which is a chemical indicator. These tests are designed to meet rigorous test conditions (e.g. based on ISO 11140-3 *Sterilization of health care products – chemical indicators – Part 3: Class 2 indicator systems for use in the Bowie-Dick type steam penetration test* and ISO 11140-5 *Sterilization of healthcare products – Chemical indicators – Part 5: Class 2 indicators for Bowie-Dick type air removal tests*). A specific cycle is programmed into the steam sterilizer to be able to conduct such a test under defined process conditions. A positive (pass) result of a Bowie-Dick test will indicate that air has been removed and full steam penetration has taken place in the test package. Failure of the test will result in the presence of air in the test package, which can be caused by poor air removal, a leakage of air during a vacuum phase or the presence of excessive air in the steam. Another example is the hollow-load ("helix") test that is used to check the air removal/steam penetration of a lumens device.

Special considerations in steam sterilization
Flash or immediate use sterilization
Immediate use (commonly known as "flash") sterilization may be defined as a process designed for the steam sterilization of patient care items for immediate use. A typical

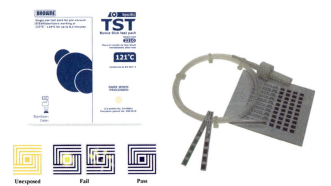

Figure 11.11 Example of air removal tests for dynamic (including vacuum-assisted) air removal steam sterilizers, including a Bowie-Dick test (left) and a hollow load (lumen penetration) test (right) with their associated chemical indicators. The Bowie-Dick test example shows examples of various fail and pass results following exposure to a steam sterilization test cycle.

example of the traditional use of flash sterilization is when an essential instrument has been dropped onto the floor during a surgical procedure, a rapid sterilization process is used to re-sterilize the device quickly before its continued use on the patient. It is common for the device to be unwrapped but this will depend on the manufacturer's instructions (which may include the use of sterilization wraps or rigid containers). Similar to any sterilization process, safe and effective immediate-use sterilization requires that all reprocessing steps have been correctly adhered to, before each cycle, during sterilization and maintained up until the point of use. Shortcuts should not be taken, as improperly sterilized (i.e. contaminated instruments) can result in serious consequences such as surgical site infections (SSIs). Each flash sterilization cycle should be routinely monitored according to a written facility policy; physical monitors, as well as chemical and biological indicators should be considered to verify that the required parameters for effective sterilization have been met. Flash sterilization of certain devices (such as implantable devices) is generally not recommended.

Good practice when using flash sterilization should include an effective cleaning process before terminal sterilization. Inadequate cleaning and lack of correct documentation regarding the process can result in increased risks of human error. The sterilizer must be maintained as per standard hospital policy and all routine sterilizer monitoring must be recorded. Typical steam sterilization times range from three to ten minutes, depending on the type of device being sterilized and the type of flash sterilizer (i.e. pre-vacuum or gravity-displacement). The manufacturer's instructions for use should be reviewed and followed at all times. It is important that staff using flash sterilization are trained in how to operate the equipment, in order to decrease the possibility of operator error during the process. Following flash-sterilization, items should be transported to the point of use in a manner that minimizes the potential for contamination; ideally the sterilizers to be used for flash sterilization should be located in the surgical suite or treatment site. Staff must wear PPE such as heat-protective gloves when handling items as the tray and the items within it will be hot. Flash-sterilized items cannot be stored, they must be used immediately. If the flash sterilizer allows the item to be wrapped with a single wrapper or other packaging, these packs must be clearly marked as being flash sterilized in order to differentiate between the flash and conventionally processed trays and sealed devices. As most immediate-used sterilization cycles will only have a very brief drying time, the device and/or any associated packaging material should be considered as being wet.

Staff should be trained on any facility policies and procedures for immediate-use sterilization based on relevant regulations, standards, and recommended practices. It is recommended that flash sterilization is only performed once all of the following conditions have been met:
• Work practices should ensure proper cleaning, inspection, and arrangement of instruments before sterilization.
• The physical layout of the department or work area ensures direct delivery of sterilized items to the point of use (e.g. the sterilizer opens into an area either within or directly adjacent to the procedure room).
• Procedures are developed, followed and audited to ensure aseptic handling and personnel safety during transfer of the sterilized items from the sterilizer to the point of use.
• Items are needed for use immediately following flash sterilization.
In most sterilizers the immediate use or flash cycle is pre-programmed to a specific time and temperature setting established by the sterilizer manufacturer. It is critical that staff check the device manufacturer guidelines to check if the device is compatible with the cycle, as the specific cycle will vary depending on the type, age and model of the sterilizer (including method of air removal). Selecting the correct cycle parameters for the devices to be sterilized is critical, if sterility is to be achieved and to prevent damage to the device. It is also important to follow the manufacturer's instructions regarding the types of devices that are suitable for a particular flash sterilizer, as in some cases instruments with lumens, power equipment and porous items cannot be processed by this method (due to potential difficulties with air removal and steam penetration); in some cases manufacturers explicitly recommend that flash sterilization is not used.

Extended steam sterilization cycles

An "extended" sterilization cycle is a cycle that is considerably longer than expected from the sterilizer manufacturer's standard cycle time. Typically steam sterilization cycles with exposure times greater than four minutes in a 134°C/274°F dynamic-air removal sterilization cycle (or indeed any typical steam sterilization cycle, see Principles of steam sterilization) are commonly referred to as extended cycles. Extended steam sterilization cycles are typically recommended in two cases:
• As defined by the device manufacturer to sterilize complex devices and their containers. Most device

manufacturers recommend standard sterilization cycle times (e.g. four minutes at 132–135°C (270–275°F) in a dynamic-air-removal sterilizer). Extended exposure times are most frequently encountered with larger orthopedic and neurological instrument sets that are considered a more significant challenge to air removal and steam penetration. Such loads are often heavier or denser, and may incorporate complex and/or difficult-to sterilize designs, such as lumened devices.

• For the inactivation of prions, when re-usable devices are known to be used in high-risk surgical procedures on patients with known or suspected prion diseases (such as CJD, Chapter 15, see the section on Devices known or suspected to be contaminated with prion material). As an example, neurological devices are often considered high risk of contamination when used on such patients. Typical recommended prion sterilization cycles include a pre-vacuum cycle at 134°C/274°F for 18 minutes and a gravity displacement cycle at 121°C/250°F for one hour. Prion sterilization with steam is considered in further detail in the following section.

The extension of sterilization times should be followed if recommended by the device manufacturer, but can create some concerns within a facility. Specific extended cycles will need to be programmed into the sterilizer and staff trained on when they are to be used. It is critical to check with the device and packaging manufacturer, before using an extended cycle, to ensure it is safe and will not have a negative effect on the product. Most stainless steel instruments may routinely undergo such extended steam sterilization times without affecting their functionality, but this may not be the case for all devices. For example, textile products, devices containing lenses and delicate instrumentation can become damaged (warped or brittle) during such cycles; further, the extended conditions of pressure and temperature can lead to premature aging of the device. Extended pressure/temperature conditions may even compromise packaging materials (if not tested for such purposes). For example, it is possible that extended exposure of packaging materials (peel pouches, wrap, etc.) to steam may break down the barrier properties of these materials, therefore this should be confirmed (in writing) with the supplier/manufacturer.

Various types of chemical indicators (CIs) and biological indicators (BIs) used to monitor defined steam sterilization processes may not be validated to be exposed in such cycles. It is important to note that such indicators should only be used under their label claims, to include their use and validation in specific steam sterilization cycles. This should be confirmed with the CI/BI suppliers.

Historically, existing CI and BI challenge packs and indicators have been designed for and labelled for use in shorter steam cycles (e.g. three or four minute pre-vacuum cycles at 132°C–135°C) and should not be used to monitor cycles that are longer. As examples:

• Chemical indicators designed to indicate shorter steam sterilization cycle times will give no assurance that longer cycle times have been achieved.

• The growth media or growth indication methods used in BIs are also designed for shorter exposure times, and may become damaged on extended exposure conditions that would fail to allow the test spores (if they survived) to grow or to identify growth.

As a final consideration, extending the steam exposure time for sterilization is more than often indicative for the need to optimize the conditioning phase of the steam sterilization cycle (see the principles of steam sterilization). Pre-conditioning should be designed to ensure that air removal and steam penetration is adequate prior to the sterilization holding phase (at the sterilization temperature and pressure). Therefore, modification of the steam sterilization cycle (conditioning phase) or the device set (into sub-sets) may be necessary to ensure adequate conditioning and sterilization in typical steam cycles.

Prion sterilization

Prions are unusual infectious agents and are considered to be highly resistant to even steam sterilization (Chapter 5, see the section on Prions and other infectious proteins). A more detailed discussion of prion decontamination of devices (including the use of sterilization techniques) is given in Chapter 15 see the section on Devices known or suspected to be contaminated with prion material. Initial laboratory investigations to study the inactivation of prions showed that longer steam sterilization cycles should be considered, to include:

• Pre-vacuum cycle at 134°C/274°F for 18 minutes

• Gravity displacement cycle at 121°C/250°F for one hour

Such extended cycles have been recommended by the World Health Organization (WHO, 2000[1]), due to the high level of resistance of prions to physical and chemical inactivation. These steam cycles (in particular 134°C/274°F for 18 minutes) have become widely recommended and used in healthcare facilities as a

---

[1] WHO infection control guidelines for transmissible spongiform encephalopathies (2000). Report of a WHO consultation, Geneva, Switzerland, 23–26 March 1999. WHO/CDS/CSR/APH/2000/3. http://www.who.int/csr/resources/publications/bse/WHO_CDS_CSR_APH_2000_3/en/

precaution against prion contamination. These are considered as extended steam sterilization cycles (see the previous section). Extended pressure/temperature conditions may not be recommended by the device manufacture (due to risks of damage) and any packaging materials may become compromised (unless specifically labelled for such use); further, only CIs and BIs should be used to monitor such processes if they have been validated and are labelled for those uses. These are important to confirm prior to considering the use of any, including prion-specific, extended steam sterilization conditions.

Other recommendations (including the WHO 2000 guidelines) have included the immersion of suspected or known prion-contaminated devices into strong chemical solutions (such as 1 N NaOH, a strong alkaline chemical) and then exposing them (in the chemical) to a steam sterilization process. Although this may be considered an effective process, this treatment is not recommended by device or steam sterilizer manufacturers due to the risks of damage and may void any manufacturer's warranty.

The initial laboratory experiments conducted to study the resistance of prions to steam sterilization did not consider the cycle of device decontamination used in healthcare facilities such as cleaning followed by sterilization. For example, many of the experiments did not test surfaces contaminated with prions or the effects of cleaning prior to steam sterilization. In recent years, these aspects have been considered in more detail with the following conclusions to date:

• Steam sterilization is an effective process to reduce the risks of prion contamination. In the absence of cleaning, standard steam sterilization cycles (such as 134°C for four minutes) can significantly reduce this risk and this is improved by extending the exposure conditions (such as 134°C for 18 minutes).
• If contaminated devices are required to be pre-treated by a steam sterilization process prior to routine cleaning, disinfection and sterilization, this should be performed under conditions where the devices are placed into water and then steam sterilized. Maintaining "wet" conditions is considered more effective than direct exposure to a normal steam sterilization process.
• Cleaning of contaminated surfaces can also reduce the risk (Chapter 15, Devices known or suspected to be contaminated with prion material), in particular when followed by steam sterilization. A note of caution is given, in that the choice of cleaning chemistry and cleaning process used is important. Specific types of cleaning chemistries and their effects on prion inactivation/surface removal are considered in Chapter 15. In some

cases, normal cleaning processes with some cleaning chemistry formulations followed by standard steam sterilization cycles (134°C for four minutes) were effective, but with other cleaning formulations it was not. There is some evidence that some cleaning chemistries can have a negative effect, reducing the ability of steam sterilization to be effective. Therefore, the cleaning chemistry should be considered in addition to the steam sterilization process. It is recommended that such decontamination processes are tested and supported in writing by the manufacturer in developing and using any facility policy for reducing the risks associated with prion contamination.

Local guidelines and standards can vary significantly from country to country, and can periodically change. It is also true that local prion decontamination recommendations may not be recommended by the device or steam sterilizer manufacturer for various safety reasons. Therefore, a facility policy (to include requirements for steam sterilization) should be developed and maintained with current data to ensure the correct handling of any known or considered high risk prion-contaminated devices (Chapter 15).

Water purity and steam quality

Water is the basis for steam and any steam sterilization process. Chemically it is a simple molecule (H_2O), but the chemistry of water and, when heated to produce its gas form (steam), can be complicated (Chapter 6, see the sections solids, liquids, gases and plasma and on mixtures, formulations and solutions). Water is rarely pure, but is actually found to have a range of different chemical, microbial and other contaminants. These include various types of dissolved materials (such as calcium, chlorine, iron, etc.) and gases (e.g. oxygen and carbon dioxide), as well as suspended materials (such as microorganisms and larger particles; Chapter 6, Table 6.3). In considering steam sterilization, two terms are frequently used in relation to water/steam:

• Water/steam purity: "purity" refers to the chemical (and microbiological) contaminants that may be present in water or steam. It is important to note that any chemical contaminants present in the water can carry over in the steam produced from that water. Depending on the chemical, this can lead to device damage as well as potential toxic effects in patients (following condensation onto a device during the steam sterilization cycle). Further, although most microorganisms in a water source will be inactivated when converted into steam (depending on the temperature and time), parts of the microorganism can remain intact and biologically active (such as endotoxins, Chapter 5, see the section on bacteria). Such toxins can also be carried over in the steam and can cause adverse patient reactions if they are deposited onto a device (during condensation).

• Steam quality: "quality" refers to the physical properties of steam to particularly include its saturation, non-condensable gases and dryness. These properties are indicative of the ability of steam to perform optimally in a steam sterilization process (i.e. provided as saturated steam and to ensure that air/non-condensable gases do not impede the penetration of steam to all surfaces of the device/load).

Water and steam purity is an important variable to understand and control (for more detailed discussion on water purity, see Chapter 15). For steam sterilization, good quality potable (drinking) water may be used to generate steam, but it is highly recommended to confirm the following purity guidelines:

• "Hardness" levels of <20 mg/L (this is typical of softened water): water hardness is defined as the concentration of calcium and magnesium in water. It is typically given as milligrams per litre (mg/L) or parts per million (ppm) of calcium carbonate ($CaCO_3$) in the water. "Hard" typically refers to water containing high levels of hardness, in excess of 120 ppm and "soft" water is considered less than 60 ppm $CaCO_3$. Therefore, softened water (preferably <20 mg/L) should be considered for steam generation. Softened water can be generated by passing the water through a water softener (Chapter 15, see the section on water quality). The levels of hardness can range considerably depending on where you live and even the time of the year. Hardness cannot be seen by the eye as the chemicals are dissolved in the water, but when the water is heated it causes the deposition of often visible water-insoluble precipitates (known as limescale, a white grainy substance consisting of chemicals such as calcium carbonate). Water hardness can cause problems by precipitating on device surfaces (known as spotting or as a fine white or otherwise colored precipitate) or building up as scale within boilers, steam generators and pipework (Figure 11.12). Over time it can cause steam generation and handling systems to fail.

• Conductivity <40 μS/cm: conductivity is an overall measurement of chemicals (particularly dissolved) in the water and is a simple method of determining the purity of the water. In this case, high levels of chemicals such as chlorides or silicates in the water can lead to device damage (e.g. rusting, seen as a brown deposit; Figure 11.13).

Consider, for example, that when chlorine is present in water and is heated it forms chlorine gas, which is very damaging to stainless steel surfaces (of the steam sterilizer and of many re-usable devices). As an estimate, a conductivity level below 40 μS/cm is equivalent to a chloride level of below 10 mg/L. If it is suspected that specific chemicals may contaminate the water source, other tests for individual compounds may be carried out (e.g. silicates, iron, copper, phosphates, etc.) using other chemical analysis methods (such as ICP-OES analysis). A similar measure to conductivity is known as total dissolved solids (TDS), which is also a measure of dissolved chemicals in the water (and should be less than 50 mg/L).

• pH is recommended to be in the range of 6–9. If the water is too acidic (<pH 6) or too alkaline (>pH 9) this can lead to damage to devices/materials, but is also not considered potable.

• Total organic carbon (TOC) <50 mg/L: total organic carbon is a measure of any organic (carbon-containing) materials in the water, including microorganisms. It is an overall indicator of water quality. One particular organic concern with steam is endotoxin, a particular type of toxin found associated with Gram negative bacteria (chapter 5, see the section on bacteria). Endotoxins can be carried in steam and if deposited at high concentrations onto a device may lead to a toxic reaction when used in a patient. Endotoxin levels are generally recommended to be <20 EU/mL (endotoxin units) and may be separately tested for.

If these specified water purity levels are higher, this may affect the safety of steam sterilization and particularly lead to device damage/build up of residues. In many cases, the water quality may need to be improved by either using specific methods to remove specific contaminants (e.g. carbon filtration for chlorine and water softener for hardness) or by providing pure water quality (by reverse osmosis (RO), deionization or distillation; Chapter 15, see the section on water quality). Reverse osmosis is generally the most practical method, but requires strict control to ensure the process is operating correctly. If the method for pure water production is correctly operating and maintained the typical levels of acceptable contaminants in steam will be:

• pH 5–7
• Conductivity ≤5 μS/cm
• Hardness ≤1 mg/L
• Total organic carbon (TOC) ≤0.5 mg/L
• Total dissolved solids (TDS) ≤0.5 mg/L

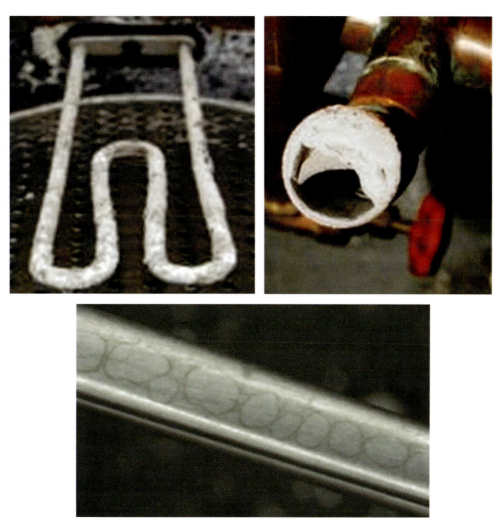

Figure 11.12 Examples of water hardness deposits associated with steam, with white scaling seen on a heating element (top left) and in a supply pipe (top right). Water hardness associated "spotting" observed on a device surface.

- Chloride ≤2 mg/L
- Silicates ≤1 mg/L
- Phosphates ≤ 0.5 mg/L
- Bacteria ≤10 cfu/mL
- Endotoxin ≤10 EU/mL

Testing of water purity can be conducted directly from the water used to produce steam (e.g. within or being fed to a facility or plant room boiler or integral steam generator) or more specifically by the collection of water from the steam being provided to the steam sterilizer (e.g. using a condenser system that rapidly cools the steam by passing it along a cold water treated surface, causing the steam to condense into water, which is then collected for analysis). The second method is optimal, as it reflects the final steam being provided for sterilization (including any potential boiler/generator feed-water, boiler treatment and supply pipework contaminants/chemicals that may be present).

A separate issue is steam quality, referring to the physical properties of steam (see the section on principles of steam sterilization earlier in this chapter). These ensure that saturated steam is provided and that air/non-condensable gases are sufficiently removed to ensure they do not impede the penetration of steam to

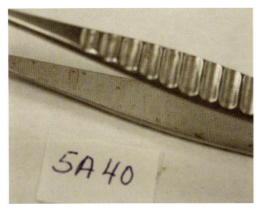

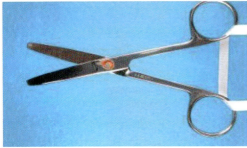

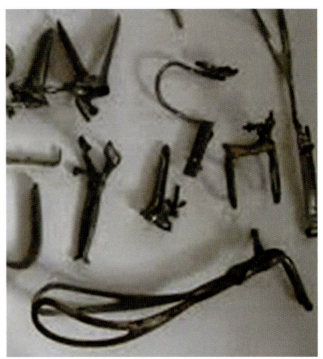

Figure 11.13 An example of minor (left) and excessive (right) rusting observed due to high levels of chlorine in steam.

all surfaces of the device/load. Three typical measurements of steam quality are:

• Non-condensable gases (NCGs): high levels of NCGs can prevent the penetration of steam to all areas of the load, similar to the presence of air. These gases are present in water and therefore their main source is water being used to generate steam, but they may also be present due to the design of the steam generation/supply system. Non-condensable gases are removed by degassing the water (by preheating the water to temperatures at or above 80°C, such as by boiling, which drive off the gases). A typical recommendation for the level of NCGs is ≤3.5% in water. This is determined using an NCG test, that determines the volume (in mL) of gas collected from a volume of water/condensed steam (expressed as a %, where 2.5% refers to 2.5 mL of NCGs in 100 mL of water).

• Saturated steam is the point at which steam forms or condenses under controlled conditions of pressure and temperature, and is considered the most efficient for sterilization (see the section on principles of steam sterilization earlier in this chapter). At a given pressure/temperature, if too little moisture is present the steam is "superheated" and is less efficient for steam sterilization (acting more like a dry heat process; see the section on

dry heat sterilization). Equally, when excessive moisture is present the steam is considered "wet" (or oversaturated) and can also lead to problems such as wet loads (requiring extended drying post-sterilization). The two tests that can be used to check that saturated steam is present are:

○ Dryness test/fraction: this tests for the amount of moisture present in steam and is typically expressed as a dryness factor. Typical recommended dryness factors range 0.90–0.99 (therefore 90–99% steam and 10–1% water); a dryness factor for healthcare (including metal) loads is often given as ≥0.95.

○ Superheat test: a temperature-based test, where when steam is taken from its line pressure and suddenly applied to atmospheric pressure the observed temperature should not exceed 25°C (≤25°C) of the normal boiling temperature at atmospheric pressure (generally 100°C and therefore should not exceed 125°C) when measured with a specific superheat test apparatus (Figure 11.14).

Examples of apparatus used for the testing of steam quality are shown in Figure 11.14. Further consideration is given to water used during the decontamination cycle, including for sterilization, in Chapter 15, see the section on water quality.

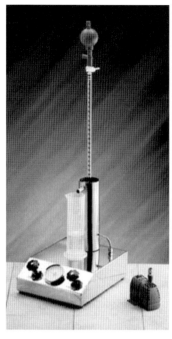
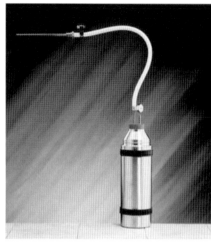
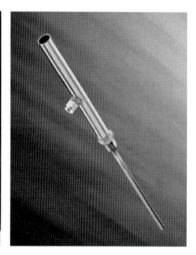

Figure 11.14 Examples of test apparatus used for testing non-condensable gases (left), dryness value/fraction (middle) and superheat (right).

Troubleshooting steam sterilization problems
Process failures

There are many different causes of steam sterilization process failures, from procedural errors that are easily remedied (like overloading) to mechanical problems that can take a sterilizer out of service. A sterilization process failure may be detected by any of the process monitoring tools used in or with the sterilizer as part of any quality control program, that is, physical, mechanical, chemical and biological. These can range from an event within a single pack (in-pack chemical indicator) or load (integrator challenge pack) or a complete sterilizer (Bowie-Dick test, biological indicator (BI) test or any of the types of parametric monitoring mechanisms within the sterilizer). Many of these are first-line (often immediate) monitoring tools that assist in detecting that the sterilization process may not have occurred correctly. Steam sterilization failures are most commonly due to human error, such as incorrect packaging material or techniques being used, improper loading and incorrect cycle selection for the load contents, resulting in an inadequate cycle temperature, inadequate time at that temperature and incomplete air removal.

In the event of a failed process indicator(s) the first step should be to quarantine the load (avoiding its accidental use in a patient procedure) and prevent the sterilizer from being used until the extent of the failure is known. It is important that a suspected faulty sterilizer should not be made operational without identifying and correcting any underlying problem. A well-planned, systematic and written procedure should be in place at a facility to address any of these potential situations, since they can occur at any time. An investigation will need to take place to clarify the failure and the sterilizer needs to be taken out of service while the investigation is taking place. This investigation is critical in assisting the supervisor in deciding whether to recall just the one load or potentially an entire day's work. The decision will be based on all the available evidence used for monitoring the effectiveness of the sterilization cycle (i.e. physical monitors, CIs and BIs). All process monitors used in parametric and routine monitoring of the sterilizer should be reviewed to assist in solving the problem.

A logical first step is to ensure that the pack/load actually passed through a sterilization cycle and that the cycle was actually initiated by the operator by comparing the cycle sequence from the print-out tape or graph recorder against

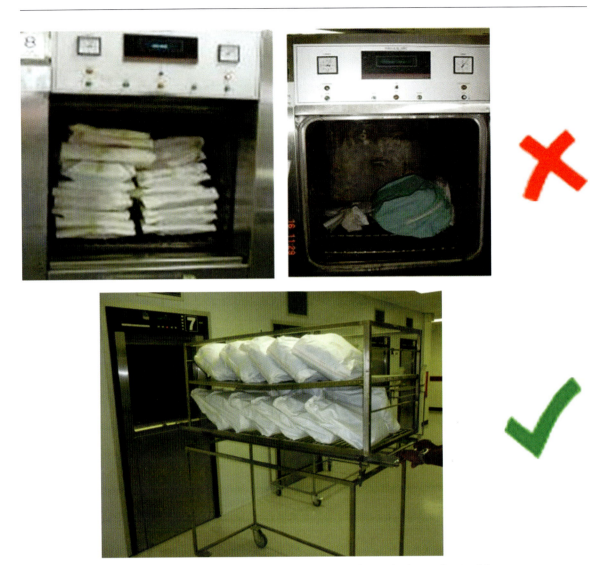

Figure 11.15 Incorrect loading of steam sterilizers. Examples of poor loading that can lead to sterilization failures.

the number of loads documented in a sterilization load log. Inspect what packaging material/wrap and indicator(s) were used to ensure that the correct steam sterilizations materials/indicators were used. It is also possible that there may have been an operator error in loading or packaging that may have resulted in sterilization failures in only one, or some of the items in the load (Figure 11.15). Always follow manufacturers' recommendations when loading the sterilizer. The basic rule to consider when loading the sterilizer chamber is that all items need to be properly prepared and arranged in a way that will present the least possible resistance to the extraction of air and the passage

of the steam throughout the load (Chapter 10, see the section on loading and unloading sterilizers). Steam sterilizers should never be overloaded (Figure 11.15). Packages should not touch the top, bottom or sides of the sterilizer as this may result in sterilization failure and "wet packs" in the case of steam sterilization (see below and Table 11.6).

A single non-responsive or inconclusive CI should not be considered definitive proof that the entire load is non-sterile. If, however, the sterilization failure is due to a procedural/human error, all affected devices will need to be reprocessed. A large percentage of sterilization failures are due to human error. Although there are many ways in which

Table 11.6 Common steam sterilization problems, causes and solutions.

Problem	Cause	Solution
Failed chemical or biological indicators	Inadequate sterilization. The fault may be with the sterilizer (mechanical or electrical), steam supply (superheat or wet) and/or load being sterilized. Always confirm that the correct indicator has been used (and used correctly) for monitoring the steam sterilization cycle in use.	Confirm the sterilizer is operating correctly. A common cause is the way the sterilizer chamber has been loaded. It is essential that packs are not too dense and are loosely loaded into the sterilizer to ensure that air is not trapped and can easily circulate.
Failed Bowie-Dick test	Incomplete air removal. Trapped air may be due to human error, mechanical failures and/or water quality. Typical causes include: • Faulty door seals/gaskets • Problems with the vacuum pump • Incorrect loading • Incorrect packaging • Incorrect cycle parameters for the load • Clogged drain • Low steam pressure or high water pressure • High levels of dissolved gases (non-condensed) in the feed-water/steam	A routine maintenance schedule should be followed to ensure the sterilizer is operating correctly, to ensure daily inspections by staff (e.g. ensuring the sterilizer chamber drain is not blocked) and maintenance of the sterilizer/utilities (such as routine maintenance of the vacuum pump and any steam/water pre-treatment).
Wet packs, where a pack/load contains an appreciable amount of moisture after a sterilization cycle	Intermittent operation (chamber cold) or jacket heating not working (e.g. steam supply line malfunctioning). Steam supply is wet. Sterilizer installation, including improper insulation of steam pipes or excess water in steam (wet steam). Insufficient drying time. Improper loading or cycle for the load. Large overweight packs/sets (in particular metals). Overloading may not only cause improper sterilization (insufficient air removal/steam contact) but may promote excessive condensation. Clogged or malfunctioning drain or steam supply systems.	Pre-warm the sterilizer before using and check steam supply valves/traps (chamber and jacket). Confirm steam supply; test steam quality (see the section on water purity and steam quality). Check that steam pipes are insulated. Review with manufacturer or consider using a drying cabinet. Review procedures and train staff on how to pack, load correctly, pack size, pack weight or pack density and proper wrapping technique. Review sterilizer manufacturer's recommendations on proper loading. Clean debris from the chamber drain daily. Ensure any associated valves/traps controlling incoming or draining steam are functioning. A preventive maintenance schedule should be established to ensure these are functional.
Material damage (e.g. rubber deterioration or textile/paper/packaging material scorching) or steam pressure is too low for the desired steam temperature	Superheated (unsaturated or super-dry) steam. This is steam at a very high temperature for its saturation pressure (see the section on Water purity and steam quality). Superheated steam can act as hot air, which is less efficient as a sterilization medium.	Test for superheated steam (see the section on water purity and steam quality). Confirm that the steam supply is correct (e.g. steam pressure, not only to the chamber but also to the jacket) and associated supply/drain valves are functioning correctly. Check calibration of pressure/temperature sensors.

(continued)

Table 11.6 (*cont'd*).

Problem	Cause	Solution
Variations in pressure	Persistent or dangerously high pressure is rare and controlled by safety valves. High pressure usually indicates a blockage (e.g. in the drain line) or a malfunctioning valves (in the steam supply or drain valves). Low pressure can be attributed to many causes, such as inadequate steam supply (e.g. boiler heater is broken or there is a clogged water/steam line/filters), leaks (chamber or associated pipework), out of calibration pressure/temperature gauges, broken/malfunctioning valves, and the presence of non-condensable gases.	Safety valve – sterilizers have a safety valve to prevent over-pressurization; this valve can get stuck open and leak. Other supply and drain valves should be checked to ensure they are functioning correctly. By observing the sterilizer as it pressurizes, steam may be detected as escaping from a particular location (e.g. around the door gasket). Particularly check the door gasket for signs of wear, cracks, chips, etc. Ensure that the sterilizer is correctly maintained/serviced according to the manufacturer's guidelines. Check steam quality.
Instrument staining	Improper instrument cleaning procedures, including incomplete removal of soil, inadequate rinsing or rinsing with water of high mineral content. Inadequate cleaning/rinsing can be detected prior to sterilization, but not always (e.g. change of color observed after steam treatment or when surfaces are dry). Poor steam purity, where any chemicals present the steam will react with or precipitate out on surfaces. Sometimes the color or types of instrument staining may help in understanding the cause (Table 11.7).	Standardized cleaning procedures and post-cleaning inspections should be established (Chapter 8). Check for any deviations. Check the water quality used in the generation of steam (including the dosing of any chemicals used in the boiler). Remember the water purity can vary seasonally and often from day to day.
Excessive rusting of stainless steel devices	Damage of stainless steel surfaces that allow for the development of FeO_2 (ferric oxide or "rust") as a reddish-brown material on the surfaces of instruments (particularly on any moving parts). This will also be observed as "pitting" or the development of small pin-holes on the surface of the device.	The main causes of rust are wear and tear on the device and the presence of high levels of chlorine/silica-based chemicals in water used to generate steam (but also from other sources). Check for the levels of chlorine/chlorides and/or silicates in the feed-water to the steam-generator. Note: chlorine is widely used for the disinfection of water. It is also considered good practice not to sterilize stainless steel instruments together in the same pack with aluminum, brass, copper or chrome-plated instruments because of the risk of "galvanic" corrosion that may result. The visual signs of rust can be removed by immersing the device in an acid-based cleaner (Table 11.7), but it should be noted that this only removes the visual signs of rust (by dissolving the ferric oxide) and does not resolve the existing damage; further, acids can further enhance the damage to the device surface.

Table 11.6 (*cont'd*).

Problem	Cause	Solution
Packaging materials show signs of staining but not the instruments	The wrap may act as a "filter" to keep various chemicals (as specified above or in Table 11.7) away the instruments. If the wrap shows signs of staining but the instruments are clean, or if unwrapped instruments are consistently dirtier than wrapped ones, steam purity/quality is the major cause of the problem.	It is likely that the sterilizer in question has a deficiency in the steam purity/quality. Review Table 11.7 for typical causes of various stains. Wet steam can particularly show these problems (as an early warning sign).

human error can play a part, the most common errors are incorrect cycle selection, overloading or improperly loading the sterilizer, failing to initiate the cycle once the sterilizer has been loaded and change in procedure or personnel. Procedural errors occur when improper sterilization procedures are being used, for example reprocessing a device in the wrong cycle or even according to a departmental procedure that does not comply with the device manufacturer or equipment manufacturers' instructions. The facility's written operating procedures should be reviewed and compared with the sterilizer and device manufacturers' instructions to ensure they are consistent. Make sure that all staff are trained on how to operate and interpret monitoring equipment, selecting the correct cycle for load contents (i.e. containment device), choosing the correct packaging materials/techniques, operating the equipment and on always following the medical device manufacturer's instructions. If the failure is due to human error and no equipment repairs are necessary the sterilizer can be immediately returned to service. If there is no obvious cause identified from this review, the investigation will need to be expanded and it may be necessary to seek outside assistance.

Once procedural errors have been ruled out, the investigation continues by reviewing all sterilizer monitoring (parametric and other indicators) that has been collected in the last 24 hours. Review any sterilizer printout tapes or records (such as computerized data collected from the sterilizer control systems(s)) to determine if the appropriate sterilization parameters have been met, that is, temperature/time/pressure. Sterilizers that have independent monitoring systems have two sets of data that can be compared: those from the control system and those from the independent monitoring system. In some cases the results from such systems need to be visually inspected for differences, while in others this is performed by the sterilizer. Overall independent monitoring systems are useful to ensure that various sensors used for controlling the process are adequately calibrated and functioning. If the physical monitoring results have changed or differ from what is expected, the sterilization process should be considered incomplete and the load(s) not released for patient use. Physical monitors provide a real-time assessment of each individual sterilization cycle and assist in the early detection of sterilizer malfunction.

The next step is to review the results of any air removal tests, the most common of which is the recommended daily Bowie-Dick (air removal) test. The Bowie-Dick test is designed to ensure that air removal is sufficient within the steam process, which is noted to be affected not only by the programmed conditioning phase of the test cycle, but also the quality of steam (see the section on water quality/purity). Steam sterilization failures often result from incomplete air removal, including poor steam quality/quantity. Inadequate air removal, sterilization temperatures and/or times will also be indicated by failed biological or chemical indicators used during routine testing of the sterilizer. Note that there are different classifications of chemical indicators, with different stringencies in their capabilities to detect a passed/failed cycle. In the case of a failed Bowie-Dick or biological indicator test, it is recommended to repeat the test (and if possible use a different product batch) to confirm the result. The indicator manufacturer's instructions should be consulted and it may also be necessary to confirm that these are performing as intended. Examples are to confirm that the indicators have been used according to their instructions and are within any stated shelf-life. If the repeated tests indicate a "pass" result suggesting that the sterilizer is operating effectively, facility procedures will need to be reassessed to identify what went wrong. In the case of a "fail" result, the sterilizer and/or the utilities that supply the equipment will require further investigation. Factors that can often affect the efficiency of the steam sterilizer include the air seal of the door of the sterilizer, the quality of the steam and the characteristics of the load. It is the responsibility of the reprocessing area manager to establish a periodic maintenance procedure to assure correct operation of the sterilizer and its utilities. Many common problems associated with steam sterilizers are due to lack of maintenance. Such malfunctions will require further investigation from a trained engineer, manufacturer or other process/equipment expert. When a mechanical failure is identified, this should immediately cause an investigation and potential recall procedure. It may be necessary to recall affected loads (prior to patient use) identified during the investigation. All such packs should be retrieved, quarantined and re-sterilized (if necessary) under the standard facility quality procedures (Chapter 14).

In the case of any inconclusive results from the inspection of internal pack chemical indicator(s), other packs associated with the same sterilizer load should be identified and inspected if possible. If an individual chemical indicator has failed, there is a possibility that the entire batch/load is also compromised. These are often identified at the site of surgical/medical use; therefore staff handling devices in these areas should be trained on the correct inspection procedures prior to patient use (Chapter 12). First verify that the correct internal chemical indicator was selected for the items that were sterilized. All other packages should be opened to check their internal indicators and then reprocessed. If no other packs have been affected this is probably a procedural failure. If all the other packs in that particular load are affected this could be a mechanical or process monitoring product failure, and further investigation will need to be done. Verify that all monitoring products are within their manufactured expiration date and have been stored properly.

If biological indicators are used as the only load control monitoring test being used, then items from all loads since the last passed biological test may need to be recalled. Similarly, if class 5 or 6 indicators or integrator test packs are used, then all items from all loads since the last passed result may also need to be recalled.

After any major repair has been performed the sterilizer should not be used until the necessary quality monitoring tests are completed in accordance with facility policy. For steam sterilizers, this will typically include Bowie-Dick tests and chemical/biological indicator tests (sometimes in multiple test cycles). If all of the test results are satisfactory and the mechanical monitoring results are acceptable, the sterilizer should be considered in good working order and can be put back into service.

There are many potential hidden process failures that can occur. These are difficult to detect and are dependent on having proper controls in place for the whole decontamination cycle. These are often the case when procedures that should take place prior to sterilization are not properly followed. Examples include incorrect cleaning methods (soil remaining on a device), detergents or other chemicals that are not correctly rinsed from devices or during laundering, damaged or malfunctioning valves associated with devices, damaged filters used with rigid sterilization containers, incorrect loading and wrapping techniques, etc., all of which may compromise sterilization. Such failures can lead to adverse patient reactions and can only be minimized as part of a quality assurance system within a facility, such as by ensuring that staff are correctly trained in device inspection. Further failures can occur when environmental conditions cause a sterilized device to become re-contaminated, such as during storage, transport and preparation for a surgical/medical procedure (Chapter 12).

Troubleshooting steam sterilization problems

Troubleshooting can be defined as the identification of problems and their cause(s) in order to prevent or minimize any negative effects. Troubleshooting requires patience and often in-depth investigation. A variety of steam sterilization problems can occur and are most often related to the quality/purity of water (see earlier section). A summary of the most common problems, causes and recommended solutions is given in Table 11.6.

A common complaint with the steam sterilization process is the gradual or sudden onset of changes in color or appearance on devices. These problems are most often associated with inadequate cleaning/rinsing of devices or water purity. Due to the varying purity of water, sudden changes in observed device color and/or damage (such as rusting) is most often associated with both of these causes. It should be noted that these effects may happen over time but may only visually develop over time. The problem may be due to water used in washer-disinfector and/or steam generation system(s). As a note, if the problem is not observed following cleaning/disinfection, but is observed following sterilization (usually on opening and inspection of the pack prior to patient use, Chapter 12), this usually indicates a problem with the steam sterilizer. These effects may be seen not only on the devices, but also on the steam sterilizer chamber walls. Common examples are given in Table 11.7.

Table 11.7 Example of problems frequently associated with color changes on devices and their causes. This list is given only as a guide and the specific cause of such problems may be due to more complicated reasons than those specified below.

Observed color	Typical cause	Solution
Brown/red residues	Incomplete removal of soil (in particular, blood). Development of rust, in particular due to the presence of chlorine in the water used to make steam. This may come directly from the feed-water (where it is used for the control of microorganisms in water distribution systems). A further common sources of chlorine in water is due to the incorrect installation/maintenance of a water softener system (used to reduce water hardness); these systems exchange (swap) hardness in the water (e.g. calcium carbonate) with sodium chloride (NaCl) and can therefore be a source of chorine if not balanced correctly. A build-up of iron deposits from water and/or supply lines (e.g. from old iron-containing pipes in water delivery/circulation systems).	Soil (material from a previous patient procedure) can be generally removed using an alkaline cleaning. Inorganic deposits (such as rusting or iron deposits) generally require treatment with an acid-based cleaner to dissolve/remove. Check the purity of the water/steam, in particular for high levels of chlorine/chlorites. High levels of chlorine can be removed by installing/maintaining an activated carbon filter. Ensure that any water softener systems are correctly installed and maintained.
Brown residues	Excessive heat (e.g. super-heat) due to the development of chromium oxide on stainless steel surfaces.	Check the steam quality, in particular for super-heat.
Fading of colored device surfaces over time (in particular aluminum-based devices)	Chlorine (and other oxidizing agents) in the steam supply or highly alkaline (pH >8) in the cleaning chemistry. These will cause a reaction with colored surfaces, causing fading over time.	Check the purity of the water/steam, in particular for pH and presence of chlorine. This is sometimes observed with the use of RO water, which naturally happens over time and may indicate a limited number of reprocessing cycles with such devices (but these effects are cosmetic only).
Orange/brown staining	Presence of phosphates (from water/steam or as a residual from the cleaning chemistry on reaction with heat). Note: orange-brown color may also come from the use of iodine/iodophor-based antiseptics on the device that should be discussed with the operating room and such practices discontinued.	Check the purity of the water/steam, in particular for phosphates. Water treatment systems should reduce these levels if present.
Black staining	Overuse of acid-based cleaner or inadequate neutralization of such cleaners during a cleaning process. May also occur due to the use of bleaching agents on devices (e.g. bleach solutions for cleaning), which should be identified and discontinued.	Ensure that acid-cleaning solutions are either correctly neutralized (as required by the manufacturer) or correctly rinsed from device surfaces.

Table 11.7 (*cont'd*).

Observed color	Typical cause	Solution
Multi-colored, "rainbow" effect	Excessive (in particular) dry heat, often associated with super-heat (see above) or excessive drying phases.	Check the steam quality, in particular for super-heat. Discuss with the sterilizer manufacturer or steam sterilization cycle development expert.
White or otherwise colored grainy precipitate	Often seen first as a build-up over time on the chamber walls (particularly close to steam entry ports into a chamber), but also in excessive cases on devices/container surfaces. Will eventually cause the failure of valves, steam generation systems and even pipework clogging in excessive cases. Due to the presence of water hardness in the water/steam. Other causes may include high levels of silica or sulfur-containing water contaminates. Also observed as spotting on device surfaces.	Check the purity of the water/steam, in particular for hardness (but also other minerals such as copper, iron and chromium that may also be present). Consider installing and maintaining water softeners for pre-treating feed-water for steam generation. Further pre-treatment may be required to reduce levels of silica- and sulfur-water contaminants if present.
Gold-tinting	High chlorine levels	Check the purity of the water/steam, in particular for pH and presence of chlorine. Chlorine levels may be reduced by installing carbon filters into the incoming water lines prior to steam generation.
Purple/blue colors	Overdosing of amines, commonly used to reduce the risks of corrosion within water/steam boilers/lines.	Review for amine-dosing systems associated with boilers/steam generators.

Steam sterilization guidelines and standards

Steam is the most widely used method of sterilization and there are many guidelines and standards associated with steam sterilization processes and equipment. The specific recommendations can vary from country to country and although there may be many similarities there are also many specific requirements that need to be locally considered. Table 11.8 lists some examples of the guidelines and standards related to steam sterilization and monitoring used worldwide, but this list should not be considered exhaustive.

Dry heat sterilization
Principles of dry heat sterilization

"Dry" heat methods are used for sterilization applications. These are based on the principles of directly applying heat or heated air for sterilization. Typical applications include the use of incinerators and dry heat ovens.

Incineration refers to "burning to ashes", where contaminated materials and devices are essentially burned to ash in specifically designed furnaces (known as incinerators) at excessive temperatures (such as >800°C). Burning (also known as combustion) is one of the oldest described methods of sterilization, but is essentially destructive. This is a commonly used method for the destruction of clinical waste materials that are no longer required (including many single-use or discarded devices). Waste can include infectious and non-infectious waste. It is also a useful method to reduce the volume of waste, even up to a 95% reduction. Incinerators can range in design and capacity, ranging from simple burners to high-capacity furnaces and batch to continuous systems (Figure 11.16). High-capacity incinerators usually consist of a feed system, a primary chamber (in which the waste is incinerated), a secondary chamber/furnace (particularly for burning off waste gases) and a cooling/feed-out

Table 11.8 Examples of steam sterilization guidelines and standards.

Guidelines/standards	Title	Description
ISO 17665-1: 2006	*Sterilization of healthcare products – moist heat. Part 1: requirements for the development, validation and routine control of a sterilization process for medical devices*	Specifies requirements for the development, validation and routine control of a moist heat (steam) sterilization processes for devices.
ISO 17665-2: 2009	*Sterilization of healthcare products – moist heat. Part 2: guidance on the application of ISO 17665 Part 1: 2006*	Provides guidance on the understanding and implementation of ISO 17665-1.
EN 285:2006+PLUS;A2:2009	*Sterilization – steam sterilizers – large sterilizers*	This European standard specifies requirements and the relevant tests for large steam sterilizers primarily used in healthcare for the sterilization of devices and accessories.
EN 13060:2004+PLUS;A2:2010	*Small steam sterilizers*	This European standard specifies requirements and the relevant tests for small steam sterilizers primarily used in healthcare for the sterilization of devices and accessories.
ISO 11138-3:2006	*Sterilization of healthcare products – biological indicators. Part 3: biological indicators for moist heat sterilization processes*	Provides specific requirements for test organisms, suspensions, inoculated carriers, biological indicators and test methods intended for use in assessing the performance of steam sterilization processes.
ISO 11140-3:2007	*Sterilization of healthcare products – chemical indicators. Part 3: class 2 indicator systems for use in the Bowie-Dick type steam penetration test*	Specifies the requirements for chemical indicators to be used in the steam penetration test for steam sterilizers for wrapped goods, for example instruments and porous materials (i.e. class 2 indicators as described in ISO 11140-1).
ISO 11140-4:2007	*Sterilization of healthcare products – chemical indicators. Part 4: class 2 indicators as an alternative to the Bowie-Dick type test for detection of steam penetration*	Specifies the performance for class 2 indicators to be used as an alternative to the Bowie-Dick type test. This type of indicator is intended to identify poor steam penetration but does not necessarily indicate the cause.
ISO 11140-5:2007	*Sterilization of healthcare products – chemical indicators. Part 5: class 2 indicators for Bowie-Dick type air removal tests*	Specifies the requirements for class 2 indicators for Bowie-Dick type air removal tests used to evaluate the effectiveness of air removal.
AS/NZS 4187:2003	*Cleaning, disinfecting and sterilizing re-usable medical and surgical instruments and equipment, and maintenance of associated environments in healthcare facilities*	General guidance on reprocessing, to include steam sterilization (in Australia and New Zealand).
ANSI/AAMI ST79:2010	*Comprehensive guide to steam sterilization and sterility assurance in healthcare facilities*	Provides recommended practice on steam sterilization in healthcare facilities in the USA. ANSI/AAMI ST 79 is a consolidation of a previous series of guidelines.
CDC/HICPAC:2008	*Guideline for disinfection and sterilization in healthcare facilities*	Recommendations on methods for cleaning, disinfection and sterilization of patient-care medical devices in the USA.
HTM 2010	*Sterilization*	Published in five parts, this guidance document for the UK includes detailed information on the design and testing of steam sterilizers.
Canada Communicable Disease Report, 1998	*Hand washing, cleaning, disinfection and sterilization in healthcare*	Guidance includes recommendation on steam sterilization.

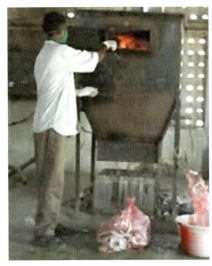
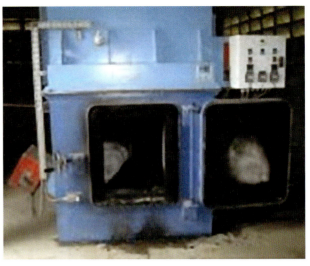
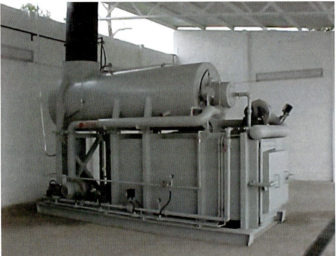

Figure 11.16 Examples of incinerators, ranging from simple burning furnaces and more complicated two-stage incinerator designs.

system. Typical temperatures for primary incineration are in the range of 400–980°C (750–1800°F) and for the secondary furnace in the 870–1100°C (1600–2000°F range). They may also include heat recovery systems that can be used to heat a water supply. Exposure times will vary depending on the volume of the load, but can be up to a number of hours. A particular concern with incineration is the release of highly toxic (even carcinogenic) and particularly persistent chemicals released on burning of plastic and other materials. These include "dioxins" as a series of fluorine-containing chemicals and various gases

such as carbon monoxide and carbon dioxide. For this reason, alternative systems such as hot-alkaline digestion and other heating/chemical treatment/shredding systems have been adopted. An example is known as electro-thermal deactivation (ETD) that employs an electrically heated oven in combination with low frequency radio waves as a rapid dry heating method, but without melting of plastics; in such systems the waste is treated and shredded to reduce volume up to 80%. Incineration and similar systems are destructive and only used for waste-disposal methods; these are not considered in further detail.

Dry heat sterilizers (also known as hot air or oven sterilizers) are rarely used clinically for the sterilization of restricted types of material, such as glassware, oils, powders and instruments that for various reasons cannot be routinely sterilized by steam (e.g. are moisture-sensitive materials/devices). Many of these items are now provided as single use materials/devices and are therefore not subjected to reprocessing. Therefore it is rare to see the use of dry heat sterilizers in clinical practice today. Dry heat "sterilizers" should not be confused with drying cabinets that are only designed for use to remove water (i.e. for drying); although drying cabinets may provide some antimicrobial effects, including restricting the ability of certain types of microorganisms to grow, such as bacteria, fungi and protozoa, they are not designed for and should not be considered for use as sterilizers.

"Dry" heat sterilization applications use air heated to a high temperature, generally in excess of 160°C for antimicrobial effects and are therefore much higher than those used for steam sterilization. There may or may not be various levels of water (humidity) present during such processes (e.g. within the load or air), but this is not specifically controlled as part of the process. It is of interest to note that the less humidity that is present, the *longer* the time required for dry heat sterilization. Therefore, the conditions for effective dry heat sterilization can depend on the amount of water present in the materials to be sterilized and in the environment/air of the sterilizer. To compensate for this variability, dry heat sterilization cycle times can be overall quite long.

Similar to all disinfection and sterilization methods, all items to be sterilized must be cleaned, dried and prepared for dry heat sterilization. Items may be wrapped with foil, packed into a closed metal container or placed unwrapped onto a tray or sterilizer shelf. Items should remain in the oven at the correct temperature for the required time, including cool-down.

The mechanisms of action of dry heat, considered to be predominantly due to direct heating and oxidation effects, are different to those observed with steam. The only parameter that is controlled during a typical dry heat sterilization process is the air temperature and it can therefore be a relatively simple process in design. A typical sterilization process will include preheating of the air and load to the desired sterilization temperatures (preconditioning), holding it at that set temperature (sterilization) and then allowing the load to cool prior to handling/patient use (cooling, typically to less than

80°C). There are enormous variations in times and temperatures in dry heat sterilization, based on sterilizer design itself and the volume, density and packaging recommendations with the load. The heating process is generally slow, and long sterilizing times are required. Sterilization times alone can range from 30-minute exposure at 180°C to six-hour exposure at 121°C, not including times for conditioning (pre-heating) and cooling the load. Common sterilization phase temperatures and exposure times include:

- 180°C 30 minutes
- 170°C 1 hour
- 160°C 2 hours
- 142°C 2.5 hours
- 141°C 3 hours

Note: there are no standard cycle times, as this will depend on the sterilizer design and indications for use. At such high temperatures (>160°C) and contact times, dry heat is traditionally considered effective against microorganisms, with the most resistant organism to such processes widely accepted to be *Bacillus atrophaeus* spores. These spores are therefore used in the design, validation and routine testing of dry heat sterilization processes. Following such long sterilization times, cooling of the load can take some time before the devices can be safely handled/used, sometimes up to eight hours, depending on the load and sterilizer design. In some older designs, the control of the sterilization process is conducted manually; under such conditions, defined load configurations should be specified in a written procedure (in collaboration with the sterilizer manufacturer), timing for sterilization should not begin until the oven/load reaches the desired temperature and care should be taken to allow the load to cool prior to handling/use.

This method of sterilization is not recommended for items that could melt or burn. These can include rubber, many plastics, elastomers, devices containing certain types of adhesives, and even some devices that may be considered heat-resistant (such as stainless steel devices that can be damaged by stress-cracking). In all cases, devices or material (including packaging), manufacturers' instructions should be reviewed to ensure that they are compatible and can be safely used in dry heat sterilization processes. Given such high temperatures (and times used), the clinical applications for dry heat sterilizers are limited.

Dry heat sterilization is considered to be penetrating over time, due to the convection transfer of heat. Convection, in this case is defined as transfer of heat by the movement or circulation of air. In comparison to steam sterilization it is also considered as having a low corrosive profile and not to be associated with many of the common water quality/purity problems often reported with steam sterilization. It is often the only option for the sterilization of moisture-sensitive materials such as powders and oils. Dry heat sterilizers are often available at low cost and are not associated with the complexity of installation/utility requirements of steam sterilizers. Dry heat is an effective method to neutralize endotoxins (Chapter 5, see the section on bacteria), unlike steam sterilization. The term "depyrogenation" refers to the specific inactivation of the toxic effects of toxins such as endotoxins, but dry heat is rarely used clinically for such purposes. Dry heat sterilizers do, however, have many disadvantages, such as the length of time required for sterilization and the restrictions on the types of materials/devices that can tolerate dry heat sterilization processes.

Design

There are two essential designs of dry-heat sterilization systems: dry heat ovens and incinerators. Incinerators designs have already been briefly introduced in the previous section on the principles of dry heat sterilization. Dry heat ovens consist of a chamber (generally made of stainless steel) within which the air is electrically heated (not unlike a kitchen oven). Such designs will typically include fans to allow for the circulation of air during the process (to optimize even heat distribution), are often conducted under slight pressure and are vented through HEPA-filters to prevent the ingress of contaminants during the sterilization process. High-efficiency particulate air can be used to assist with cooling during the sterilization process. Sterilizers can be designed for batch sterilization (similar to other sterilizers, where a load is placed into the sterilizer, sterilized and then removed) or as a continuous design (as a tunnel or conveyor system). Batch sterilizers are generally used for packaged materials, while continuous systems are for non-packaged items. The sterilizer design should have calibrated thermometer(s) or temperature gauge(s) to make sure that the designated temperature is reached, distributed and maintained for the desired time. Overall, the sterilizer may be automatically (microprocessor) controlled or operated manually. It is recommended that any sterilizer process records (manually or automatically produced by the sterilizer) should be maintained as verification that the process was correctly completed.

Standards and guidelines

Table 11.9 lists some examples of widely used guidelines and standards relating to dry heat sterilizers, sterilization processes and monitoring used worldwide.

Table 11.9 Examples of guidelines and standards considering dry heat sterilization.

Guidelines/standards	Title	Description
ISO 20857:2010	*Sterilization of healthcare products – dry heat – requirements for the development, validation and routine control of a sterilization process for medical devices*	Specifies requirements for the development, validation and routine control of a dry heat sterilization process for devices (including for de-pyrogenation).
ISO 11138-4:2006	*Sterilization of healthcare products – biological indicators* *Part 4: biological indicators for dry heat sterilization processes*	Provides specific requirements for test organisms, suspensions, inoculated carriers, biological indicators, and test methods intended for use in dry heat sterilizers.
ANSI/AAMI ST40:2004	*Table-top dry heat (heated air) sterilization and sterility assurance in healthcare facilities*	Provides guidelines for dry heat sterilization in USA healthcare facilities.
HTM 2010	*Sterilization*	Published in five parts, this guidance document for the UK includes detailed information on the design and testing of dry-heat sterilizers.
AS/NZS 4187:2003	*Cleaning, disinfecting and sterilizing re-usable medical and surgical instruments and equipment, and maintenance of associated environments in health care facilities*	General guidance on reprocessing, to include dry heat sterilization (in Australia and New Zealand).

Radiation

Radiation and various forms of light can have disinfection and sterilization properties (Chapter 6, in the section on light, radiation and the electromagnetic spectrum). Low energy radiation methods, such as UV and IR light are used for various disinfection applications (Chapter 9, in the section on radiation). High energy radiation sources are actually widely used as sterilization methods, but not for re-usable device reprocessing or for routine use in healthcare facilities. High energy radiation sources and generators are more widely used for the sterilization single-use materials within healthcare facilities such as bandages and types of single-use devices.

Radiation sterilization is mostly used for contract sterilization of single-use devices and materials that are then supplied to a healthcare facility pre-sterilized and discarded following use. They all consist of exposing a load to a given dose of radiation (over time). Typical radiation technologies include:

• γ-radiation: this form of radiation is released from unstable forms of certain types of elements (Chapter 6, see the section on Light, radiation and the electromagnetic spectrum) known as "radioactive isotopes". Examples include ^{60}Cobalt and ^{137}Caesium. Being unstable, they breakdown (or "decay") over time to release energy (in the form of γ-radiation) that is a very powerful antimicrobial (and also the basis of radioactive power generation!).
• X-ray radiation: also a source of high energy radiation (X-rays, being less energized than γ-radiation, Chapter 6, see the section on Light, radiation and the electromagnetic spectrum), but in this case it is generated from specific X-ray producing tubes/systems.
• E-beam radiation. A different form of radiation (β-particles or "electrons") that are generated and focused in systems known as "accelerators", also producing a powerful antimicrobial effect.

Specific facilities are designed to ensure the safe handling/production of radiation and its use for sterilization. For this reason, they are not covered in detail. The various different forms of radiation were identified in Chapter 6 (in the section on light, radiation and the electromagnetic spectrum).

At the time of writing, there are no specific guidelines or standards regarding the routine use of radiation for sterilization of re-usable devices in healthcare facilities. There are, however, a number of industrial standards that may be referenced if applicable (Table 11.10).

Filtration

Filtration is commonly used as a physical mechanisms of disinfection and sterilization, especially with gases (e.g. air) and liquids (such as water). For this reason, it is often used as a part of various device sterilization processes. Examples include:
• For the introduction of air during steam and low temperature gas sterilization methods. The most commonly used filters are HEPA filters of various grades. Typically these filters have the capacity to retain particles down to a 0.5 to 1 μm range (thereby removing most bacteria), but this will depend on their specific design. They can also cause removal of smaller particles due to attachment to/interaction with the filter material.
• As part of the treatment of water used for rinsing of devices following liquid chemical sterilization. Examples include sterile water filters (0.1–0.2 μm), reverse osmosis (RO) systems and sterile water filter/UV-light combination treatment systems, depending on their design and integration as part of the sterilization process/sterilizer.
Filters are used to physically remove various microorganisms due to their size. This is discussed in further detail in Chapter 9, in the section on filtration. The use of filters as part of a sterilizer design needs to be controlled

Table 11.10 Examples of radiation sterilization standards used for industrial purposes.

Guidelines/standards	Title	Description
ISO 11137-1:2006	*Sterilization of healthcare products – radiation* *Part 1: requirements for development, validation and routine control of a sterilization process for medical devices*	Specifies requirements for the development, validation and routine control of a radiation sterilization process for medical devices. It covers radiation processes employing irradiators using the radionuclide ^{60}Co or ^{137}Cs, a beam from an electron generator or a beam from an X-ray generator.
ISO 11137-2:2006	*Sterilization of healthcare products – radiation.* *Part 2: establishing the sterilization dose*	Specifies methods of determining the minimum dose needed to achieve a specified requirement for sterility.

to ensure their safe and effective use. This will include the design of the filter(s) and how they are used/tested within the process, as well as maintenance/replacement recommendations. In such cases, care should be taken to follow sterilizer manufacturers' instructions.

Chemical sterilization

Ethylene oxide gas

Ethylene oxide (C_2H_4O), also known as oxirane or more commonly as EO/ETO, is a colorless gas at 20°C and atmospheric pressure. It is possible to smell ETO at about 500 ppm of the gas in air, described as a sweet, almond-like, odor, but at lower concentrations is essentially odorless. Note that in gas, 500 ppm is approximately (but not exactly) equal to 500 mg/L, therefore these levels are within the range used for sterilization (see the next section on the principles of ethylene oxide gas sterilization). It dissolves easily in water, alcohol and most organic solvents. Ethylene oxide is one of the most widely used industrial chemicals in the manufacture of detergents, polyester and anti-freeze. It is actually one of the most used organic chemicals in the world, but mostly for industrial applications; examples include its use in the manufacturer of various other chemicals such as plastics, glycols (e.g. used as anti-freeze) and detergents. Ethylene oxide is also one of the most commonly used antimicrobial chemicals for low temperature sterilization and as an alternative to steam process. It is widely used for industrial sterilization (e.g. for single-use devices provided sterile and even for certain types of foods) and, although to a much less extent, in hospitals or contract sterilization facilities for sterilization of re-usable, heat-sensitive devices. As a biocide, it demonstrates broad spectrum antimicrobial activity, including against bacterial spores, when controlled as part of a sterilization process (including the chemical concentration and presence of high humidity). Its mechanisms of action are by a process called alkylation, which attacks the various different types of macromolecules (such as protein) leading to the loss of structure and function, resulting in death. Ethylene oxide is used to sterilize items that are heat or moisture sensitive. The ability to process plastics and complex products of diverse material composition (as well as other types of chemicals such as glutaraldehyde and peracetic acid) accelerated the development and evolution of many of these types of devices, including flexible endoscopes. Ethylene oxide readily permeates commonly used packaging materials, porous materials and various types of devices (including lumened devices) at low temperatures; it is also

Table 11.11 Examples of ethylene oxide gas sterilization processes, highlighting the gas concentration, relative humidity range, temperature and typical exposure times for sterilization (based on US-FDA approved sterilization cycles).

ETO concentration (mg/L)	Temperature		Relative humidity (%)	Exposure time (hours)
	(°C)	(°F)		
700–900	37–38	98–100	50–80	4–4.5
700–900	55	131	50–80	1
550–650	55	131	30–70	2
350–450	55	131	30–80	7.5

used to sterilize materials such as paper and types of fabrics. Further, ETO is generally considered non-corrosive and non-damaging to a variety of materials, including those used in devices and packaging systems. But on the negative side, it can be flammable and explosive in the presence of air (at or above 3% air), is irritating and even carcinogenic (associated with causing cancer). Therefore close control of the use of ETO is important for staff and patient safety.

Principles of ethylene oxide gas sterilization

Ethylene oxide sterilization requires the correct chemical concentration, water (humidity) level, temperature and contact time to be controlled during any such process (Table 11.11):

• Ethylene oxide concentration: typically ranges from 400 to 1200 mg/L. In general, the higher the concentration the more efficient the sterilization process, but it is also considered that concentrations greater than ~800 mg/L do not appear to provide any further increase in activity against bacterial spores.

• Temperatures can vary, but for most hospital applications this will be 30–65°C (86–149°F), with higher temperatures found to be more efficient than lower. The temperature range of such processes are generally limited to at or below 55°C as higher temperatures are considered damaging to many types of materials/devices (that recommend temperatures of <60°C/140°F).

• Humidity (or the "relative humidity", which is the amount of water in air at a specific temperature), is recommended at 40–80%. Lower and higher levels may be recommended depending on the sterilizer/process manufacturer. Note: 100% relative humidity is considered water "saturated" at a given temperature (see Chapter 6).

• Exposure times, which will depend on the ETO concentration, temperature and humidity, as defined by the

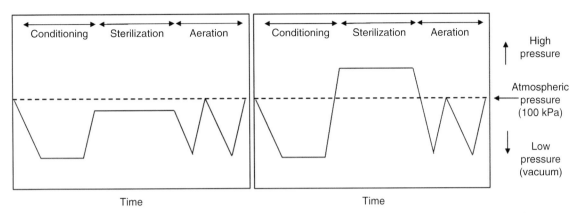

Figure 11.17 Examples of ethylene oxide sterilization processes. On the left is shown a sterilization cycle under vacuum (negative pressure), specifically the gas exposure phase of the cycle (sterilization), and on the right a pressurized (positive pressure) cycle.

manufacturer to meet an SAL of 10^{-6} or equivalent (see Basic principles of sterilization).

Overall, these are the minimum, required variables for sterilization to be achieved. Individual sterilization processes are defined and verified to be effective within these ranges using bacterial spore preparations of *Bacillus atrophaeus* (previously known as *Bacillus subtilis* sub-species *niger*). *B. atrophaeus* is considered the most resistant organism to ETO sterilization processes.

Similar to other sterilization processes, there are various different phases of the process to ensure that these conditions are achieved within the types of loads that are being sterilized, as well as to ensure that such loads are safe for use following sterilization. A typical ethylene oxide sterilization process will therefore include (Figure 11.17):

• Conditioning, to ensure the load is correctly humidified, heated and mixed with ETO gas to meet the defined conditions for sterilization. In some cases, although rare, pre-conditioning may be conducted in a separate chamber to preheat and humidify the load prior to placing into the ETO sterilizer. It is also important during conditioning to ensure that air is adequately removed for two reasons: as air can inhibit the penetration of humidity/ETO to all surfaces within the load and that ETO is explosive in the presence of as little as 3% air. This is generally achieved by pulling the air out of the chamber/load using a vacuum-pump ("drawing a vacuum" to a pre-determined low pressure). Steam is also introduced (or generated directly within the chamber from water) under these conditions to act as both a heating and humidification mechanism; remember from the discussion on steam (see Principles of steam sterilization), that while steam can be generated at higher temperatures by increasing

the pressure, it can also be made at lower temperature under lower pressures. In this way, steam (under vacuum/low pressure) can be used to pre-condition the load prior to sterilization. Steam introduction and air removal may be assisted by repeated pulses of pulling a vacuum and introducing steam to given controlled pressure set-points. Generally, as a final part of the conditioning cycle, ethylene oxide gas is then introduced into the chamber and allowed to diffuse within the load. As ETO is a gas at temperature above ~11°C (~52°F) and at atmospheric pressure, in accordance with the gas laws it can be maintained as a liquid at lower temperatures or higher pressures. Ethylene oxide is therefore generally provided as a liquid in single or multiple use pressurized canisters (Figure 11.18). The canister is provided to a delivery system within or associated with the sterilizer (e.g. an example of a single use canister loaded within the sterilizer chamber as shown in Figure 11.18); the gas is then generated during the process (under vacuum or negative pressure, Figure 11.17) by heating (e.g. at 60–70°C). Ethylene oxide can be provided as 100% preparation, typically in single-use canisters or vials containing low volumes of ETO (e.g. 10–100 mL). Such canisters are designed for specific sterilization processes, as defined by the manufacturer. But because of the flammable nature of ETO in the pure form, ETO preparations are also provided mixed with an excess of inert gases such as carbon dioxide (CO_2) or hydrochlorofluorocarbons (HCFC) as non-flammable blends. Examples include 10% ETO, 90% HCFC (can be commonly referred to as 10–90) or 8.5% ETO, 91.5% CO_2. In general, these preparations are usually provided in larger canisters for use in multiple ETO sterilization cycles. Conditioning is complete when the required conditions of temperature, humidity and ETO concentration are achieved.

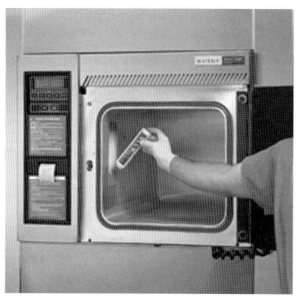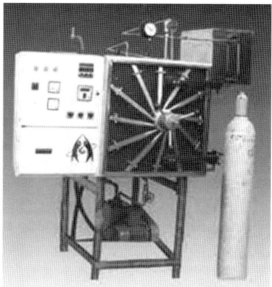

Figure 11.18 Examples of ethylene oxide sterilizers and supply canisters/tanks (providing liquid ETO under pressure). The example on the left shows a canister (100% ETO) being placed into a sterilizer chamber. On the right is a larger sterilizer provided with an ETO blend canister.

• Sterilization, where the temperature, humidity and ETO gas concentration is maintained within the sterilizer for the defined time (e.g. to provide a SAL of 10^{-6} as defined by the manufacturer). It is typical for processes using 100% ETO to be maintained under a vacuum (negative pressure) and when ETO blends are used as the sterilant supply that loads are exposed to under pressure; however, the specific process variables will vary depending on the manufacturer and cycle definition. In both cases the processes are designed to ensure adequate distribution and penetration of the gas. Typical cycle conditions are summarized in Table 11.11.

• Aeration: ethylene oxide is removed from the chamber and load by one or a number of vacuum pulses (sometimes including the aid of steam or heat to improve aeration times). The gas is passed through a system (e.g. abater or catalytic converter) to break down the gas safely into water and carbon dioxide. Safe aeration of the load is the longest part of a typical ETO sterilization cycle; depending on the load materials and size, this can be typically 8–12 hours (depending on the aeration process, including the temperature) but may even be longer. An example of an aeration cycle would be 12 hours at 50°C (122°F), although device manufacturers should provide information supporting the safe aeration cycle conditions for their specific device types. Aeration can be achieved in the

sterilizer itself (depending on the type of load and sterilization process defined by the manufacturer) and/or more commonly in a separate aeration chamber/cabinet that holds the load at a constant air flow and temperature (e.g. 35–60°C) to aid in the removal of ETO toxic residues.

As discussed, there are essentially two main types of ETO sterilization processes: those that use ETO blends and those using 100% ETO. They both have advantages and disadvantages:

• One hundred percent ETO: generally provided in single-use ETO cartridges used directly within the sterilizer. These require no additional supply tanks, valves or fittings that could leak on providing ETO to the sterilizer. Such sterilizer designs ensure that the used cartridges are safely aerated with the load, rendering them non-hazardous and safe to discard (in a safe manner according to the gas manufacturer/supplier instructions and healthcare facility policy). One canister is typically used per sterilization cycle. Sterilizer chambers are, however, limited in size but do operate under negative pressure (vacuum); therefore if a leak did accidentally occur the gas should remain in the chamber and not vent into room as room air is drawn into the chamber.

• Ethylene oxide blends: generally provided as multiple-use gas tanks, which can offer greater flexibility in the number of types of cycles that can be programmed with the sterilizer. Such blends are safer in handling and storage, due to their non-flammability; but it is important to ensure that they are connected correctly to the sterilizer and that the connection system does not leak during use or over time. Sterilizer designs can be smaller or larger in design, being able to accommodate smaller or larger loads respectively (as specified by the manufacturer). Sterilization cycles using blends are most often designed to operate under pressure, which may increase the risk of leaking from the sterilizer during the processes; as with all sterilizer designs, routine maintenance and periodic servicing according to manufacturers' instructions should minimize such risks.

Ethylene oxide sterilization processes are used as low temperature alternatives to steam sterilization. Ethylene oxide, under the correct exposure conditions (particularly temperature and humidity), is a reliable and well-appreciated sterilizing agent. As it is a very stable gas, it demonstrates good penetration capabilities into loads and specifically challenging devices (such as long-lumened or porous instruments); however, it is important to note that the antimicrobial effects are dependent on the presence of the gas and humidity (therefore also the removal of air). Ethylene oxide demonstrates exceptional device and material compatibility. Overall, these benefits are due to the non-reactive nature of ETO, with various types of metals, plastics and other materials (including various types of sterile packaging materials and containers); despite this, it is recommended to only use packaging materials that are labelled for use with ETO sterilization processes. Typical loads can include temperature-sensitive materials and devices, including flexible endoscopes and plastic-ware.

When handled properly, ETO is a reliable and safe agent for sterilization, but the risks of gas emissions and residues of ETO present hazards to personnel and patients. A safe work environment must be maintained for employees when working with ETO. Many countries have strict regulations in place governing the safe use of ETO. Adequate ventilation, air exchanges and environmental monitoring are required. Ethylene oxide is a toxic gas even at very low concentrations, being listed as a carcinogen (cancer-associated). As an example, the typically recommended average exposure limit over an eight-hour day is 1 ppm, but the short-term exposure limit is actually only 5 ppm for 15 minutes; remember that under these conditions the gas cannot be detected by smell. The first safety limit is often referred to as the time weighted average (TWA), referring to the personnel exposure concentration measured over a specific period of time, usually eight hours. Personnel exposure is usually expressed as a TWA based on environmental exposure, measured by wearing a personal monitor (Figure 11.19). These recommended safety levels are periodically reviewed and may change depending on the individual country or region. Further terms that are used include:

- Permissible exposure limit (PEL), the maximum ETO exposure allowed per worker. It is the employer's responsibility to ensure that employees are not exposed to airborne concentrations of ETO in excess of this concentration. The required maximum exposure level is usually set at 1 ppm over a typical eight-hour working day.
- Excursion limit (EL) refers to workers' short-term exposure limit. No more than four exposure periods within this range are permitted within an eight-hour work day. This exposure is typically task related (transferring load to aerator, removing indicators from un-aerated load, changing cylinders, performing maintenance, etc.).

Low concentrations can lead to irritation of the eyes and mucous membranes, with higher concentrations being more damaging to health, as well as posing a flammability risk. Ethylene oxide installation requirements can vary regionally, but generally require a dedicated exhaust, emission controls, enclosed controlled ETO sterilizer/aerator room and monitoring systems. Gas manufacturer/suppliers' instructions (including safety sheets) should be consulted regarding ETO storage conditions. These will include storage in a well ventilated area under controlled conditions (including temperatures, flammable gas safety cabinets, etc.; Figure 11.20).

The levels of ETO present at any point in time and over time can be reliably monitored using a range of sensor systems (Figure 11.19). These include personal monitors that are recommended to be worn (as badges or pins) during a normal working day near to the "breathing zone" (on a lapel or upper pocket, as shown in Figure 11.19). The monitoring discs are collected and sent to an external laboratory for analysis, which provides a final result of the exposure to ETO during the time worn (within a range). They have the advantage of providing information regarding the actual exposure to ETO over a period of time within an area, but the results are not available until after the analysis (sometimes over days or weeks after being worn). Therefore, as additional safety precautions, real-time monitors or sensors are also recommended; these can range from being simple hand-held monitors (providing a digital display of the ETO concentration) to wall-mounted systems of varying complexity. It is common for such systems to provide

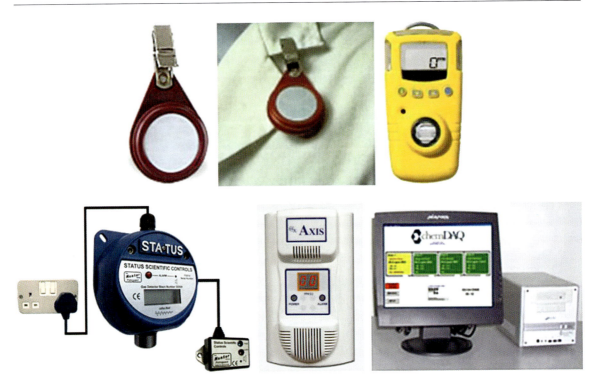

Figure 11.19 Ethylene oxide gas sensors and monitoring equipment. These include personal monitors (top left), handheld and wall-mounted sensors (top right) and (bottom) sensor examples.

visual (flashing light) or audible (siren) alarms at various warning or danger levels. Procedures should be in place and staff trained on the emergency procedures (including evacuation and area re-entry) to take place in the event of an alarm. Correct installation and maintenance of such systems are therefore important. In some countries, the results from personal monitoring and any excursions (including investigations and resolutions of any problems) are required to be maintained (archived) with personal history files.

Policies must be in place to ensure that sterilization loads are adequately aerated prior to storage and/or direct patient use. Even low levels of ETO remaining on devices or within packaging can lead to patient and staff toxicity risks. For example, ETO can be released over time from exposed loads within a storage area and, if not adequately ventilated, can cause toxicity problems to staff working in that area. In addition to ETO gas residuals, the gas can react with other chemicals present in/on the load and can form other toxic chemicals. For example, in preparation for sterilization, it is recommended that residual soil or excess liquids should not be present as they will not only hinder sterilization efficacy, but may also result in further harmful residuals being formed. These include:

• Water and ETO can generate ethylene glycol residuals.
• Saline and ETO can generate ethylene chlorohydrin, which is also a toxic chemical.

Therefore, efficient aeration is not only required to remove residuals of ETO, but also any other toxic by-products. This is initially conducted within the sterilizer (during the aeration phase of the cycle) and may be completed by further, extended aeration with the sterilizing chamber or in a specially designed aeration chamber. Aeration is achieved by holding the load at a given temperature and time, under a controlled number of air exchanges per minute (e.g. 4–6 air volume changes/minute). Aeration may also be assisted by drawing a vacuum within the chamber and pulsing steam/air into the chamber during the aeration process. The aeration requirements (time, temperature, number of air pulses/changes, etc.) should be specified by the manufacturer and specified for different types of loads. Staff should consider the correct aeration conditions not only for the devices, but also any other associated sterile packaging materials. If using a

Figure 11.20 A gas safety cabinet and typical warning signs used for ETO gas storage.

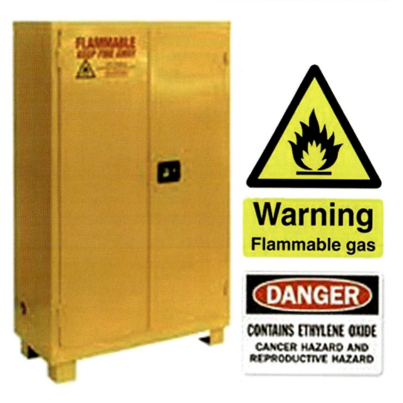

separate aeration chamber, the contents of the sterilizer need to be safely transferred to the aeration cabinet after completion of the sterilizer cycle (including initial aeration). Before transferring items it is important to confirm that the aerator has sufficient room to handle the load and is turned on (and working!) at the appropriate temperature. Typical aeration conditions (specified as a time/temperature relationship) are:

- 8 hours at 60°C (140°F)
- 10 hours at 54°C (130°F)
- 12 hours at 49°C (120°F)
- 20 hours at 38°C (100°F)

It is important to note that the overall aeration time/ conditions will depend on the ETO sterilization process and aeration system used (including the air exchanges provided), the thickness of the sterile barrier systems used, the design and weight of the load, the size and arrangement of packages in the sterilizer/aerator or aeration cabinet, and the number/types of ETO absorbent materials within the load or being aerated at any given time.

Due to the required balance of efficacy and safety requirement with ETO sterilization processes, it is important to ensure that ETO sterilizer and/or aerators are not overloaded or contain materials/load descriptions that have not been defined as suitable for this process by the manufacturer. With the long times associated with such sterilization processes, there is often a tendency to attempt to maximize load capacity, but this can lead to inefficient sterilization and safety (toxicity) risks.

Typical sterilizer design

Similar to steam sterilizers (see the section on steam sterilization), there are a variety of sizes and designs of ETO sterilizers (Figure 11.21). They range from benchtop to large capacity sterilizers. Most systems widely used in hospitals are similar to small steam sterilizers, consisting of a sterilization chamber, associated piping system (including air venting and a vacuum pump), associated control system and gauges (where applicable), and a steam (or humidity) supply. In addition, the sterilizers will have an associated ETO gas supply system, as well as a method of breaking down the residual ETO as it is being removed from the chamber. Two essentially different types of systems are commonly used: traditional chamber-based systems (which may apply the ETO sterilization under pressure or vacuum; Figure 11.17) and sterilization-in-a-bag type systems.

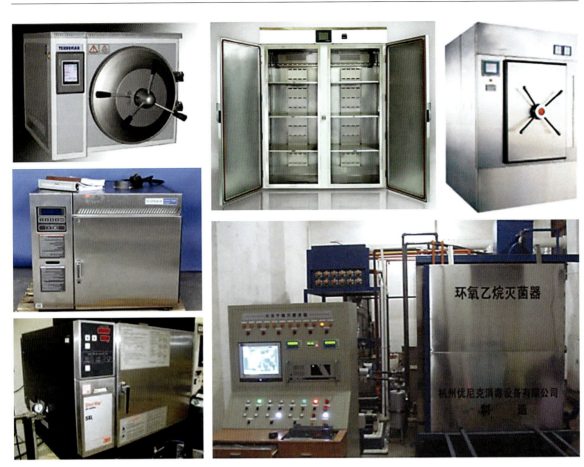

Figure 11.21 A variety of ethylene oxide sterilizer designs. Smaller sterilizer designs are shown on the far left and larger on the right. Note that all but one of the sterilizers (middle, top cabinet) shown are considered traditionally designed sterilizers, where a load is placed into the chamber and exposed to the process. The cabinet-based sterilizer is an example of a single dose or sterilization-in-a-bag type application, where the devices and a supply of ETO gas/humidity are placed into specially designed and sealed bags, and the sterilization process conducted within the bag but held within the exposure cabinet. Both designs can range in size, shape and sterilization cycle development.

The basic design of a traditional chamber-based ETO sterilizer is shown in Figure 11.22. The chamber is designed to handle the required pressures associated during the process, including low pressures for vacuum-based stages of the process and high pressures for such pressurized ETO processes. In some cases the chamber is also jacketed to allow for greater temperature control. Ethylene oxide sterilization chambers are more typically designed as single-door designs, although double-door designs are also available. In some designs, fans may also be present within the chamber to assist in the circulation of ETO gas/humidity and air during the process.

The chamber associated pipework allows for the introduction of humidity (usually in the form of steam, which can both heat and humidify the load), ETO gas, air and their safe removal. Ethylene oxide gas is generated by passing the provided liquid ETO over a heated surface and then introducing it into the chamber. The chamber is usually associated with a vacuum pump that allows low pressures (e.g. during air removal) to be applied within the chamber. As ETO is a toxic chemical, the exhaust of the gas during the process is rendered safe by passing it through an abater/catalytic converter system, which degrades the gas into carbon dioxide and

Figure 11.22 The basic design of a traditional, chamber-based or batch-type ETO sterilizer.

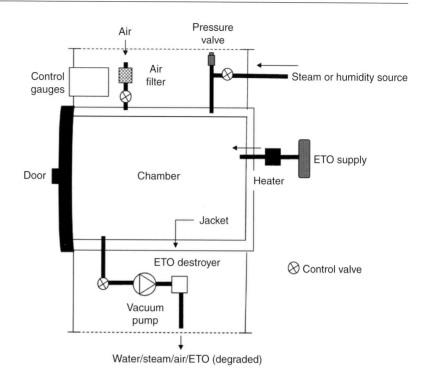

water (both naturally present in air). The whole process is controlled and monitored by a control system (which can be of varying complexity), including a recording system that records the variables of the process conducted. In these designs, the load is prepared, placed into the chamber and sterilized in a batch-type process; the load is only released following the completed cycle and may or may not be subjected to extended aeration as part of a separate cycle within the same chamber or in a separate aeration system (as described earlier).

Alternative, cabinet-based sterilizer designs are also used that provide a chamber for the control of heat and provision of sterilization utilities (e.g. air, water supply or exhaust system). In such designs, the sterilization process is actually conducted within specifically designed plastic bags (generally made of heavy-duty plastics such as low-density polyethylene, LDPE). These are often referred to as single-dose or sterilization-in-a-bag type applications, where the devices to be sterilized and a supply of ETO gas/humidity are placed into specially designed and sealed bags, and the sterilization process conducted within the bag but held within the exposure cabinet (for

conditioning, including heating, and aeration control of the process). The cabinet is not sealed, but allows the placement of a number of sterilization loads at different times into the chamber, depending on its capacity design. The chambers can range from single (bench-top) to multiple (large, standing cabinet) load designs. One hundred percent ETO is used, provided in ampoules (e.g. containing 5 or 20 mL of liquid ETO) specifically designed for a given bag capacity (e.g. 7 or 35 L capacity, respectively) or similarly, for larger sizes, provided within ETO-containing cartridges. The load is placed into the bag containing the ETO source and, in some designs, a water supply (for humidification), heat-sealed and then placed into the holding chamber. Bag designs often allow for their connection to the utility supply/aeration system contained within the sterilizer cabinet design. Such sterilizer designs have the advantages of using less ETO gas, often with minimal installation requirements and are often considered safer than the multiple cycle, gas tank systems described above. But they are also often restrictive in load capacity (and load type), can require longer exposure times and close attention of staff to ensure that the bags are correctly sealed during the process.

Table 11.12 Ethylene oxide sterilization guidelines and standards.

Guidelines/standards	Title	Description
ISO 11135-1:2007	*Sterilization of healthcare products. Ethylene oxide. Part 1: requirements for development, validation, and routine control of a sterilization process for medical devices*	Specifies requirements for the development, validation and routine control of an ethylene oxide sterilization process for medical devices.
ISO/TS 11135-2:2008	*Sterilization of healthcare products – ethylene oxide – part 2: guidance on the application of ISO 11135-1*	This is a guidance document on the application of ISO 1135-1 for ETO sterilization.
ISO 11138-2:2006	*Sterilization of healthcare products – biological indicators. Part 2: biological indicators for ethylene oxide sterilization processes*	Provides specific requirements for test organisms, suspensions, inoculated carriers, biological indicators and test methods intended for use in ethylene oxide gas sterilization processes.
ISO 10993-7	*Biological evaluation of medical devices. Part 7: ethylene oxide sterilization residuals*	Specifies allowable limits for residual ethylene oxide (EO) and ethylene chlorohydrin (ECH) on ETO-sterilized devices.
ANSI/AAMI ST41:2008	*Ethylene oxide sterilization in healthcare facilities: safety and effectiveness*	Guidelines on the safe and effective use of ETO for sterilization in the USA.
AS/NZS 4187:2003	*Cleaning, disinfecting and sterilizing re-usable medical and surgical instruments and equipment, and maintenance of associated environments in healthcare facilities*	General guidance on reprocessing, to include ethylene oxide sterilization (in Australia and New Zealand).
HTM 2010	*Sterilization*	Published in five parts, this guidance document for the UK includes detailed information on the design and testing of ETO sterilizers.
Canada Communicable Disease Report, 1998	*Hand washing, cleaning, disinfection and sterilization in health care*	Guidance includes recommendation on ETO sterilization.

Standards and guidelines

Table 11.12 provides a list of useful guidelines and standards regarding sterilization with ETO.

Formaldehyde gas

Formaldehyde (CH_2O), also chemically known as methanal, is a gas at room temperature and atmospheric pressure. It is generally provided as a white solid polymer (a molecule consisting of repeated single sub-units) known as paraformaldehyde (consisting or 8–100 repeated units of formaldehyde) or as a liquid (e.g. formalin solutions consisting of 34–40% of formaldehyde dissolved in water, often containing other chemicals such as methanol as chemical stabilizers). Formaldehyde is widely used in the chemical industry to make a variety of other chemicals such as resins (adhesives), plastics and paints. It has been traditionally used as a disinfect-

ant for a variety of applications, including as a gas for area/room fumigation and in liquids as a preservative (e.g. formaldehyde-releasing agents) and even as an antiseptics (e.g. for wart treatments). Formalin (formaldehyde solutions) are used in some hospital pathology departments for the treatment and mounting of tissue samples for microscopic investigations (in a discipline known as histology), but are rarely used as solutions or in formulation for disinfection or sterilization applications. This section primarily considers the use of formaldehyde gas for sterilization of re-usable devices, particularly for hospital and dental use. Humidified formaldehyde gas is used on its own, or in combination with other biocides (such as alcohol), for low (less than 60°C), intermediate (60–80°C) and even high temperature (e.g. at 134°C) application as alternatives to steam sterilization. They can therefore be used for temperature-sensitive devices/materials (which is their predominant use) or for temperature-resistant devices, depending on their design, process and manufacturer claims. Formaldehyde gas is widely appreciated as a broad-spectrum antimicrobial, including activity against bacterial spores. The most-resistant microorganism to formaldehyde is considered *Geobacillus stearothermophilus* spores and these are therefore used in the development and routine testing of formaldehyde gas sterilization processes. Its mechanisms of action appear to be predominantly due to its toxicity to cells and viruses, by reacting with the various types of molecules that give them structure and function, such as proteins and nucleic acids; formaldehyde reacts directly with these structures and can even cause them to cross-link to each other leading to loss of the structure/function for viability. In this sense, formaldehyde is a considerably toxic chemical. Depending on the exact process used, formaldehyde-based processes are considered very gentle on devices and materials due to the general lack of reactivity of the chemical with many of these surfaces; in particular the humidified formaldehyde gas-only processes are considered non-damaging to materials, devices and packaging. Despite this, some process conditions can be damaging to certain types of materials and devices; these should be specified by the process manufacturer. The main disadvantages of formaldehyde sterilization processes can include longer cycles times, requirements for extended aeration and particularly the associated toxicity of the chemical. Formaldehyde is toxic, being an irritant and is considered carcinogenic even at low exposure concentrations. Therefore, similar to the discussion with ETO (see the section on ethylene oxide sterilization), formaldehyde sterilization processes should be closely controlled; monitored and maintained to ensure that they are used safely.

Principles of formaldehyde sterilization

Formaldehyde gas requires the correct gas concentration, water (humidity) level, temperature and contact time for sterilization. Formaldehyde gas processes are found to be optimized when condensation of formaldehyde in solution in water is formed on the surfaces to be sterilized; a similar condensation process is required for sterilization with high temperature formaldehyde-alcohol based processes. Formaldehyde gas only processes are commonly referred to as low temperature steam formaldehyde (LTSF). The variables of these processes include:

- Formaldehyde gas concentration: this can vary significantly from process to process, but is generally in the sporicidal range of 5–50 mg/L. The gas is most commonly made by heating a liquid supply of formalin (ranging from 2 to 40% formaldehyde in solution). In some sterilizer designs, other chemicals may also be used as part of the antimicrobial process, such as high concentrations of ethanol (70% ethanol with ~0.25% formaldehyde in water).

- The temperature of the process can also vary significantly between manufacturers and in specified sterilizer cycles. The typical range is 50–80°C (122–176°C), depending on the specific process. Temperatures above 60°C, although considered "low temperature" in comparison to steam sterilization, may have limited application for certain types of devices. The best way to attain and maintain such temperatures, in combination with the high humidity requirements for formaldehyde sterilization, is by using low temperature steam (steam provided under vacuum, and as typically used for ETO-based processes; see the section on ethylene oxide sterilization). There are limited types of sterilizers that use much higher temperatures (132°C) in combination with lower concentrations of formaldehyde.

- High humidity levels are required for optimal formaldehyde sterilization. The required humidity levels are often cited at greater than 70% and up to 100%, but in most modern formaldehyde sterilizers 100% humidity at the required temperature is specified as being the optimal for sterilization, in particular to allow liquid formaldehyde to condensate onto surfaces to ensure its antimicrobial effects.

- The contact time is specified by the manufacturer to meet at least the minimal requirements for sterilization, such as a sterility assurance level of 10^{-6}. Typical sterilization times range depending on the process conditions, with shorter exposure times generally specified for higher temperature cycles (such as 65°C for 30 minutes and 80°C for 10 minutes).

There are essentially two types of formaldehyde-based sterilization processes: those based on LTSF sterilization and alternative high temperature formaldehyde/alcohol sterilization processes. Low temperature steam formaldehyde processes have been well described but are not widely used, with the exception of certain countries in Europe, Asia, the Middle East and South America. These are commonly larger types of sterilizers, often designed to provide low (formaldehyde gas) and high (steam) sterilization cycles within the same chamber design (see

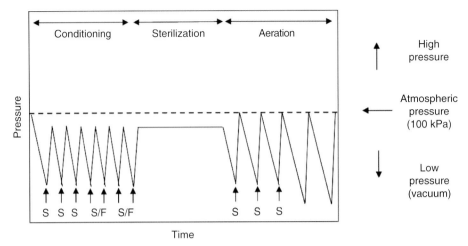

Figure 11.23 A typical low temperature steam formaldehyde (LTSF) sterilization process. The cycle can be described as three phase: conditioning, sterilization and aeration. The introduction of steam is indicated by S and steam/formaldehyde by S/F. Multiple steam, steam formaldehyde and air introduction pulses can be specified by the manufacturer depending on the sterilization process.

steam sterilization). Low temperature steam formaldehyde sterilizers are used for lower temperature sterilization of a variety of devices, including flexible/rigid endoscopes (and accessories), plastic materials (e.g. diathermy or other types of electrical cables) and other heat-sensitive materials/devices. High temperature formaldehyde/alcohol chemical processes are even less used, such as small table-top types of sterilizers for small dental and medical clinics. A typical representation of such a process is shown in Figure 11.23.

A typical LTSF process will have three main stages:
• Conditioning: the conditioning phase is programmed to achieve air removal, heating, humidification and formaldehyde gas distribution in the load as a requirement for sterilization. The load is first pre-treated by a series of low pressure (vacuum) pulsing, followed by the introduction of steam. This is to ensure air removal and steam penetration (for humidification and heating). Following these pre-treatment pulses, a similar series of vacuum pulses with the introduction of formaldehyde gas and steam is conducted to ensure that the formaldehyde gas/humidity requirements are obtained within the load. The gas is generally made from a liquid formaldehyde solution (e.g. ranging from 2 to 40% in water) that is heated and introduced into a chamber with steam to a pre-specified pressure setting. The number of formaldehyde pulse injections will depend on the specific cycle (e.g. up to ten pulses).

• Sterilization: formaldehyde is a relatively stable molecule and is held at the pre-conditioned state for the length of the sterilization cycle (which can range from 10 to 60 minutes, or even longer). During this time the formaldehyde concentration, temperature, pressure and humidity are considered to be constant, where the temperature can be maintained by a heating mechanism from the walls of the sterilizer chamber (as used with a jacketed chamber; see the section on typical sterilizer design). Formaldehyde sterilization is generally conducted under low pressure, which will also prevent formaldehyde from leaking from the chamber.

• Aeration (also known as "desorption" or post-treatment conditioning): during this stage the load is treated to remove formaldehyde (or other associated) residues. This can be achieved by a series of vacuum pulses within the chamber, followed by the introduction of steam as a flushing mechanism and/or by similarly pulling a vacuum and pulsing with air. The example shown in Figure 11.23 shows a series of vacuum/steam pulses followed by a series of lower (deeper) vacuum and air pulsing. Such aeration cycles are developed to be efficient for the specified applications, although in the case of some types of materials/loads, extended aeration of the load may be required prior to transport and direct patient use. The formaldehyde gas residues from the chamber are commonly removed from the air by condensation (cooling) and are diluted/flushed to the drain with water.

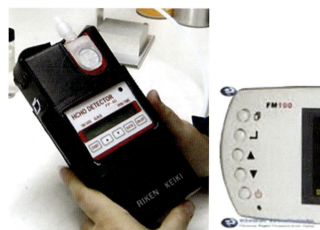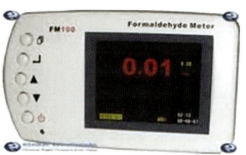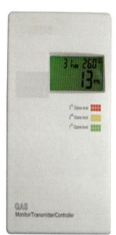

Figure 11.24 Various types of formaldehyde gas sensors.

Formaldehyde is considered biodegradable over a couple of hours in the environment. Following the process, the load may also need to be dried and may be assisted within the chamber by a series of vacuum pulses under controlled temperature or performed in a separate drying cabinet.

The other type of formaldehyde sterilizers are the high temperature chemical sterilizers combining heat (at 132°C), formaldehyde (at low concentrations, ~0.25%) and ethanol (72%). In these processes, the formaldehyde/ethanol liquid is heated to 132°C under pressure (138 kPa) to cause it to vaporize, be held in the presence of the load for the required exposure time and then aerated to remove the chemical residues. In more modern and safer sterilizer designs, during aeration the air is passed through specific types of filter to remove any associated harmful chemicals/residuals.

Formaldehyde is known to be a toxic, irritating and allergenic chemical; it is also referenced to be a suspected carcinogen, but this is often debated as it is also a naturally occurring molecule in the body. Considering toxicity risks, tight controls are recommended regarding the safe use of formaldehyde. For example, the recommended full day's (eight-hour) working limit is 0.5 ppm (also known as the maximum allowable concentration, MAC), with a maximum limit of 1.1 ppm over 15 minutes (noting that 1 ppm is ~1.2 mg/cm^3 of formaldehyde in air). Formaldehyde has a pungent odor that can be detected by smell at ~0.05 ppm, with nose and eye irritation being sensed at 0.01 to 1.2 ppm (depending on the person). A variety of different types of sensors, handheld

and wall-mounted, can be used for the routine or contact monitoring of formaldehyde gas in a given area (Figure 11.24). These can be designed to be specific to formaldehyde or may be used to detect multiple types of gases.

Typical sterilizer design

Formaldehyde gas-based sterilizers can be provided in a variety of sizes, but in most cases bench-top sterilizers are used in limited applications for high-temperature formaldehyde/alcohol-based processes and larger capacity sterilizers for low temperature steam-formaldehyde (LTSF) systems (Figure 11.25). The essential designs of formaldehyde sterilizers are similar to those described for ETO-based processes (see ethylene oxide sterilization) and are summarized in Figure 11.26.

The chamber is usually constructed of stainless steel and, depending on the process, may be designed to withstand high pressure (i.e. a pressure vessel, similar to that described for steam sterilizers. Although this may not be required for low temperature formaldehyde gas sterilization, many designs are provided as dual process sterilizers being used for both high temperature (steam) and low temperature (formaldehyde gas) sterilizers. In such cases, a rapid cooling and/or heating system may also be provided with, or programmed into, the sterilizer design to allow for alternate high or low temperature processes to be chosen without the need of extended pre-cooling or heating prior to placing a load into the sterilizer; note: a cold chamber can cause excessive condensation to

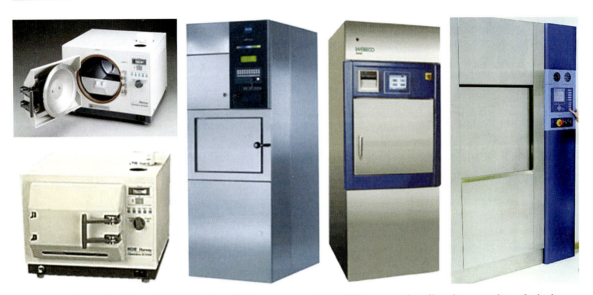

Figure 11.25 Examples of formaldehyde-based sterilization processes. On the left are examples of bench-top sterilizers for high temperature formaldehyde/alcohol processes and on the right are larger LTSF sterilizers.

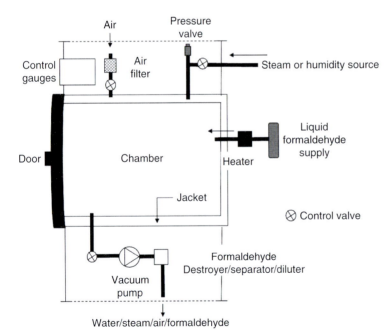

Figure 11.26 The basic design of a formaldehyde sterilizer. A chamber jacket may or may not be present, the sterilizer chamber may be a single or double-door design and formaldehyde supply may be mixed with other chemicals used as part of the process.

occur within a load during a high temperature steam sterilization process and initial high temperatures within the chamber could cause some damage to certain types of loads designated for low temperature steriliza-tion. For high temperature formaldehyde-alcohol sterilizers, these are required to be pressure vessels as the process is dependent on providing steam under pressure.

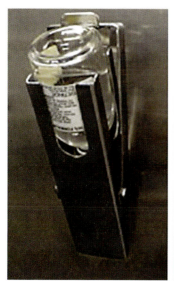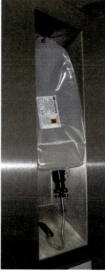

Figure 11.27 Examples of liquid formaldehyde solution delivery systems, including a formaldehyde solution containing a multiple dose glass bottle (left) and a plastic bag (right).

Steam, for humidification and load heating, is provided to the chamber either from an external source (house steam supply or separate, local boiler) or through an integrated electrically heated steam generator within the design of the sterilizer itself. Formaldehyde-containing solutions are provided in single or multiple-dose containers, being supplied to a heater to generate formaldehyde gas at the required stages of the programmed sterilization cycles (Figure 11.27).

Sterilizer designs will include an air vent, where air entering the chamber will pass through a HEPA filter to prevent the ingress of bacteria and other microorganisms during the process. The associated pipework will also include a vacuum pump, to be able to provide the necessary low pressure requirement within the chamber for any applicable cycle stage (both in high or low temperature applications). Formaldehyde residues removed from the chamber are often simply diluted in water and flushed to drain; formaldehyde is generally considered unstable in the environment, being degraded over a number of hours into products such as water (H_2O) and carbon dioxide (CO_2). Alternative systems may include formaldehyde destroyers that degrade any formaldehyde residuals prior to release into the environment. The full sterilizer processes/cycles will be microprocessor controlled and may be associated with various process gauges, recorders and/or cycle printers.

Standards and guidelines

Some examples of guidelines and standards regarding formaldehyde sterilization are given in Table 11.13.

Hydrogen peroxide gas (including plasma processes)

Hydrogen peroxide (H_2O_2) is a liquid at ambient temperature and atmospheric pressure. It is commonly used as a bleaching agent (e.g. for paper and hair), as a propellant and industrially for the manufacturing of other chemicals. Its antimicrobial properties have been appreciated for many years, being used as an antiseptic, disinfectant and sterilant. At the same time, it is often considered as a "safe" biocide, for example being recognized as GRAS ("generally recognized as safe") in the USA. As a disinfectant it is used in liquid (as direct solutions in water or as part of a formulated mixture with other chemicals) or in gas form (Chapter 9, in the section on peroxygens) for device or general surface disinfection applications. For sterilization applications it is predominantly used in gas form. Hydrogen peroxide gas (or vapor) is generated by heating liquid peroxide; the temperature required will vary depending on the concentration of peroxide in the water, with examples being under atmospheric pressure at 108°C (226°F) with a 35% peroxide and 114°C (237°F) with a 50% peroxide solution. In accordance with the gas laws (Chapter 6), this can be achieved at low temperatures under vacuum (low pressure) conditions. In associated sterilization processes, this is typically achieved by flash heating (e.g. using a heated surface or other heating source) a given volume of 50–60% liquid hydrogen peroxide. Pure samples of peroxide in water are very stable, but when generated into gas it has a relatively short life and in particular with reaction on various surfaces, including devices and microorganisms. Note that a vapor and a gas are chemically similar, with the distinction being that a vapor is a gas that can readily revert back into its liquid form (condense) under the right conditions (e.g. at a given temperature/pressure and depending on the concentration of the gas). In this sense, hydrogen peroxide and water gases are both considered vapors, while ethylene oxide and formaldehyde in their own rights are considered "true" gases, as they have a preference to be in gas form under ambient temperature/atmospheric pressure. Hydrogen peroxide gas, depending on the process, may be used under condensed (oversaturated; gas and liquid present) or under-saturated (gas only) conditions for sterilization applications. The specific conditions within a given sterilization process may not be known or described.

Table 11.13 Examples of guidelines and standards for formaldehyde sterilization processes.

Guidelines/standards	Title	Description
ISO 25424:2009	*Sterilization of medical devices – low temperature steam and formaldehyde – requirements for development, validation and routine control of a sterilization process for medical devices*	Specifies requirements for the development, validation and routine control of a low temperature steam and formaldehyde (LTSF) sterilization process for devices.
ISO 11138-5:2006	*Sterilization of healthcare products. Biological indicators. Part 5: biological indicators for low-temperature steam and formaldehyde sterilization processes*	Specific requirements for test organisms, suspensions, inoculated carriers, biological indicators and test methods intended for use in assessing the performance of sterilization processes employing low-temperature steam and formaldehyde as the sterilizing agent.
EN 15424:2007	*Sterilization of medical devices. Low temperature steam and formaldehyde. Requirements for development, validation and routine control of a sterilization process for medical devices*	Requirements that will enable the demonstration that a low temperature steam and formaldehyde sterilization process has appropriate microbiocidal activity.
EN14180:2003+A2:2009	*Sterilizers for medical purposes. Low temperature steam and formaldehyde sterilizers. Requirements and testing.*	Requirements for the design and performance to formaldehyde sterilizers.
ISO 14937: 2009	*Sterilization of healthcare products. General requirements for characterization of a sterilizing agent and the development, validation and routine control of a sterilization process for medical devices.*	Specifies general requirements for the characterization of any sterilizing agent and for the development, validation and routine monitoring and control of a sterilization process for devices.
BS 3970-5:1990	*Sterilizing and disinfecting equipment for medical products. Specification for low temperature steam disinfectors.*	Particular requirements for equipment used for disinfection or sterilization of heat-sensitive products using formaldehyde.
HTM 2010	*Sterilization*	Published in five parts, this guidance document for the UK includes detailed information on the design and testing of formaldehyde sterilizers.
AAMI/WD-2 ST58	*Chemical sterilization and high-level disinfection in healthcare facilities*	Guidelines for the selection and use of chemical sterilizing agents and high-level disinfectants (HLDs) that have been cleared for marketing by the USA-FDA for use in hospitals and other healthcare facilities.

Hydrogen peroxide gas is a very powerful antimicrobial, being much more effective than liquid preparations at lower concentrations (e.g. 0.0000–0.001% in gas form are typically used in comparison to 2–6% or higher for liquid-based applications). Depending on the concentration and contact time, peroxide gas is considered an effective antimicrobial, including rapid bactericidal, fungicidal, cysticidal, virucidal and sporicidal activity. In addition, the gas form (but notably not the liquid form, with the exception potentially of high concentration, >60% peroxide) has been shown to be effective under certain conditions against prions, toxins (including bacterial endotoxins; see Chapter 6, section on bacteria) and to penetrate over time through organic soils (including blood). *Geobacillus stearothermophilus* spores are considered the most resistant organism to hydrogen peroxide gas and are therefore used for determining the minimal sterilization process conditions (e.g. in determining the conditions for a demonstrated minimum SAL of 10^{-6}) and for routine monitoring of the process (where biological indicators are used; see the section on Process monitoring).

The mode of action of peroxide gas is due to its activity as an oxidizing agent, being considered to have effects on various molecules that make up microbial structure/

function, including proteins, nucleic acids and lipids; it has been reported that the specific mechanisms of action of liquid peroxide are distinct from gaseous peroxide, but the overall effects are antimicrobial.

In addition to being an effective antimicrobial the gas can be safe for use on most device and material types, including electrical components and electronics, although this will vary depending on the process conditions (e.g. exposure time, concentration, temperature, etc.). Depending on the sterilization application/process, negative effects can include loss of color (bleaching) over time, loss of activity on contacting certain types of materials (e.g. paper, wood and brass/copper, thereby losing antimicrobial activity) and damage to some types of materials (particularly adhesives). Hydrogen peroxide gas has a good safety profile, but is considered toxic even at concentrations as low as 1 ppm over time. Being unstable, it rapidly breaks down in the environment.

Principles of hydrogen peroxide gas sterilization

Hydrogen peroxide gas sterilization activity is primarily dependent on the gas concentration and exposure time, but is also affected by the process temperature.

• Hydrogen peroxide gas concentration: hydrogen peroxide has been shown to be sporicidal at as low as 0.1 mg/L gas concentrations, but typical concentrations used for sterilization processes are set at a higher range (e.g. 5–10 mg/L); however, the initial concentration of gas introduced into a chamber will degrade over time (particularly in the presence of a load for sterilization) and therefore the sterilization cycle should be developed at the lowest concentration found in the presence of a worst case load for the manufacturer-defined process conditions. As the concentration increases, the sporicidal activity increases (contact time for antimicrobial activity decreases), with a typical log reduction for bacterial spores (of *Geobacillus stearothermophilus*) being ten minutes a 0.1 mg/L and one minute at 1 mg/L. Temperatures can impact the activity of the gas in two ways. First, increased temperatures can improve the sporicidal activity of the gas but have the negative effect of degrading the peroxide quicker over time (into water and oxygen, both ineffective as antimicrobials). Second, in accordance with the gas laws, maintaining peroxide in gas form is dependent on the temperature (therefore at lower temperatures peroxide gas will condense to revert to its preferred liquid state); in addition to temperature, this will also vary depending on the pressure and the presence of humidity (water in gas form). Hydrogen peroxide gas does not appear to have the same requirement,

as defined with other antimicrobial gases, for high humidity levels to ensure sporicidal activity. Humidity is, however, always present as peroxide gas is generated from liquid peroxide solutions at 50–60% in 50–40% water, and will increase as peroxide degrades into water and oxygen during the exposure process. It is therefore typical that pulses of hydrogen peroxide gas are introduced and held in the sterilization chamber for a specific period of time, then removed and replaced with a fresh pulse of peroxide gas for the desired contact time and number of pulses.

• Contact time: the overall contact time for sterilization will depend on the conditions defined by the manufacturer in the design of the specific process. Typical exposure times for sterilization can typically range from 10 to 30 minutes, depending on the process, with various levels of overkill (e.g. at or over an SAL of 10^{-6}).

Similar to other physical and chemical sterilization processes, a number of phases are defined during a typical cycle in order to ensure that the load is prepared for sterilization, sterilized and rendered safe for patient use (Figure 11.28). These include:

• Conditioning: this stage is designed primarily to remove air from the load, which may be simply facilitated by drawing a deep vacuum (low pressure, for example 0.053 kPa, equivalent to 0.0005 bar, 0.0077 psi or 0.4 Torr). During this phase the load may also be further preconditioned by heating (within the chamber maintained as a given pressure) and/or drying. In general, drying is not necessary, as according to most manufacturers' instructions with these sterilization processes, loads should be pre-dried before placing within the chamber as excessive moisture can lead to cycle failure. Note: hydrogen peroxide gas, like other gaseous or low temperature sterilization methods, is not used to sterilize liquids such as water. Conditioning may be enhanced, in particular air removal and drying during this phase by pulsing the vacuum levels or by adding other heating methods (such as the generation of plasma during this phase, which is employed in some sterilizer designs).

• Sterilization: hydrogen peroxide gas is generated from liquid hydrogen peroxide solutions (typically in the 50–60%) range. Examples of different methods of liquid peroxide supply to sterilizer designs are shown in Figure 11.29.

Gas is generated from liquid by vaporization, the rapid heating of liquid by dropping it onto a hot surface (a heating block, which can be of various designs), and then introduced into the chamber that is already under vacuum to allow rapid penetration of the gas. The

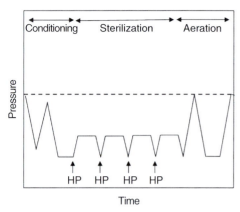

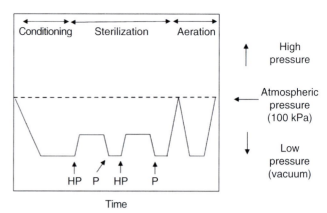

Figure 11.28 Examples of hydrogen peroxide gas sterilization processes. Two examples are shown, with hydrogen peroxide gas alone (left) and peroxide gas utilizing plasma generation (right). On the left, a pulsing conditioning cycle is shown, followed by a four-pulse sterilization phase with the introduction of peroxide gas, exposure and then removal (by pulling a vacuum) in each pulse and aeration (by applying a vacuum to the load, assisted by heat). On the right is a similar cycle, with a simpler conditioning cycle, a two-pulse peroxide gas exposure (with exposure to peroxide gas, removal and plasma generation in each pulse), followed by aeration.

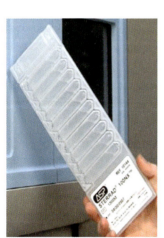

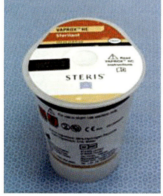

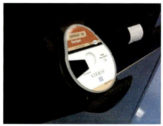

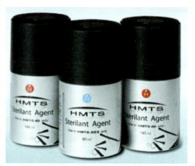

Figure 11.29 Examples of liquid hydrogen peroxide supply methods used in different types of peroxide gas sterilizers. All designs shown provide sufficient liquid hydrogen peroxide for multiple, respective sterilization cycles. In the centre is a supply cartridge system (top centre) and when placed into the sterilizer delivery system (bottom centre).

introduction of the gas causes a rise in pressure within the chamber. The temperature at which hydrogen peroxide "boils" into a gas (boiling point) will depend on its concentration in water, for example 108°C (226°F) with 35% peroxide and 114°C (237°F) with 50% peroxide; as the peroxide gas degrades at a higher temperature, this can be minimized by vaporization at lower temperatures under low pressures. Some systems will use alternative heating sources to heating blocks to generate the gas, such as the minimal use of plasma generation (see below) on the liquid as an energy source. As hydrogen peroxide gas degrades over time, including on contact with the load, it is generally held for a programmed exposure time, residual gas is removed by re-pulling a vacuum within the chamber and then a further pulse of hydrogen peroxide gas is introduced. In some processes (known as gas plasma), a plasma is generated on any remaining liquid/gas within the chamber following the re-drawing of a vacuum and prior to introduction of fresh peroxide gas (Figure 11.28); the concept of plasma generation is discussed below, but it is used as a method to break down peroxide residuals. The number of pulses can typically range from two to four and exposure times can vary, but this will depend on the sterilization process and will be specified by the individual manufacturer (and for each cycle defined).

• Aeration: this phase is designed to remove any hydrogen peroxide (gas or liquid, if present as part of the process) residuals from the load. This is usually conducted in the heated chamber by pulling (and/or pulsing) a vacuum within the chamber/load; aeration may also be assisted by the generation of a plasma during this phase.

Many types of hydrogen peroxide gas sterilizers are commonly referred to as gas plasma sterilization systems. These describe the use or generation of "plasma" at some stage (or stages) during the process of sterilization. As introduced in Chapter 6 (see the section on solids, gases, liquids and plasmas), there are essentially three states of matter: solids, liquids and gases, depending on the energy provided to it. In true chemical-physical terms, plasma is essentially a gas that has been further energized (or ionized; see the section on solids, gases, liquids and plasmas). Plasma is therefore considered the fourth state of matter, being generated when sufficient energy is provided to a gas (e.g. hydrogen peroxide or indeed any gas) to break the gas molecule into its basic chemical parts. In the case of hydrogen peroxide (H_2O_2), this will essentially be hydrogen (H) and oxygen (O) in various reactive and unstable forms such as $^{\bullet}OH$ (the "hydroxyl radical"; note the position of the $^{\bullet}$), OH^-, O_2^-

and H^+, etc. This creates a very reactive mixture of chemicals/species, as well as releasing energy (in the form of light, such as UV light) that can actually combine to provide a potent antimicrobial effect. When the energy source is then turned off, the molecules will recombine to include various stable species particularly water (H_2O) and oxygen (O_2). For the above reasons, plasmas have been the focus of much research into their application as antimicrobial processes in their own right. Despite this, to date, plasmas have not been used alone for their antimicrobial effects in standardized sterilization processes; these are specifically discussed later in this chapter as new developments in low temperature sterilization. Their actual role in hydrogen peroxide gas sterilization processes has been the subject of much debate. In these systems the primary antimicrobial effects appear to be due to hydrogen peroxide gas alone; although the generation of plasma during the cycle may have a role as an antimicrobial, to date it has been shown to be minimal. Plasma generation does, however, play an important role as part of these processes. For example, the most widely used hydrogen peroxide gas plasma systems are the STERRAD® systems (Figure 11.30). Depending on the specific design and processes provided, plasma is used as a heating source (e.g. during conditioning) and primarily as a method of degrading residual peroxide (into water and oxygen) that remains following exposure to hydrogen peroxide gas. An example of such a process is shown in Figure 11.28, where following the introduction and exposure to hydrogen peroxide, the majority of the gas is removed by pulling a vacuum in the chamber and only then is the plasma generated; in such process conditions the plasma has been shown to have little antimicrobial effects as part of cycle but is an effective way of removing toxic residuals. Non-plasma systems use other methods for ensuring that such residuals are safely removed as part of the sterilization process. Since the initial development of plasma systems, particularly in recent years, there has been a range of alternative hydrogen peroxide gas plasma systems developed. These may use plasma in a similar manner, as discussed previously, but also as a method of generating peroxide gas from a liquid source (at lower energy levels), as a heating mechanism, as a drying method (to remove water from the load prior to exposure) and/or for enhancing aeration. In all cases, the sterilizer manufacturer should provide details regarding the specific sterilization cycle conditions/processes used.

An interesting topic regarding the development of hydrogen peroxide (or indeed other degrading biocide-based)

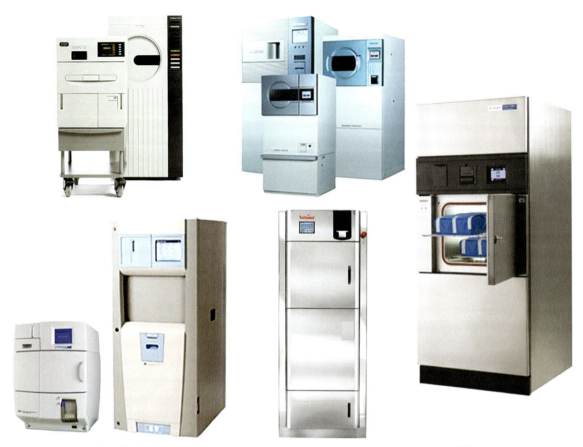

Figure 11.30 Examples of hydrogen peroxide gas sterilizers. They can be considered as using plasma or not as part of their sterilization processes. On the far left are examples of the STERRAD® series of plasma sterilizers (with older type systems shown above and newer NX™-based processes below), various other designs of plasma sterilizers (centre) and an example of a peroxide gas-only system (the V-PRO series that do not use plasma).

gas processes is the ability to ensure that the gas can adequately penetrate the load and individual devices. As already described above, the conditioning phase of such processes should be designed to ensure the adequate removal of air from the load/chamber prior to exposure. This can be a particular challenge in many situations, similar to the use of other gases used for sterilization (including steam in some cases). For example, liquids such as water cannot be sterilized using hydrogen peroxide gas; this is particularly important when significant water residuals remain on a surface and can hinder the penetration of the gas to the surface. In many sterilizer designs the presence of water can be indirectly detected by the process conditions being controlled by the sterilizer (in particular the ability to draw low pressures/vacuum within the chamber); in such designs

this can cause the cycle to abort or be extended to ensure drying has occurred prior to sterilization. A further issue is to avoid the use of various types of materials that could significantly absorb and/or break down the peroxide, with an example being paper or other cellulose-based materials. Such materials can be used as packaging materials for steam sterilization but when a significant amount of this material is present in a peroxide gas sterilizer it acts like a sponge to rapidly reduce the available gas concentration required for activity. Therefore, such materials should be avoided, with only packaging material recommended by the sterilizer manufacturer being used. As a further precaution, chemical indicators (CIs) specific to the sterilization process should be used to ensure that the correct concentration of peroxide is present in the load. A final consideration is the penetration of gas through a lumen of a device, such as rigid and flexible endoscopes (see Chapter 4). Lumened devices provide a challenge to all types of sterilization processes, due to the residual air that can remain within the lumen, impeding the penetration of the gas. In all hydrogen peroxide sterilizer designs, the lumen penetration limitations are generally defined by the manufacturer. These are traditionally based on the diameter and length of the device lumen, but will also depend on the number of lumens and type of material the lumen is made from (e.g. plastic or stainless steel). Such claims can often be confusing and may be regularly updated and changed based on the manufacturer and/or local regulatory approval. Various methods can be used to improve lumen penetration, such as pressure/vacuum pulsing mechanisms, number and process type of hydrogen peroxide exposure pulses, longer peroxide exposure conditions and increased peroxide concentrations. As an example, the newer series of STERRAD NX processes provide a different sterilization process to the traditional STERRAD series, in that as part of the process the hydrogen peroxide gas is concentrated concentrated and then exposed to the load; this is achieved by forming hydrogen peroxide gas from the liquid supply, removing the water (by a selective condensation process), and applying the concentrated gas to the load. Under these conditions it is shown that lumen penetration is improved, as defined by the manufacturer. Note that in many hydrogen peroxide sterilizer designs different sterilization processes are provided for various types of loads, including non-lumened devices, stainless steel-containing or rigid lumened devices and flexible endoscopic devices; therefore care should be taken to ensure that staff are correctly trained on which cycle is correct for different types of loads. Overall, given the range of sterilizers and associated sterilization processes available, close attention should be paid to the manufacturer's instructions, particularly limitations on device/packaging materials and claims of sterilization with lumened devices.

Similar to all sterilant gases, hydrogen peroxide is considered toxic. It can be noxious at low concentrations (e.g. 5–10 ppm), and a recommended safety level within an area is typically defined at 1 ppm over a typical eight-hour working day; a recommended short-term exposure limit is also defined at no more than 75 ppm for 15 minutes. Note: typical sporicidal concentrations of hydrogen peroxide gas are in excess of 75 ppm and for sterilization processes are generally greater than 1000 ppm. Handheld and wall-mounted sensors are available for monitoring such low level safety concentrations within a given area, and can include alarm systems that trigger a warning when excessive levels of peroxide gas are detected. Hydrogen peroxide gas is short-lived, rapidly degrading in the environment to water and oxygen; it is therefore often considered safer for use as a sterilization agent than alternative ETO or formaldehyde processes. Liquid hydrogen peroxide can also present a safety risk, particularly at the concentrations used in sterilization processes. Remember, at low concentrations (e.g. 3%) peroxide can be safely used on the skin and hair, but at higher concentrations (such as in the 30–60% range) it can burn the skin and at even higher concentration (e.g. >80%) is used as a rocket propellant! As with all chemicals, it should be handled with care. Liquid peroxide delivery systems can be designed to ensure that there is minimal risk on exposure, to include being tamper-proof and to be empty following use in a sterilizer design. Some sterilizer designs can also provide a mechanism for the safe disposal of expired peroxide containers/delivery systems prior to placing in normal waste; others may require special handling and chemical disposal precautions. In addition, if any suspicious liquid is detected in the chamber or on a load following a sterilization cycle, it should always be suspected as being hydrogen peroxide and may be present at relatively high concentrations. In such cases the load should not be used, only handled with gloves and the sterilizer investigated to ensure it is operating correctly.

Typical sterilizer design

Hydrogen peroxide gas-based sterilizers can be considered as two design types: those that use and those that do not use plasma as part of their design (Figure 11.30). Although these sterilizers can provide a variety of different and unique sterilization processes, their basic designs are very similar (Figure 11.31). The chamber is typically made of aluminum but other types of metals/materials can be used, is designed to be able to withstand and maintain vacuum conditions. Single or double-door versions are available, which can be manual or automated for opening/closing. A chamber jacket may be present to optimize heating within the chamber. In gas plasma sterilizer designs, the plasma sources may be located within the chamber (along the walls), built into the chamber walls and/or, depending on its use during a particular process, at a remote location from the chamber (e.g. as a method of vaporization or in destroyer designs). Depending on the specific design, when plasma is generated within the chamber it is recommended that the load

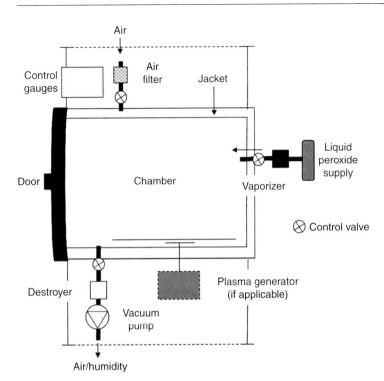

Figure 11.31 Typical basic design of a hydrogen peroxide gas sterilizer. The plasma source is only used on those designs that utilize plasma as part of the sterilization process and can include the generation of the plasma within and/or remote to the chamber. A vaporizer or other heating mechanism can be used to generate the gas at the appropriate stages of the programmed cycle.

(and particularly metal objects) are not allowed to touch the walls of the chamber/door due to risks of arcing (sparking) during the cycle. A hydrogen peroxide gas generation system is included, providing the gas during the required stages of the cycle. This will include a system of peroxide liquid delivery, vaporization (at a specific temperature and pressure) and injection into the chamber. In addition, the chamber is connected to a vacuum pump for removal of air and/or peroxide gas; it is typical for the gas to be broken down (e.g. by passing through a catalytic converter) prior to being released into the immediate environment. Air can be introduced into the chamber, passing through a HEPA filter. The complete system is under microprocessor control, including various different types of sensors for process control (such as temperature, pressure and volume sensors).

Standards and guidelines
Table 11.14 provides a list of standards and guidelines associated with the use of hydrogen peroxide gas sterilizers. It should be noted that at the time of writing a range of newer guidelines are under development due to

the increased use and range of such sterilizers for healthcare applications.

Liquid peracetic acid
Peracetic acid (PAA, CH_3COOOH, also known as peroxyacetic acid) is a liquid at atmospheric pressure and ambient temperature. It is widely used industrially for the manufacturing of other chemicals/materials and is particularly used for disinfection and/or sterilization of surfaces in a liquid form. Gaseous peracetic acid-based sterilization has been described in the past (e.g. PAA plasma sterilization processes) but has not been commercially successful to date (such applications are considered briefly under other processes). It is supplied in a liquid form (5–37% PAA in water) and is always found in the presence of its breakdown products (referred to chemically as being in equilibrium with) water, hydrogen peroxide and acetic acid (Figure 11.32). For example, 35% peracetic acid will contain 40% acetic acid, 18% water and 7% hydrogen peroxide, with the concentrations of water and acetic acid increasing as the PAA degrades or is used up. The acetic

Table 11.14 Standards and guidelines applicable for hydrogen peroxide gas sterilizers.

Guidelines/standards	Title	Description
ISO 14937: 2009	*Sterilization of healthcare products. General requirements for characterization of a sterilizing agent and the development, validation and routine control of a sterilization process for medical devices*	Specifies general requirements for the characterization of any sterilizing agent and for the development, validation and routine monitoring and control of a sterilization process for devices.
ISO 11138: 20xx	*Sterilization of healthcare products – biological indicators. Part 6: biological indicators for hydrogen peroxide vapour sterilization processes*	Specific requirements for test organisms, suspensions, inoculated carriers, biological indicators and test methods intended for use in assessing the performance of sterilizers and sterilization processes employing hydrogen peroxide vapor as the sterilizing agent.
ISO 18472:2006	*Sterilization of healthcare products – biological and chemical indicators – test equipment*	Specifies the requirements for test equipment to be used to test chemical and biological indicators including for hydrogen peroxide gas processes for conformity to the requirements given in ISO 11140-1 for chemical indicators, or the requirements given in the ISO 11138 series for biological indicators.
ANSI/AAMI ST58: 2005	*Chemical sterilization and high-level disinfection in healthcare facilities*	Provides guidelines for the selection and use of liquid chemical sterilants (LCSs)/high level disinfectants (HLDs) and gaseous chemical sterilizers that have been cleared for marketing by the US Food and Drug Administration (FDA) for use in hospitals and other healthcare facilities.
AS/NZS 4187:2003	*Cleaning, disinfecting and sterilizing re-usable medical and surgical instruments and equipment, and maintenance of associated environments in healthcare facilities*	General guidance on reprocessing, to include low temperature sterilization (in Australia and New Zealand).

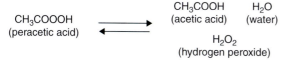

Figure 11.32 Typical components of a PAA-based solution shown in equilibrium.

acid component gives these preparations a strong "vinegar" odor (note: household vinegar contains 4–8% acetic acid), which can be quite noxious at high concentrations.

As an alternative to such commercial solutions, PAA can also be generated by combining other chemicals in water such as sodium perborate or sodium percarbonate with acetylsalicylic acid, or tetraacetylethylenedi-amine (TAED) with hydrogen peroxide. When supplied on its own such solutions can have a very low, acidic pH (e.g. pH 2.5) and under such conditions are considered very corrosive. For this reason PAA is not used on its own but as part of a formulation (mixture of chemical) for disinfection and sterilization applications. The formulation effects can be designed to optimize the antimicrobial activity of PAA and minimize any negative effects, such as potential damage to surfaces; as an example, PAA-based disinfectants/sterilants generally have a pH within the 5–8 range. These can range considerably in antimicrobial efficacy, safety, device compatibility and practical applications. They are widely used for high-level disinfection applications (in particular as alternatives to traditional aldehyde-based disinfectants such as glutaraldehyde; Chapter 9), but some

PAA-based processes have been designed for liquid chemical sterilization applications. These are further considered in this section.

Peracetic acid is an oxidizing agent and has been shown to affect the structure/function of various molecules, including protein, lipids and nucleic acids, which are essential to microbiological structure and function; these effects culminate to cause cellular death or loss of viral infectivity. Peracetic acid is considered an effective biocide with well-described broad spectrum activity; it is considered particularly effective, depending on the concentration present, even in the presence of organic/inorganic soil that can often interfere with the activity of liquid/gas-based processes.

Peracetic acid liquid sterilization processes are very rapid (less than 30 minutes) and safe for use on water immiscible instrumentation, but do not allow for sterile storage of the devices following sterilization. For this reason, they are often referred to as "just-in-time" or immediate use processes, where the device is immediately used for the medical/surgical procedure following sterilization.

Principles of liquid peracetic acid sterilization

Although PAA is widely used as a disinfectant/sterilant, only a limited number of processes have been developed to date that provide sterilization claims (e.g. in compliance to ISO 14937; see the section on Basic principles of sterilization). Liquid chemical sterilization with peracetic acid-containing formulations is dependent on the peracetic acid concentration, formulation (including variables such as pH), temperature and contact time.

• Peracetic acid concentration: typical PAA concentrations range from 800 to 3000 mg/L. At such concentrations PAA can be shown to provide a SAL of 10^{-6}, depending on its formulation and exposure temperature. The most resistant organism to PAA has been shown to be *Geobacillus stearothermophilus* spores, which are therefore used to design and test such sterilization process. Higher concentrations are known to be more effective than at lower concentrations, but lower concentrations are often compensated for by the effects of higher temperatures. Peracetic acid has the potential to degrade over time, with the rate of degradation depending on the water quality, presence of soil, temperature and formulation. This should clearly be factored into the development of any associated sterilization process, to ensure that the minimal SAL is achieved under worst case test conditions (such as lowest PAA concentration).

• Formulation refers to the combination of ingredients, including active (antimicrobial) and inert ingredients, into a product for its intended use. Peracetic acid-based formulations will include ingredients such as buffers (for pH control), anti-corrosives (to prevent damage to surfaces), chelating agents (to aid in control of chemical contaminants in water) and surfactants (e.g. to aid in penetration and even cleaning). In some formulations PAA can be used to enhance cleaning from a surface, but this may not always be the case and should be supported with experimental evidence.

• Temperature plays an important role in enhancing the activity with PAA. Peracetic acid-based processes can typically range from room temperature (20–25°C; 68–77°F) to 50–60°C (122–140°F), where the higher the temperature the greater the antimicrobial activity. For example, at about 1000 mg/L PAA the typical time to kill one log of *G. stearothermophilus* spores (the D-valve) at 30°C can be about five minutes (depending on the formulation), while at 50°C it is about one second. Therefore, at 50–55°C a SAL of 10^{-6} can be theoretically provided in less than 12 seconds.

• Exposure time for sterilization will depend on the SAL requirements, the PAA concentration, formulation and temperature. It is typical for a significant level of overkill (greater exposure time under these defined conditions) to be provided in excess of the SAL (as seen in other sterilization processes). Typical sterilization processes will operate at ~2000 mg/L PAA, 50–56°C for 12 minutes and ~2000 mg/L PAA, 46–55°C for six minutes.

A typical PAA sterilization process will consist of three phases: sterilant preparation, sterilization and rinsing. In sterilization processes designed to date, the PAA formulation is delivered in a single-dosed cup design (e.g. shown in Figure 11.33). Each cup is designed with two compartments, an upper area containing liquid PAA (typically at 35%) and a lower, dry, solid-containing compartment with the other ingredients of the formulation. These cups are usually provided with a limited shelf-life (typically 6–9 months). The formulation cup is placed into the sterilizer design and on initiation of the process the sterilant is prepared by mixing both compartments with water and heating to the desired sterilization temperature. The sterilant is then flowed through and over the load to be sterilized for the required sterilization time and within the defined temperature range. The external parts of the device(s) are sterilized by immersion in the sterilant, but special consideration is required for any lumened device. These are sterilized by flowing the sterilant solution through the respective lumens, for which purpose specific connectors are provided to allow the device lumens to be connected to the sterilant pumping systems within

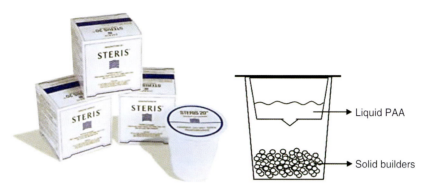

Figure 11.33 An example of a PAA sterilant formulation delivery system. The examples shown are known as STERIS 20™ or S40™. The single-use cup design (on the left) consists of two compartments (shown on the right, as a cup within a cup design), consisting of an upper liquid PAA compartment and a lower area containing the dry components of the formulation. The cup components are mixed with water during the sterilization process to provide the final sterilant.

the process design (examples are shown in Figure 11.34). Such connectors are designed for use with a defined individual and/or series of endoscopes; they should be designed to ensure that the correct flow is achieved through the lumen(s), as well as around the connection points to the endoscope to provide sterilization for the complete device.

Following the sterilant exposure, the devices are rinsed with the appropriate (sterile) quality of water (e.g. sterile filtered water and/or otherwise treated, such as with UV light) and for the process defined number of rinse cycles (typically 2–4 rinses, depending on the process). To date, two such PAA sterilization processes have been developed, known as the STERIS SYSTEM 1® and SYSTEM 1 E™, being similar in sterilizer/process design (see below). It is important in the sterilization of lumened devices to ensure that the correct lumen connectors are used in accordance with manufacturers' instructions, including confirming that connectors have remained attached during the process.

Peracetic acid is a toxic, caustic and irritating chemical, both on its own and in formulation. The greatest risk is with handling concentrations greater than 10% (such as in cup delivery systems that contain ~35% PAA), although such cup systems are designed to minimize any risks of direct exposure. The final formulation is only mixed with water when placed within the sealed sterilizer design (see below) and, following sterilization exposure, is discarded directly into the drain and rinsed away with water as part of the overall process. Despite this, it is always good practice to use gloves and eye protection, as PAA will burn the skin at concentrations of ~3% and can cause eye damage at even lower concentrations (~0.3%). The cup is vented, to prevent pressurization during the degradation of PAA over time, and should be stored in a well ventilated area. Peracetic acid itself, even at lower concentrations when diluted for use (the final, mixed formulation in water), has a strong, acrid, vinegar-like odor that is irritating to the eyes and mucous membrane. At the time of writing, there is no defined safety (permissible) level/limit for PAA, but it is recommended that it is handled and used in well ventilated areas so as to minimize any risks. In all cases, it is recommended as a precaution to use PPE when handling PAA or using PAA-based sterilization processes to include safety glasses and gloves. Safety training should always be given according to a written procedure, on the correct emergency procedures in the case of an accidental spill of PAA-based sterilants and/or sterilizer malfunction within a given area.

Typical sterilizer design

An example of a PAA-based sterilization system is shown in Figure 11.34; the most widely used systems to date are the STERIS SYSTEM 1® and SYSTEM 1 E™, which are similar in essential design, but are also distinctly different processes. A typical design example is shown in Figure 11.35.

The sterilizer load is placed within the chamber, according to manufacturers' instructions; note that there is no packaging system for the devices being placed directly into the chamber for sterilization. Different types of insert tray systems are designed to support the various types of loads, ranging from general instrument trays to those specifically designed to accommodate larger

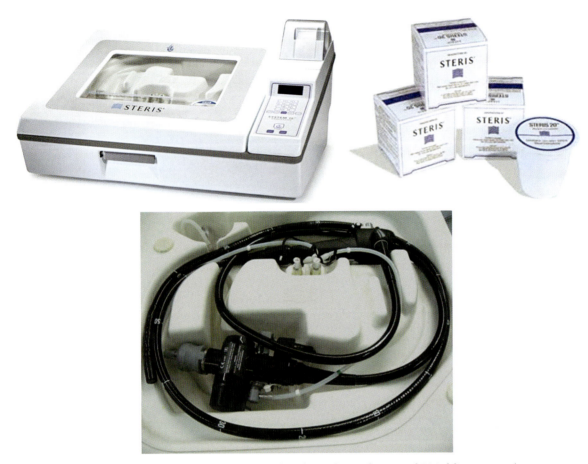

Figure 11.34 An example of a PAA sterilization process, including the sterilizer and associated PAA-delivery system (cup, on top right). The other accessories (below) include the support trays (placed into the sterilizer to support the devices) and the connector systems (required to connect internal lumens of any device to the flow system of the sterilizer).

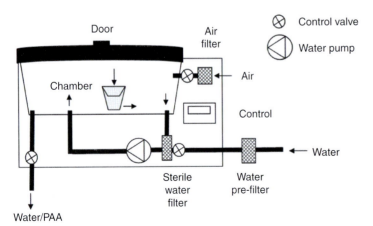

Figure 11.35 Typical design of a PAA-based sterilization system. Such systems are designed to be top loading and have a single door.

flexible endoscope designs (Figure 11.34). Devices that contain internal lumens (rigid and flexible endoscopes) are connected to the sterilizer flow system using a series of connectors specifically designed for each type/series of devices (Figure 11.34). The sterilizer is sealed, by closing the lid and initiating the sterilization process. Potable water (typically in the 42–55°C range) is taken into the system through a series of pre-filters (which can vary depending on the water quality), but ultimately through a sterile water filter. In some designs this will be a designated, final 0.2 μm sterile water filter, while in others this will include pre-treatment with a UV-system and then be followed by a final dual 0.1 μm sterile water filter. The water is heated to the desired sterilization temperature, while the two-component sterilant is dissolved and mixed to give the final use dilution for sterilization (at ~2000 mg/L PAA). The sterilization phase is controlled at the defined temperature range and time (50–55°C for 12 minutes or 46–55°C for 6 minutes). All parts of the load and internal sterilizer design are exposed to the sterilant, to include the sterile water filter, followed by a drain. The final rinsing stage will include two or four sterile water rinses (fill, rinse time and drain), depending on the

defined process. The full cycle is controlled by a microprocessor and associated sensors for process control. In addition, these systems have programmed diagnostic cycles to be conducted every 24 hours that perform a series of self-tests to confirm proper functioning. The total process time is <30 minutes and will vary depending on the process.

Standards and guidelines
Table 11.15 provides a list of standards and guidelines associated with the use of liquid peracetic acid sterilizer.

Other processes
The most widely used chemical sterilization processes worldwide have been described above, but there is constant development of new types of chemical sterilization processes. These may or may not become available at various locations around the world, depending on local regulations and their commercial success. These can be based on any chemical that has the ability to demonstrate broad-spectrum (including sporicidal) antimicrobial activity, are developed for use as part of a sterilization process (e.g. providing an SAL of 10^{-6}, see the section on

Table 11.15 Standards and guidelines applicable for liquid peracetic acid sterilizers.

Guidelines/standards	Title	Description
ISO 14937: 2009	*Sterilization of healthcare products. General requirements for characterization of a sterilizing agent and the development, validation and routine control of a sterilization process for medical devices.*	Specifies general requirements for the characterization of any sterilizing agent and for the development, validation and routine monitoring and control of a sterilization process for devices.
ISO 11138:1 2006	*Sterilization of healthcare products. Biological indicators. General requirements.*	General requirements for production, labeling, test methods and performance requirements for the manufacture of biological indicators.
ANSI/AAMI ST58: 2005	*Chemical sterilization and high-level disinfection in healthcare facilities*	Provides guidelines for the selection and use of liquid chemical sterilants (LCSs)/high level disinfectants (HLDs) and gaseous chemical sterilizers that have been cleared for marketing by the US Food and Drug Administration (FDA) for use in hospitals and other healthcare facilities.
CDC/HICPAC: 2008	*Guideline for disinfection and sterilization in healthcare facilities*	Recommendations on methods for cleaning, disinfection and sterilization of patient-care medical devices in the USA.
AS/NZS 4187:2003	*Cleaning, disinfecting and sterilizing re-usable medical and surgical instruments and equipment, and maintenance of associated environments in healthcare facilities*	General guidance on reprocessing, to include low temperature sterilization (in Australia and New Zealand).

basic principles of sterilization) and meet healthcare requirements for safety and device compatibility. Note that the use of the term "sterilization" and how any such sterilization processes are regulated in a particular region can vary; for example the use of a "sporicidal disinfectant" or "sterilant" does not necessarily ensure that sterilization is achieved and/or maintained during a given process. At a minimum such processes should be required to meet the requirements of various international standards, with particular emphasis on the essential requirements defined in ISO 14937 *Sterilization of healthcare products – general requirements for characterization of a sterilizing agent and the development, validation and routine control of a sterilization process for medical devices.* A number of existing or developing sterilization technologies are briefly discussed in this section.

There are many new hydrogen peroxide gas (particular gas plasma) sterilization systems. The essential components of such sterilization processes and sterilizer designs have been discussed earlier. The individual sterilization processes provided in these sterilizer designs will vary widely and close attention should be given to the exact process conditions, the claims made with each individual design and any required regulatory approvals to allow any sterilizer to be legally sold within a given country/region. Processes can range in hydrogen peroxide gas concentration, saturated or unsaturated gas conditions (i.e. liquid/gas or just gas peroxide exposure), exposure temperatures, pressures (vacuum levels), presence/absence and specific use of a plasma phase at various parts of the cycle, etc. Each system should be considered unique, even though they may have similar trade names or claim equivalency to other existing systems.

Ozone, similar to hydrogen peroxide and peracetic acid, is a potent antimicrobial chemical. It is a gas at room temperature and atmospheric pressure, being easily formed from oxygen (e.g. present in air at ~21% or provided as oxygen gas within an area) by applying energy in the form of a UV light or electricity (e.g. by creating a corona discharge). Also, it is a very unstable biocide quickly breaking down to oxygen again, particularly on contact with various surfaces. It is used as a deodorizer/disinfectant (in air and water) and has often been investigated as a method of sterilization due to its potent antimicrobial activity at relatively low concentrations. For sterilization activity, humidified ozone is required and at a typical concentration of 50–100 mg/L. The most resistant organism to ozone-based sterilization processes is considered to be *Geobacillus stearothermophilus* spores, which are used in the development and routine testing

of such sterilizer designs. Examples of ozone-containing sterilization processes that have recently been developed are shown in Figure 11.36.

Ozone-based sterilizer designs and sterilization processes, in particular the STERIZONE®125L, is similar in many respects to those described for hydrogen peroxide gas systems, with the exception that very high humidity control is also required. The sterilizer consists of a chamber (to hold the load), an ozone generator, humidifier and a piping system incorporating a vacuum pump. The process is conducted under vacuum (low pressure), within the temperature range of 30–36°C (86–97°F) and consists of three phases: conditioning, sterilization and ventilation. During conditioning a vacuum is drawn in the chamber to remove air and the load is humidified by the introduction of water through a humidifier. Ozone, similar to ETO and formaldehyde, requires high levels of humidity (optimally just below saturation at 90–95%) for antimicrobial activity. Following conditioning, low pressure is re-drawn (at 0.01 kPa, approximately equivalent to 0.0001 bar, 0.001 psi and 0.075 Torr), humidity is controlled within the 85–100% range and ozone is introduced into the chamber at an initial concentration of 85 mg/L. Ozone is generated from medical grade oxygen (that can be provided from a facility supply or directly from an oxygen gas tank) through a corona discharge-based generator (as the energy source) and allowed to diffuse within the chamber for a given exposure time. Similar to hydrogen peroxide gas, the concentration of ozone is reduced within the chamber during the exposure time (dependent on the load). A vacuum is then re-drawn in the chamber and this exposure phase (vacuum, humidity and ozone introduction) is repeated. Therefore a total of two ozone exposure pulses are conducted for each cycle. During sterilization, the ozone is degraded when removed from the chamber by passing it through a catalytic converter. The final phase is ventilation, when a vacuum is reapplied to the load to remove ozone residuals, also broken down through the converter and then returned to atmospheric pressure to release the load. The total cycle time is at least 4.5 hours, and may be longer depending on the load. No additional aeration is found to be required, due to the instability of ozone. Despite this, ozone is a respiratory irritant at low concentrations (e.g. at 0.01 ppm) and can have more serious health consequences at higher levels. Typical safety levels that are recommended are at 0.1 ppm over a typical eight-hour working day (weighted average) and a short-term exposure limit of no more that 0.3 ppm over 15 minutes. Ozone detectors, including personal monitors, handheld

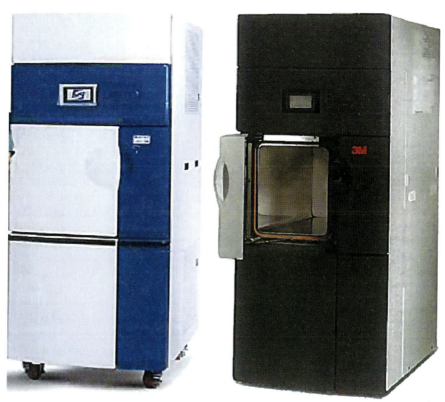

Figure 11.36 Example of humidified ozone gas chemical sterilization processes. The STERIZONE® 125 L sterilization system (right) utilizes humidified ozone gas alone for sterilization and the OPTREOZ™ 125-Z system (left; also known as the STERIZONE® 125 L+) utilizes a mixture of hydrogen peroxide and ozone gas.

and room/area mounted sensors are available for safety monitoring. It is recommended that ozone sterilizers are installed in well ventilated areas (e.g. with ten or more air volume changes per hour). These designs of ozone sterilizers claim to have low running/maintenance costs but require intermediate cycle time (shorter than ETO but longer than hydrogen peroxide gas systems). There are some limitations on material compatibility (to include aluminum, brass and polyurethane), as well as not being used to sterilize liquids, textiles and cellulose-based materials (including paper packaging systems).

A newer version of the ozone sterilizer is known as the STERIZONE® 125L+ system (or also as OPTREOZ™ 125-Z; Figure 11.36). These sterilizers provide a completely different sterilization process, based on hydrogen peroxide gas and ozone gas together. It is also a vacuum-based process, but at a higher temperature of 40–42°C and of similar sterilizer design to the ozone sterilizer. A major difference is that hydrogen peroxide gas is generated from a hydrogen peroxide solution (at 50%) during

the process and mixed with ozone during the sterilization cycle. Further, at the time of writing, there are three cycles available (ranging from 46 to 100 minutes long) that are chosen depending on the sterilizer load (e.g. lumen or non-lumen device within the load). The overall process is also distinct from the ozone system. The cycle has a much shorter conditioning phase, consisting of drawing a deep vacuum (at a pressure of 0.13 kPa, equivalent to 0.001 bar, 0.019 psi and 1 Torr) only, and then entering the sterilization phase, consisting of a number of hydrogen peroxide/ozone gas exposure pulses (two to four depending on the cycle). During each pulse, the peroxide gas is introduced first into the chamber under vacuum and then ozone gas is added, followed by an exposure time and then re-drawing of the vacuum. A similar catalytic converter system is used to break down any ozone/peroxide gas residuals before venting into the room. In this system design, ozone is present at a much lower concentration (depending on the cycle, within a range of 2–10 mg/L) and it is claimed that the antimicrobial effects are due to a combined action of peroxide/ozone gas. Finally, the ventilation stage consists of two pulses of drawing a vacuum and using oxygen gas to purge any remaining ozone/peroxide gas from the load. The claimed benefits of this sterilizer, in comparison to the ozone design, are having a shorter cycle time and greater lumen penetration capability.

There are other types of gases that have been or are being investigated for use in sterilization processes. These include the use of PAA gas, chlorine dioxide (not to be mistaken for chlorine gas, being separate chemicals) and nitric oxide. These could include single or multiple biocide-based processes. In an example, a plasma-PAA sterilization process (similar to hydrogen peroxide, gas-plasma systems described in the section on hydrogen peroxide gas, including plasma processes) had been developed but is no longer commercially available. Other gas plasma systems are also under investigation. As outlined in Chapter 6 (in the section on solids, liquids, gases and plasmas) plasma can be made by applying energy to any gas. Gas plasma processes based on the generation of plasma within oxygen, nitrogen, helium and argon or combinations of these gases (as examples) have shown potent antimicrobial activity. In all these cases, it is expected that sterilizer and sterilization process designs will be similar to the other low temperature gas processes discussed earlier in this section. For example, PAA, chlorine dioxide and nitric oxide are all found to require high humidity levels for optimal antimicrobial activity. Equally, such processes will need to ensure the correct balance of antimicrobial efficacy, safety and device compatibility for routine clinical use.

There is also a similar range of liquid chemicals that could be further developed as true sterilization processes. These are based on many processes already in use as disinfectants, such as liquid PAA formulations, oxidized water, chlorine, liquid hydrogen peroxide and liquid applications of chlorine dioxide and ozone (Chapter 9, see the section on chemical disinfection). An example is the use of various systems of chlorine-generation systems (also known as "activated", "electrolyzed" or "super-oxidized" water applications; see the section on halogens). These operate by passing electricity through water (generally containing a low concentration of salt (NaCl, sodium chloride), to produce active chlorine species (primarily HOCl, but also Cl_2 and OCl^-). Such processes can produce liquid preparations with powerful antimicrobial activity, including sporicidal activity. While their use to date has been as sporicidal disinfectants, future developments could include their optimization as part of sterilization processes in compliance to the applicable standards. Further examples include the use of various gases (or even gas plasmas) that are introduced into water or liquid chemical preparations for antimicrobial applications such as with chlorine dioxide, water and different types of gas plasmas.

Process monitoring

Process monitoring or low temperature sterilization processes will include a similar series of tests as previously described, such as parametric, biological indicator, chemical indicator and process control devices (PCDs; see the section on the basic principles of sterilization earlier in this chapter). These quality control indicator systems are used in combination with recommended practice guidelines and standards. These will specifically include:

- Parametric monitoring should include the key process conditions required for sterilization, to include cycle or sterilant exposure time, temperature, pressure and even the concentration of the sterilant (if applicable). Printout reports from the sterilizer design can provide useful information about each sterilizer cycle performance. In some sterilizer designs, independent control systems may also be available (as an option) or installed to verify the calibration of key controlling sensors (e.g. temperature and pressure).
- Biological monitoring (using biological indicators, BIs) can also be used to verify the efficacy of a sterilization process. Examples of the types of bacterial spores used to monitor chemical sterilization efficacy are given in Table 11.16. Biological indicators can be provided in a variety of designs, but are most widely used as self-contained designs and may include an additional chemical indicator.

Table 11.16 Types of bacterial spores used for testing and monitoring of chemical sterilization methods.

Sterilization process	Test bacterial spores
Ethylene oxide	*Bacillus atropheus*
Hydrogen peroxide gas (including gas plasma)	*Geobacillus stearmthermophilus*
Low temperature steam-formaldehyde gas	*Geobacillus stearmthermophilus*
Liquid peracetic acid	*Geobacillus stearmthermophilus*
Ozone	*Geobacillus stearmthermophilus*

- Chemical indicators (CIs) are widely used to assess if critical physical parameters of the given chemical sterilization process have been met. It is important to note that these indicators can vary in their classification and therefore their ability to indicate a successful sterilization process (see Table 11.4). Similar to steam sterilization, some CIs are used as external indicators giving an immediate result after the sterilization cycle and may provide an early indication of a problem in the process. Examples include various types of sterilization tapes or often indicators integrated into packaging materials (similar to steam sterilization tapes). Such indicators do not show that sterilization has been achieved but rather that the item has been exposed to a given sterilization process. Internal chemical indicators are designed to be used inside packages as a pack control to assist in confirming that the chemical sterilization process has been efficient within the load; these indicators will also vary in their specificity and sensitivity, depending on their classification and labeling. These are most commonly multi-parameter indicators that monitor at least two of the critical parameters of the sterilization process.
- Process challenge devices (PCDs) are used in low temperature sterilization as challenging or worst-case tests for sterilant penetration within the sterilizer. These generally consist of a barrier system (e.g. an absorbent pack or a lumened device), inside which a biological and/or chemical or indicator is placed as a penetration challenge (see the section on Basic principles of sterilization). Process challenge devices can be used to test empty or full sterilizer loads.

Parametric release of the load is also possible with low temperature sterilizers, depending on their design and manufacturers' claims (Basic principles of sterilization). Similar to steam, a low temperature chemical sterilization process requires evidence that the sterilizer has performed the necessary cycle parameters to ensure sterilization. Parametric release for chemical sterilization will therefore require an in-depth knowledge and control of the sterilization parameters. These variables require continuous

(and preferably independent) measurements and documentation, to include time, temperatures, pressures, relative humidity, chemical concentrations, etc. (dependent on the defined sterilization process). Similar to other sterilization process (including steam), parametric release of loads may depend on final verification of an internal chemical indicators (in specific packs) prior to patient use.

In addition to quality control monitoring of low temperature sterilization, personnel monitoring is often recommend or even required (according to local regulations) with some chemical sterilization methods. This is due to the staff health and safety risks associated with working with even low concentrations of chemical sterilants during work. While low temperature sterilization processes such as ethylene oxide, formaldehyde and ozone can be used effectively to kill a wide range of microorganisms these same sterilants may pose a serious health risk to personnel, working in and around the process, if they are not closely monitored to ensure that permissible or safety exposure limits are not exceeded. Even with standard compliant equipment, ventilation systems and well established work practices, accidental leaks of toxic sterilant gases can and do happen and personnel working in these areas must be protected. In some cases strict guidelines and recommendations are given regarding "safe" levels of chemical sterilants, while in others these may not be defined. In some countries, "Immediately dangerous to life or health" (IDLH) exposure limits have been defined for airborne contaminants such as gases (Table 11.17). It is important to note that the concentration at which some chemicals can become a significant health risk can be much lower than those sensed by humans (e.g. smelt, tasted or giving signs of irritation). The IDLH is defined as the concentration at which a chemical in a given area is likely to cause death or immediate/delayed permanent adverse health effects or prevent escape from such an area. For example, the IDLH value currently set for ethylene oxide is ~800 ppm, hydrogen peroxide is 75 ppm, and ozone at 5 ppm. A further important exposure limit

Table 11.17 This table gives some examples of acceptable IDLH and TWA-PEL limits for chemical sterilant gases.

Sterilant	IDLH (ppm)	8 hr TWA PEL (ppm)	15 min TWA PEL excursion limit (ppm)
Ethylene oxide	800	1.0	5
Formaldehyde	20	0.75	2
Hydrogen peroxide gas plasma	75	1.0	n/a
Ozone	5	0.1	n/a

that is often referenced is the eight-hour time weighted average (TWA). Time weighted average or permissible exposure limit (TWA/PEL) values are based on the cumulative average concentration over a typical eight-hour/day, 40-hour/week to which a worker can be safely exposed (in this case, as defined by the American Conference of Government and Industrial Hygienists, ACGIH). They are intended to provide an exposure rate that most employees can safely and continuously be exposed to without significant adverse effects on their health. As an example the PEL limit of ETO is 1 ppm (but a 15-minute exposure limit of 5 ppm is also given as the maximum ETO exposure level for 15 minutes that an employee may be exposed). The eight-hour PEL thus represents an exposure limit that should provide a safe work environment based on chemical toxicity and injury as well as longer term risks from cancer, etc. The PEL for ETO and hydrogen peroxide is similar, 1 ppm for both gases. The eight-hour PEL for formaldehyde (0.75 ppm) and ozone (0.1 ppm) are lower. Exposure to extremely low concentrations of ozone, for example, can cause an inflammatory response (including cough, shortness of breath, tightness of the chest, a feeling of an inability to breathe (dyspnea), dry throat, wheezing, headache and nausea) in the respiratory tissue that can persist for up to 18 hours.

Various personnel and environmental monitoring system are available which give immediate indication of concentration in the work area so that workers can be protected from acute and chronic exposure.

Troubleshooting

Given the range of chemical sterilization processes and sterilizer designs, troubleshooting problems specific to each type are considered outside of the scope of this chapter. Despite this, many of the typical problems (in particular process failure indicators) described in the troubleshooting of steam sterilization are applicable to chemical sterilization processes (see the section on troubleshooting steam sterilization problems). Process indicators specific for the chemical sterilization process, which include chemical, biological, process control device and parametric indicators that indicate failed results can often result from procedural issues, such as:

• Devices incorrectly prepared and placed into the sterilizer. A typical example is with some vacuum-gas processes that require devices to be dry prior to placing them into the sterilizer.

• Incorrect indicator or process control device used with the load.

• Overloading or incorrect loading of a chamber.

• Wrong cycle chosen for a particular application in a sterilizer design.

Various indicators can also detect mechanical or other sterilizer faults, which are based on their design, and include:

• Loss of pressure (high or low), indicating a leak in the sterilizer (e.g. a failed door gasket).

• No sterilant present within the cycle.

• Temperature not achieved within the sterilizer chamber.

As discussed for troubleshooting steam sterilization process failures, a well-planned, systematic and written procedure should be in place at a facility to address any of these potential situations as they may occur at any time. This procedure should be developed with the assistance of the sterilizer manufacturer and/or as recommended in their instructions for use or any associated training provided.

Some common failures or problems associated with chemical sterilization processes will include:

• Failed sterilization indicators: ensure that the correct indicators (chemical, biological and those associated with process control devices) have been used and that the correct procedures have been used concerning the use of sterilizer (e.g. packaging, loading, etc.). In the absence of any specific procedural fault identified, the load should be considered non-sterile, the sterilizer locked from use and investigated according to manufacturers' instructions. Independent parametric control sensors/systems may be available in the sterilizer design and where a fault is identified the sterilizer should be locked out from use and investigated according to manufacturers' instructions.

• Self-diagnostic tests: many chemical sterilizers have self-diagnostic cycles/tests that are recommended to be performed periodically. Examples include sterilizer leak tests and filter integrity tests. Failure of such tests indicates an error in the operation of the sterilizer and should be investigated according to manufacturers' instructions.

• Gas detection: various types of sensors are available to detect concentration of gases above safety levels. Gas concentrations above safety levels indicate significant health risks to staff and inadequate control of the sterilization process (e.g. failed door gaskets, leaking gas tanks/feed-line systems). The sterilizer should immediately be locked out from use and then investigated by trained staff/service providers. Excessive gas level can also indicate inadequate aeration of a load during or following a sterilization cycle. These should be immediately investigated as significant safety risks to staff and patients. Typical causes can include overloading of the sterilizer, insufficient aeration for particular types of devices/loads and the use of the wrong packaging materials. Gas detection can pose a serious safety risk and will vary depending on the type of gas used for chemical sterilization.

• Moisture detection: the presence of significant levels of water on device surfaces prior to chemical sterilization may or may not be detected by the sterilizer design. Failure to dry devices before processing can lead to inadequate sterilization or, in sterilizers with detection systems, to delays in reprocessing of loads.

• Incompatibility or device damage: damage to devices can occur for various reasons during the reprocessing cycle, including the use of chemical sterilants. It is good practice to ensure that all devices are examined to be fit for use directly prior to their use on patients (Chapter 12). Suspected damage to a device following chemical sterilization should be reported to the sterilizer and device manufacturer for further investigation. It may be necessary in such cases to discontinue use of the sterilizer for these devices until the investigation is completed to ensure the device(s) are compatible with the process.

12 Storage and distribution

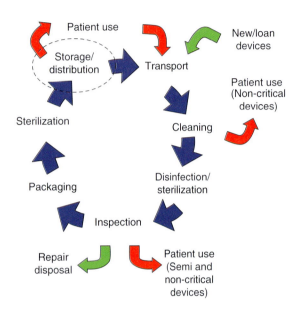

Introduction

Device reprocessing or decontamination is designed with one main goal in mind: to ensure that a device is safe and "fit for purpose". This applies to all re-usable devices, ranging from non-critical to critical (Chapter 1). It is important to remember that despite the various stages of device reprocessing and efforts to render a device clean and disinfected/sterilized this can all be compromised through inadequate handling and storage of these devices/surfaces prior to patient use. Therefore, the storage (if applicable) and distribution of re-usable devices is an essential step to complete the reprocessing cycle.

In cases of non-critical and even semi-critical devices that are cleaned and/or disinfected, it is recommended that these are used immediately for their intended patient application. These devices are not generally packaged to prevent recontamination and are considered in more detail in the next section. Similarly, in the case of immediate use (or "flash") sterilization or liquid chemical sterilization processes (that are designed for just-in-time availability of a sterile device), the device(s) should be delivered directly for immediate use; these devices are not protected and should not be stored.

In this chapter special consideration is given to the storage and distribution of re-usable devices that have been packaged and sterilized. These devices are ready for immediate use on a patient or can be stored in the correct manner and made available for a patient procedure at a future date. Various types of rigid and flexible sterile barrier systems/materials have been designed for such purposes (Chapter 10); however, these systems can become compromised during storing and handling. Adequate storing and distribution procedures should be specified for each facility. For example, environmental control of the conditions of any designated storage and distribution area should ensure that the integrity of all sterile materials and products is maintained. Items should be stored in a well ventilated, where possible air conditioned (no open windows), and restricted access area. Ensure that these areas are always kept clean and dust-free. Packaged materials should be protected from getting wet and from being damaged during storage. It is the responsibility of the reprocessing staff to ensure that items are stored correctly and are not compromised by improper storage and handling practices.

Best practice for maintaining sterile packs is to minimize handling and to store and transport correctly. It is important to consider appropriate facility flow (e.g. from a reprocessing area, to storage area and to point of use with a patient) when developing a storage and transportation system. The less an item is handled the less likely it is to be compromised (potentially recontaminated).

A Practical Guide to Decontamination in Healthcare, First Edition. Gerald McDonnell and Denise Sheard.
© 2012 Gerald McDonnell and Denise Sheard. Published 2012 by Blackwell Publishing Ltd.

Handling of non-packaged or non-sterilized devices

Non-packaged and non-sterilized devices can include:
- Non-critical and semi-critical devices or surfaces that have been disinfected (high, intermediate or low-level disinfection; Chapter 9): these may have been reprocessed by thermal or chemical disinfection methods. They are non-packaged (not reprocessed within a sterile barrier system designed for storage/transport following the reprocessing cycle). As a result, the surfaces of these devices can easily become recontaminated when handled, transported or exposed to air.
- Critical devices that have been sterilized but not contained within a sterile barrier system: examples include the sterilization of devices in an immediate use or "flash" steam sterilization cycle or within a liquid chemical sterilization process that is labelled as a "just-in-time" process. Such devices may be sterilized, but can become recontaminated during handling, transport or exposure to air over time.

In these cases, at the point of disinfection or sterilization completion (if applied correctly) the device(s) should be used immediately. It is important that such devices are aseptically handled and presented for patient use to minimize any risks of cross-contamination. Many guidelines recommend a minimum time from which they have been processed before they have to be used on patients. For example, some European guidelines recommend the use of flexible endoscopes on patients following high-level disinfection for up to three hours after the device has been reprocessed. Such recommendations are based on the correct handling and storage of the device prior to use. Inappropriate handling and/or storage could allow the device to be recontaminated during any interim time. Overall, a facility policy should be in place that describes the safe handling of any non-packaged or non-sterilized devices prior to patient use. This will include:
- Disinfection/sterilization methods to be used.
- Handling and/or storage procedures following reprocessing, including any minimum or maximum times within which the device can be used.
- Handling of devices that have been compromised (even if only suspected) or that have been held/stored for greater than the allowable time.

For heat disinfected or steam sterilized devices it is important to ensure that the devices are allowed to cool to at least ~50°C or less (cool to touch) before handling or patient use, to prevent condensation which may affect sterility of the pack; this may require up to an hour to ensure, depending on the device/set. Low temperature chemical disinfected/sterilized devices can be used immediately, ensuring that any residual chemicals have been correctly rinsed in accordance with manufacturers' instructions. A common cause of patient-associated toxicity reactions are residual disinfectants remaining in or on devices when clinically used. Similarly, contaminated rinse water can lead to toxic reactions (due to the presence of chemical contaminants) and patient infections (due to the presence of microorganisms). A typical example is with flexible endoscopes that are often reprocessed as semi-critical devices by being cleaned and high-level disinfected (Chapter 15, in the section on endoscopes and other lumened devices). Flexible endoscopes are manufactured with various types of plastic (often porous) materials and can have one or more internal lumens. It is difficult to ensure that these materials and lumens are safely reprocessed. Common problems include inadequate cleaning, disinfection, recontamination (following disinfection, such as with contaminated rinse water) and insufficient rinsing. Residuals can therefore include cleaning chemistries, disinfectants and chemical/microbial contaminants from the rinse water. Bacteria present in rinse water and remaining in/on the endoscope following disinfection can pose a risk to patients. These risks increase significantly when bacteria are allowed to grow within the lumens of these devices if they are stored wet (even with a low level of moisture remaining within the endoscope lumens). Residual water can remain within these channels, even if reprocessing was conducted within a washer-disinfector or automated endoscope reprocessor that may have lumen purging/drying claims. In some areas, specific drying cabinets are employed to assist in the drying and storing of flexible endoscopes following reprocessing (Figure 12.1). Such cabinets are generally designed to flow HEPA-filtered air through the various device lumens for the purpose of drying. When stored in such a manner, the manufacturer may recommend that the devices are safely maintained to prevent recontamination and bacterial/fungal growth in or on the device. Such storage cabinets and any associated testing data should be carefully examined with the manufacturer to ensure they are safe for use in accordance with any facility policies. Staff training is important to make sure that these storage cabinets are correctly used and maintained. Note that some transport systems for flexible endoscopes are essentially designed as rigid containers with dust-covers, to prevent contamination of the device during transport to a site of patient use; these are not

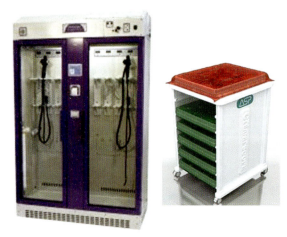

Figure 12.1 Examples of temporary storage methods used for flexible endoscopes. On the left is a storage cabinet, designed to flow HEPA-filtered air through the endoscope lumens to aid in drying. On the right is a covered transport system used to transfer contaminated/reprocessed endoscopes from one area to another (using different colored systems for contaminated and reprocessed scopes).

sterile packaging systems and do not imply that the device can be safely stored prior to patient use. Care should be taken to read and understand any manufacturer instructions provided with these systems.

Sterile storage environment and layout

A designated area should be defined for the storage of packaged, sterilized items. Ideally, there should preferably be a physical separation between the storage area and the rest of the reprocessing area. This will reduce any risks of mixing of sterile and non-sterile items, as well as cross-contamination. If this is not possible, extra care is needed to ensure that air and traffic always flows from clean to dirty areas of the facility. Access to the area should be clearly defined with traffic controlled to minimize the movement of airborne contaminants. No through traffic should be allowed, with only staff allocated to the "clean side" being allowed access to the storage area.

The storage area should be well lit, easy to clean and arranged in a way that will make it easy to identify packs with minimal handling. The maintenance (cleaning and disinfection) of work surfaces, floors, shelving and transport equipment is important. Light fittings, pipes

and air conditioning ducts, which can collect and shed dust should not be overlooked when cleaning. Surfaces in contact with sterile goods should be as clean as possible to minimize contamination. Care should be taken to use cleaning/disinfection chemistries that will not damage packaging materials. It is not necessary to keep surfaces disinfected, but they should be visually clean. Cleaning of the sterile storage area should be planned in such a way as to minimize handling of sterile packs – as excess handling can increase the risk of damaging the packaging materials.

The storage system should be designed to meet the specific needs of the facility. As long as the system conforms to the facility policy, hygiene, infection control and security requirements, a manager should be free to lay out and maintain the storage area in the best way possible to meet the needs of the facility. Sterile packs should be arranged to allow them to be easily identified for their intended use. Shelving systems and sterilization baskets are most often used (Figure 12.2). The type of shelving used for sterile storage should protect the sterile packs, allow for easy stock rotation and be easy to clean, as well as allowing air to circulate around packs. Sharp edges or parts can pose a staff safety risk as well as causing packaging materials to rip.

Storage conditions can affect the integrity of a sterile pack, with the following guidelines given:
- The correct choice and use of packaging material.
- Reduce exposure to environmental factors such as light, air, temperature, humidity and sources of water.
- Minimize handling within the storage area.
- Controlled transportation to the place of intended use.
Water and air can be a major source of cross-contamination. Examples include an overly humid environment, direct exposure to sunlight and high temperatures over time may degrade the packaging material and increase the risk of contamination. High humidity may also cause condensation to form on packaging and enhance the capability of microorganisms to enter sterile packs. Likewise, very dry conditions may cause packaging materials to dry out, become brittle and lose their barrier function. Ideal environmental temperatures should be controlled at 18–22°C (65–72°F) and relative humidity should be 35–50%. Air supply to the storage areas should be clean and dust free, and may require filtration. Ideally, the sterile storage area should be maintained under a positive pressure with ~13 air exchanges per hour or positive pressure to surrounding areas, in order to reduce the possibility of airborne contamination from air outside the storage area.

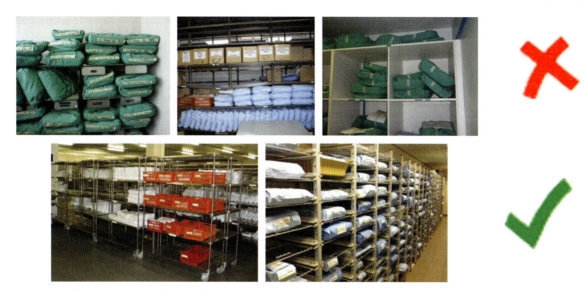

Figure 12.2 Shelving systems used for sterile pack storage. The top panel shows some storage conditions that may cause damage to device loads. The bottom panel shows examples of adequate storage conditions.

Storage and handling of sterile, packaged devices

Sterility maintenance should be viewed as a quality management process as possible events that may compromise sterility will vary from one facility to another. Each reprocessing facility should have policies and procedures in place for the labelling, storage, handling and rotating of sterile packaged materials in the storage area. This can include other facility sterile supplies that are also used for patient surgical/medical procedures.

Shelf-life refers to the period of time during which a sterilized item is considered safe to be used. Guidelines regarding sterility shelf-life can vary from country to country, and particular attention should be paid to instructions for use that are given by the packaging system/material manufacturer. Traditionally packaged re-usable devices were considered to be sterile for a given storage time (e.g. up to four weeks), after which if the pack was unused it would be recalled for reprocessing. Internationally, this is no longer considered to be valid or warranted. An alternate system, known as "event related sterility", is more practical and now being widely used. This system defines the sterility of a pack as being dependent on events that may occur during the handling, transporting and storage of the item. As an example, if the pack has remained intact and has been stored correctly the devices within should be expected to remain sterile, unless otherwise specified by the packaging manufacturer. Sterile packaged devices can become compromised depending on the quality of packaging material used, the storage conditions, conditions during transport, and the amount of handling. The greatest risk to a sterilized pack is damage to the packaging materials. Events that can compromise sterility can include:

• Holes or torn wrappers
• Securing tapes or locks that have been tampered with or removed
• Broken or incomplete seals on laminated pouches
• Items that have been dropped onto a dirty surface
• Exposure to blood, body fluids or any type of moisture
• Moving of items from one area to another
• Elastic bands or tapes used to bundle items and causing tearing
• Excessive temperature or pressure conditions, for example through exposure to sun

Sterile items should be arranged so that handling is reduced and they are easy to locate. They can be organized to suit the facility, for example alphabetically, by procedure, by discipline or numerically using stock codes. Efficient labelling of shelves and sterile packs facilitates easier location and identification of sterile packs making access easier and more efficient. A good tracking system (Chapter 14) will also make identification and location of packs easier. Packs should be stored away from direct sunlight and water and should not be stored next to or under sinks, on the floor or windowsills where they are likely to get wet or damaged. Common sense dictates that storing sterile items on the floor or too close to the floor, in a moist area, or not covering shelves to protect packs from dust will compromise sterility. Sterile packs should be stored at least 25 cm/8–13 inches above the floor, 45 cm/18 inches below the ceiling or sprinkler heads and at least 5 cm/2 inches from outside walls to allow for air circulation in the room and to prevent contamination during cleaning.

There should be enough shelving and cupboard space available to store all sterile goods without having to stack them tightly or on top of one another. Shelving should be designed in a way that makes it easy to see the number of packs in storage at a glance. Shelving should be slatted, easily cleaned and allow air to circulate around stored packs. Spacing of shelving and packs must also be planned to prevent packs from being touched, bumped or leaned on by cleaning staff or when packs are retrieved for distribution. Packs should not overhang the shelving. Shelving should be made of an easy-to-clean material, preferably not wood. Freestanding or mobile shelving provides a practical solution for handling the flow of products in and out of storage and cleaning. It allows staff to access all sides of the storage area for rotation of sterile packs. Open shelving units are more commonly used as it is convenient and less expensive than closed shelving units. Open shelves (wire-mesh or bars) allow dust to pass through making them easier to clean than solid shelves. If open shelving units are used, it requires special attention to traffic control, housekeeping and environmental ventilation. A barrier should be created between the floor and the bottom shelf. The disadvantage of open shelving units is that sterile packs are more vulnerable to accidental physical and environmental hazards.

Closed shelving units or covered cabinets are often used for seldom-used items. Closed cabinets should have doors, preferably with a lock. When items are stored in closed cabinets, dust is limited, handling is discouraged, and inadvertent contact with sterile items is minimized.

Packs should be stored in a way that allows for easy handling in order to prevent injury. Personnel should avoid compromising the sterility of the item by not dragging, crushing, bending, compressing or puncturing the package. Larger, heavier packs may be stored in transport trays to prevent tears in the wrappers during handling. Heavier packs should be placed on lower and middle shelves, with lighter, easier to handle packs on higher shelves. Shelf liners may be used on shelves if tears on the bottom of packs are a problem. Tears usually occur as a result of heavy packs, especially, instrument trays, being "dragged" off the shelf. The edges of the metal trays and weight of the instruments increase the negative effects of friction, causing packaging to catch and tear. Burrs or sharp edges on the shelves may also damage sterile packs. When removing sterile packs from the shelf, both hands should be placed underneath the pack and the pack lifted to avoid dragging and tearing or snagging the wrapper.

When packing shelves do not squeeze packs into tight spaces, bend, stack, compress or fold them as this can tear the packaging and potentially rupture closures and seams, if the air inside the pack is forced out. When a pack is compressed air is forced out of the pack creating a void, when the source of compression is released, that is, the weight on top of the pack is removed, a suction is created which may potentially "suck in" contaminated air.

Rigid sterilization container systems should only be stored on shelves or racks designed to hold the weight and configuration of the containers. If containers need to be stacked due to space constraints, it is important that manufacturers' stacking guidelines are adhered to and that the containers are firmly seated on top of each other, and can be easily removed. Staff should be instructed not to hold rigid containers by only one handle, as this can lead to injury, damage to instruments and increased risk of dropping.

Cardboard boxes should not be used as storage containers because they can release paper fibers into the environment, cannot be easily cleaned and sometimes have rough edges which can make holes in packaging and may contain mold. It is recommended that any shipping cartons are not brought directly into the sterile storage area because they serve as reservoirs for contamination during transport.

If sterilized packages are likely to be exposed to excessive environmental challenges (e.g. transport to another location) or multiple handlings before use, dust covers or containers may be used to protect the packs. These covers/containers are designed to protect the pack against outside elements. Dust covers should be applied and sealed, immediately after the cooled pack is removed from the sterilizer cart and prior to storage/shipping.

Inventory control

An inventory control and cycling system is important to ensure the efficient use of devices within a facility. A number of stock control systems are available and should be chosen to meet the requirements of the facility. It is good practice to ensure that devices do not stay in a sterile storage area for extended periods of time and that similar device sets are equally used. This requires close coordination between staff in the reprocessing area, storage area, involved with transport and at the site of patient use (e.g. in the operating room).

The longer a sterile pack has been exposed to the environment and been handled the more likely it is to be compromised. Therefore, a common stock rotation system works on a "first in, first out" (FIFO) principle. Rotation of stock is important to ensure that "older" sterilized supplies are used before "newer" supplies. Examples of such systems are:

• From left to right: older sterilized supplies are kept to the left of the storage area/rack. New supplies are added to the right side, moving older supplies to the left. Staff should be instructed only to take supplies from the left for distribution.
• From top to bottom: old supplies are removed and distributed from the top of the stock area. New supplies are added to the bottom shelves and moved up as supplies are distributed.
• From front to back: older supplies are placed at the front of the shelf and should be first to be distributed. Newer supplies are added to the back of the shelf, pushing older supplies forward.

Transport of sterile packaged items

Various methods can be used in the transport of sterile packaged items to their point of use. This can range from hand carriage (in particular where a decontamination area is located close or adjacent to a point of use), to the use of trolleys and other transport systems for taking items to a remote location (within a facility or at a different facility). Similar considerations to those discussed for the storing of sterile packaged devices (see the section on storage and handling of sterile packaged devices) should be given to any immediate or remote transportation in order to reduce any risks of cross-contamination.

Hand transport

Appropriate hand transportation of sterile packs will generally include supporting with both hands under the pack. Avoid cradling packs or carrying them under the arms. When carrying sterile packages containing instruments, the package should be kept away from the body and parallel with the floor in order to avoid shifting of the instruments. Good body mechanics should be used when transporting any items to prevent injury (e.g. lifting from the knees rather straining the back).

Trolley systems

When instruments are to be taken from one area to another, trolley systems should be considered (Figure 12.3). Both contaminated and sterile supplies should be transported in separate dedicated covered or enclosed trolleys with a solid bottom shelf (Chapter 7, in the section on transportation post-procedure). The solid bottom shelf prevents

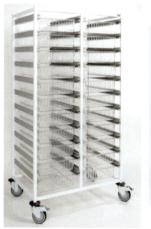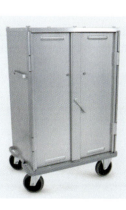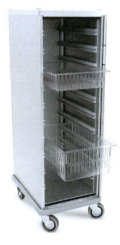

Figure 12.3 Examples of closed and open trolleys for sterile good transport.

contamination on the floor being picked up by the wheels of the trolley and redeposited onto sterile packs. Unintentional contact with staff and other sources of contamination along the transportation route can be avoided if covered or enclosed carts are used for transportation of such items. All transport vehicles (motorized or manual) should be constructed of materials that allow for a proper decontamination (cleaning and disinfection) process; this is particularly important if the same vehicle will transport alternating sterile and soiled items. If re-usable covers for carts or other transport vehicles are used, they should have a re-sealable opening and should be cleaned after each use. Trolleys should be cleaned and dried after each use, because even though they are used with sterile items, contamination can be picked up during transport. It is important to wash the outside tops and bottoms of shelves on trolleys used to transport sterile packages. Loaded transport vehicles should never be left unattended or in an unsecured location. If plastic or paper bags or boxes are used to contain and transport items, they should be placed in a container in such a way that would prevent them from being crushed, damaged or contaminated.

Packages should be placed securely in a flat position, not placed on top of each other and should not extend beyond the edge of the cart shelf or table surface, to prevent accidents.

Dedicated lifts (elevators)

Where appropriate, separate, dedicated "clean" and "dirty" lifts (elevators) can be used to transport sterile items directly from the reprocessing dispatch area to a point of use (e.g. OR suite) or from the point of use back to the dirty receiving area of the reprocessing area (Figure 12.4). Such systems can provide a fast, direct transport system between the two areas, with minimal

handling. This can only be done if there is a direct vertical link between the area where the devices are used and a reprocessing area on two separate floors. Preferably the lift should lead directly into the storing/dispatching area of the reprocessing department or to an access corridor in close proximity to this area.

The main advantage of a dedicated lift (elevator) is to increase transport operational efficiencies and lower instrument turnover time when the two areas are on separate levels. A dedicated dirty lift (elevator) may also assist in reducing the potential for cross-contamination of items being transported in a common patient/visitor/staff/service lift (elevator), but may not prevent airborne transmission of pathogenic microorganisms. A dedicated clean lift (elevator) will only remain clean if proper cleaning procedures of the cabs, floors, ceiling and walls are performed on a regular basis, something that is not generally done in most facilities. Poor lift (elevator) maintenance and housekeeping of the hoist-ways and pits can lead to an accumulation of waste, water, oil, dirt and dust in the hoist-way and pit, creating an ideal breeding ground for mold and other potentially infectious microorganisms.

If a dedicated "clean" lift is used to transport clean or sterile items from the reprocessing dispatch area, the lift should be located in a designated "clean area" of dispatch and the point of use. The same lift should not be used for transporting contaminated and sterile items. A dedicated "soiled" lift should be available to transport soiled items from the point of use to the "dirty" receiving area and a dedicated "clean" lift should be used to transport sterile items separately. A possible disadvantage of dedicated lifts may be that longer queue times are experienced as a result of waiting for the respective dedicated soiled or clean lift (elevator). In the case of sterile items there is also the potential for condensate to occur on plastic or

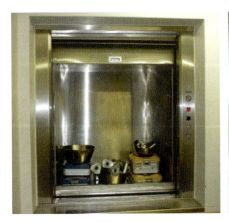 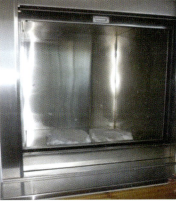

Figure 12.4 Examples of lifts used to transport items to and from a reprocessing area. In this case, a dedicated lift is shown for soiled items (left) and sterile items (right).

metal surfaces that are moved from air-conditioned areas such as theatres and the reprocessing area to non-air-conditioned environments such as lifts (elevators) and then back to another environment.

Transport to another facility

In some cases, reprocessed (including sterile) goods will need to be transported to a different off-site facility for further storage and/or patient use. In these cases, it is recommended that transport vehicles are completely enclosed with all items (clean and/or dirty) securely packed and separated in order to protect them from damage and contamination during transport. The vehicles used for transport should be able to completely separate clean and reprocessed/sterile items from contaminated items (Chapter 7, Figure 12.5). Reprocessed items being transported by road should

preferably have a dedicated drop-off unloading area and procedures in place for separation from any loading area for dirty items. Ideally the delivery area should lead directly to a dedicated receiving area to minimize handling.

External transport vehicles should have a routine cleaning and maintenance program. If applicable, carts should be secured during transportation within the vehicle to prevent damage or cross-contamination. Vehicles should be designed in such a way as to allow for ease of loading and unloading. Many vehicles carrying high volumes of devices have a tail lift fitted to facilitate the loading of trolleys. Environmental conditions should be regularly assessed for temperature and humidity changes, which may affect the load during transport; for example in very hot areas vehicles may need to have a temperature control.

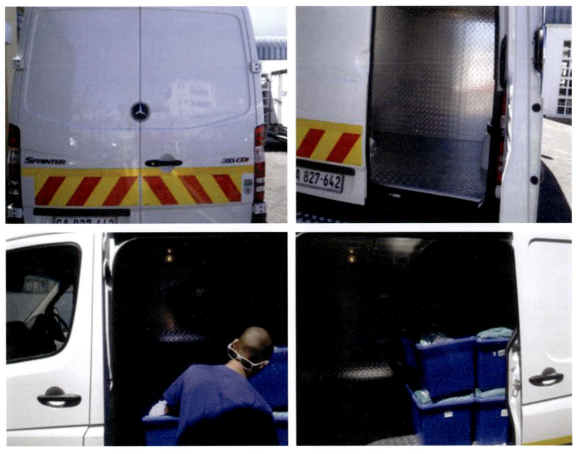

Figure 12.5 Example of a dedicated transport vehicle separating clean and dirty items. The sterile items go into the back of the vehicle (top panel), which is separated from the front by a metal divider. The dirty items (in bins) go into the front of the transport vehicle through a sliding side door.

Guidance at the point of use

Sterile packaged or otherwise reprocessed items should be inspected at the point of use. First, the external condition of any packaging should be inspected (Figure 12.6). Conditions under which a product may be considered unsterile or otherwise compromised include:
- Incorrectly wrapped
- Damaged or opened
- Punctures, holes or tears
- Signs of moisture or stains, including if still wet after a sterilization cycle or that may have come into contact with water during storage

- Obvious signs of external contamination where packs might have been placed or dropped on a dirty surface
- Have no indication of having been through a sterilizing process (e.g. an external chemical indicator not present or has not changed to a defined color)
- Broken seals, including tamper proof locks on rigid containers are broken/missing
- Excessive dust
- Evidence of crushing
- No labeling or no production and/or expiration date

Finally, when the packaging is opened at the site of use (Chapter 3, in the section on the operating room (OR)/procedure room) by the medical/surgical staff, they must check that the device/set is fit for use, to include:

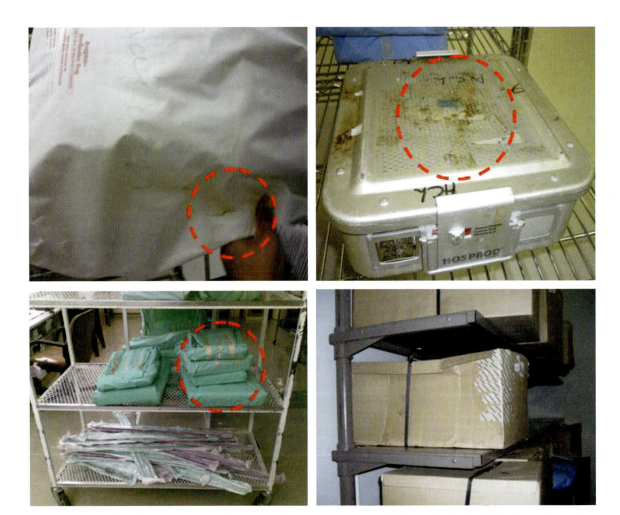

Figure 12.6 Examples of damaged, sterile packaged goods that may be compromised. Torn packaging (top left), dirty rigid container (top right), inadequate transport/storage (compressed packs, bottom left) and inadequate packaging (bottom right).

Table 12.1 Standards and guidelines for the storage and distribution of devices prior to patient use.

Guidelines/standards	Title	Description
AS/NZS 4187:2003	*Cleaning, disinfecting and sterilizing re-usable medical and surgical instruments and equipment, and maintenance of associated environments in healthcare facilities*	Section 9 provides guidelines of the storage and handling of reprocessed items
ANSI/AAMI ST79:2010 & A1:2010	*Comprehensive guide to steam sterilization and sterility assurance in healthcare facilities*	Sections 8.9.1 and 8.9.2 cover storage facilities for steam sterilized items
Association of periOperative Registered Nurses (AORN), 2011	*Perioperative standards and recommended practices*	Standards and recommendations for peri-operative practice including decontamination and storage
DIN 58953-9 (2010-05)	*Sterilization – Sterilgutversorgung – Teil 9: Anwendungstechnik von Sterilisierbehältern*	German advice on the shelf-life of sterilized devices
CDC (Centers for Disease Control) HICPAC Guidelines (2008)	*Guideline for disinfection and sterilization in healthcare facilities*	Provides guidance on storage and handling of disinfected and sterilized goods
AAMI ST58 (2005)	*Chemical sterilization and high-level disinfection in healthcare facilities*	Includes guidelines for device storage and transport following disinfection/sterilization
Association for Perioperative Practice (AfPP), 2011	*Standards and recommendations for safe perioperative practice*	Standards and recommendations for peri-operative practice including decontamination and storage
Canada Communicable Disease Report, 1998	*Hand washing, cleaning, disinfection and sterilization in healthcare*	Guidance includes recommendation on storage and transport
AFNOR NF S98-030 (2008)	*Enceinte de stockage des endoscopes thermosensibles*	Standard for flexible endoscope storage cabinets
Institute of Decontamination Sciences (IDSc)	*Standards and practice guidance standards and practice guidance document revised edition 2011*	Sections 4.8 processed goods storage and 4.9 distribution and storage

• Any associated internal chemical indicators (where these are used) have changed to the defined color, as described by the manufacturer (Chapter 14).

• All devices in a set are present and operational for the procedure. The staff may check for any signs of damage at this stage. For example, rusting may have occurring during storing due to the effects of sterilization (e.g. presence of chlorine or other chemicals in steam; Chapter 11, in the section on troubleshooting steam sterilization problems) or if devices have been stored wet. Another example is damage due to inadequate handling during storage/transport of the device/device set.

• All devices are present in a set and in accordance with a checklist.

• No recalls have been requested by the reprocessing department (Chapter 14).

It is essential that the devices are handled correctly and aseptically during a procedure set-up and immediately prior to use to ensure that they are safe for patient use (Chapter 3, in the section on the operating room (OR)/procedure room). Inadequate handling at this stage can compromise the entire reprocessing cycle and patient safety.

Standards and guidelines

Correct storage and distribution of devices and materials is important to maintain the safety of reprocessed devices, including sterile packaged instruments throughout the storage and transportation. Table 12.1 provides a list of standards and guidelines that are used worldwide.

13 Safety

Introduction

"Safety" may be defined as the condition of being protected from danger, harm or injury. Everything we do on a daily basis, both private and professional, has potential safety risks. Work safety practices are designed to reduce these risks to a minimum while at work. Reprocessing facilities can pose numerous safety issues, including physical activity (lifting, pushing-pulling), use of chemicals (including liquids, gases and even radioactivity), handling of contaminated waste/devices, handling of sharp instruments, etc. Safety in reprocessing facilities is therefore a particularly important aspect to consider. It is impossible to eliminate all safety risks, but these can be reduced by understanding the hazards, establishing facility policies to reduce them, providing regular training to staff and from the dedication of staff/management to maintain safe working practices. Safety is therefore the responsibility of everyone, staff and management alike. The goal of safety management should be to reduce these risks of danger and injury where possible and to be prepared to cope with emergencies. Essential precautions such as safety policies, training, emergency procedures, waste policy and even possible evacuation are an integral part of safety management. Although it is possible to reduce healthcare worker exposure to hazards, it is largely dependent on training and staff compliance with procedures. Most accidents are avoidable with correct staff training and compliance.

Types of workplace safety hazards

Healthcare facility staff can face a wide range of hazards on the job. These include:

- Microbiological risks, in particular the risks of being directly exposed to various different types of pathogenic microorganisms (Chapter 5).
- Chemical risks, from the various types of chemicals used for cleaning, disinfection and sterilization. Chemicals are a significant safety concern, be they in solid, liquid or gas form (Chapter 6). These can range from short to long-term health effects.
- Device risks: many surgical and medical devices are sharp (Chapter 4) and can damage the skin, eyes and mucous membranes. Sharp injuries are particularly common during device reprocessing and are an even greater concern when pathogenic microorganisms may be present.
- Equipment risks: these may include the risks of burns (e.g. from the internal surface of a steam sterilizer or accidental release of steam into a working area), injury to the hands (e.g. crushing) or feet (from dropping). Any moving part of a piece of equipment is a particular safety hazard.
- Physical health, including ergonomics (or human factors), such as posture on sitting or standing while working, correct design/use of loading carts, minimizing risks from bending/moving articles and overall well-being while working in a reprocessing environment.
- Emotional health: although often underestimated in comparison to other safety risks, emotional health issues such as stress should also be considered.

Health and safety must be at the forefront of all decisions and policies within a reprocessing facility. The overall safety of employees and patients is the ultimate responsibility of the facility management team. But equally, all healthcare workers must be made aware of potential hazards associated with day-to-day activities, be trained in practices that will prevent injury and accidents, and be responsible in ensuring that they following best practices.

A Practical Guide to Decontamination in Healthcare, First Edition. Gerald McDonnell and Denise Sheard.
© 2012 Gerald McDonnell and Denise Sheard. Published 2012 by Blackwell Publishing Ltd.

Microbiological risks

Microbiological safety risks are particularly concerned with pathogenic (or disease-causing) microorganisms. These have already been introduced in Chapter 4 (in the introductory section), with particular examples including:

- Viruses, such as hepatitis B (causing liver disease), HIV (causing AIDS, a disease of the immune system) and norovirus (causing gastroenteritis).
- Bacteria, such as *Staphylococcus aureus* (wound, skin and other infections), *Escherichia coli* (gastrointestinal and other diseases) and *Mycobacterium tuberculosis* (causing a respiratory disease known as tuberculosis).

The problem with microorganisms is that they cannot be seen, but they are often deadly. Although individuals that are infected may be diagnosed (or known) to have a particular microbial disease, many more will be "carriers". Carriers may not know they have an infection (not showing signs of disease) or may be immune to or protected from the microorganism, yet are a hidden source of pathogenic microorganisms. Similarly, many microorganisms may be relatively harmful to healthy individuals, but can be a particular concern to sick (in particular immunocompromised) individuals. Microorganisms can also be picked up in a variety of ways, including through the air and surface contacts such as the hands, environmental surfaces and re-usable devices (Chapter 4, in the section on the manufacturing process).

An important concept to understand is the principle of "standard precautions" (formerly referred to as univer-

sal). The concept assumes that all blood and body substances are potential sources of infection, independent of any known or perceived risk to a patient. Typical examples of precautions used throughout the facility will include wearing of personal protective equipment (PPE), hand hygiene and safe injection practices or handling of any sharp materials (such as needles; Figure 13.1).

Blood-borne pathogens are an important part of this concern and are defined as disease-producing microorganisms spread by contact with blood or other body fluids contaminated with blood from an infected person. Notable examples of blood-borne pathogens are the viruses HIV and hepatitis B. There is no need to know if the patient is infected with a particular microorganism as it is automatically assumed that they and any associated body fluids pose a risk. Devices used for surgical and medical procedures should therefore always be considered contaminated and handled appropriately. It is good practice to ensure that the same precautions are used if blood is obviously present or not. Standard precautions are ultimately about the safety of healthcare workers, but equally apply to the patient, by ensuring that a standard reprocessing cycle is conducted on all reprocessing devices. It is a system of barrier techniques and safety procedures routinely used by healthcare workers, to prevent cross-contamination and the spread of infectious diseases when caring for patients, reprocessed devices and dealing with healthcare waste.

The role of infection prevention and control in healthcare facilities has already been introduced as procedures

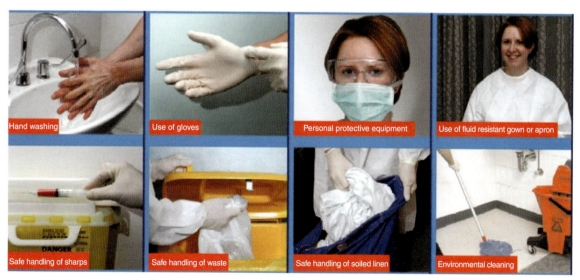

Figure 13.1 An example of a healthcare facility's standard precaution recommendations.

and practices to reduce the risks of microbial, in particular pathogen, transmission (Chapter 4, see the section on instrument marking). These include standard precautions that are as equally important in reprocessing areas as they are in working directly with patients. Examples include:

- Use of personal protective equipment (PPE), such as gloves, masks and eye protection.
- Frequent hand washing, particularly immediately on leaving a reprocessing area.
- Covering cuts and abrasions when coming into contact with patients or handling contaminated materials.
- Routine surface disinfection in the immediate vicinity of patients (high-risk touch surfaces in particular), including manual cleaning or soiled device sorting areas.
- Cleaning up known spills of blood and other body fluids.
- Reducing accidental cross-contamination such as by rubbing the eyes and touching the nose/mouth.
- Safe handling and decontamination of re-usable devices. Clearly the greatest risk will be during the transport of soiled devices, sorting and cleaning of devices. Adequately disinfected (preferably to a high level) devices can be considered safe for further handling (e.g. packaging for sterilization or transfer to a patient for use).
- Use of sterile disposable materials on patients.
- Safe handling of contaminated waste. The safe collection and disposal of needles (hypodermic and suture) and sharps (scalpel blades, lancets, razors and scissors) is an important example (see the section on device and equipment risks). The risk of infection following a needlestick injury with needle from an infected patient is estimated to be 0.3% for HIV, 3% for hepatitis C and 6–30% for hepatitis B. This includes safe hospital waste management and disposal, which is discussed in more detail in the section on waste management.
- Immunization of staff against known risks (for example against hepatitis B).

Strictly speaking, once standard precautions are in place, there should be no need to designate a set of instruments or other materials as being of greater or less risk. Despite this, facilities may decide to have particular warnings or handling procedures in place when devices are known to be used on patients with particular diseases. Such policies should be carefully considered and minimized, as it may often be the case that these diseases or associated pathogens are present but undiagnosed in a given patient. A current exception is the handling and reprocessing of devices and materials used on patients with known (or highly suspected to have) prion diseases (Chapter 6, see

the section on prion and other infectious proteins). Due to the unusual nature of these agents and particularly their resistance to cleaning, disinfection and sterilization, special precautions and procedures are recommended at this time (these are considered in further detail in Chapter 15, in the section on devices known or suspected to be contaminated with prion material).

Microbiological safety will not only apply to patients and staff, as there may also be risks to facility visitors and to the general public. Visitor safety will be a consideration in infection prevention and control, to include various precautions, depending on where the visitors will be and what they will do during their visit. Hand hygiene is always good practice (before and after visiting a hospital or clinic) and risks can also be reduced by the routine disinfection of various high-touch surfaces (such as bedrails, telephones, light switches, etc.). Visitors to a reprocessing facility should be aware of any risks and follow facility policies just like any staff (such as the use of PPE). This is particularly important for any person visiting the department for work, including engineering or biomedical personnel (either facility staff or external contractors).

An effective facility policy should be in place to reduce microbiological risks, including high-risk areas such as when dealing with patients, occupational exposure to blood or other body fluids, reprocessing of devices/materials and waste disposal. In addition to the specified standard precautions and procedures, guidelines should also be given to staff regarding what to do when things go wrong. Examples include a blood or body fluid spill, needlestick or sharps injury with a contaminated device and accidental swallowing or eye contact with soiled materials. This should include the immediate first aid required, reporting mechanisms, procedures to be followed (e.g. may include post-exposure, anti-infective prophylaxis such as taking antibiotics) and follow-up testing, provision of support and counselling (if applicable).

Chemical risks

The principles of chemistry and chemicals have been introduced in Chapter 6. A variety of chemicals in solid, liquid and gas form can be used in a healthcare facility and particularly in a reprocessing area for cleaning, disinfection and sterilization. Chemicals are a significant safety concern and can range from short to intermediate and long-term health effects. As a general statement, all chemicals can do you harm under the right conditions. Some of these are obvious, such as strong acids and alkalis can give a direct, quick and even serious burn when placed on the skin or eye. Others will be more subtle, with some extreme cases leading to increased allergic reactions (sensitization), toxic effects or damage over time and carcinogenicity ("cancer-causing", where a carcinogen is a cancer-causing agent/chemical). Any chemical used during reprocessing should be respected and the necessary precautions should be taken to limit exposure. Nearly one third of all occupational diseases are thought to be related to chemical exposure in the workplace. Toxic chemicals can cause health effects in humans if they are swallowed, contact the skin or if vapors are inhaled.

In considering chemical safety, there are at least three considerations:

• Personal safety
• Patient safety, that can be associated with chemicals remaining on a device surface (e.g. not being rinsed away) or that could damage the device
• Environmental safety, a growing concern internationally
Personal safety is the responsibility for each employee or worker in the area to ensure that any chemicals are correctly handled. It is the responsibility of supervisors/managers to ensure that staff are aware of any safety risks and have been given the correct training and equipment to minimize those risks. Note: this will also apply to visitors to the reprocessing area, as many chemical accidents happen to those in the vicinity of someone using a chemical.

In establishing and maintaining good personal safety practices when using chemicals (as for other risks) it is recommended to conduct a risk analysis (see the section on reducing safety risks and risk analysis). This would include identifying chemical risks in a given area, deciding and introducing measures to reduce risk (including staff training), and ensuring that these measures are maintained.

For each chemical product, it is good practice (if not a legal requirement in most countries) for safety information to be provided with the product. This is usually provided with the product, including the product label and associated material safety data sheets (MSDS). All chemicals used in the workplace should have an accompanying MSDS, specifying risks and precautions that need to be taken when dealing with these substances. The information on material safety data sheets will typically include:

• Product and chemical identification
• All active constituents as well as hazardous ingredients
• Specific health hazards
• Precautions for use at application strength, including any exposure limits

• Potential reactions with other chemicals/environmental conditions (e.g. temperature)
• Safe storage and handling information
• Emergency procedures
Material safety data sheet examples are shown in Figure 13.2. It is the worker's responsibility to be aware of possible risks and personal protective equipment that should be used. Staff should be aware of and be able to recognize a variety of standardized warning symbols that can be used to denote certain health risks associated with the product (Figure 13.3).

In general, the most effective way to reduce the risks associated with any chemical in use is to provide training, use personal protective equipment (PPE) and to periodically audit that safety practices are being followed in a department. Training is the first step, to allow any chemical user to understand their risks, so that they can appreciate how PPE or other safety precautions can reduce those risks. Personal protective equipment includes equipment such as gloves (Chapter 5, in the section on protect yourself and co-workers), safety glasses or goggles, face shields and disposable aprons (Figure 13.4). Note, for example, that safety glasses are usually designed to protect the eyes from splashes from the front as well as from the sides.

The final step is safety auditing; auditing can be defined as an evaluation or review of practices based on established procedures. When safety policies and procedures are put into place it is important to review over time that they are being followed. Audits can be defined at intervals, in cases where they are expected or, more beneficially, unexpected; they help establish that safety is important in a given area and that staff/management are committed to it.

Some chemicals are considered of higher risk than others and may require even tighter controls. Examples include the use of various types of gases, such as ethylene oxide (for sterilization; Chapter 11, in the section on chemical sterilization) or aldehyde-based liquid disinfectants like glutaraldehyde (Chapter 9, in the section on chemical disinfection). Ethylene oxide gas, for example, is considered flammable/explosive at concentrations of ~3% gas in air, can be lethal at 800 ppm and is considered a carcinogen (cancer causing) over time. For this reason, reasonably tight controls and monitoring systems are strongly encouraged to be used in areas using the gas for sterilization. Special facility design or handling equipment (e.g. dedicated ventilation) may be required based on manufacturers' guidelines and local health and safety requirements.

MATERIAL SAFETY DATA SHEET

Issue Date: 6/01
Issue Date: N/A
Supersedes: 2/1.00

SECTION I - CHEMICAL PRODUCT

Identity: **Disinfectant Powder Cleanser**
Brands: **COMET Disinfectant Cleanser with Chlorinol (Professional Line)**

Hazard Rating: 1

Health: 1
Flammability: 1
Reactivity: 1

4=EXTREME
3=HIGH
2= MODERATE
1=SLIGHT

Emergency Telephone Number: - 1-800-332-7787 or call Local Poison Control Center

SECTION II - COMPOSITION AND INGREDIENTS

Ingredients/Chemical Name: Bleach, cleaning agents (calcium carbonate, sodium carbonate, anionic surfactants), quality control agents, perfume, color. Comet Disinfectant Cleanser with Chlorinol contains no phosphorus.

Hazardous Ingredients as defined by OSHA, 29 CFR 1910.1200.

Chemical Name	Common Name	CAS No.	Recommended Limits	Composition Range	LD50/LC50
Calcium carbonate	Limestone	1317-65-3	ACGIH TWA: 10mg/m³ (total dust) / 5 mg/m³ (respirable dust) OSHA PEL: 15mg/m³	60-100%	NA/NA
Silica, quartz	Quartz (naturally occurring component of limestone)	14808-60-7	ACGIH TWA: 0.1mg/m³ (respirable dust) OSHA TWA: 0.1 mg/m³	0.1-1%	9 g/kg/NA

SECTION III - HAZARDS IDENTIFICATION

Health Hazards (Acute and Chronic)

Ingestion: Mild mucous membrane irritant. May result in gastrointestinal irritation with nausea, vomiting and diarrhea.

Eye Contact: Mild eye irritant. Direct contact with eye may result in superficial, temporary irritation similar to those produced by other household detergents.

Skin: Mild skin irritant. Prolonged skin contact or direct contact with eye may result in superficial, temporary irritation similar to those produced by other household detergents.

Inhalation: Mild respiratory irritant. Unusually high exposures may cause coughing or irritation of nose and throat.

Health 3
Fire 1
Reactivity 0
Personal Protection J

Material Safety Data Sheet
Carbamide peroxide MSDS

Section 1: Chemical Product and Company Identification

Product Name: Carbamide peroxide

Catalog Codes: SLU1123

CAS#: 124-43-6

RTECS: Not available.

TSCA: TSCA 8(b) inventory: Urea peroxide

CI#: Not available.

Synonym: Oxygel; Peroxgel; Urea peroxide; Urea Hydrogen Peroxide; Carbamide Peroxide, USP

Chemical Name: Carbamide Peroxide

Chemical Formula: CH4N2O H2O2

Contact Information:
Sciencelab.com, Inc.
14025 Smith Rd.
Houston, Texas 77396
US Sales: **1-800-901-7247**
International Sales: **1-281-441-4400**
Order Online: ScienceLab.com
CHEMTREC (24HR Emergency Telephone), call:
1-800-424-9300
International CHEMTREC, call: 1-703-527-3887
For non-emergency assistance, call: 1-281-441-4400

Section 2: Composition and Information on Ingredients

Composition:

Name	CAS #	% by Weight
Urea peroxide	124-43-6	100

Toxicological Data on Ingredients: Urea peroxide LD50: Not available. LC50: Not available.

Section 3: Hazards Identification

Potential Acute Health Effects: Very hazardous in case of skin contact (irritant), of eye contact (irritant), of ingestion, of inhalation. Hazardous in case of skin contact (corrosive), of eye contact (corrosive). The amount of tissue damage depends on length of contact. Eye contact can result in corneal damage or blindness. Skin contact can produce inflammation and blistering. Inhalation of dust will produce irritation to gastro-intestinal or respiratory tract, characterized by burning, sneezing and coughing. Severe over-exposure can produce lung damage, choking, unconsciousness or death. Prolonged exposure may result in skin burns and ulcerations. Over-exposure by inhalation may cause respiratory irritation. Inflammation of the eye is characterized by redness, watering, and itching. Skin inflammation is characterized by itching, scaling, reddening, or occasionally, blistering.

Potential Chronic Health Effects: CARCINOGENIC EFFECTS: Not available. MUTAGENIC EFFECTS: Not available. TERATOGENIC EFFECTS: Not available. DEVELOPMENTAL TOXICITY: Not available. Repeated exposure of the eyes to a low level of dust can produce eye irritation. Repeated skin exposure can produce local skin destruction, or dermatitis. Repeated inhalation of dust can produce varying degree of respiratory irritation or lung damage.

Figure 13.2 Examples of the front pages of two material safety data sheets (MSDS). Note: the MSDS will generally be a number of pages long.

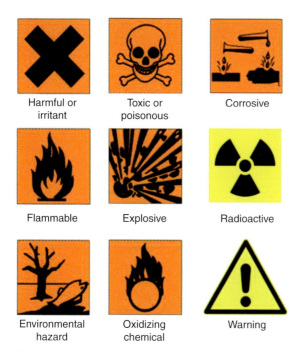

Figure 13.3 Examples of widely used internationally standardized chemical safety warning symbols.

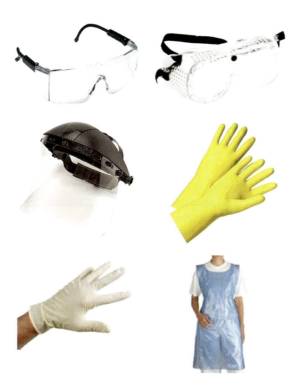

Figure 13.4 Various types of PPE, personal protective equipment.

In addition to personal safety, there are chemical risks to patients and to the environment. Patient chemical risks should be minimized by correct use and removal of chemicals used for reprocessing or used to maintain the device. Patient risks will include direct or indirect safety concerns. A direct concern is where a chemical is mistakenly used and left on a device prior to use in/on a patient; in these cases, toxic effects can be observed in the patient leading to health consequences. Examples can include overuse of the chemical (e.g. not diluted correctly) and inadequate rinsing (to remove the chemistry after use). Many chemical disinfectants, for example, require multiple cycles of water rinsing (sometimes up to 5–6 rinses in fresh water, each time) to adequately remove toxic residues of the chemistry. Indirect effects are due to damage by the chemical to the device; this damage, over time, can lead to problems in the safe use of the instrument on a patient.

Environmental safety issues concerning the use of chemicals is a growing concern internationally, with many countries putting restrictions on the types of chemicals that can be used. The main concerns are those regarding chemicals that are not easily broken down in the environment and can therefore lead to accumulation in environmental sources (such as water, the air and plants/animals). It is the responsibility of the manufacturer (e.g. to ensure they are complaint with any local or regional regulations), as well as the healthcare facility (e.g. local regulations on the disposal of certain types of chemicals down public drain or sewer systems).

Device and equipment risks

Surgical/medical devices and associated equipment can also present a range of safety risks to staff and patients alike. These may be considered as:

• General device/equipment risks: examples include sharp devices or needlesticks, as well as hot surfaces (e.g. the internal chamber of a steam sterilizer or thermal washer-disinfector). Many surgical and medical devices are sharp (Chapter 4) and can damage the skin, eyes and mucous membranes. Examples include various types of forceps, needles, scalpel blades and scissors routinely used in surgical/medical procedures. Sharp (or "percutaneous") injuries are particularly common during device reprocessing and are an even greater concern when pathogenic microorganisms may be present (e.g. during sorting and cleaning of soiled devices or other materials, Chapter 7, in the section on post-procedure sorting, and during waste disposal, and later in this chapter the section on waste management). An effective sharps injury prevention program should concentrate on prevention and should include training on

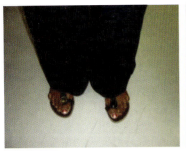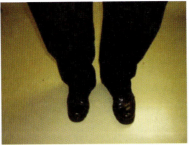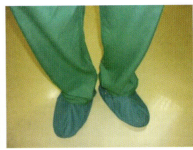

Figure 13.5 Protective footwear: on the left would be considered *inappropriate* (although comfortable) footwear; center and left are more protective, considering risks of chemical, infectious or weight-associated risks in a reprocessing area.

prevention of such injuries. It should also advise on measures to take in the event of a sharps injury, such as immediate washing, encouraging free bleeding of puncture wounds and reporting of the incident to management. A further risk to the skin/eyes is from burns, both from heat (e.g. from the internal surface of a steam sterilizer or accidental release of steam into a working area) and chemicals (e.g. on accidental release of chemicals during an automated chemical disinfection process; chemical risks are further considered in Chapter 6).

• Mechanical risks: examples will include injury to the hands (e.g. crushing) or feet (from dropping). Any moving part of a piece of equipment (e.g. washer-disinfector and sterilizer doors, as well as automated loading-unloading equipment) is a particular safety hazard. This will not only apply to staff/visitors but may also affect device safety (where a device is damaged due to inadequate equipment maintenance or use). Consideration may need to be given to the use of correct footwear (in particular to protect from mechanical and spill risks; Figure 13.5).

• Electrical risks: many devices and reprocessing equipment are driven by electric power. The combination of water and electricity is a particular safety hazard, as is the correct maintenance of equipment/devices. Any such risks should be clearly identified by the device/equipment manufacturer in their instructions for use. Electrical risks can also be caused by staff or bad equipment installation (Figure 13.6).

• Environmental considerations: this is a developing but important topic. It can consider the utility consumption (water, electricity, etc.) of devices/equipment but more particularly concerns the handling of devices/equipment on decommissioning. Regulations are developing on the safe disposal of such items, including electronic and material handling requirements.

It is important to ensure that these risks are considered and policies/procedures put in place to ensure any risks

are reduced to a minimum. Staff training is particularly important in such cases. This will include clear designation of responsibilities, and in particular on troubleshooting equipment malfunction. Untrained staff should not be allowed to investigate the mechanical/electrical components of equipment, but this should be the responsibility of designated internal or external engineering or biomedical specialists. Regarding mechanical, electrical and environmental safety, any risks should be clearly identified by the device/equipment manufacturer in their instructions for use. It is the manufacturer's responsibility to reduce any such safety risks during the design and routine testing of any device/equipment. It is equally the user's responsibility to ensure that any designated safety risks are understood and that devices/equipment are operated and handled correctly. The age and maintenance of older equipment is a particularly high risk, as the older the equipment the more likely it will go wrong (and the less likely that the equipment is compliant to the latest guidelines and regulations); such equipment should be closely monitored and maintained to ensure optimal and safe use.

Physical and emotional health

Physical health is an important consideration in any work environment, to reduce any unnecessary physical stress or risk of injury on the body (short or long term) from any repetitive and/or periodic actions such as lifting, pulling, pushing, etc. Ergonomics (also known as human factors) is a broad subject that considers the understanding of human-equipment interaction and design to minimize any safety risks, and optimum use of equipment. Safety risks included in this subject will include:

• Posture on sitting or standing while working (Figure 13.7)

• Minimizing risks from bending, picking up or moving articles from one area to another (Figure 13.8)

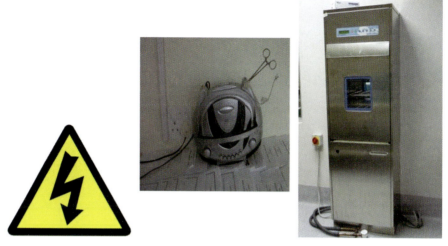

Figure 13.6 Electrical risks: a typical electrical hazard sign (left) and examples of potential electrical risks (right). Note that the picture on the far right is a washer-disinfector not in use (feed-water lines shown at the front), but is plugged into an electric source; the free lines would also pose a tripping hazard to staff.

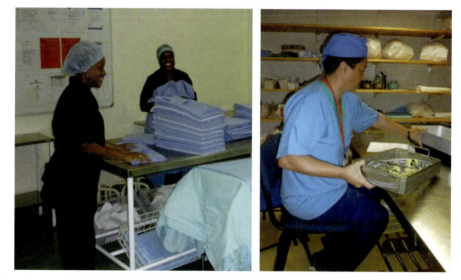

Figure 13.7 Standing or sitting close to a work surface at the right height and with a straight back can help reduce the risks of injury.

- Correct design/use of loading carts (pulling/pushing; Figure 13.8)
- Overstretching into, up to or down to a particular area (Figure 13.7)
- Safe operation of equipment and accessories according to instructions for use
- Minimizing risks with any mechanical moving parts
- Overall well-being while working in a reprocessing environment

For example, back or neck injuries account for nearly 50% of workplace compensation claims in healthcare facilities. The most common causes of back injury are heavy lifting, over stretching, postural stress (on sitting/standing) and repetitive job performance. The primary

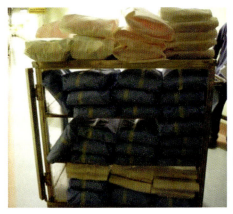 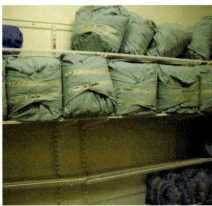

Figure 13.8 Pushing or pulling overloaded or heavy transport carts or lifting heavy loads (in the case of storage) can be safety concerns.

approach to reducing back injury should be training and reducing manual lifting and load bearing tasks.

Examples of practices to reduce ergonomic risks will include:

• Training on safe lifting, moving, pulling and pushing techniques. When particular high risks are identified, these should be reduced, such as by reducing the allowable weight loads/packs/sets tools to aid in reaching into equipment/areas to retrieve items or the introduction of motorized transport carts. The allowable weight of an instrument set should be based on whether personnel can comfortably carry the set; as an example, some guidelines recommend set weights of no more than 12 kg (~25 US pounds in weight), but even this may be considered too heavy for some individuals. Remember that the introduction of a method to reduce one risk may itself lead to another risk!

• Height adjustable workbenches and chairs, which allow a person to adjust to the right posture position when sitting or standing (Figure 13.9). The same will apply to height adjustable sinks or ensuring that the sink design is not too deep to allow for manual cleaning.

• Correct organization of workbench materials. All materials, such as in a packaging area to include packaging materials, indicators, etc., should be located within easy reach. A similar concept should apply to device sorting or a manual cleaning area. This will not only allow for good ergonomics but also efficient work practices (see Chapter 14).

• Wrist supports at every computer location.

Although often underestimated in comparison to other safety risks, emotional health issues such as stress should also be considered. Stress can be defined as the feeling of being under too much pressure. It is not always a bad thing,

as pressure can be motivating, improves performance and even increases productivity; however, excessive or prolonged pressure on an individual or group of employees can lead to unhealthy stress. Stress symptoms can range depending on the person and situation, but can include difficulty in sleeping and increased mistakes. These situations should be closely monitored in staff before they become serious. Suggestions to improve emotional health will include:

• Adequate facility design, including good lighting (preferably natural light), adequate ventilation and comfortable humidity/temperature conditions.

• Sufficient staff to cope with the demands on the reprocessing department.

• Introducing policies and procedures to protect staff from difficult situations. Examples include a policy regarding being asked to reprocess a device not provided with reprocessing instructions or to skip stages of a defined decontamination cycle due to surgical/medical needs. A simple suggestion in both of these cases is to have a form that needs to be signed by an authorized person (which may include a senior member of surgical/medical staff or infection prevention/control) that assumes any legal risk for such a breach of policy.

• Fair and legal working practices, such as intolerance of abuse (verbal and physical), frequent breaks, reasonable working hours and allowable vacation. Investment into staff, both financially and emotionally helps to retain good quality and trained staff.

• Including staff in department decisions and quality improvement exercises (see Chapter 14, in the section on personnel management).

• Being a good personnel manager and encouraging teamwork (see Chapter 14).

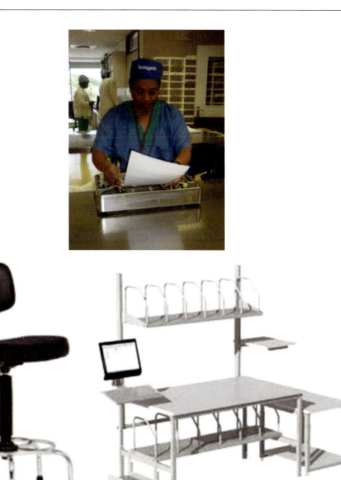

Figure 13.9 Height adjustable chairs and workbenches: the recommended correct posture position while sitting is shown as an example.

Reducing safety risks and risk analysis

It is important to understand the risks associated with any working environment and especially when things can go wrong. Risk analysis can therefore be an important tool to identify and reduce any safety concerns. Risk analysis has already been introduced in the reducing risks during the reprocessing cycle (Chapter 14, in the section on process risk analysis). The same concepts are applicable to safety and are further considered in this section.

There are four steps to consider in establishing and maintaining good and safe practices are:

• Identify and understand any safety risks (microbiological, chemical, device, equipment, physical and emotional) in a given area.

• Decide what are the highest risks and what precautions are necessary to reduce these risks.

• Introduce and train on any procedures or control mechanisms to prevent or control the risks.

• Ensure that procedures/measures are used, are maintained (e.g. by auditing) and optimized over time.

The first two steps are assisted by completing a safety risk analysis within the reprocessing area, as previously described in Chapter 14, in the section on process risk analysis. This allows for a structured and teamwork exercise to consider any risks and their priority. The introduction of any control measures may range from training, to new or existing PPE, new equipment or tools, etc. Many of these may require minimal or significant investment, therefore management should be involved in understanding any safety risks and recommendations from a risk analysis; where a specific investment cannot be made, alternative measures should be identified and introduced. The final step is equally important, as safety procedures are only as good as the people that use them. It is therefore essential to ensure that staff (and visitors) follow all safety rules and instructions within an area. Managers should lead by example. They should carefully follow the rules themselves and should have a zero tolerance of any staff/visitor (despite their job description) not following safety standards within an area. It is also recommended that a periodic audit of safety measures should be conducted within the area. Audits can be scheduled to be expected (e.g. every month) or unexpected, but either way staff should be aware that they will occur. The audit may be conducted by a manager, designated member of staff or an external person (e.g. an infection prevention nurse or facility safety officer). Be careful to investigate any reasons for lack of compliance to specified safety measures. For example, certain types of PPE may be uncomfortable to wear and alternatives may be identified with the help of staff to improve compliance. As in all cases, frequent, deliberate and/or repeated refusal to follow rules and policies within a department or area, including safety measures, may require disciplinary action.

Reducing safety risks in a work environment should be a constant goal. Continuous improvement should be encouraged. This will include full investigations of any near or actual incidents, with a re-evaluation of any applicable or associated safety measures. The initial risk analysis can be periodically reviewed to ensure it is up to date (e.g. if new chemicals or equipment have been introduced) or if any further improvements can be made.

Overall, risk analysis and management can help to create a "safety culture" within any reprocessing area or facility. For example, research has shown that frequent management visits to work areas and regular "safety rounds" convey a message to employees that safety is important. Another safety strategy is publishing results in the work area that highlight how many accidents have occurred or even been avoided. These are simple, yet effective methods to encourage safe working practices in any area.

Specific safety considerations

Waste management
Introduction
Waste management is an important society problem, but particular attention is given in this section to the safe handling and disposal of healthcare waste. This can include a wide range of materials and contaminants such as:

- General paper, plastic or other used packaging wastes
- Patient materials, including blood, other body fluids/wastes and even body parts
- Various chemicals (used or expired)
- Damaged, old or expired devices or equipment
- Used single-use devices (needles, catheters, sharps, etc.)
- Pharmaceuticals
- Radioactive materials, etc.

Healthcare facilities are encouraged to dispose of waste (hazardous or non-hazardous) in a responsible and legal manner in order to avoid risks to individuals and the environment. It is therefore essential that each facility has a waste disposal policy in place for the segregation and handling of medical waste from the point of generation to any treatment and safe disposal. An audit of what waste is generated by a facility is necessary to understand the types and volumes of waste generated so that an appropriate waste management policy can be put into place.

Most countries will have legislation regarding waste management and its enforcement. The legislation may stand alone or be part of a more comprehensive document (e.g. total healthcare management). Such laws are usually complemented by policy documents and technical guidelines. These policies/guidelines should specify the requirements for the treatment of different waste categories, segregation, collection, storage, handling, disposal and transport of waste, responsibilities and training requirements. They will also take into account any resources and facilities (e.g. incinerators) available in a particular area and any cultural aspects that may apply.

Management and treatment options should at all times be aimed at protecting the healthcare worker, patient and the general population, while at the same time minimizing environmental exposures. Individuals that may be put at risk and potentially exposed to infection, pollution, toxic hazards and injury by incorrectly managing waste include:

- Medical staff: doctors, nurses, technicians, etc.
- Patients receiving treatment in healthcare facilities as well as their visitors
- Support services staff: laundries, waste handling and transportation services; sanitary staff and hospital maintenance personnel
- Workers in any waste disposal facilities
- The general public: scavengers, children playing with items found in the waste outside the healthcare facilities when it is directly accessible to them (e.g. syringes) etc.

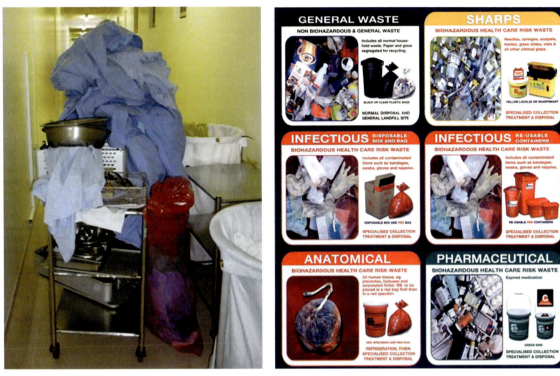

Figure 13.10 A typical example (left) of surgical waste requiring segregation at point of use/reprocessing as part of facility waste management. Examples of segregated wastes are shown on the right.

Waste segregation and types

Waste management is a specialized activity requiring well-equipped and adequately trained staff. The greatest impact of a waste management system is at the point of use. In general, healthcare waste is approximately 80% general (non-hazardous) waste and 20% hazardous waste that may be infectious, toxic or radioactive. The majority of hazardous waste (75%) can be considered as being potentially infectious (e.g. soiled materials, used devices or body parts), while the remainder may include various chemicals, pharmaceuticals, genotoxic waste, and radioactive matter.

The key to effective management of healthcare waste is segregation at point of use (Figure 13.10). For example, infectious materials should be separated from non-infectious materials as they will be handled differently during disposal. Segregation and clear identification of wastes reduces disposal costs and assists in protecting the environment. The World Health Organization (WHO) describes hazardous healthcare waste in the following ten categories:

1. Infectious: may be potentially or known to contain pathogens. Examples include discarded medical materials or equipment that have been in contact with body fluids such as feces, urine, blood, sputum or other body fluids.

2. Highly infectious: defined as specific high concentrations of microbial agents, including laboratory cultures and certain body fluids.

3. Pathological: human tissues or fluids, for example body parts, blood and other body fluids. Such waste will also be considered infectious, but may be handled separately.

4. Pharmaceutical: unused pharmaceuticals, such as vaccines and drugs, that have been opened, spilt or have expired.

5. Chemical: potentially hazardous chemicals discarded during the decontamination process, laboratory reagents, unused concentrated expired disinfectants, solvents, etc.

6. High content of heavy metals (such as cadmium and mercury): will include broken mercury-containing thermometers and blood-pressure gauges. As chemical wastes, they are recommended to be handled separately.

7. Pressurized containers: full or emptied containers or aerosol cans with pressurized liquids, gas or powdered materials.

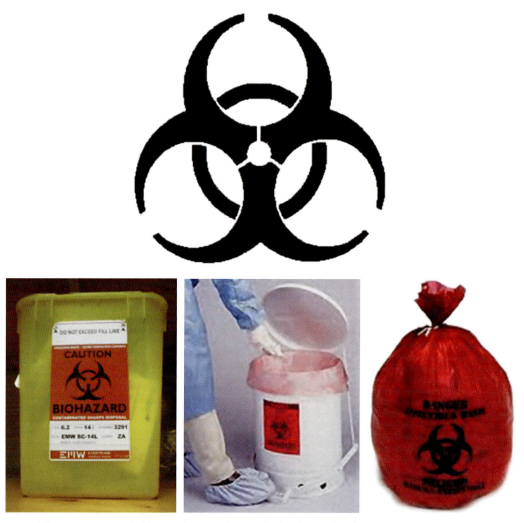

Figure 13.11 The international symbol for an infectious substance (top) and examples of its use on waste containers/bags.

8. Sharps: any medical equipment that could puncture the skin, for example needles, infusion sets, scalpels, knives, blades and broken glass.

9. Genotoxic/cytotoxic: classified as highly hazardous, mutagenic, teratogenic or carcinogenic chemical waste, such as cytotoxic drugs used in cancer treatment. Cytotoxic/genotoxic drugs have the ability to reduce/stop the growth of fast growing cells and are used in chemotherapy for cancer treatment. Feces, vomit or urine from patients treated with these drugs should also be treated as cytotoxic.

10. Radioactive: from the use of radiation (Chapter 6, in the section on light, radiation and the electromagnetic spectrum) in medical applications, such as for cancer therapy and imaging. This is typically low level radio-active waste, often including radioactive forms of chemicals such as cobalt, technetium, iodine and iridium.

Segregation should always be at point of use and is the responsibility of the waste producer. The easiest and most effective way of identifying the categories of waste is by sorting into color-coded and correctly identified plastic bags or containers. In addition to color coding the following practices are recommended:

• General, non-hazardous, healthcare waste should be disposed of as regular, domestic (household) waste. It can be collected in washable containers or cardboard containers lined with black or clear plastic bags. Care may need to be taken with certain types of materials; an example is with aerosol containers or batteries that should not be mixed with general waste destined for incineration.

• Infectious waste should be marked with the international infectious substance symbol (Figure 13.11). Bags and containers are generally colored red, yellow or orange. Colored bags should be supported in washable containers or cardboard containers lined with a red or yellow plastic bag. Small amounts of chemical or pharmaceutical waste may be collected together with infectious waste. It is recommended that infectious waste should, whenever possible, be sterilized as soon as possible by steam (autoclaving). Special handling may be required for waste materials considered to be "highly infectious", in particular, large volumes or high concentrations of infectious waste.

• Cytotoxic waste should be collected in strong, leak-proof containers clearly labelled as cytotoxic (Figure 13.12). Waste containers/bags are often colored purple.

• Sharp wastes are generally collected together, regardless of whether or not they are known to be contaminated/infectious. Containers (Figure 13.13 and usually designated as biohazardous) should be rigid, impermeable, tamper proof and covered so that they safely retain the sharps and any residual liquids that may be present (e.g. from syringes).

• Chemical (non-cytotoxic) and pharmaceutical solid waste should be collected in brown plastic bags or waste containers. Large quantities of liquid/solid/gas chemical waste should be packed in chemical resistant containers with the identity of the chemicals clearly marked on the containers and sent to specialized treatment facilities. Hazardous chemical wastes of different types should never be mixed, with reference to their respective MSDS (see the section on Chemical risks). Some wastes that are known to contain a high content of heavy metals (e.g. cadmium or mercury) may need to be collected and treated separately. Large quantities of obsolete or expired pharmaceuticals stored in hospital wards or departments should be returned to the facility pharmacy for safe disposal.

• Radioactive waste, where applicable, should be collected in a lead box, labelled with the radioactive symbol (Figure 13.14). Waste bags or containers are usually colored yellow. Low-level radioactive infectious waste (e.g. swabs, syringes for diagnostic or therapeutic use) may be collected in bags or containers for infectious waste, but may require special handling in compliance to local/regional requirements.

Staff should refrain from correcting segregation mistakes by removing items from a bag or container after disposal. If general and hazardous wastes are accidentally mixed, the mixture should be treated as hazardous.

Waste transport and storage

Accumulation of waste is a significant health risk to any facility. Waste should be collected and removed, according to the facility policy on a regular basis. It is recommended that waste containers/bags should not be overfilled. For example, when bags are ¾ full they should be closed with plastic cable ties or another method and placed into larger containers or liners in a designated intermediate storage area (if applicable).

Such storage areas should be close to the wards/departments, not accessible to unauthorized persons (such as patients and visitors) and be correctly labelled/signed as being a storage areas (Figure 13.15).

Any optimum storage area should have an impermeable, hard-standing floor with good drainage; it should be easy to clean and disinfect, with an accessible water supply for cleaning purposes. The area should be protected from outside elements, inaccessible for animals/insects/birds and not situated in close proximity to certain areas (e.g. fresh food stores, food preparation areas or patient waiting areas).

Transport of waste to a designated central storage area should be performed using a wheelie bin or trolley that is easy to load and unload, has no sharp edges that could damage waste bags or containers and be easy to clean/disinfect. Ideally, transport bins should be the same color as the corresponding bags and be covered. General waste should be transported separately from the collection of other hazardous wastes to avoid potential cross contamination or mixing. Waste should be transported along designated routes avoiding patient care, visitor and clean areas where possible.

The central storage area should follow the same guidelines as outlined above for any intermediate storage area. It should be sized according to the volume of waste generated by the facility as well as the frequency of collection. As a general rule, storage time should be minimized and not exceed 24–48 hours, especially in countries that have a warm and humid climate. Further external transport (e.g. for incineration) should be done using dedicated vehicles. The transportation should always be properly documented and all vehicles should carry a consignment note from the point of collection to the treatment facility.

Terminal waste disposal and the environment

Waste has a huge impact on the environment, potentially leading to pollution and even contributing to climate change (e.g. from greenhouse gas emissions). The amount of waste materials is increasing and becoming

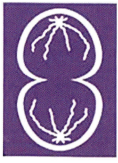
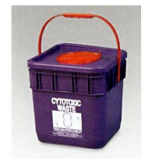
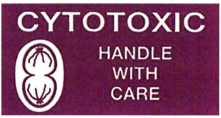
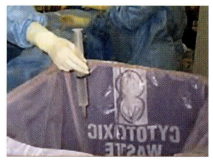

Figure 13.12 The international symbol for a cytotoxic hazard and examples of its use on waste containers/bags.

more complex, in particular with technological advances. An example is with complex mixtures of materials, including plastics, precious metals, electronics and hazardous materials that can be difficult to dispose of safely. Each year in the European Union alone it is estimated that three billion tonnes of waste is generated – with 90 million tonnes of it hazardous. This amounts to about six tonnes of solid waste for every man, woman and child per year! Healthcare is a significant contributor to this concern. Most healthcare waste is either incinerated, or dumped into landfill sites, with both these options creating environmental concerns. Landfilling not only takes up more and more valuable land space, but also causes air, water and soil pollution, discharging carbon dioxide (CO_2) and methane (CH_4) into the atmosphere and chemicals and pesticides into the earth and groundwater. This, in turn, is itself harmful to human health, as well as to plants and animals. It is therefore important to highlight that the most important step in waste disposal is the separation of waste at source of generation. This will help to minimize the various types of wastes which are designated for disposal in accordance with the facility and local policies.

The general public can be affected either directly or indirectly through the dumping of waste in uncontrolled areas, such as by contaminating soil and underground water supplies. Controlled areas are generally known as "landfill". Landfill is one of the most widely used methods of terminal waste treatment and the least desirable option. Landfill is a specially engineered site for disposing of solid waste on land, constructed so that it will reduce hazards to public health and safety. It is usually a large hole in the ground, such as an old quarry or mine. It may also be an area where rubbish is piled above ground and covered, creating a hill, which is then naturally covered (such as with grass) in a process known as land-raising. Such waste is generally compacted to the smallest practical volume and covered with soil to minimize any risks (including public health and safety). Landfills are generally used for the disposal of non-hazardous solid wastes. Landfills can have significant complications, including the production and release of methane and other "greenhouse" gases into the air. Landfill gas is produced from the breakdown of organic material in waste. Typically it consists of 50–60% methane (CH_4), 30–40% carbon dioxide (CO_2) and 10% nitrogen (N_2). If not controlled it can also build up in the landfill mass and cause explosions. A further complication is the leaching of hazardous materials into natural water sources.

Incineration (burning to ash) of wastes has been widely practiced for many years (Chapter 11, in the section on dry heat sterilization) and has many advantages. For example, it reduces waste volume to a minimum of ash and is also considered safe for the terminal treatment

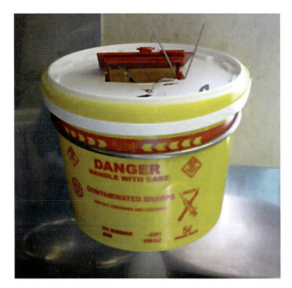 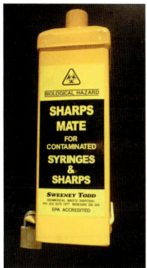

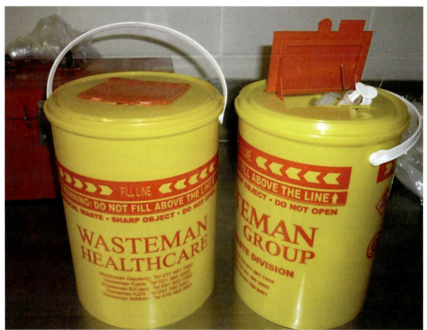

Figure 13.13 Examples of sharp disposal containers. Note that the picture on the left shows the *inappropriate* use of the container, with items protruding from the lid.

(sterilization) of infectious, hazardous waste. Historically all hazardous/infectious healthcare waste was incinerated, but with the increasing volume of plastic wastes such as polyvinyl chloride (PVC) that releases toxic substances such as dioxin (a bio-accumulative toxin) on incineration, this is no longer encouraged. In the last few years there has been growing controversy over the incineration of healthcare waste. The incineration of materials containing chlorine can generate dioxins and furans, which are classified as possible human carcinogens and have been associated with a range of other adverse health effects. Dioxins and furans are

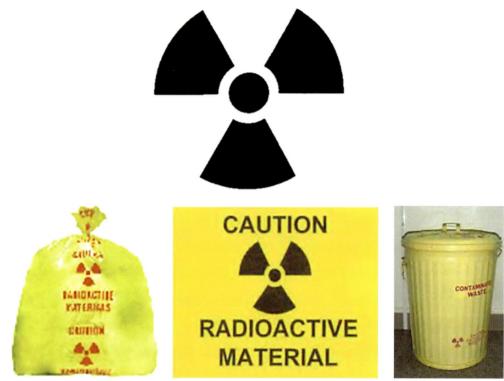

Figure 13.14 The international symbol for radioactivity and examples of its use on waste containers/bags.

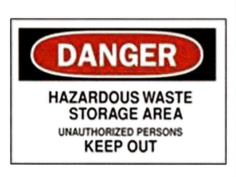
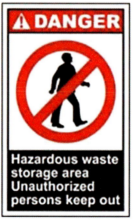
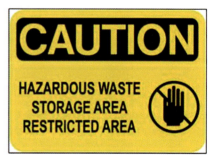

Figure 13.15 Examples of hazardous waste storage area signs.

persistent substances that do not readily break down in the environment and that can bio-accumulate (e.g. reaching the food chain). The risk of dioxin/furan release is higher at lower incineration temperatures (<800°C; 1472°F). Most human exposure to dioxins and furans is through the intake of food. Modern incinerators are recommended to be used that work at 800–1000°C (1472–1832°F) and include special emission-cleaning (chemical filtering) equipment that can ensure that only insignificant amounts dioxins and furans are produced.

More environmentally friendly alternatives are becoming available, such as autoclaving of infectious waste, chemical treatment and microwaving, and may be preferable under certain circumstances.

Overall, healthcare waste should be disposed of in accordance with all relevant national legislation, including regulations related to waste in general, environmental protection and air quality, and prevention/control of infectious disease. Environmentally friendly waste management is based on three principles:

• Waste prevention: if the amount of waste generated is lowered, this lessens any hazards by reducing the presence of dangerous substances in products, automatically simplifying disposal.

• Recycling and re-use: if waste cannot be prevented, as much as possible should be recovered, preferably by recycling.

• Improving final disposal and monitoring: where possible, waste that cannot be recycled or re-used should be safely incinerated, with landfill only used as a last resort.

Examples of international agreements that include these principles include:

• The Basel Convention, a global agreement ratified by approximately 160 member countries in an attempt to deal with the problems and challenges posed by hazardous waste. The key principles of the convention are environmental health and safety protection. They include the reduction of hazardous waste, disposal of hazardous waste as close to the point of generation as possible and to minimize movement of waste.

• Stockholm Convention on Persistent Organic Pollutants, a global treaty that protects human health and the environment from persistent organic pollutants (POPs). Persistent organic pollutants are defined as chemicals that remain intact in the environment for long periods. The key principle of this convention is that it is the duty of any organization that generates waste to dispose of the waste safely.

Accidental spillages/leakages

It is recommended that all healthcare facilities have an emergency spillage procedure in place stating what precautions must be taken and what procedures to follow in the case of an accidental spillage of hazardous waste (chemical, infectious, etc.). The procedure will depend upon the physical characteristics and volume of materials being handled, their potential toxicity, and the potential for release to the environment. A major consideration for reprocessing areas should be in the handling or accidental spillages, considering the use of various types of chemicals (solids, liquids, gases) and/or materials in these areas.

Before drafting a policy, it is strongly recommended to review what chemicals are present and their associated material safety data sheets (MSDSs), as well as other references/guidances for recommended spill clean-up methods and materials (including personal protective equipment such as respirators, gloves, protective clothing, etc.). Spill control procedures and control materials/kits should be readily available for any reasonably anticipated chemical spills. Place spill control materials and protective equipment in a readily accessible location within or immediately adjacent to the area where the chemicals are used. Chemical spill procedure guidelines will vary depending on the chemical risk, but in general the following should be considered:

• Management notification and who will be responsible for determining the nature of the spill and coordinating the necessary clean-up actions.

• Evacuation procedure of the contaminated area, if applicable.

• Immediate first aid and decontamination procedure for the eyes and skin of exposed personnel.

• Protective clothing/equipment should be worn by personnel involved in the clean-up.

• Measures to be considered to limit the impact of the spill. Examples include protecting floor drains or other means for environmental release. Spill "socks" and other absorbent materials may be placed around drains, as needed.

• Methods to neutralize or disinfect the spilled or contaminated material if indicated.

• Methods to collect all spilled and contaminated material. For example, sharps should never be picked up by hand; brushes and pans or other suitable tools should be used. Spilled materials and any disposable, contaminated items used for clean-up should be placed in the appropriate waste bags or containers.

Fire

Healthcare facility fires are especially dangerous, as they not only require staff to evacuate the area, but there is also the need to evacuate patients (many of which may be bedridden/immobile). A fire emergency is defined as an uncontrolled fire or imminent fire hazard, the presence of smoke or the odor of burning, the uncontrolled release of a flammable or combustible substance, or a fire alarm sounding.

The most common fire hazards in hospital settings are: patients/staff smoking, compressed gas cylinders, solvents and faulty equipment. The widespread use of combustible liquids presents a major problem. Many liquids or gases used, including in reprocessing areas, may be flammable or combustible and can be ignited by a spark or static electricity. As an example, a liquid may be classified as flammable or combustible depending on its flash point (the temperature at which it gives off enough gas to form an ignitable mixture with air, e.g. at or above 37.8°C (100°F). Examples of particularly flammable liquids include most alcohols, benzene, acetone and "combustible" liquids such as some lubricating oils, ethylene glycol and carbolic acid. For a fire to ignite, oxygen (in the air), fuel (the liquid or gas) and an ignition source (e.g. spark) are needed. To prevent fires caused by liquid chemicals, consider the following guidelines:

• Restrict the amount of flammable liquids in the working area.
• Carefully read manufacturers' instructions and material safety data sheets (MSDSs).
• Store large amounts of flammable liquids in a metal cabinet.

Many types of gases are used in healthcare settings, for example oxygen, anesthetic gases and sterilizing gases (e.g. ethylene oxide and hydrogen peroxide). Although oxygen is labelled as non-flammable it is an oxidizing gas that will aid combustion. Most gas cylinders are flammable as they are all under pressure and can present a fire risk. Such cylinders must be handled with care.

They should be secured and stored in a well-ventilated, fireproof, dry area at a temperature not exceeding the gas supplier recommendations. Cylinders should be handled carefully (never drop or bump) and stored away from boilers/hot water pipes/flammable solvents, open flames, etc.

Electrical equipment malfunctions are a further major cause of fires. Equipment that is not maintained or incorrectly grounded is often the root cause. Because healthcare facilities have many damp areas electrical maintenance and safety is vitally important.

Where evacuation from an area or facility is needed due to a fire, general regulations require that a fire alarm signal is given continuously and fire safety signage is in place to assist with evacuation and/or fire fighting. All staff must be familiar with an emergency exit plan. Signs (Figure 13.16) are needed to:

• Warn of hazards.
• Identify safe routes for escape.
• Indicate the location of fire equipment.
• Give instructions.

If a fire is initiated or discovered the following is recommended:

• Alert people in the area of the need to evacuate.
• Activate the nearest fire alarm.
• Call for assistance and leave the area immediately, if you are not a trained fire fighter.
• Close doors behind you.

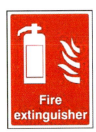 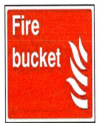 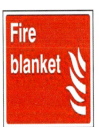 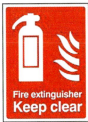 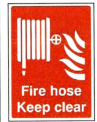 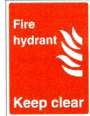

 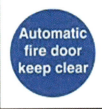 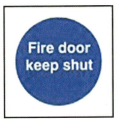 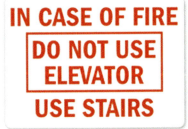

Figure 13.16 Examples of fire-associated signs.

• Do not attempt to use elevators.

• Assemble at the area designated in your emergency action plan and remain there until instructed that it is safe to re-enter the building.

Overall, a policy should be in place that describes the necessary preventive and action procedures in the case of a fire. It is important that area managers keep a record of any particular safety risks (including chemical, infectious or equipment) for the information of emergency personnel (e.g. fire officer). Staff should be trained on this policy and periodic drills should be made of the evacuation procedure.

Disaster planning and management

A disaster is defined as a sudden and usually massive accident, mishap or natural occurrence. Examples include nuclear accidents, hotel and high-rise fires, terrorist attacks, aviation accidents, bomb blasts, riots and industrial explosions, as well as natural disasters such as floods, tsunamis, epidemics, droughts and tornados. In such situations healthcare facilities are immediately affected, with significant demands being placed on personnel, resources and facilities. Facility disaster management plans are designed to best deal with such situations, which should include any reprocessing areas (both existing and temporary, based on the facility needs).

The aim of a disaster plan is to provide maximum benefit to the maximum number of affected people with the available staff and resources. This involves coordinated planning of all departments within a healthcare facility as well as coordinated outside community assistance. During a disaster, healthcare systems will be confronted with increased demands and decreased availability of resources. Local or regional health care systems best understand their own needs and resources and are therefore recommended to develop specific disaster medical capacity and capability plans, including reprocessing areas.

Disaster planning should reflect any local or country-specific regulations and guidances. Every healthcare facility should have a collaborated and coordinated crisis plan, including protocols, checklists, and signs to facilitate efficient hospital management and minimize chaos during emergencies. These equally apply to reprocessing areas, where the increased needs for medical equipment and supplies will be demanded. Protocols within the reprocessing area during disasters should be simple, concise, realistic, workable and located in an easily accessible place to all staff. Contingency plans may be necessary, such as alternative methods of cleaning, disinfection and sterilization that may not be optimal but sufficient to reduce any cross-contamination risks under a disaster situation.

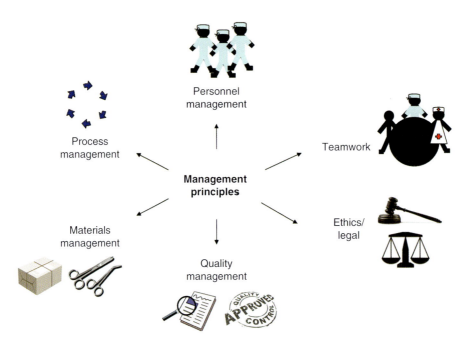

14   Management principles

Personnel management

Process management

Management principles

Teamwork

Materials management

Quality management

Ethics/ legal

Introduction

The term management refers to getting things done through planning, organizing, leading and coordinating of activities. It not only refers to managing people (personnel management and teamwork), but also ensuring that an area of responsibility is managed correctly (including process, materials and quality management). Any reprocessing area provides an essential supply to a healthcare facility, and it is the responsibility of the area manager and staff to ensure the safety and adequate supply of devices for medical/surgical needs. Managing is about being organized and pro-active, being able to anticipate and adapt to an ever changing and increasingly diverse environment with numerous challenges. Effective managers and management systems are proactive and make things happen, as opposed to ineffective managers/ systems that may only react to problems (i.e. crisis manage) and can lead to problems. Management is therefore not only the responsibility of an individual head of department or area manager, but takes a team effort to ensure that the overall process is efficient.

It is the responsibility of a manager to create and maintain an internal environment that enables others to work efficiently and effectively. Basic management skills include problem solving and decision making, planning, meeting management, delegation and most importantly

A Practical Guide to Decontamination in Healthcare, First Edition. Gerald McDonnell and Denise Sheard.
© 2012 Gerald McDonnell and Denise Sheard. Published 2012 by Blackwell Publishing Ltd.

effective communication. The key responsibilities of every manager involve:

• Planning: a systematic approach to setting and achieving the goals of the department and deciding how tasks will be completed.

• Organizing: making sure that the necessary resources are available to carry out the plan, that is, staff, technology, facilities, equipment, raw materials, information and budgets, etc.

• Directing: involves ensuring training, mentoring, leading and generally overseeing staff and others that may be involved in achieving the set goals.

• Controlling: ensuring that the overall departmental performance matches the plan and therefore the surgical/medical needs.

A manager cannot be effective without having the dedication of their co-workers (both within and outside a department under their control) and efficient management processes in place. The reprocessing area is a dynamic area, often with increasing demands, and is therefore dependent on a team environment with staff cooperation at all levels. Reprocessing area personnel need to work collaboratively with surgical and medical staff to ensure that the demand for sterile or otherwise reprocessed devices is met. In order for the area to keep up with changing technology, regulations and demands, individual staff members must excel at their specific jobs and work together as a team. Teamwork is particularly important because without it reprocessing can be inefficient and even increase the risks of mistakes being made. With the right teamwork, efficient management processes can be put in place and optimized over time. These will include management of the decontamination process, material/device supplies and quality, to ensure compliance with local and international regulations and standards.

Personnel management

Skilled and dedicated staff are often rightly considered the most valuable resource to any reprocessing area. Safe decontamination in a busy department can be labor intensive and relies heavily on having the right people. Staffing resources should be decided by considering customer (medical/surgical) demands, available decontamination equipment and the flexibility of the available staff. This can range from existing medical/surgical staff as part of their job description, to a fully dedicated reprocessing team. Device reprocessing is important for staff and patient safety, therefore these tasks should not be underestimated or designated to existing staff that are already overwhelmed by other responsibilities. Reprocessing area staff can be dedicated to this specific role or may be responsible for many different tasks, depending on the size and needs of a facility. If the department has employees that don't have adequate skills or training quality may be compromised. Targeted recruitment and training of the workforce should be identified to ensure quality and consistent processes. Designating the right time and staff to the process can have many benefits in patient safety, the care of equipment/devices and job satisfaction.

Personnel organization

Most reprocessing roles or specific jobs are part of larger organizations that can vary from a few to thousands of people. Examples include a small dental facility with one or two dentists and dental nurse assistants, to large hospital systems with dedicated departments. All will have some kind of personnel organization, ranging from various managers, heads of departments and business owners to supporting staff, including technicians. Despite the size of the organization, each level should have clearly designated roles and responsibilities. Examples in this case of a reprocessing facility will include:

• Department manager: this position requires a highly skilled individual manager who should have an understanding of reprocessing services and management. This person will be responsible for managing staff, the department processes and the overall functioning (including budgeting) of the reprocessing area. The department may include multiple areas, such as operating areas, endoscopy departments, associated supplies and infection control/prevention.

• Section manager: generally qualified in the field of reprocessing services and is responsible for the day-to-day management of staff/service, as well as staff training and ensuring standards are maintained.

• Team leader/supervisor: supervisors are an important part of the management team since they are the representatives of management in closest contact with the people who actually produce the work. They are very much first-line managers and should be regarded as such by both senior management and employees. Each part of the reprocessing area (e.g. dirty or clean areas) may have a team leader that is skilled in the functions of that area and is responsible for overseeing training and the running of that particular area.

• Technician/operator/assistant operator/entry level operator: depending on how long they have been working in the area these staff can have different levels of expertise, but should all be trained at the same level. They may have specific roles (e.g. packaging or cleaning) or be capable of moving from role to role. They work together as a team in carrying out the actual reprocessing work. The key responsibilities of a technician's job can include:

- Following department policies and procedures
- Collecting and transporting soiled items from wards and theaters
- Manual and/or mechanical cleaning of devices
- Device packaging
- Safely operating all types of equipment, such as washer-disinfectors, ultrasonic cleaners, sterilizers
- Cleaning and maintaining all equipment according to manufacturers' recommendations
- Monitoring and maintaining accurate records of the decontamination process
- Interpreting and maintaining accurate records of quality test results, such as Bowie-Dick tests, biological indicators, physical tests, etc.
- Maintaining tracking and traceability records
- Overseeing sterile storage and dispatch procedures
- Transportation to site of use (e.g. operating room or ward)

In a larger organization, career development and growth is an important consideration. Career growth can be defined as progressing through different stages of a job, where, as you grow and become more competent, you are introduced to new challenges, activities and responsibilities, as well as learning new processes, ultimately leading to a job which has more duties and receives more compensation. Career growth and personal development also encompasses acquiring educational and practical qualifications. For in-house training to be successful it must generate commitment from the participants and this can be achieved by linking to personal and career development.

Skills and knowledge requirements

Decontamination has become a specialized profession and is recognized, in most parts of the world, as a specialty in its own right. Reprocessing departments play a specific and important part in the running of any healthcare facility, requiring highly qualified personnel, highly technical equipment and standards. Working in such departments can be challenging, demanding and varied. Historically, reprocessing responsibilities fell within existing nursing structures and responsibilities; this is no longer always the case and is more often managed by a specific, independent and highly skilled manager, trained specifically in reprocessing medical devices and ensuring the supply of safe medical supplies. Depending on the country, there are many structured training programs that consider reprocessing as a unique discipline and allow for career development.

It is the responsibility of the top management of any healthcare facility to make sure that staff education and training is appropriate to their specific functions and this includes decontamination and reprocessing. It is the reprocessing area manager's responsibility to identify specific developmental and training needs of all staff in the department in order to ensure patient safety, quality and an efficient process. Considering the range of chemical, microbiological and equipment risks to staff and patients, it is essential that all personnel involved with device/material reprocessing have an in-depth knowledge of the full decontamination process and are adequately trained. Initial and regular (refresher) training are of equal importance. This will not only reduce any safety risk, but can also be an important cost saving to a facility by improving efficiencies and reducing accidents.

It is recommended that those working in a reprocessing area have a good general education, including numeracy and literacy skills, to ensure compliance with area procedures and processes (including use of equipment, tools and chemicals). An ability to follow detailed instructions and work quickly and precisely is an advantage. Good communication and teamwork skills are also highly regarded in this area of work. A training program should be aimed at improving the skills and abilities of the technician. All new technicians should be required to undergo routine induction training in hospital policies and procedures related to safe work practice. Regular additional or refresher training should also be considered (and is often mandated in different countries) to ensure staff are kept up to date on facility policies, procedures and standards. Training for staff in reprocessing areas can be broad and should include:

- Basic microbiology (including infection prevention/control), chemistry and anatomy
- Essentials of device types and designs
- Department policies, procedures and standards
- Awareness of legal and ethical requirements
- Health and safety issues, such as safe work procedures
- Personal hygiene, personal protective equipment and dress codes in order to protect the individual, colleague and the patient from harm
- The various steps in the decontamination process
- Specific procedures applicable to their area of work (e.g. disassembly, cleaning, disinfection, packaging, use of equipment, etc.)

• Safe operation of chemicals and equipment
• Accidents, incident reporting and emergency procedures
The most important measure of competence is that an individual understands why they are doing what they are doing. Examinations can be a useful tool to check the success of any staff training, skill or knowledge.

Personnel management tips

Managing people is a skill and often does not come easily. Some managers can have a natural ability to manage people and situations, while others only gain this ability over time and with experience. These skills not only apply to the management of individuals that may be under direct supervision, but also to individuals in other departments/ areas and even to senior managers/superiors! There are many management styles, approaches and recommendations. Some simple guidelines to managing people include:

• Focus on your common goal: staff/patient safety and ensuring efficient medical/surgical equipment supplies. Consider setting targets, including departmental, group and/or individual goals/objectives. These will encourage ownership and continuous improvement.
• Build relationships: working environments are all about people and individuals. Individuals make things happen and deserve respect. Building relationships does not mean making friends but does build mutual respect. It is helpful for managers to understand what motivates their staff. This can be different for each person, and may include monetary compensation, formal recognition, benefits, promotion, extra time off, etc.
• Be sensitive to the diversity of your staff. Take into consideration age, gender, language and cultural differences. These factors influence how you should communicate and manage the various individuals.
• Managing people and processes does not mean doing all the work yourself. Learn to delegate responsibility and encourage responsibility. Staff should be responsible for their actions; admit your own mistakes and encourage staff to do the same. Everyone makes mistakes, but everyone should also learn from them. Discuss and rectify mistakes quickly and with respect.
• Build a team spirit: encourage staff to work as a team, including team goals and responsibilities. This is equally important in and outside the reprocessing area.
• Develop your staff: encourage leadership and ensure training is adequate to meet current and future demands. Set goals and praise (or even celebrate) success.
• Set standards and lead by example. Encourage staff to be part of setting these standards and optimize existing processes within a department. The more you involve staff the more ownership and pride they will have in their roles.
• Be honest, ethical and fair. Enjoy your work and others will enjoy it with you.
• Managers will have their own unique style of managing people, but there are three basic management styles. The autocratic manager is very controlling and makes all the decisions. A participative manager allows the staff to be involved in decision making, but this manager still makes the final decision. A laissez-faire manager leaves all the decision making to the staff and is generally an ineffective manager. Each style has advantages and disadvantages, and a manager often needs to adjust his/her style to the circumstances and the individuals s/he is dealing with. In an emergency situation, for example, the manager will need to be autocratic. Overall, an effective manager will make use of all management styles depending on the situation.
• Decision making is an important part of everyday life and an important skill in management. There is only one thing worse than making a decision and that is not making a decision! In making a decision, try to follow a series of steps, including:
  ○ Gathering information
  ○ Understanding the problem
  ○ Looking at alternatives
  ○ Choosing an alternative and implementing it
  ○ Evaluating the results or outcome of that decision

Teamwork

Introduction

Teamwork is about a group of interdependent individuals, often with different abilities, talents, experience and background, working together to achieve a common goal. Teams can be specific to certain reprocessing areas or contain a wider range of skilled workers from different departments and possibly different organizations. Working together as a team within any reprocessing department has already been highlighted in the section on personnel management; however, it should be remembered that the reprocessing department can depend on others within the healthcare facility and likewise other departments depend on the efficiency of the reprocessing cycle. Consider, for example, the dependency of a modern reprocessing area on support engineering or biomedical staff to ensure the efficient operation and maintenance of equipment, but with surgical and medical staff demanding the immediate availability of sterilized devices for a patient procedure. Device and material reprocessing is one of the cornerstones of infection prevention and control within a facility, requiring close cooperation. Less obvious, yet important, staff members that may be involved can include finance and legal/quality representatives to understand budgets (today and future) and risks that could affect the operation and even reputation of the facility. The goal of a team approach to reprocessing is to ensure optimal and efficient reprocessing for all concerned, including the patient. Any such team needs a leader, whose challenge is to gain the trust and cooperation of all involved and to encourage them to work together as a team. A smart leader, which may or may not be the manager of the reprocessing area, will use all of these available resources in order to get the job done.

Effective communication is generally the key to these collaborative teams succeeding. If team members do not communicate effectively amongst themselves the task will not be accomplished. Communication can be achieved in many ways, but open discussion and agreement as part of a team should be considered as the most beneficial. Consider regular meetings, speaking face to face or using the telephone rather than writing letters or emails: emails can be a great way to send messages but a poor way to communicate. Irrespective of how smart or educated any one individual is in the team, the combined talents, expertise, experience and ideas of the group will always be more effective. Great team members should consider themselves part of the whole process/goal, with positive attitudes, willingness to listen to others and belief in themselves to play their role. A team must have operating ground rules, policies, procedures, principles and values in order to function efficiently.

Team leadership

To enable team success, a leader should be nominated who is able to lead effectively through their example, motivation and delegation. Unfortunately, not all managers are considered effective leaders. The behaviour of leaders and management will generally be similar throughout the organization; therefore focusing on providing an efficient service within a reprocessing area can have greater effects throughout a facility. If team members are treated as valued members of the team and with respect, no matter what position the team member occupies, they will be motivated to do the same to others. If team members feel that their efforts aren't recognized they become de-motivated and less inclined to do a good job. The personnel management skills and tips (in the section on personnel management tips) equally apply to managing a team under direct supervision and to a wider multidisciplinary team. Consider the following guidelines in managing any team:

• Define what the team is trying to achieve and make sure the team agrees.
• Make sure that all team members are aware of and understand the team rules (policies, procedures, ethics, etc.).
• Know what skills each member of the team has to offer.
• Ensure that all team members are capable and trained to do their specific job.
• Manage the team fairly.
• Delegate responsibilities (see below).
• Give recognition and praise where it is due; it motivates people.
• Deal directly with any conflict and differences of opinion.
• Enforce agreed policies and positively discipline team members who break these rules.
• Represent and support the team.

Delegation is one of the most important team management skills – and one of the easiest to get wrong. It is defined as empowering individuals or groups to take responsibility for certain tasks or goals. Delegation can help individuals and teams to be more effective and efficient, but also motivates and develops staff (including new leaders). Poor delegation can cause frustration, de-motivation and failure to get the task done. Delegation is not about telling someone what to do, but rather about empowering and enabling others to take control of tasks/goals and holding them accountable for the outcome. This can be particularly effective if team members understand, are involved with and agree with the goal. If team members are required to think about the task/goal, consider alternatives and make choices, the work becomes more challenging, with the added advantage of motivating the team member to succeed. For effective delegation consider the following points:

• Define what has to be achieved, particularly with the team member (even better if it is their idea).
• Ensure the chosen person is trained and able to perform the activity.
• Explain what is expected and agree on a timeline.
• Make resources available, if required. Consider people, location, premises, equipment, money, materials, other related activities and services.
• Offer support and encouragement, but do not interfere, unless the outcome is critical.

- Periodically review to let the person know how they are doing.
- Congratulate when they are doing well and offer advice when not. Do not try to fix their problems! It may appear quicker or easier for you, but it does not help either of you in the long term. You must be willing to absorb the consequences of failure, and pass on the credit for success.

Team communication

Effective communication is at the core of any successful team and organization. One of the first signs that a team is not working together is a lack of communication. Effective communication should concentrate on the basics, that is, listening, speaking, questioning, sharing information and mutual respect. When successful, it improves morale and the overall performance, reducing the opportunity for confusion and conflict.

Communication moves in both directions, downward and upward. Downward communication is the way that management communicates with employees. Every employee needs to know how the organization functions, what the organization's mission statement, values and goals are. Employees should be aware of all the up-to-date personnel policies and procedures. Managers should have regular face-to-face meetings with employees recognizing and celebrating major achievements. This helps employees perceive what's important, gives them a sense of direction and fulfilment, and let's them know that management is aware of their contributions. All employees should receive at least annual (yearly) performance reviews from their managers, regarding their performance, their goals for the future, accomplishments, needs for improvement, and management plans to assist the employee to accomplish the improvements. Upward communication can be equally important, from employees to various different levels of management. This can be done informally or formally at an individual level or at team meetings; it is important to use these opportunities to discuss any current concerns and ideas from employees.

The reprocessing area often deals with an interdisciplinary team that includes representatives from various departments (see the section on an introduction to teamwork). Communication outside the department can therefore be as important as inside. The reprocessing area should develop communication patterns, between the individuals involved and their respective departments; these should be meaningful, direct, open and honest. Be clear and precise about the direction of the department, its intentions, expectations and values. It is recommended

to focus on one issue at a time, using facts rather than judgements, that is, say what you mean and mean what you say. Effective communication is only possible in an atmosphere of trust and openness. As for internal teams, if other team members do not understand or agree to your goals then you can expect that the message will be lost.

It may appear simple, but there are three components to effective communication:
- Sender
- Message
- Recipient

Before communicating with others the sender needs to be aware of what they want to communicate, that is, what message must be understood by the recipient. Remember, communication is a two-way process and in order to communicate effectively, both parties need to take turns at listening. When communicating with staff members, ask them to explain what you have just told them, to make sure that you conveyed the correct message and that they understood the message clearly. The sender sets the tone of the communication; if the sender is aggressive the recipient will more than likely ignore the message and even respond aggressively. The expectations that you communicate will shape the response that you get; if the recipient does not understand the meaning of the message that the sender has tried to impart, the communication has failed. Remember that face-to-face or phone conversations are better to resolve issues quickly and effectively. Other methods, such as emails, can also be effective, in particular in providing information to a larger group of interested team members. Within any organization, an email should be considered as an official document within or provided outside a facility, and can have even legal implications; they will reflect on the sender, their department and even the organization. Care should also be taken to ensure that what is written is necessary, accurate, concise, professional and inoffensive.

Change management

Change is a fact of life; we may not be able to control change, but we can choose how we will respond to change. Change should be embraced and seen as an opportunity to do things differently, to grow and to develop new strengths. If change is to be effective the team should be involved in planning the changes and decision making from the beginning; if the team is involved they are less likely to resist change. Change can be disruptive, but forces the group to make choices. A good team leader will anticipate change and prepare the team to face the challenges. It is their role to challenge, motivate and empower the team through the change(s), whilst maintaining the dynamics of the team. Sharing the group, department or facility vision of the future with employees, defining their role and what they need to achieve, as well as the benefits of change to them, will encourage employees to embrace change.

Conflict management

Disagreements and conflicts, both personal and professional, are a normal occurrence, but how we deal with them can be successfully managed. The basic principle of conflict management is about understanding that not all conflict can be resolved, but it can be managed in a way that will decrease the impact on the team. The most common reasons for conflict among members of a team are:

• Lack of time or resources, which can either be perceived by a team member or be real
• Feelings of unfair treatment
• Gender and generational based differences
• Cultural differences
• Lack of role clarification and communication to team members
• Ineffective leadership

Conflict is natural and inevitable, but is often a symptom of problems and the need for change. Conflict in itself is not the problem; unresolved, destructive conflict that is not dealt with and erodes the team is the real problem. This is a responsibility of a team leader and should be taken seriously. An effective "conflict manager", must be aware of some conflict management skills and be able to use communication effectively to resolve or minimize the conflict. These include:

• Do not ignore conflict: manage it.
• Set team and individual goals, ensuring adequate resources (staff, equipment, etc.) are available. Getting staff to work together and to depend on each other can be helpful to diffuse disagreements.
• Hold regular staff or team meetings to discuss goals and problems.
• Build a team spirit and working relationships.
• Set team rules, including mutual respect. These may include already defined facility expectations, such as gender, social and racial equality. When rules are broken be quick and firm to reprimand.
• Consider having an anonymous suggestion box.

Resolution of conflict is dependent on effective communication and compromise when possible between the two "warring parties". Underlying issues need to be openly expressed and addressed, with the goal of gaining a mutual agreement. The outcome should be mutually satisfactory, but often with neither party feeling that they have been completely satisfied. Sometimes an excellent compromise is when neither party feel completely fulfilled. By discussing issues related to conflict management, teams can establish an expected protocol to be followed by team members when in conflict.

Effective teamwork

As an example of an effective team, let's look at a professional soccer team. The aim is not only to win a game, but also to win the league. In order to win the league you have to be the best. In order to be the best you have to have the best team, not just the best players. A great team works together as one unit, producing fast, creative, wise, decisive and consistent results. All team members must be aware of what they are trying to achieve and aware of what rules need to be adhered to. These rules give the team a sense of stability, in knowing what to expect. A soccer team needs rules on how to manage it and play the game. These rules are usually defined by the football authorities and tradition (i.e. if the goalkeeper is hurt the ball is kicked out of play). The team will also have its own rules regarding how many practices a player can miss, how many red or yellow cards are acceptable, etc.

In order to score goals against the opposing side all members of the team have to work together and contribute; it is difficult for ten players to win against eleven. The team is only as strong as its weakest link. If players are injured or suspended the entire team is affected. If one person forgets his/her role or does not perform adequately, the opposing team could score a goal. Team members need to monitor each other and be accountable to each other.

A team that wants to be great (world class) needs to stop every once in a while and look at how it is doing. Losing should not shut the team down. The team must learn from failures, re-focus and move forward. If a team loses they should look for mistakes, identify weaknesses and work on the weaknesses. Improvements can only be made if problems are identified. It is not a good sign if players start skipping practice, arriving late or unprepared for games or are being sent off. These are signs of the team starting to break down. In order to prevent this, the team will need to be reassessed regularly. The team manager is crucial in developing a winning strategy. For optimum production the manager will need to constantly observe the team and look at ways of working together more effectively by:

• Identifying differences and problem areas
• Deciding if it is time to do things differently
• Helping the team develop through training
• Bringing in new players or even coaches

Finally, when the team goal is achieved, there is pay-off for all team members. In soccer this will include the end of season bonuses, but also the sense of achieving the best, which all depends on how the team is playing. If the team is playing well and winning then the stadiums will be full and supporters are happy. They will continue to support and invest in the team. The supporters will expect the team to maintain a certain high standard, to change with the times and meet their expectations. The better the team the more supporters (everyone loves a winner), the more investors the club will attract. If a team is doing badly players and supporters tend to look for more exciting clubs.

Ethics and legal responsibility

All reprocessing area workers have a legal and ethical responsibility to safely prepare devices and materials for patient use. The patient, their family/friends and the healthcare facility depends on this and this should be clearly understood by each individual involved in the decontamination process. The word "ethics" is derived from the Greek word *ethos*, which means "the sum of good values of a character". Aristotle, the Greek philosopher, is thought to have been the father of ethics. A person is said to be ethical, when they respect others, follows the rules and values life and the community. Being ethical is essentially being fair or doing the right thing. This means understanding the situations from another person's perspectives – not just your own.

Legal responsibility refers to understanding and following the laws of any region, state, country or area in which you belong. This can often be complicated, changing and different from region to region. Legal responsibilities can include:
- Civil laws deal with relationships between people and protecting their rights. Examples are:
  ○ Negligence (malpractice): this can lead to injury (including infection) to you, other workers and to patients (e.g. not reporting a defective piece of equipment/device or intentionally providing a non-sterile device for a critical procedure).
  ○ Defamation: providing false or inaccurate statements about a person that could damage their reputation. Included under defamation are statements that are spoken ("slander") and/or written ("libel").
  ○ Assault and abuse: physical, verbal or mental abuse can include hitting, swearing and gender, sexual and racial abuse.

○ Invasion of privacy: this includes revealing personal or private information about a person without their consent. This could include employee or patient information.
○ Occupational health and safety: most countries have strict regulations regarding employers providing safe working environments and employees following safe working practices/procedures. This includes the correct provision and use of PPE (see Chapter 5 and 13).
- Criminal laws deal with actions against a person, property or society with intent. Many of the examples given under civil laws may also be considered as criminal, depending on the nature of the act. These many include:
  ○ Health laws, specifically directing facility leadership to provide safe care to patients. Facility management and/or an individual may be directly responsible for the negligence in the care of patients (e.g. infection transmission) or leading to staff accidents, with serious civil and criminal legal consequences.
  ○ Stealing equipment and materials.
  ○ Illegal disposal of chemicals or wastes.
  ○ Deliberate damage to persons or property.
  ○ Accepting bribes, directly or indirectly, including money or gift that alters the behaviour of the recipient (e.g. using a new product or influencing the acquisition of equipment/supplies).

Employees should be aware of the facility and personal legal responsibilities and understand the long-term consequences of negligence, omissions, and unlawful and unethical behaviour. The facility's legal responsibilities should be based on current regulations and laws applicable to their region, state, country and/or region. Employees must also be knowledgeable about the law, as in certain situations they may be involved in writing or modifying facility guidelines. For example, various regions, states, countries and/or regions may periodically introduce or adopt various regulations, standards and guidelines that directly affect the reprocessing area. To clarify:
- A regulation is a rule or order issued by a country, community or administrative agency, generally under legal authority and has the force of law.
- A standard is a document that specifies the minimum acceptable characteristics of a product or material, issued by a standards organization (e.g. ISO, International Organization for Standardization and CEN, European Commission for Standardization). Standards may or may not have legal stature within a given country.

• A guideline is a document used to communicate recommended procedures, processes or usage of particular practices. In general, guidelines do not have legal stature, but are often considered best practice at the time of writing.

In some cases, the correct adoption of the various regulations, standards and guidelines within a facility or department will be periodically audited by independent bodies and can have significant consequences (including closure, legal penalties, loss or reputation, etc.). Examples include in the USA by the Joint Commission (http://www.jointcommission.org), under the European Parliament and the Council of the European Union Medical Devices Directive (Directive 93/42/EEC) by a number of notified bodies and in the UK by the Quality Care Commission (http://www.cqc.org.uk).

Process management

Introduction

Decontamination is a process that includes various resources and requirements such as personnel, materials, equipment, utilities, quality, etc. These resources must be effectively managed in order to provide an efficient, effective and quality service. Resource and process management can be a delicate balancing act. When managing the whole process, an effective manager will consider the reprocessing area as a service centre with a number of customers, who at any given time will require prompt service. The manager needs to bear in mind that the service centre is limited by available resources and can only serve a limited number of customers at any given time. If the system becomes congested, due to inadequate resources, that is, instruments, personnel, space, equipment, the service will be delayed. The reprocessing area is generally arranged in a sequential series of steps (transport, sorting, cleaning, sterilization, etc.), which means that if there is a hold-up in one area it will impact on all the other areas. If a new device/set arrives and the service resources are fully engaged or not available, they will have to enter a queue and wait until the service facility becomes available. This queuing could present a particular challenge when items are urgently needed, such as for emergency procedures where a surgical device set is not available. Therefore, in addition to the "normal" process, special consideration may need to be given in the cases of such emergencies to allow for the safe reprocessing of these sets/devices to meet the demand.

It is important in both routine and emergency cases that a safe and effective process is in place. This process should consider all device types (critical, semi-critical and non-critical) and their requirements for reprocessing (including handling, cleaning, disinfection and/or sterilization). A facility reprocessing system should be established, with consideration given to any local regulation, standards and guidelines. It is recommended that the same process and policies/standards are applied across the whole facility, even if reprocessing is conducted in a centralized area and/or at smaller reprocessing areas. The best facility policies will consider the needs of all involved departments or individuals affected by the process, therefore they are best developed by a facility team. It is then up to the reprocessing unit manager, working with their support team, to ensure the optimal running and efficiency of the department.

Process improvement

Once a process is in place, the team should constantly be looking at ways to improve its effectiveness and efficiency. Many methods can be used to improve established processes. Commonly used methods include:

• Lean, a management philosophy that looks to constantly identify and reduce waste (time, money or resources) from a process. Lean manufacturing was initially developed in car manufacturing, but lean principles can be applied to any process, including reprocessing. It focuses on identifying wastes during a process (e.g. any unreasonable work, such as handling of device from one area to another, availability of associated supplies and increased safety risks) and how it handles changing demands (e.g. increased or decreased demands from operating rooms or failed quality indicators). Lean focuses on a number of key areas in any such process, including: transport or moving devices/supplies from one area to another; inventory control; motion of people/equipment; downtime; underproduction; overproduction (excessive inventory); and defects or failed quality indicators (such as device rejections due to inadequate cleaning or failed chemical indicators). The identification of waste leads to a team approach to reduce it, which is monitored for success/failure over time.

• 6-sigma (6σ), a similar guideline to increase effectiveness, but particularly uses mathematical analysis and specially trained individuals to lead/guide the effort. It involves improving processes by identifying and minimizing causes of mistakes/errors and variability.

An example of such an approach is known as the acronym DMAIC: define (the problem or goal), measure (process indicators by collecting data), analyze (to identify root causes), improve (the process) and control (to continually monitor the success of the changes and the process).

• Total quality management (TQM) is a further management philosophy for improving process quality. It is based on the simple concept that all those involved in the process should ensure its success, including suppliers, reprocessing staff, other department representative (including "customers"), management, etc. Total quality management encourages wider teamwork to establish and improve process quality, including many aspects of management, such as materials/personnel management, feedback, analysis and leadership.

Although these methods use different approaches, they all have similar basic concepts in optimizing any process:

• Establish a cross-functional team that is involved in and dependent on the process.

• Understand the "customer's" needs (in this case, the surgical/medical staff using reprocessed devices/materials) and the limitations of the process (e.g. washing or sterilization process times).

• Use some quantitative methods to monitor the process. Examples can include cleaning rejection rates, failed sterilization indicators at the site of use, device damage, turnaround times, etc.

• Identify a limited number of key areas to improve the process and decide, as a team, on the best ways to improve.

• Collectively make changes to improve the process.

• Monitor the success/failure of the changes and continue to improve the process.

Process risk analysis

It is important to understand the risks associated with the process going wrong. Risk analysis can therefore be an important tool in the device/material reprocessing procedures. It can be used not only to reduce risks in any process, but also in identifying important areas for process improvement. A typical risk analysis will consist of two steps:

1. Review current process/procedures and identify key risks in each area. Examples include devices not available for a patient procedure, insufficient cleaning, failed disinfection/sterilization conditions and damage to packaged goods on transport to a site of use.

2. Evaluate the risks, their significance and determine any action items for risk reduction.

Teamwork is the best approach in performing a risk analysis. Those typically involved may include: reprocessing staff, nursing and/or other surgical/medical staff ("the customer"), equipment/device/consumable manufacturers, infection prevention/control, health and safety officers, equipment maintenance/engineering and facility management. The team should assist in the identification of risks from their perspectives. This can be an extensive list; for this reason, at the start it may be better to focus on one part of the process (e.g. transport, disinfection/sterilization, etc.) and particularly if process analysis or complaints have focused on that aspect. The team should then consider rating the level of risk on an agreed scale (Figure 14.1). Such analysis allows for any risks to be graded from high to low, allowing the team to identify the more significant risks and consider action to reduce them.

There are many different methods, guidelines and standards that can be used in conducting risk analysis. An example is ISO 14971 (2007) *Medical devices – application of risk management to medical devices.*

Recall

A recall situation is important to consider as part of a decontamination process. Recall is the retrieving of unsafe supplies that have been stored or even already issued for patient use. All reprocessing facilities should have a written recall policy in place stating when and how items will be recalled. Examples of such situations could include failed indicator tests (biological or chemical), washer or sterilizer malfunctions, or if sterile packs are known to have been compromised. In the event of such process failures, items known or suspected to have been affected must immediately be recalled for reprocessing. In addition, any equipment or processes will need to be closely evaluated, including putting equipment (sterilizers, washers, packaging, sealing equipment, etc.) out of operation.

It is recommended when a recall is required that the details are documented, to include any known causes, affected items, retrieved and reprocessed items, and if any items have already be used on patients. As it becomes apparent that items need to be recalled, reprocessing personnel will immediately notify users and retrieve the supplies from storage or directly from users as soon as possible. A recall is usually authorized by the most senior staff member on the shift, or according to the facility policy. The reprocessing failure may be due to problems identified in the reprocessing area, site of device use or even from patient information (e.g. infection, toxic reaction or

Hazard scale

		5 Death or total systems loss	4 Major injury or illness	3 Lost time, injury or illness	2 First aid incident	1 Very minor, little consequence
		Catastrophic	Critical	Serious	Marginal	Negligible
5 Likely to occur frequently	Frequent	25 = Re-think	20 = Re-think	15 = Re-think	10 = Reduce	5 = Inform
4 Likely to occur several times	Probable	20 = Re-think	16 = Re-think	12 = Reduce	8 = Reduce	4 = Inform
3 Sometimes	Occasional	15 = Re-think	12 = Reduce	9 = Reduce	6 = Inform	3 = Inform
2 Unlikely but possible	Remote	10 = Reduce	8 = Reduce	6 = Inform	4 = Inform	2 = No action
1 Very unlikely assumption that it will never occur	Improbable	5 = Inform	4 = Inform	3 = Inform	2 = No action	1 = No action

Likelihood scale

Figure 14.1 An example of a matrix that can be used to grade risks identified in a process. Each identified risk is scored from 1 to 5 on its likelihood to occur (on the left) and the severity of the hazard (on the top). Overall, the risk is scored by multiplying the numbers on each scale (likelihood × hazard). The final score dictates if the risk is low (e.g. <2) or high (>15), therefore requiring action or not (in this example four different levels or grades are defined).

complication). Affected departments should be advised verbally as soon as possible, with a follow-up, written confirmation stipulating which items/trays from a particular batch are suspect and should be returned. Departments should be requested to check their stocks, used and unused for any suspected items. Recalled items should be labeled "under quarantine" whilst in transit back to the reprocessing area, where they can be safely handled/discarded; this will depend on the cause of the recall and should be in accordance with the facility policy.

A recall should be conducted by an authorized team. This will at least include reprocessing staff, medical/surgical staff and particularly any facility infection prevention/control representative. Infection prevention/control should assess any risks to patients that may be affected by suspected items. Team members may include other staff, such as hospital management, legal and engineering/biomedical representatives, as well as external suppliers/manufacturers, depending on the risks to patients and to resolve any identified problems. As a final note, the cause of the recall should be fully investigated, a report written and every effort made to reduce the risk associated with a re-occurrence.

Materials management

Materials management refers to purchasing and managing of supplies and equipment to enable the reprocessing department to operate effectively. A department manager may manage this directly with suppliers or with the assistance of other departments such as purchasing or finance specialists. This may include the various supplies specific for reprocessing (e.g. cleaning/disinfection chemicals, indicators, equipment, packaging materials, etc.), but also the various devices required for surgical/medical use in the facility. Two aspects of materials management are particularly considered: inventory management and tracking/traceability.

Inventory management

Inventory management applies to every item used in the decontamination process, from raw materials to finished goods. Efficient inventory control will ensure that the reprocessing area has the correct amount of stock in the correct place at the correct time to meet the needs of the facility. Everything used to reprocess various items,

Table 14.1 Advantages and disadvantages of holding too little of too much consumable/device inventory in a reprocessing unit.

Too little stock	Too much stock
This just-in-time (JIT) system aims to reduce costs by cutting stock to a minimum. Items are ordered when they are needed and used immediately.	Easy to manage, there will always be sufficient stock.
Stock doesn't expire.	Stock may expire – first in, first out (FIFO) system will need to be in place to ensure that perishable/expired stock is used before expiry.
Less storage space is needed.	Larger storage area is needed.
Makes it difficult to deal with emergencies.	Easy to deal with emergencies.
Run out of stock if there's a problem with suppliers or a sudden rush on supplies.	There is little risk of running out of stock.
Generally costs less to a facility.	Generally costs more to a facility.

provide a service and run the department is considered to be inventory:

- Capital equipment – these are generally fixed items such as washer-disinfectors, sterilizers, trolleys, tables, etc.
- Consumables – items that are used and replaced, that is, stationery, disposables, chemicals, packaging materials, etc.
- Devices – both a reserve supply of particular instruments that are in constant use (these may be directly managed by the reprocessing department or another group, e.g. operating room staff and surgeons) and reprocessed devices/device sets (e.g. sterile packs) that are ready for use.

Inventory control refers to the monitoring and recording of stock at each site of use, including how much stock to keep on hand, when to buy, how much to buy, controlling loss (e.g. due to damage/waste) and managing shortages and back orders. There are many methods for controlling inventory, all designed to provide an efficient system for deciding what, when and how much to have or order. Effective inventory management is particularly important in the supply of consumables and devices (new and reprocessed). In these cases it is about having just the right level of stock. What this level is will depend on factors such as the reliability of supply and how steady the demand/use is. When deciding on what level of stock to hold the following questions should be asked:

- How reliable is the supply, what is the lead time and are alternative sources available?
- Can demand for processed items be accurately predicted?
- What are the cost implications for holding or not holding essential inventory?

- What is the minimal functional stock level – can you identify a minimum stock level, and re-order when stock reaches that level? This is known as the re-order level.
- Is there an alternative, back-up supplier?

There are advantages and disadvantages to holding too little and too much inventory (stock) (see Table 14.1).

Effective inventory management will enable the department to accurately track all materials and processed items, to meet or exceed facility expectations. It can ensure consistency of supply and better understanding/controlling of costs.

Tracking and traceability

Inventory management can be optimized using some sort of tracking system. This can be manual or automated (computerized), depending on the facility and available technology. Tracking and traceability of reprocessed (and also single-use) devices is an important topic to consider for modern reprocessing departments and healthcare facilities.

The aim of a tracking system is to keep instruments moving efficiently and accurately to/from a reprocessing site and point of patient use. The loss or misplacement of devices can be a major cost to healthcare facilities. Understanding the complete instrument inventory assists in controlling costs and scheduling patient procedures. An efficient tracking system assists in inventory monitoring, control and associated replacement costs. In addition, some tracking systems can allow the reprocessed devices to be tracked with any decontamination evidence and direct use on a patient, which may be useful evidence in cases of patient infection/toxic reaction or a recall (see the section on recall). The ideal tracking system should have the capability to track instruments through the entire reprocessing cycle (including introduction to the facility), reduce instrument loss, maximize employee productivity, enhance staff training and education, optimize instrument inventory and utilization, and reduce surgical/medical team downtime. Historically, there have been no specific requirements or standards for marking and tracking of devices, but in many cases this is being considered as necessary in the short or long term. Presently, device sets can be easily identified (marked by various means) and tracked through a facility, but there is a growing need to ensure that individual devices can also be tracked in the future. This is sometimes specified to be done in certain countries/regions.

Unique identification codes

Many different coding systems (homemade and supplied) could be used to mark individual devices or device sets. In recent years, efforts have been made to harmonize coding systems and the GS1 (EAN) coding structure is often recommended for such healthcare applications. This system has already been adopted by different countries for implementation.

GS1 (EAN) (formerly the EAN.UCC System) was formed when the Uniform Code Council (UCC) joined the European Article Numbering (EAN). This system was introduced to enable manufacturers to eliminate duplication, provide tracking and tracing capabilities, facilitate maintenance, and provide item management. The coding system is specific, while a variety of existing data/number carriers can be used, including 2D data matrix, bar codes and radio frequency identification (RFID) for identification and tracking. Many codes used on devices/sets are identical in design to those used on foods and other goods (in particular bar codes and 2D data matrixes).

GS1 standards use a unique set of identification numbers for products, manufacturers/companies, locations, services and customers. These identification numbers are further sub-classified into groups, with the two more applicable to reprocessing being:

• GTIN: global trade item number. The foundation of the GS1 system, it is used to uniquely identify each product or item, that is, products and services that are sold, delivered and invoiced at any point in the supply chain.
• GIAI: global individual asset identifier. Used to identify any fixed asset of an organization, which includes all property of a business that will not be consumed through use (like capital equipment and devices).

GS1 identification numbers all include a GS1 company/enterprise prefix, a unique number assigned to the asset manufacturer or owner. No matter where a business is based or what language is used, GSI codes are unique and can be easily understood. The GIAI is the part of the GS1 system of standards typically used for the identification of re-usable devices. The GIAI provides a format to encode both the GS1 company prefix and the individual device number or serial identifier (Figure 14.2). The combined GS1/GIAI reference cannot exceed 30 digits. The benefits of this is that they are unique and allow tracking from the manufacturer to its repeated use on patients.

Coding or marking methods

For devices that require decontamination, etching or other permanent marking of individual instruments is possible. It should be noted that various marking or etching systems could be used, but it is important that they do not interfere with the safe use or reprocessing of a device. Consider, for example, the device being damaged, providing an area that could collect soil/hide microorganisms or even a marking tag falling off into a patient during a surgical procedure. It is preferable that the coding/marking is provided by or at least approved by the device manufacturer.

Automatic identification and data capture (AIDC) is the use of machine-readable codes to identify, quickly and accurately, an item or process. Typical examples include bar codes, data matrices and radio frequency identification (RFID). Bar codes are defined as an image of lines (bars) and spaces. This sequence of vertical bars and spaces represent numbers and other symbols. A bar code symbol typically consists of five parts: a quiet zone, a start character, data characters (including an optional check character), a stop character, and another quiet zone. A data matrix is a more advance bar code, using two-dimensional symbols, an array of dark and light squares of data housed within a distinct L-shaped pattern. They can encode product data in much smaller spaces than is possible with bar codes; they are therefore preferred on devices/materials due to the limited availability of printing space. Data matrix symbols are read by two-dimensional imaging scanners or vision systems. Finally, radio frequency identification (RFID) is a more advanced technology that transfers data (using radiowaves) between a reader and an electronic tag attached to a device/material (see Figure 4.3) for identification and tracking. An RFID tag usually contains at least two parts, one for storing/processing information (not unlike a computer chip) and the other for receiving/transmitting information (such as an antenna). The tag may be visible

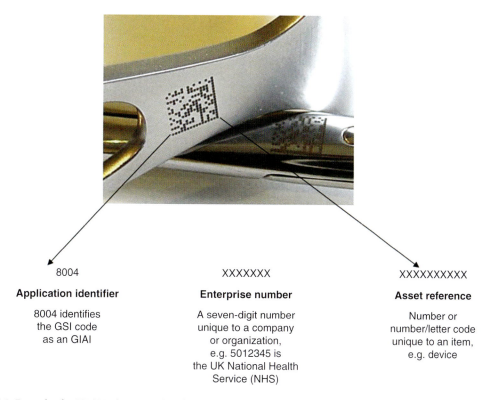

8004	XXXXXXX	XXXXXXXXXX
Application identifier	**Enterprise number**	**Asset reference**
8004 identifies the GSI code as an GIAI	A seven-digit number unique to a company or organization, e.g. 5012345 is the UK National Health Service (NHS)	Number or number/letter code unique to an item, e.g. device

Figure 14.2 Example of a GSI (GIAI) unique identification code for a re-usable device.

on the surface of a device or integrated into the device design (invisible to the eye).

It is optimal if the device/material is marked by the manufacturer and integrated into the device design. This is not always possible or provided today; therefore various types of marking methods may be used. They include:
• Adhesive labels: examples include pre-printed adhesive dots with 2D bar codes. They generally have limited data capacity.
• Laser etching: creating a mark where material is removed from the surface (etching or engraving).
• Laser annealing: creating a high contrast mark of no discernible depth. This is an alternative to etching/engraving as it does not damage the device.

Code scanning/identification

A typical code scanner uses a laser beam that is sensitive to the reflections from the lines, space thickness, variations, etc., in the bar code. The width and spacing of the bars in a bar code, for example, represents information that the scanner translates into digital data that is transferred to a computer, where it is decoded, recorded and processed. Depending on the technology used, each instrument needs to be picked up and scanned individually with a handheld or hand-assisted scanner (Figure 14.3). The use of RFID technology is an easier option as individual items can be automatically detected.

Quality management

Quality can be defined in many ways, but is essentially a measure of meeting an expectation or a standard. From a reprocessing point of view this will be providing devices/materials that are consistently safe and effective for patient use. Quality should therefore meet or exceed the needs of a "customer's" expectations (in this case anybody using the device, including facility staff and patients). Quality is therefore a standard that a facility should expect and define, based on their own and their customers' needs. A facility may expect the highest quality, but this can only be achieved by having the highest quality system/process in place that will include any reprocessing area. This will include defining, maintaining and measuring best practices in conformance with facility and other reference policies/standards.

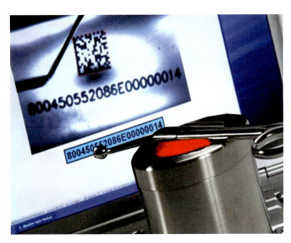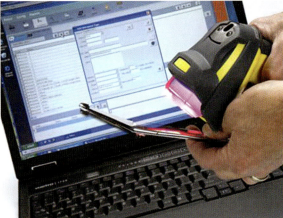

Figure 14.3 Examples of surgical instruments being scanned for identification using a fixed or handheld scanner/reader.

In order to achieve quality, a quality management system needs to at least define:
- Who is responsible for the job
- Why the job must be done
- When to do the job
- Where to do the job
- How to do the job
- What procedures to follow
- How to monitor the success/failure of the job

Quality management has two main components:
- Quality control (QC): a process that defines and ensures the consistency of all factors involved during the reprocessing cycle. The basic goal of quality control is to ensure that the products, services or processes provided by the reprocessing area meet specific requirements, are dependable, satisfactory and of an acceptable standard. This will therefore include management, management processes, staff knowledge/training/competency, equipment/materials, etc. Failure to meet these quality standards will result in unhappy customers and wasted materials, money and time. Quality control depends on various measures/tests/inspections to allow devices/materials to be released, thereby reducing the risk of unsafe supplies.
- Quality assurance helps to ensure quality. It implies that the necessary precautions have been taken to ensure that the entire provision of a product or service is within specifications. This usually requires that the whole cycle of reprocessing is optimized and monitored to reduce any risks. It will include various monitoring methods to ensure the process is working correctly and periodic auditing/checking of the process.

It is recommended that a reprocessing area should have a quality control process in place that will at least include written policies/procedures, requirements for staff training (including periodic training), maintenance of equipment/supplies and methods of ensuring quality control/assurance. This may be defined by various guidelines and standards by a facility, regionally or even internationally. Examples of such standards include:
- ISO 9000 series of standards, such as ISO 9001 (2008) *Quality management systems – requirements*. These provide general guidance on establishing and maintaining quality management systems.
- ISO 13485 (2003) *Medical devices – quality management systems –requirements for regulatory purposes*. This is a more specific version of the ISO 9000 series that applies to medical devices. Although this standard is applicable to device manufacturers, it may also be considered in some countries as being necessary for reprocessing departments, as they are providing a process of supplying a device for patient use (e.g. sterile device). The standard describes the requirements for the development, implementation and monitoring of a quality management system; this includes the requirements for the process itself, as well as for management and resources (such as staff, equipment, facilities, etc.).

A component of a quality control system is periodic auditing, where inspections are made of the processes, procedures and people within a department. Audits can be very detailed, and conducted by a department manager or independent person/group (from the same facility or by external groups, sometimes defined by local governments/agencies).

The remainder of this chapter will consider the various methods of monitoring quality control/assurance associated with a reprocessing department. Monitoring is a series of routine observations, providing evidence that the correct conditions were present in each and every item processed. Specific monitoring methods are carried out to show the extent of compliance to a formulated policy and/or standard (Table 14.2). Further details on particular process monitoring aids are given in the following sections, specifically cleaning, disinfection and sterilization.

Monitoring cleaning

The most important and practical method to monitor the effectiveness of any cleaning process is by carefully inspecting the cleanliness of instruments and materials. Visual inspection relies on the individual's eyesight and can be enhanced by inspecting in a well lit area and/or by use of a magnifying lens.

Care should be taken, where possible, to inspect areas of the device where soil may become lodged or is difficult to clean, such as a box joint on hinged instruments (e.g. forceps, Chapter 4, in the section on instruments for cutting and dissecting). Although visual inspection has the advantage of being relatively quick and easy to perform, it is known to be variable, non-quantitative and dependent on the vigilance of the staff inspecting the devices. Also, certain types/levels of soil may not be as easily detected by the naked eye. Despite these disadvantages, visual evaluation of the device cleanliness is currently considered best practice during reprocessing.

There are recommendations in some countries that visual examination should be complemented by other detection methods to confirm cleaning efficacy. It is proposed that over time such methods will become widely used, in particular as they become more practical for routine use in a reprocessing department. Many are already in use, particularly for laboratory investigations. These include microbiological and biochemical tests:

• Microbiological tests are based on the detection of microorganisms, directly or indirectly on a surface. A direct method is by taking a microbiological sample (e.g. by swabbing or extraction) from the device surface; the sample is then sent to a microbiology laboratory to determine how many bacteria are present. Such methods are limited, in that they can only be used to determine certain types of live bacteria (and potentially fungi) and require specifically trained staff (in strict aseptic technique and microbiology methods). Further, the results may or may not correlate with a defined level of cleanliness on a device (e.g. to include alive/dead organic and inorganic materials; Chapter 5). Overall, such methods are not considered practical for the routine testing of cleaning efficacy in a reprocessing department. An indirect method may include the use of a chemical marker that is found in microorganisms. An example is in the detection of a chemical known as ATP (adenosine triphosphate). Adenosine triphosphate is a chemical that is found in most living cells (such as bacteria, fungi and human cells); it is used for chemical transfer of energy in cells that respire (the process of converting nutrients into cell energy). The presence of ATP can therefore be used as an indirect marker for the presence of bacteria/fungi. In addition, as ATP is present in human cells, it may also be used as a biochemical marker for cleaning efficacy (see below).

• Biochemical tests (Figure 14.4). Essentially, any molecule that is present in human cells may be used to indicate the presence/absence of human and microbial soil. These will include proteins, carbohydrates, lipids, nucleic acids and other molecules that make up cellular structure/function. Other such indicators could be the presence of certain types of chemicals in specific soils, such as in blood, or more generally the presence or level of carbon present (as all organic molecules, including proteins and lipids include carbon; Chapter 2). To date, the most widely used biochemical indicators include protein, blood and ATP:

  ○ Protein is one of the most important molecules in the structure and function of cells (microbiological, human, plant, etc.) and viruses (Chapter 2). Protein detection methods have therefore been widely used to test for residual soil, significantly below the levels that can be directly seen by the eye. A variety of chemical reaction-based methods (such as those based on Biuret or ninhydrin reactions) are used to detect protein and/or peptides (smaller proteins structures). Easy to use protein-detection kits have become widely used for testing cleaning efficacy in reprocessing departments (examples are shown in Figure 14.4). As an example, a swab is used to sample the device surface and the swab is then treated with the chemical ninhydrin that reacts with most protein/peptides to give a purple color on heating; the presence of purple indicates the presence of protein above a detection level (usually defined by the kit manufacturer). At the time of writing, there is discussion ongoing regarding the level of protein detection that should be considered as indicating "clean". A recommended level is $\leq 6\,\mu g/cm^2$ of device surface.

Table 14.2 Examples of various monitoring methods used in a reprocessing area. This should not be given as an exhaustive list.

Reprocessing area	Monitoring
Cleaning	Manual: • Volume of water and cleaning chemistry • Water temperature • Frequency of water/chemistry changes • Rinsing • Visual or biochemical cleanliness Automated: • Ultrasonic power • Spray arm movement and non-blocked jets • Chemistry delivery • Process variables (temperature, pressure, flows rates, etc.) • Soiling and cleaning indicator tests • Visual or biochemical cleanliness Presence and use of PPE
Disinfection	Process variables (temperature, pressures, chemistry delivery, etc.) Equipment independent monitoring/process data collection Chemical indicator pass/fail Number and method of rinses (chemical disinfection) Sensor calibration Presence and use of PPE
Packaging	Visually check for cleanliness/residues/damage Rejection policy (presence and compliance) Check all instrument sets against a list to identify missing items Presence of in-pack chemical indicators Heat sealer efficiency/operation Visual damage to packaging (e.g. staining, wetness)
Sterilization	Process variables (temperature, pressures, chemistry delivery, etc.) Sterilizer print-out and/or data collected Sterilizer sensor calibration and equipment maintenance Pressure leak tests Biological and chemical indicators (internal and external) Process control device testing, including B-D tests for pre-vacuum steam sterilizers Gas sensors and calibration Gas or liquid storage conditions (internal and external); check that all packs have external chemical indicators before loading into a autoclave Items removed are intact, dry and undamaged Failed indicator policy Water or steam quality/purity
Storage	Stock rotation Damage of packaging materials Area humidity/temperature
Handling/ transport	Check all instrument sets against a list to identify missing items Cleaning/disinfection frequency of carts
Site of patient use	Check all instrument sets against a list to identify missing items Visual examination of device cleanliness/damage Aseptic technique Checking in-pack chemical indicators

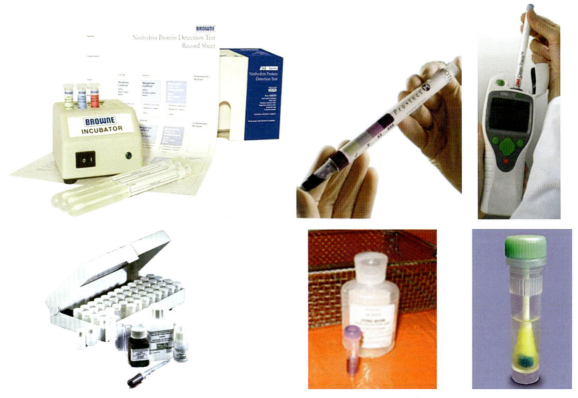

Figure 14.4 Various types of soil detection kits. On the left and center are various types of protein detection kits (including swab-based tests). On the far top right is an ATP-based test (with detector) and bottom right a qualitative residual blood test.

○ Blood can be detected using hydrogen peroxide, due to the action of enzymes found in blood cells that break down peroxide to release oxygen, shown as bubbling. Similar but more sensitive tests are based on a swab test that turns green/blue in color in the presence of blood/hemoglobin. Unlike protein, blood may not always be present on a soiled device but is a very common soil component in the use of many surgical/medical instruments.

○ Adenosine triphosphate (ATP), a molecule found in actively respiring cells as described above, has also been used as an indirect indicator of the presence of contamination on a surface. These include test swab or strip-based tests that give a color change on reaction with ATP at a certain level of detection ("qualitative") or a fluorescent (light-generating) reaction that is read using a handheld sensor/detector to give a quantitative level of ATP (Figure 14.4).

Care should be taken to read and understand the instructions for use provided with residual soil detection kits to ensure their correct application and interpretation. It should also be remembered that cleaning tests do not guarantee that a device, set or load is clean, only that the surface tested passes or fails a cleaning indicator test.

Manual cleaning processes can be considered very variable, depending on the operator, cleaning method, attention to detail, etc. Despite this, some quality controls can be used to reduce risks. Examples include standardizing the volume of water used in a sink (measuring and indicating the amount of water in a sink to a defined level) and an automated pump method to ensure the volume of chemistry used is in compliance with manufacturers' label claims, etc.

Modern washer-disinfectors can provide greater control and cleaning assurance. Monitoring tests can include:

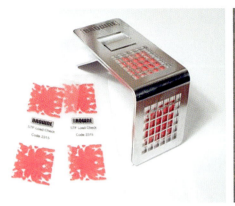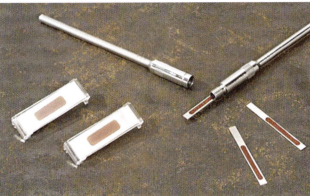

Figure 14.5 Examples of cleaning indicators.

• Parametric tests: test monitoring of key parameters that have been specified as being required for the automated cleaning process. This will include the cleaning phases (pre-cleaning, cleaning, rinsing), time, temperature, pressure, draining, chemistry dosing volume, etc. Some washer-disinfectors (in particular those in compliance with ISO 15883-1 *Washer-disinfectors: general requirements, terms and definitions and tests*) have independent sensors and separate process control sensors to confirm many of these important parameters; the data from these systems may need to be manually or automatically checked (by the washer control/computer system) to verify the correct process conditions. In addition to automated tests, various manual quality assurance tests can be specified, including checking drains, spray arm/nozzle circulation and lack of blockages, etc. (Chapter 8).

• Cleaning indicators: these are designed to provide a standardized challenge to a cleaning process (Figure 14.5). They are ready-to-use indicators with soil dried onto representative surfaces. Cleaning indicators can be used to test for the efficacy and reproducibility of cleaning in a washer/washer-disinfector. They may be used during installation and/or periodic testing of a washing process, but can also provide a routine test (e.g. daily or on every load) to check on cycle performance. There are currently no standards that define the design of such indicators, but they do specify their performance.

• Cleaning test soils: test (or simulative) soils are designed to represent patient soils that may be present on device surfaces following surgical/medical use. There are many types of test soils that are used for the development or routine testing of cleaning processes. Many are

country-specific, the recipes and associated test methods have at the time of writing been listed in ISO TS 15883-5 (2005) *Washer-disinfectors: test soils and methods for demonstrating cleaning efficacy*. These can be prepared with basic laboratory equipment. In addition, some commercially available test soils are available (Figure 14.6). Soils are composed of many materials, such as defined proteins, starch, egg yolk, etc., and some contain pigments so that they can be detected more easily during visual inspection. The test soils are applied manually (e.g. by brushing) to the instruments, washer chamber walls and any associated racks, and then dried for a specified time prior to testing. The instruments are then examined for traces of this soil following a cleaning cycle. Over time it is expected that future, international test soils will be described, including the requirement for pass-criteria in the use of the test soils to test any cleaning process.

Additional monitoring tests may be recommended, depending on the washer technology. These will specified by the manufacturer and/or in local/regional guidelines. For example, ultrasonic washer tests can include:

• Cavitation energy: ultrasonic cleaning uses ultrasonic (sound) waves, generally in combination with a cleaning chemistry, to cause the disruption and removal of soil from surfaces. When ultrasonic waves are applied within a liquid it causes "cavitation", the production and collapse of small bubbles along the surface of the device. This process can be confirmed using a color-change indicator that is designed to indicate the correct energy and other conditions (Figure 14.7).

• Aluminum foil test: this is used to test the ultrasonic efficiency in various locations in the washer. Strips of

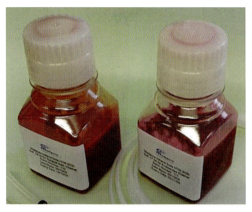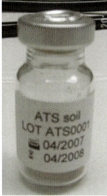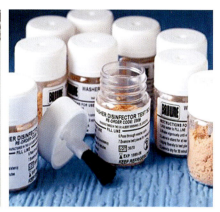

Figure 14.6 Examples of cleaning test soils.

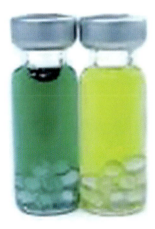

Figure 14.7 An example of an ultrasonic cavitation test. The indicator is provided as a green liquid (left) and changes color to yellow on exposure to defined ultrasonic conditions.

aluminum foil (e.g. 10 cm × 20 cm) are suspended at various locations within the ultrasonic bath (Figure 14.8). The ultrasonic bath is turned on for a typical cleaning cycle and the foil removed/inspected. All foil samples should be perforated and eroded to about the same degree.

Monitoring disinfection

The main method of monitoring thermal (heat) disinfection is by measuring and/or confirming temperature and exposure time. This may be conducted manually or in automated systems (washer-disinfectors, pasteurizers, etc.). Similar to cleaning processes (see the section on monitoring cleaning), modern washer-disinfectors will include independent monitoring systems to verify the correct disinfection conditions, in accordance with ISO

15883-1 *Washer-disinfectors: general requirements, terms and definitions and tests*) and other parts (Chapter 9). Process monitoring sensors will require periodic calibration. Periodic testing may also include the use of temperature monitoring equipment to verify the temperature distribution in the disinfection chamber over time.

Chemical disinfection can be more challenging. These are often best controlled in automated systems. ISO 15883 compliant washer-chemical disinfectors will also include various parametric measures of the process, in particular in compliance to Part 1, Part 4 (*Requirements and tests for washer-disinfectors employing chemical disinfection for thermo-labile endoscopes*) and Part 7 (*Requirements and tests for general purpose washer-disinfectors employing chemical disinfection for bedframes, bedside tables, transport carts, etc.*). These will include systems to confirm the correct chemical dosing, temperatures, pressures, flow rates, etc., during the process. Some systems may also include chemical disinfectant sensors that monitor the concentration (directly or indirectly) during the process. Manual chemical disinfection is also widely used and it can be more difficult to ensure a quality process due to the inability to validate a manual process. Suggestions will include the use of timers, recording sheets on the use of the disinfectant (in particular with re-usable chemical disinfectants) and verifying rinsing methods (number, time per rinse, etc.).

In both automated and manual chemical disinfection process, it is recommended that chemical indicators are used that are specific for the type of disinfectant, usually specified by the disinfectant manufacturer (Figure 14.9). Chemical indicators are discussed in further detail in the section on monitoring sterilization.

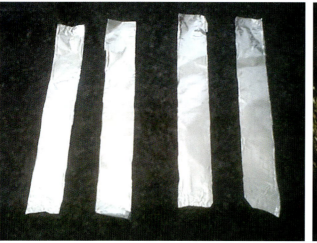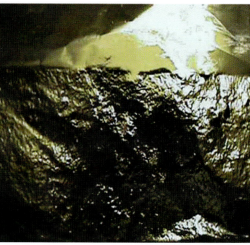

Figure 14.8 Ultrasonic bath aluminum foil test. Test strips are shown before (left) and a close-up of one strip after (right) exposure.

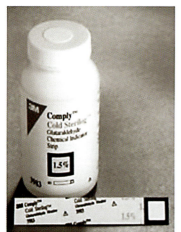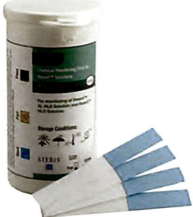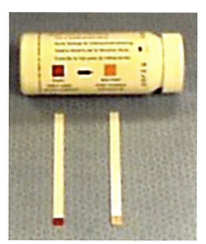

Figure 14.9 Examples of disinfectant chemical indicators.

Monitoring sterilization

The requirements for monitoring the various types of physical and chemical sterilization methods can vary from country to country. There is no practical method that can confirm a sterile device, but various methods can be used to verify that a defined sterilization process has been achieved within a device set or load. These will include a variety of parametric and indicator-based tests, usually specified by guidelines/standards and/or the sterilizer manufacturer. An example is with steam sterilization, where process monitoring within a sterilizer is based on the concept of "parametric release", that is, a declaration that the product is sterile, based on records

demonstrating that the process parameters were delivered within specified tolerances. In the case of steam sterilization, the critical parameters are attainment of minimum values of time, temperature and presence of moisture, but of course other variables can affect the efficacy of the process (such as air removal, pressure, water/steam quality, etc.; Chapter 11, see the section on steam (moist heat) sterilization). Therefore, a combination of steam sterilization monitoring and validation methods is employed, to include:

• Parametric monitoring (e.g. time, temperature, pressure)
• Biological indicators

- Chemical indicators
- Process challenge devices (PCDs), such as the Bowie-Dick test and hollow-load test (to test air removal/steam penetration)

Many of these monitoring methods (for physical and chemical sterilization methods) have already been introduced in Chapter 11, in the section on the basic principles of sterilization, and are further considered in the following sections. These are given as a guide; local guidelines/standards and manufacturers' guidelines should be consulted to determine the minimum requirements for the routine monitoring of any sterilization process.

Parametric monitoring

This refers to the monitoring of the important parameters that have been specified as being required for sterilization to be achieved. Steam is a useful example, as its successful application for sterilization is dependent on reaching the correct temperature (that can only be achieved by steam under pressure; Chapter 11). Therefore, the physical monitoring of the temperature and time of the process are good indicators that the process has been correctly applied. Others will include various types of air detector systems, as effective air removal and steam penetration are important considerations for steam sterilization. For a chemical sterilization process, this may include the concentration (directly or indirectly) of the sterilizing agent(s), humidity levels, temperature, pressure and other process variables, depending on the sterilization process. Overall, these various types of sensors can be used for monitoring the effectiveness of the process and can provide this information immediately for inspection/control.

Sterilizers have various gauges, sensors, timers, recorders, and/or other devices that monitor their function. These are all required to be periodically maintained and/or calibrated (in accordance with manufacturers' instructions). Some will have independent monitoring systems (separate to their control sensors) and may have various alarm systems that are activated if the sterilizer fails to operate correctly. Monitoring records for each cycle should be inspected and maintained, as dictated by local guidelines or regulations. The details of sterilizer designs can vary considerably; therefore close inspection should be made of the provided operator manuals.

Typically, at the end of a cycle, and before the items are removed from the sterilizer, the sterilizer records (printouts, collected data, etc.) are examined to make sure that the process conditions have been achieved, and then signed by the person inspecting the record for future confirmation before releasing the load (Figure 14.10).

Although parametric monitoring can provide assurance that the sterilization process has been applied, there are limitations associated with each sterilizer design. Therefore parametric monitoring is most often complemented by other tests, such as those based on chemical and biological indicators (see below).

The term "parametric release" refers to the release of loads as being "sterile" and ready for patient use, without the specific need for inspection of other chemical/biological indicators. This concept originated in the pharmaceutical industry, where a very high level of product and process understanding, change control and documentation is demanded. Parametric release has traditionally been used for many industrial sterilization processes (in particular, steam, ethylene oxide and radiation) and requires a high level of consistency and control of all steps of the process. Parametric release has been also applied to the reprocessing of devices/materials, but has not (as yet) been accepted in all regions. An effective parametric release program requires a quality management system to be in place (see the section on quality management). The system needs to be well designed and maintained, following various guidelines and standards (such as ISO 13485 (2003) *Medical devices – quality management systems – requirements for regulatory purposes*). The quality management system should be documented to include policies, standard operating procedures, safe work instructions, test measurement protocols and reference documents, as well as a quality plan, applicable to all of the elements of the sterilization process. An important part of the system is the definition, monitoring and maintaining of parametric release criteria with the sterilization process. This will need to be defined with the sterilizer manufacturer and may or may not be capable depending on the sterilizer design. Once defined, the entire process must be tested (validated) and documented to ensure that it will consistently yield the defined sterilization process. This will include:

- Installation qualification (IQ): the process of obtaining and documenting evidence that equipment has been provided and installed in accordance with its specification.
- Operational qualification (OQ): the process of obtaining and documenting evidence that installed equipment operates within pre-determined limits when used in accordance with its operational procedures.
- Performance qualification (PQ): the process of obtaining and documenting evidence that the equipment, as installed and operated in accordance with operational

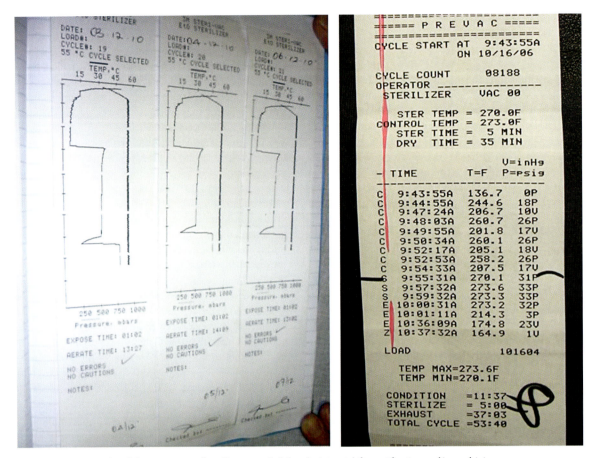

Figure 14.10 Examples of the inspection of sterilizer recorded data (print-outs) for verification and/or archiving.

procedures, consistently performs in accordance with pre-determined criteria and thereby yields a product meeting its specification.

Chemical indicators (CIs)

Chemical indicators (CIs) are generally used in combination with parametric monitoring to ensure the consistency of a sterilization process. They are defined as test systems (usually in the form of test strips) that reveal a change in one or more pre-defined process variables based on a chemical and/or physical change resulting from exposure to a process. They are generally provided as color-change indicators and are widely used in monitoring sterilization processes. The ISO 11140-1 *Sterilization of healthcare products – chemical indicators* standard classifies indicators into six basic types, according to their intended use or performance criteria (Table 14.3).

The various classes of chemical indicators are considered in more detail below, with consideration for how they are typically used in a reprocessing area.

Process indicators

A process indicator is the most basic of chemical indicators and is most commonly placed on the outside of a package to verify that the package has been exposed to a sterilization process. Such an indicator should be clearly visible on the outside of the sterilized package. This helps differentiate sterilized from unsterilized items (Figure 14.11). Process indicators are available as tapes, labels or are printed onto sterile packaging materials.

These indicators are affixed onto the outside of the package or rigid containers, once they have been assembled for sterilization (Figure 14.11). They may also be provided as an integrated part of the packaging material. Following exposure, the process indicator should be checked to ensure

Table 14.3 The classification of chemical indicators[1].

Class	Indicator type	Description
Class 1	Process indicator	These are simple indicators to demonstrate exposure to a process and also to distinguish between processed/unprocessed units. They are generally used outside packaging to indicate it has been exposed to a sterilization cycle. A common example is steam sterilizer (autoclave) tape.
Class 2	Indicators for use in specific tests	Used to indicate a specific type of test, generally established in another standard. Examples include the Bowie-Dick test (for confirming air removal/steam penetration into a porous load) and hollow-load tests (for testing sterilant penetration into a lumen). These are generally routine tests.
Class 3	Single variable indicators	Designed to respond to only one critical process variable (e.g. concentration of a biocide).
Class 4	Multi-variable indicators	Designed to respond to two or more of the critical variables (e.g. temperature, time and concentration of a biocide).
Class 5	Integrating indicators	Designed to respond to all critical variables of the process and are generally similar in performance to a biological indicator (e.g. indicators containing bacterial spores used to test sterilization processes).
Class 6	Emulating indicators	Designed to react to all critical variables for a complete specified cycle. The indicator performance is matched to the critical parameters of the sterilization cycle.

[1] Defined based on ISO 11140 *Sterilization of healthcare products – chemical indicators*.

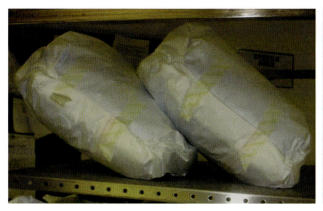 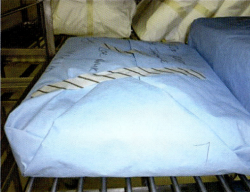

Figure 14.11 Example of the color change with a class 1 (process) chemical indicator, in this case for steam sterilization. The packs on the left (unsterilized) are clearly differentiated from those on the right (sterilized).

that it has changed color according to the manufacturer's instructions, prior to release for patient use or storage.

In-pack/internal chemical indicators

These are mainly supplied as test strips and are generally placed inside packs to be sterilized. Different classes of CIs may be used, such as ISO 11140 classes 3, 4, 5 or 6.

This will depend on how many critical process variables are to be monitored and any local guideline/standard requirements. An in-pack chemical indicator can detect sterilizer malfunction or error in packaging or loading of the sterilizer. It is recommended that the CI is placed in the package, instrument tray or rigid container in an area that is considered to be the least accessible to

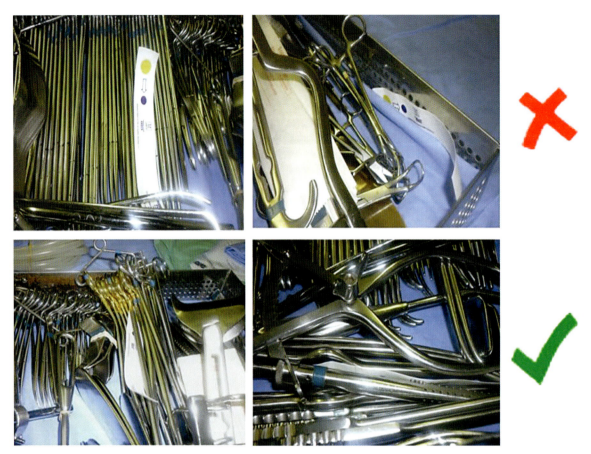

Figure 14.12 Positioning of chemical indicators within a load. The lower locations are optimal.

sterilant penetration. This may not always be in the centre of the package (Figure 14.12).

In-pack chemical indicators cannot be examined until the pack is opened at the site of use. Therefore, it is important that surgical/medical staff are trained on the correct monitoring and interpretation of the chemical indicator result. The associated pack/devices should not be used in the case of a failed indicator. Any non-responding or partially responding indicator, signifies a failed sterilization process, and the contents of the package should not be used. A facility recall (see the section on Recall) should be initiated in such cases.

Biological indicators (BI)

Biological indicators are defined as test systems containing viable microorganisms providing a defined resistance to a specified sterilization process. Various examples are shown in Figure 14.13. Biological indicators

contain bacterial spores, of various types that are considered the most resistant microorganisms to their respective sterilization processes (Table 14.4).

Biological indicators contain a known population of bacterial spores (e.g. 10^5 or 10^6) and are supplied in many ways including:

- Sealed vials or ampoules (in suspension).
- Placed onto a carrier material (e.g. paper or a stainless steel disc) and provided as:
  - Dry spore strips or discs in envelopes. These are required to be recovered, transferred to growth media and incubated following exposure. Note, close attention to aseptic technique (microbiological handling methods to prevent cross-contamination) is required.
  - As a self-contained system incorporating a growth media and typically a chemical indicator. These require no specific handling precautions following exposure,

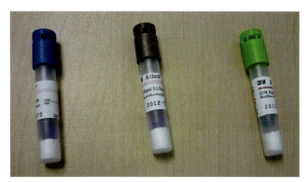

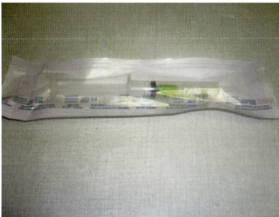
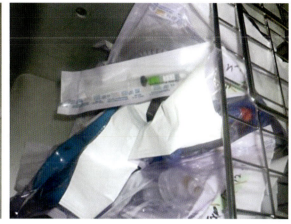

Figure 14.13 Examples of biological indicators (BIs), in this case color-coded according to their use in specific types of sterilization processes. These include blue (flash sterilization), brown (steam sterilization), and green (ETO). Below is an example of a BI test. In this case, a BI (self-contained) is placed into a syringe and a peel-pouch as a challenge within the full load.

Table 14.4 Sterilization methods and types of bacterial spores used in BIs for routine monitoring. These microorganisms are widely accepted and used for the testing of their respective sterilization method.

Sterilization method	Bacterial spores
Steam under pressure	*Geobacillus stearothermophilus*
Humidified ethylene oxide	*Bacillus atropheus*[1]
Hydrogen peroxide gas (with or without plasma)	*Geobacillus stearothermophilus*
Liquid chemical peracetic acid	*Geobacillus stearothermophilus*
Humidified formaldehyde	*Geobacillus stearothermophilus*
Dry heat	*Bacillus atropheus*[1]

[1] Previously known as *Bacillus subtilus*.

but ensure that the spore strip/carrier is exposed to the provided, internal growth media and then incubated (as described by the BI manufacturer)
• Included in specially designed challenge packs (known as process challenge devices, see below).

A BI is designed to be able to show growth or no growth following incubation of the BI on exposure to a sterilization process. Growth would be a fail result and no growth a pass result. This can take time, with the incubation time ranging from one day (24 hours) to seven days, before the result is known. Some BI designs (known as "rapid-read") include an indirect, chemical indicator of this final result, such as a color change (based on a change in pH in the growth media) or the presence of enzyme activity (indicated by the production of light), both suggesting that spore growth is occurring; in both cases, these early indications are considered preliminary and require verification of growth/no growth for the final result, and must be verified at a later stage according to manufacturer guidelines.

Biological indicators are often recommended to be performed on a regular basis (e.g. daily or weekly) in each sterilizer. In some countries, BIs are required to be tested with certain types of sterilization loads (e.g. when including implantable devices). Similar to CIs (see previous section), BIs should be placed in the chamber/load in a least favorable position for sterilization (Figure 14.13).

After sterilization, retrieve the BI (allowing cooling if applicable), check any associated chemical indicators (if provided) and, if CI passes, ensure that the BI is incubated at the correct growth conditions for the indicator. These instructions will be provided by the BI manufacturer and may require specific handling to ensure aseptic technique (to prevent cross-contamination). Self-contained BIs are preferred in such cases as they require minimal handling post-exposure; in these cases, a media-containing vial is crushed or otherwise exposed to the spore carrier following exposure. The incubation conditions will depend on the BI instructions and can vary depending on the manufacturer and types of spores. For example:

• *Geobacillus stearothermophilis* spore-containing BIs (such as for steam and hydrogen peroxide gas processes) are typically incubated at 55–60°C for 24 hours to 7 days.
• *Bacillus atrophaeus* – containing BIs (such as those used for ETO sterilization processes) are typically incubated at 35–39°C for 48 hours to 7 days.

It is important to note that bacterial spore growth requires specific temperatures and incubation time; therefore these variables should be closely controlled. These conditions can be tested by using another BI that has not been exposed to the sterilization process (i.e. a positive control); if this BI fails to show growth then there is a problem with the method (e.g. not following manufacturers' instructions), the batch of BIs or incubation conditions.

As described above, a preliminary result (presence or absence of bacterial growth) may be provided depending on the BI design. Such "chemical" indicators may include the release of acid (which changes the color of the media) or other indicators of spore germination and growth.

The final result will be determined following the full incubation conditions, as defined by the manufacturer. A negative (pass) result is defined as being the lack of growth following exposure to a sterilization process, while a positive (fail) result is the presence of growth.

Specific sterilization monitoring tests

A variety of specific sterilization tests may be defined depending on the sterilization process. They are generally designed as routine tests and are therefore not used for testing in-packs; some tests are designed to only be tested in specified sterilizer cycles defined for that purpose. Many of these tests are described in various guidelines/standards, while others are development by manufacturers specifically to test a sterilizer design. They often incorporate chemical and/or biological indicators under some challenging test condition. Examples are process challenge devices (or PCDs). These are designed to be able to provide a specific challenge (e.g. penetration challenge) for a sterilization process, being used as a more robust or worst-case method to monitor the performance of that process.

An example is a hollow load (or helix) test described for testing steam sterilization. Similar tests are also described for other gas sterilization processes. The hollow load test consists of a length of tubing, with one end open and the other closed; the closed end is designed to hold a chemical or biological indicator. The test simulates a worst case challenge for sterilant penetration through a long lumened-device. An important example of a specific test for steam sterilization is the Bowie-Dick (B-D) test.

The Bowie-Dick test was developed in 1963 by Dr J. Bowie and Mr J. Dick in order to detect problems with air removal/steam penetration in a pre-vacuum sterilizer, particularly within a "porous" load represented as a pack of towels. The test works by being able to trap air within it and therefore preventing the penetration of steam. If the sterilizer's air removal stage is working properly (Chapter 11), the air is removed and replaced with steam. The steam then reacts with the special indicator ink on an internal test sheet and changes color evenly to show that all the air has been removed. If, on the other hand, all the air is not removed from the test pack, the air/steam mixture will not have the right temperature or moisture content to change the test sheet and a failed result is observed.

The original B-D test required a standard test pack consisting of 25–36 washed, all cotton towels. The towels are folded in half, three times, to provide eight thicknesses, each with an area of 300 mm × 225 mm, and stacked one above the other to form a stack approximately 270 mm high. The exact number of towels often depended on how often they had been used. The indicator was then placed on a piece of paper in the middle of the stack and the whole stack wrapped to keep it in place. In most situations, commercially made single-use test packs are used. It is recommended that any B-D test packs are checked for compliance to established standards (e.g. ISO 11140-3 *Sterilization of healthcare products – chemical indicators – Part 3: class 2 indicator systems for use in the Bowie-Dick type steam penetration test*). Specific manufacturers' instructions (both provided by the B-D test and the steam sterilizer) should be followed to ensure the correct use and interpretation of the test. It is important that the Bowie-Dick test pack is placed *on its own* on the bottom shelf of the sterilizer over the drain and close to the door, as this is likely to be the coolest part of the sterilizer. The reason that the Bowie-Dick test must be run on its own is that if the sterilizer contains other packs as well, these can also trap air within them which will decrease the sensitivity of the test. A Bowie-Dick test is typically designed to be run for specific test cycle conditions (e.g. 3.5 minutes steam sterilization), where other cycle conditions (e.g. longer exposure times) will invalidate the results.

If the B-D test result is unsatisfactory (fails), the sterilizer should be taken out of use and the fault investigated (this may require testing by a designated test person). It is important that the sterilizer and the associated steam supply are at full operating temperature before carrying out the test. A warm-up cycle will not only ensure that the sterilizer chamber and jacket are at the correct temperature, but it will also purge the steam supply of any moisture and non-condensable gases, for example CO_2, which build up when the sterilizers are not being used (e.g. overnight). All water contains a certain amount of non-condensable gases, but the colder the water the higher the concentration of gases. When the steam supply is not active, the temperature of the steam drops, leading to a build-up of water in the supply system. As this water cools it absorbs non-condensable gases. The first cycle on the following day can therefore contain unusually high levels of non-condensable gases as they are flushed out of the system. It is recommended that if, after carrying out a warm-up cycle, the Bowie-Dick test fails, a second Bowie-Dick test should be performed. This is to ensure that the first fail was not simply further contaminants still being flushed out of the steam supply. If the second Bowie-Dick test also fails, then the cause must be investigated in more detail. It is important to remember that the chemical indicators used in Bowie-Dick tests may deteriorate in storage due to contamination or unsuitable conditions; therefore, any test shelf-life and test conditions should be finally verified to ensure an accurate pass/fail result.

15 Special interest topics

During the development of this book, a number of areas were highlighted as requiring further consideration. This chapter considers these aspects in further detail, with cross-references to other chapters and sections of the book.

Water quality/purity

Water is an essential component during decontamination, including its use for cleaning, rinsing, disinfection and sterilization (see Chapter 6, in the section on solids, liquids, gases and plasma for an introduction to the chemistry of water). Examples of the use of water can include:

- Dilution of concentrated cleaning and liquid chemical disinfection/sterilization solutions to provide "use dilution" for particular applications
- Rinsing of devices/materials to remove patient soils and chemical residues during and following cleaning and chemical disinfection/sterilization methods
- Thermal (hot water) disinfection
- Thermal (steam) sterilization
- Humidification of loads as a conditioning requirement for some low temperature sterilization process (e.g. ETO and formaldehyde)
- Hand washing with bland soaps or antiseptics

It is important to note that water, as we receive it for drinking or other purposes is rarely "pure", but is actually found to have a range of different chemical, microbial and other contaminants (Table 15.1). These can include various types of chemicals that are dissolved or other materials suspended/floating in the water. Most of these cannot be seen, but can play an important role in device decontamination. Water contaminants can vary depending on the water source (reservoir, lake, water table, etc.), any purification steps (e.g. to render it safe for drinking),

how it is transported to and within a facility and if any further treatment is done within the facility. Facility treatments can include the addition of antimicrobial chemicals (such as chlorine) or the removal of certain contaminants (such as the use of chemical/microbial filters, UV treatment or water "softening"). The quality or purity of the water will also vary over time, in particular between seasons. For clarification, on the discussion of steam sterilization (Chapter 11, in the section on water quality and steam purity), water "quality" refers to the physical properties of steam (e.g. saturation, non-condensable gases and dryness), while "purity" refers to the chemical (and microbiological) contaminants that may be present. Elsewhere within the book both terms are used interchangeably to refer to the chemical and microbial contaminates in the water.

Examples of various negative effects of water quality include (Figure 15.1):

- Device and equipment damage: a common example is rusting (or the development of "rust", chemically known as ferric oxide, FeO_3) on stainless steel surfaces. Rust is seen as a reddish-brown material on the surfaces of instruments (particularly on any moving parts). This will also be observed as "pitting" or the development of small pin-holes on the surface of the device. Rusting is a visual sign of surface damage. One of the most common causes of premature rusting of stainless steel devices is due to the presence of a high concentration of chlorine in the water, particularly when the water is heated. Another is the presence of high levels of silicates. High levels of chlorine and water at unusually high ("alkaline") or low ("acidic") pH can also lead to device/instrument/equipment damage such as bleaching (loss of color) and decay of anodized aluminium.
- Chemical deposits: water hardness (scale, lime scale or calcium/magnesium carbonate) is a particular concern and is often detected by the presence of "spotting" or a

A Practical Guide to Decontamination in Healthcare, First Edition. Gerald McDonnell and Denise Sheard.
© 2012 Gerald McDonnell and Denise Sheard. Published 2012 by Blackwell Publishing Ltd.

Table 15.1 Examples of components that can be found in water. Some components are dissolved (or in solution) with water, while others are suspended (floating in or on water).

Component	Examples
Water	Pure water (H_2O)
Dissolved components	
Inorganic materials	Calcium (Ca), magnesium (Mg), chlorine (Cl_2)/chloride (Cl^-), silicates (molecules with SiO_4^{-4}), sodium (Na), nitrates (molecules with NO_3^-), iron (Fe)
Organic materials	Pesticides and herbicides, for example trihalomethanes, trichlorethylene and polychlorinated biphenyls (PCBs)
Gases	Oxygen (O_2), carbon dioxide (CO_2)
Suspended components	
Inorganic materials	Calcium carbonate ($CaCO_2$), clay, silt, silica
Organic materials	Endotoxins, proteins, fats, oil
Microorganisms	Bacteria, viruses, protozoa

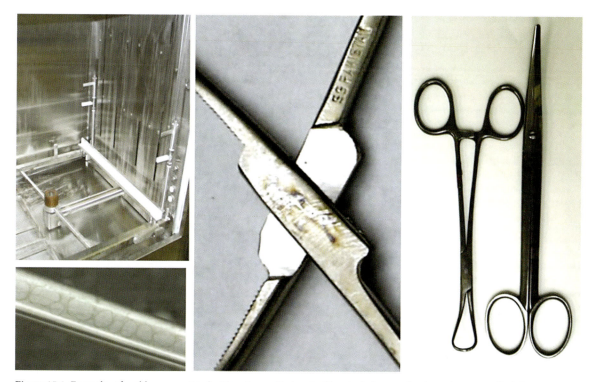

Figure 15.1 Examples of problems associated with water quality/purity. They include water hardness deposition (far left, seen as white precipitate in a washer-disinfector and "spotting" on a device surface), rusting (centre) and staining (black staining on stainless steel devices, on the right).

white, grainy deposit on surfaces (Figure 15.1). Hardness (or scale) refers to the concentration of calcium and magnesium ions in water (measured chemically as parts per million (ppm) or milligrams per litre (mg/L) $CaCO_3$).

Water can have high concentrations of hardness (e.g. over 400 ppm) without being seen, but such high concentrations will precipitate out as a salt when heated. It may also be otherwise colored (e.g. appearing more green or brown due to the presence of other metals such as copper in the water that precipitate with the hardness). When water is dried any chemical component(s) will remain on the surface and these deposits can also have negative effects.

• Staining of devices, materials and equipment: in addition to the rusting (red/brown) and hardness (white, grainy) stains discussed above, other examples include:

  ○ Multicolored stain (often seen as a rainbow effect, including yellow, brownish, blue and violet) covering large areas or drop-shaped or irregular, insular shapes are usually due to increased content of silicates in water.

  ○ Orange-brown staining, often due to high levels of phosphates in the water.

  ○ Black staining: acidic (pH <6) water.

  ○ Gold-tinting: high chlorine levels.

  ○ Purple/blue staining: high levels of amines in water (note that many of these effects may be due to various treatments of water within a facility, e.g. amines are often added to water boilers and steam generators).

• Inefficient cleaning: various chemicals can negatively impact the ability of a cleaning chemistry to work, reducing cleaning efficacy. Another example is the increased production of foam (e.g. in a washer-disinfector) that can reduce cleaning and cause damage to the equipment over time.

• Patient toxicity: examples include complication of eye and other microsurgical techniques from various water components left on the device during reprocessing. These can include chemical (such as the various deposits discussed above) and microbial/biochemical (e.g. bacterial endotoxins; Chapter 5, in the section on bacteria) contaminants.

• Patient infections: bacteria and other microorganisms present in water can remain on a surface (e.g. introduced following chemical disinfection of a semi-critical device), can multiply (in the case of bacteria) and lead to patient infections (depending on the use of the device). A typical example is in the reprocessing of flexible endoscopes (in the section on endoscopes and other lumened devices), where water is used to rinse away chemical residues prior to patient use.

Three basic steps are recommended to reduce the risks of water quality associated problems:

• Test and review water quality at the site of use. It is important to understand the quality of water at the site of use (such as delivered to a sink, equipment or machine). Water will enter a facility, but various treatments may occur (even periodically without prior knowledge, a particular concern in larger facilities). A

typical example is the addition of chlorine (or other chemicals) to the water to be able to control bacterial levels (e.g. *Legionella*, a common bacterial contaminant in water that can lead to a lung disease). High levels of chlorine can have a significant impact on device/equipment safety, leading to damage and increased costs. The transfer of water through a facility can also lead to contamination sources, such as in older facilities that have lead or copper pipework. Also consider that there may be different sources of water, such as cold, hot and "treated" or "purified". These can be different and should be individually tested.

• Identify potential water quality problems and introduce methods to reduce their impact. A summary of typical chemical water quality problems and suggested methods of reducing their levels is given in Table 15.2. Microbial contamination can also be a concern in water used for final rinsing of chemically disinfected devices and even in water used for thermal disinfection/sterilization. These include:

  ○ High levels of bacteria or other microorganisms. Disinfection can be compromised by rinsing with contaminated water and may lead to patient infections. The microbiological quality of water is generally tested by estimating the quantity of viable, aerobic bacteria. An example of recommended levels of bacterial contamination is:

    – <1 cfu/mL: satisfactory

    – <1–9 cfu/mL on a regular basis: acceptable, indicates that bacterial numbers are under reasonable control

    – 10–100 cfu/mL: unsatisfactory, investigate the potential problem and/or repeat testing

    – >100 cfu/mL: unacceptable, out-of service until quality is improved

These levels may or may not be acceptable depending on the use of the device or water (e.g. as discussed in Chapter 9, in the section on flexible endoscopes). Country-specific recommendations regarding the levels of microbial contamination in water may be specified for some device (e.g. flexible endoscope) reprocessing applications.

  ○ High levels of bacterial endotoxins. These may be present at high concentrations in the water due to the presence of Gram negative bacteria (such as *Pseudomonas aeruginosa*). Endotoxins are a class of toxins present in a microorganism, but released only on cell disintegration (Chapter 5, in the section on bacteria). High levels of endotoxin can lead to toxic reactions in patients (specifically fever and more serious complications). They are particularly heat resistant (even by boiling or

Table 15.2 Examples of common chemical water quality problems and how they may be addressed. Lower specifications may be recommended for certain applications (e.g. for heat disinfection or sterilization, Chapter 11, in the section on water quality and steam purity).

Water quality indicator	Suggested warning levels[1]	Intervention
Hardness[2] mg/L ($CaCO_3$ equivalent). Generally the following terms are used: "Soft" water: 0–60 mg/L "Moderately hard" is 60–120 mg/L "Hard" water: >120 mg/L	≥150 mg/L, although lower levels may be suggested for heat disinfection/sterilization methods (e.g. ≤20 mg/L).	Softening: a technique that removes hardness (calcium/magnesium) by replacing with another chemical (e.g. NaCl, common salt). May also reduce other chemical levels such as iron (Fe).
Chlorine mg/L	≥120 mg/L: during cleaning chloride concentrations greater than 240 mg/L chlorine can be very damaging to surfaces. Equally, at higher temperatures chlorine can be more aggressive at even lower concentrations (10–120 mg/L).	Activated carbon filtration: this can reduce chlorine (and chlorine containing chemicals such as chloramines) as well as some organic materials.
Conductivity (or resistivity) μS/cm^{-1} Measure of the concentration of "ions" and therefore various metals and molecules in solution. Will include iron, copper, chlorine and manganese.	≥100 μS /cm^{-1}. For example, a conductivity level at 40 μS/cm^{-1} is equivalent to a chloride level of 10 mg/L, but this will also be affected by the presence of other chemicals.	Specific chemical contaminants may be removed/reduced by boiling or (as an example) carbon filtration. More efficient processes include deionization, distillation or reverse osmosis.
Total dissolved solids (TDS) mg/L.	Generally recommended to be <100 mg/L; a similar measure to conductivity.	Specific chemical contaminants may be removed/reduced by boiling or (as an example) carbon filtration. Better processes include deionization, distillation or reverse osmosis.
pH: a measure of how alkaline (high pH) or acidic (low pH) the water is.	Water should not be lower than pH6 or higher that pH9 and should generally be in the neutral (6.5–7.5) range for potable water.	Will involve further investigation to identify the source of the acidity/alkalinity, given the typical range of potable water.
Total organic carbon (TOC) mg/L, a measure of any organic (carbon-containing) materials in the water, including microorganisms.	Generally recommended at <1 mg/L during disinfection and steam sterilization processes.	May be reduced with certain types of filtration methods (including activated carbon) or may require more efficient processes include deionization, distillation or reverse osmosis

[1] Remember, "≥" means "greater or equal to", ≤ is "less than or equal to" and ≈ is "approximately equally to".
[2] The official units of measurement for hardness are mg/L ($CaCO_3$ equivalent), but others include parts per million (in this case 1 ppm is ≈ 1 mg/L), German degrees (°dH, defined as 10 mg calcium oxide per litre of water and ≈17.8 mg/L $CaCO_3$), and French degrees (°f; defined as 10 mg/L $CaCO_3$).

steam sterilization). The levels of endotoxin that may cause a toxic effect are often debated, but a conservative estimate are levels >200 EU/mL water. Despite this debate, final rinse water (or disinfection water) is recommended to be ≤20 EU/ml. In some countries levels in rinse water or in steam are recommended to be ≤0.25 EU/mL (note: this reflects the typical levels that should

be present if a pure water system, such as reverse osmosis, is used to treat the water).

• Monitor the water quality over time. As highlighted previously, water quality will change periodically and sometimes dramatically. Also, uncontrolled water treatment methods can themselves cause problems if not maintained correctly. Therefore, routine monitoring is suggested. In some countries and for some applications, this is often mandated. Monitoring can include a simple or more complex series of assays (tests) and can vary depending on the use of the water. For example, water used for cleaning, thermal disinfection and steam sterilization can be monitored by periodically checking the pH, conductivity, chlorine and hardness levels. Equally, water used for the terminal rinsing of devices may need to be periodically checked for microbial and even endotoxin levels.

Methods for the analysis of water quality have already been discussed in Chapter 6, in the section on other common chemical measurement methods. In some cases, such as monitoring of pH, conductivity, chlorine and hardness levels, simple test kits or equipment can be used to directly monitor water quality on site. In others, specific laboratories are required for analysis (such as inductively coupled plasma – optical emission spectroscopy, ICP-OES, analysis for testing the levels of different chemicals and bacteria/endotoxin testing). The method

of water collection for such analysis is important to consider. The wrong sampling method or equipment (such as water collection bottles) can be a source of contamination and provide inaccurate results. For example, specific types of water collection bottles will be required for chemical analysis. For microbial analysis, the water bottle should be sterile and those collecting the sample should be trained in aseptic technique; these samples should also be refrigerated on collection and transport to a test laboratory.

The specific recommendations for the quality/purity of water at various different stages of device/material decontamination can vary from country to country. A guideline on these recommended levels of contaminants is given in Table 15.3, but this list is not exhaustive and is given only as a guide. Some of the more widely used methods of water treatment or purification are (Figure 15.2):

• Water softening: a technique that removes hardness (calcium/magnesium) by replacing with another chemical

Table 15.3 A guideline for recommended levels of water contaminants at various stages of a decontamination process. Consideration should also be given to any local guidelines and standards for water quality. Note that chemical and equipment manufacturers may specify requirements for water quality greater or lesser than the ranges given in this table.

Parameter	Units	Cleaning	Disinfection	Rinsing (post-chemical disinfection)	Steam	Pure water[1]
pH		6–9	6–9	6–9	6–9	5–7
Conductivity	μS/cm	<100	<100	<100	<40	5
Hardness	mg/L	<150	<150	<150	<20	<1
Total dissolved solids (TDS)	mg/L	<100	<100	<100	<50	<0.5
Total organic carbon (TOC)	mg/L	n/a	n/a	n/a	<1	<0.5
Bacteria	cfu/mL	n/a	n/a	<10^2	n/a	<10^2
Endotoxin[3]	EU/mL	n/a	n/a	<20	<20	<10

[1] Pure water by reverse osmosis (RO), distillation or other water purification method. Other indicators include chloride <2 mg/L, silicates. <1 mg/L and phosphates <0.5 mg/L.

[2] <1 cfu/mL: satisfactory.
<1–9 cfu/mL on a regular basis: acceptable, indicates that bacterial numbers are under reasonable control.
10–100 cfu/mL: unsatisfactory, investigate the potential problem and/or repeat testing.
>100 cfu/mL: unacceptable, out-of service until quality is improved.
Some guidelines recommend specific testing for certain types of microorganisms such as mycobacteria and legionella.

[3] In some guidelines the safe level of endotoxin is described as 0.25 EU/mL; the scientific basis for these levels are often debated, although pure water by RO or distillation should provide this level if designed and maintained correctly.

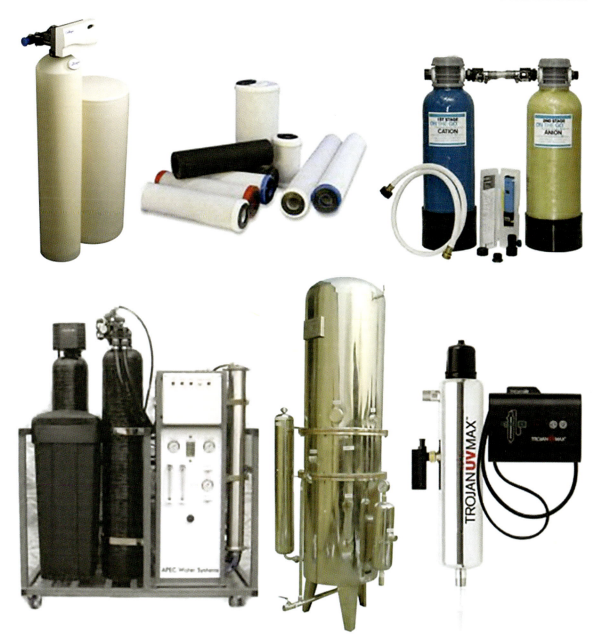

Figure 15.2 Examples of various types of water treatment or purification methods. Top, left to right: water softener, activated carbon filters, deionizer. Bottom, left to right: reverse osmosis, distillator, UV light.

(e.g. NaCl, common salt). This may also reduce other chemical levels such as iron (Fe).

• Filtration: filters are used to remove various water contaminants based on their size. The use of filtration as a disinfection method, for the removal of microorgan-

isms and the theory of filtration, is discussed in further detail in Chapter 9, in the section on filtration. Filters can also remove chemicals/materials by binding or neutralizing these materials. An example is with activated carbon filtration, used to remove chlorine (and chlorine containing chemicals such as chloramines) as well as some organic materials or "green sand" for removal of iron or manganese. Reverse osmosis, as a water purification method is based on a method of filtration.

• Distillation: a process that involves the heating of water to make steam and its condensation back into water, to separate the water from its contaminants (see Chapter 6 for more details). The process needs to be controlled, as some contaminants can transfer over in the steam and be included in the condensed water.

• Deionization: a process that removes various "charged" chemicals from water by exchange (removing in exchange for other, innocuous chemicals). An efficacy process for any charged chemicals, but not for uncharged chemicals/materials.

• Reverse osmosis (RO): a filtration (membrane)-based method that is based on filtration and contaminant rejection. It is widely used for the generation of pure water, but requires constant maintenance and control to ensure expected water quality output.

• UV light disinfection: UV refers to wavelengths of light that have a higher energy level just above visible light (specifically in the 10–400 nm wavelength range). These lights are commonly used to reduce microbial contamination in water (Chapter 9, in the section on radiation). Other methods of microbial disinfection can include the addition of various types of chemicals such as chlorine and silver/copper (Chapter 9).

• In addition to antimicrobial chemicals added for disinfection purposes, other chemicals may be added for specific purposes to include:
  ○ Acids or bases/alkali to modify water pH
  ○ Bisulfite (e.g. sodium bisulfite) for removal of chlorine
The addition of one chemical for a particular reason can lead to problems elsewhere in the decontamination process, so any decisions to add or modify various chemical treatments should be considered with the decontamination facility.

Overall, water is an essential component of most decontamination processes and can affect the safety/efficacy of these processes. Control and monitoring of water quality/purity is highly recommended to ensure process effectiveness and device safety.

Endoscopes and other lumened devices

Endoscopy refers to any procedure using a device (known as an endoscope) to look inside the body, for medical, diagnostic and surgical reasons. The various different types of endoscopic procedures have been introduced in Chapter 3 (in the section on introduction to endoscopic procedures), including their use in robotic surgery. They are used for viewing, diagnosis and surgical procedures. These devices are traditionally sub-classified into two types of devices, known as rigid and flexible endoscopes.

The various designs and features of these devices have been introduced in Chapter 4, in the section on endoscopy. Rigid and flexible endoscopes are notoriously difficult to safely decontaminate. For this reason they are the most common types of re-usable devices associated with cross-infection in patients. This is due to their complexity in design, including the presence of one or many internal lumens (cannula). Flexible endoscopes are becoming even more complicated as they become used for a wider array of medical and surgical uses. Once used for simple diagnostic purposes, flexible endoscopes are now being used for more elaborate procedures including micro-surgical techniques. In addition, many other associated devices and accessories are often used in conjunction with the endoscope; some of these will be single use and some are re-usable.

As semi-critical or critical devices (Chapter 1, in the section on goals of decontamination and the spaulding classification), endoscopes (and any re-usable accessories used with them) should be decontaminated in the appropriate manner, similar to any other device. However, they are often considered separately and reprocessed in a separate area of a healthcare facility from other devices due to their medical/surgical use, facility design, recommended methods of reprocessing and complexity of their design. It is often found that safe decontamination practices are not followed with endoscopes. Typical errors will include:

• Inadequate training of staff in the handling and decontamination.

• Failure to prepare the endoscope for reprocessing (such as disassembly or performing a "leak test").

• Failure to clean and disinfect/sterilize all internal lumens.

• Failure to clean and disinfect/sterilize important parts of accessories used with the device (such as valves; Figure 15.3).

• Taking short-cuts in reprocessing steps, such as not exposing the device to a chemical disinfectant for the manufacturer's recommended exposure time. These are often demanded by clinical need.

• Use of contaminated water in rinsing (post-chemical disinfection).

• Inappropriate storage of the device prior to patient use.

As a first step, it is important to consider the clinical use of the endoscope. Devices used for critical

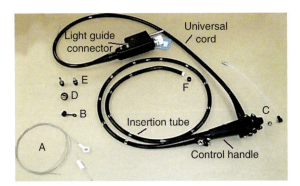

Figure 15.3 A flexible endoscope with various accessories. Included are cleaning brushes (A), biopsy valve cap (B) and valves are indicated at E (in this case two valves are used during the patient procedure).

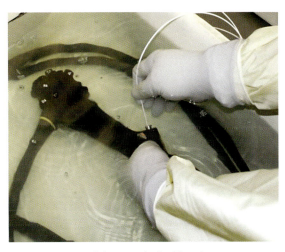

Figure 15.4 Manual cleaning of a flexible endoscope.

procedures (contacted sterile areas of the body, including blood contact) should be cleaned and sterilized, while those used for semi-critical procedures (where the device could contact mucous membranes or non-intact skin) should at a minimum be cleaned and disinfected (high level; Chapter 1, in the section on goals of decontamination and the Spaulding classification). Written procedures should therefore be in place that describe the policy procedures for the safe reprocessing of endoscopes and their accessories. Procedures should consider decontamination recommendations provided by the endoscope manufacturers and any cleaning, disinfectant and/or sterilization process/equipment/chemistry manufacturer used for reprocessing. Staff should also be trained in these procedures and in understanding the significance of any deviation to patient safety. Recommended procedures should include:

• The appropriate handling of devices, to ensure they are not physically damaged during cleaning. These devices have internal optic/fiberoptic systems that can be easily damaged by mishandling. Flexible endoscopes, for example, have a minimum bend radius (how tightly they can be coiled) that is usually defined by the device manufacturer.

• Preparation of the device for reprocessing. These are specifically considered in Chapter 8 (in the section on endoscopy). Preparation will include device disassembly, such as removal of various parts/accessories (e.g. flexible endoscope valves). Flexible endoscopes need to be prepared for immersion in water to protect electrical components that may be present, prior to cleaning. This may include the use of soaking caps (placed over the light

guide connector end) and performing a leak test. During a leak test the internal compartment of a flexible endoscope is pressurized with air to test that there are no holes that would allow water to enter this area and damage the internal workings (Chapter 8, in the section on endoscopy).

• Cleaning of the device, including external and internal (lumen) parts. Manual cleaning is often recommended by the device manufacturer, even if automated cleaning systems are available or used. Manual cleaning consists of brushing and/or flushing the various internal lumens with a cleaning chemistry, followed by rinsing with water in accordance with the recommendations from the chemistry manufacturer (Figure 15.4).

Depending on the device design, semi-automated irrigation systems or ultrasonic baths may be used to assist in the cleaning process. Ultrasonic irrigation baths are often used for cleaning of rigid endoscopes, as an example, but not all endoscopes will be compatible with ultrasonics. It is also important to consider any accessories used as part of the device. An important example is flexible endoscope valves (Figure 15.3).

• Disinfection of temperature-sensitive endoscopes can be achieved by manual immersion or using automated systems using a variety of liquid chemical disinfectants (these are discussed in further detail in Chapter 9 and specifically in the section on flexible endoscopes). Liquid chemical and gaseous sterilization systems may also be used, depending on the sterilization system manufacturer's claims (see Chapter 11, in the section on chemical sterilization, for a discussion on these systems). Low or

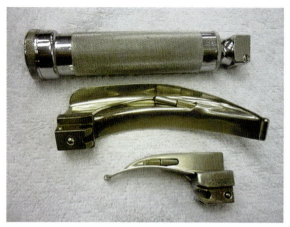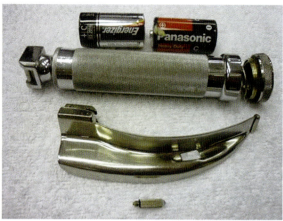

Figure 15.5 Laryngoscopes: on the left is shown the handle (top) and two alternatively used blades (bottom). On the right is a disassembled laryngoscope, including (from top to bottom) the batteries, handle, blade and small lamp.

high temperature sterilization systems may be used for both rigid and flexible endoscopes, where they are tested and recommended (Chapter 11).

• Following liquid chemical disinfection or sterilization, rinsing of the device should be performed manually or in a programmed/validated automated system. All internal and external surfaces should be safely rinsed in accordance with the disinfection/sterilant manufacturer's instructions. This is to ensure that no chemical toxic residual remain and the device is safe for patient use. In some cases, up to five or six rinses in fresh water may be required. The quality of water is important to consider to ensure safe rinsing (this topic is considered further in Chapter 9 in the section on flexible endoscopes). In some cases, following gaseous sterilization methods (e.g. with ethylene oxide or formaldehyde) devices may require extended aeration to similarly ensure that no toxic residuals (the sterilization gas or by-products) remain on the device.

Drying and any potential storage of the device is a further consideration. For gaseous (flexible/rigid scopes) or high temperature (rigid scopes) sterilization methods, the devices are sterilized in sterile barrier systems and should be stored in accordance with facility policy (Chapter 12, in the section on storage and handling of sterile, packaged devices). Devices that are not terminally packaged may require drying prior to storage and/or the use of a drying cabinet (Chapter 12, in the section on handling of non-packaged or non-sterilized devices). This is particularly important for disinfected

devices, as low levels of bacteria can be allowed to grow on storage, in the presence of water (e.g. in a lumen) and over time.

A specific type of endoscope that is often overlooked is the laryngoscope (Figure 15.5). These are a specific example of a semi-critical device that can be found at various locations within a healthcare facility. Laryngoscopes are used in operating rooms, wards and emergency rooms to assist with intubation (procedure to assist breathing, where a tube is inserted through the mouth into the trachea) and insertion of scopes.

As semi-critical (and even sometimes critical) devices, they should be appropriately decontaminated between patients. During reprocessing it is important that they are disassembled, cleaned and at a minimum high-level disinfected according manufacturers' instructions. Immediately after use, the laryngoscope blade should be rinsed in clean tap water or wiped down to remove any residue. In some designs the blade is disposable and this should be done safely in accordance with facility policy.

Decontamination of the blade and handle are considered separately. Before cleaning re-usable blades, check that the light bulb in the laryngoscope is working (by switching on/off) and then disconnect the blade from the handle prior to removal of the light carrier. Manually remove any debris trapped between the lamp carrier and the blade, then reassemble, making sure that the lamp is sufficiently tightened before submerging in water/chemistry for cleaning. Submerging the blade in water with the lamp removed can lead to damage to the internal electrical circuit. The handle, internal batteries and base cap should be disassembled; the handle should only be immersed for cleaning if batteries are removed and the handle base cap is securely replaced. Laryngoscopes can be cleaned manually or in an automated cleaner according to the manufacturer's instructions; in general, ultrasonic cleaning is not recommended. During manual cleaning, external surfaces of the handle should then be gently cleaned with a soft brush or sponge. Following cleaning, the devices should be rinsed and disinfected/sterilized in accordance with the device manufacturer's instructions. For sterilization, laryngoscope blades and handles should be wrapped but unattached. Many designs, but not all, are recommended to be steam sterilized. Standard battery handles are usually not compatible with steam sterilization; compatible handles are typically identified by the term "autoclave" written on the handle. If in doubt, refer to the specific laryngoscope manufacturer's instructions. Following decontamination, the device should be reassembled and tested prior to use. This will include lifting the blade, checking the light source is working and making sure the lamp's glass envelope is clean. The device should be maintained clean and dry prior to use. Wrapping the reassembled laryngoscope can protect it from contamination until the item is to be used. A re-sealable plastic bag or other impermeable wrap may be used as the covering because the laryngoscope will not, in this case, be considered sterile. Wrapping the blades in a designated sterilization wrap is not recommended because this may lead the user to think that the blade is sterile.

Single-use devices (SUDs)

The various different types of instruments and devices were discussed in Chapter 4, including their classification (in the section single use and re-use instrumentation definition). An important example was the designation of a device as being for single use or re-use. A re-usable device is designed to be used many times on different patients, being provided with detailed instructions on how it can be safely reprocessed between each patient. A single use device (SUD) has been designed by a manufacturer to be used on a single patient only and then discarded. The emphasis here is on a single patient, where a device may be used multiple times on the same patient, depending on its design and manufacturers' instructions.

Figure 15.6 The internationally recognized symbol for a single-use device.

The internationally recognized symbol for a SUD is shown in Figure 15.6.

Although a SUD has not been designed to be reprocessed, in many parts of the world healthcare facilities will decide to reprocess such devices and allow them to be used on other patients. The decision to reprocess a SUD should not be taken lightly. In some countries, re-use of SUDs is considered illegal, while in others it is accepted if the correct procedures are used to ensure that the device is safely reprocessed without adding any additional risk to another patient/user. Although the benefits may appear to be reducing costs and environmental considerations (less waste for incineration or otherwise disposed), risks will include damage (seen and unseen) to the device (which can lead to adverse patient effects), toxicity and infection concerns, and legal considerations. Any decisions regarding the reprocessing of SUDs should be taken at the highest level of any healthcare facility, in collaboration with infection prevention/control and written approval by management.

Single-use/disposable items are widely used in healthcare, including for simple wound care, catheterization and radio-diagnostics. They are often used for minimally invasive procedures and in the accident/emergency departments as a cost effective alternative to reprocessing similar instruments. The types of disposable instruments used most frequently include suture sets, dressing forceps and nursing scissors. More complex examples used in neurosurgery can include disposable instruments which are routinely used for brain biopsies. By having a stock of sterile, packed items ready for use, medical or surgical staff can always have supplies in stock. Many of these can be expensive and in some cases the whole set may not be specifically used during a particular procedure (or not even used, but opened), giving the concern that the device/set may appear wasteful to discard.

Legally, SUDs are not designed to be reprocessed and the manufacturer will inform the buyer that the device is for single use only by labelling accordingly. The manufacturer is not obliged to give reasons as to why the item has been classified as single use. When the manufacturer attaches the symbol for one-time use only to a device, it may mean that the device concerned can only be used once, but it may also mean that the manufacturer has not identified adequate reprocessing guidelines and the possible re-use of the device. What should be made clear is that if any harm is caused to the patient on re-using the device, the healthcare facility alone has to bear the consequences. Reprocessing of SUDs is not recommended or covered by the manufacturer's legal declaration of conformity to any local/international regulations, and attempts to do so will nullify the manufacturer's warranty. While the legal assessment of such cases remains controversial, it is clear that the liability and penalty risks involved should be borne by those reprocessing the device.

When reprocessing a single use device, in the absence of guidelines, it is important that the reprocessor considers all the requirement of a safe reprocessing cycle:

• Removal and inactivation of microorganisms to the defined level of safety (e.g. on non-critical, semi-critical or critical devices and the defined requirements for cleaning, disinfection and/or sterilization).

• No associated toxicity, as adverse patient reactions may include chemical toxicity linked to residual soil materials (e.g. due to inadequate cleaning), chemical residuals (from cleaning, disinfection, sterilization, or even water residuals) or other contaminants (e.g. on handling the device).

• Device compatibility, ensuring that no damage (seen or unseen) is done to the device or its intended purpose.

For example, complex disposable devices are sometimes constructed in such a way that they cannot be disassembled for effective cleaning. Many single-use items are manufactured from plastics that contain plasticizer oil compounds to preserve flexibility and inhibit or prevent the "drying out" and cracking of the plastic over time on storage. Some of these plasticizers can be removed from the plastic during reprocessing, which is why the device may only be guaranteed by the manufacturer for single use. Equally, the effects of steam or other sterilization techniques on a device may not be obvious (e.g. stress-cracking, leaking, residual sterilization chemical, etc). Therefore, it must be assumed that reprocessing SUDs constitutes a potential hazard to the patient's health, as deterioration in the quality of the product cannot be ruled out.

When the decision to reprocess a single-use device is made in a facility, the facility is responsible for ensuring that the reprocessed device has the same level of safety as a new device. This will require a defined re-use protocol that has been confirmed to be safe, effective and thereby minimizes any risk to a patient. Reprocessing staff must have enough knowledge or information on the device to show that any decontamination steps (including cleaning, disinfection and sterilization, if applicable) will not damage the quality of the SUD or result in any material (mechanical, geometric, optical, electrical and biocompatible) defects to the device, which may compromise the patient's safety. Unfortunately, this information is not always readily available from the manufacturer and cannot be ascertained through visual inspection of the SUD alone. Overall, the points to consider will include:

• It may not be illegal but is it ethical to re-use single-use items? Does the patient need to be informed (e.g. if the procedure is being directly paid for by the patient/insurance provider)?

• What are the legal implications?

• Why is the product being re-used? Is it economics or is there no alternative re-usable item available? What are the cost benefits?

• Who decides if the device can be safely and effectively reprocessed? Has management approved the practice?

• What are the effects of reprocessing methods (cleaning/disinfection/sterilization) on the materials used to manufacture the device? Do the people making the decision have enough knowledge to decide if it can be safely reprocessed?

• Can the device be safely and effectively reprocessed?

• How many times can each individual device be safely re-used, and how will this be tracked?

Items with limited re-use are different and must not be confused with single-use items. Limited re-use devices are designed for re-use but the number of times it can be used/reprocessed is limited by the manufacturer. Examples are certain types of diathermy leads (that may have a limited life cycle of 100 cycles), diathermy scissors or certain types of minimally invasive surgical instruments. It is important that the use of these devices is tracked through the number of times they are used in/on patients and reprocessed. A specific standard operating procedure should describe the limited number uses, how these will be recorded, how the items will be reprocessed, what checks will need to be made and how they will be disposed of when the life is deemed to be over.

Loan devices, sets and implants

For various reasons, there are many times when healthcare facilities need to loan or rent instrumentation for specialized surgery or surgical implants from a supplier, an individual (e.g. a surgeon) or a neighbouring facility. The term "loan" device/set can be defined as any device or group of devices that may be used by a healthcare facility for patient procedures, but are not part of that facility's device inventory. This includes surgeons' special instruments, specialized instruments belonging to surgical manufacturers and instruments borrowed from other healthcare facilities, all of which will eventually be returned to the supplier/owner. Typical examples include orthopedic and neurosurgical procedure sets. These may be provided as a set on a fee-per-use basis or as a mixture of re-usable and single-use (implant) devices for particular procedures (where the facility is charged when an implant is used). It is important that the same reprocessing procedures and controls apply to the use of these devices/sets, irrespective of where they come from.

The management of loan sets and implants for specialty procedures is important to consider. There are many advantages and disadvantages to this practice. Device sets are often prohibitively expensive and unaffordable to most facilities, with the only option being to loan items from the supplier. This is often a practical way to have such sets available for patient use, without the high investment costs. Unfortunately, however, the facility using such instrumentation is not likely to have knowledge of, or control over the item's history (including prior use/reprocessing). A further concern is that loan items/sets will not be available when needed for a patient procedure, and may even require reprocessing before use. Load devices/sets can be provided directly from the supplier/manufacturer or from another healthcare facility, and may or may not be correctly reprocessed for direct patient use.

Policies and procedures must be in place to manage, control and track any loaned instrumentation from the time they are received by a facility until they are returned to the lender. In the absence of effective procedures and controls confusion can arise, equipment can be lost and, most importantly, patients, employees and the facility itself can be placed at unnecessary risk. Ideally, a standardized loan agreement should be in place between the device manufacturer/lender and the facility department/borrower. The agreement should include procedures and policies, created in collaboration with both parties, to include costs, ordering, transport, receipt, pre-procedure processing/preparation, post-procedure processing, dispatch and transport out of a facility. Instrumentation supplied from the lender should include a transport/loan list that identifies the items being delivered (including quantities, if applicable) and a copy of the device manufacturer's written handling and reprocessing instructions. Ideally, the loaned set should be checked and reprocessed by the facility, but this is not always necessary and should be reviewed with the loaner. On receipt, the facility staff using, reprocessing and otherwise handling the instrumentation must be informed of all specifics related to the loaner agreement, including the number of instruments/trays and the specific surgical/medical case for which items will be used. The manufacturer's reprocessing instructions should be included for each loaned device and, when applicable, must be followed carefully as the item is prepared, cleaned, disinfected and/or sterilized. Procedures for transporting instruments to and from the facility are also important; for example sterile instruments should ideally be packed in locked, secure, tamper proof containers to help reduce the possibility of cross-contamination and damage during transport (Chapter 12, in the section on transport of sterile packaged items).

Accountability should be clearly stated and agreed, to include the responsibilities of both the lender and facility staff. Facility staff members who are involved in handling any aspect with the device/set must be trained by the manufacturer or designated member of staff. It must be remembered that accountability includes from time of receipt and continues after the surgical procedure is completed until the loaned set is returned to the owner.

Recommendations on the use of loaned devices/sets include:
• A contract should be in place between the supplier and facility.
• The facility should have a written policy regarding the use of loaned devices/sets.
• Unless otherwise agreed with the supplier, all loaned instrumentation should be considered contaminated when they are received. As contaminated, they should be handled appropriately in accordance with facility policies.
• Area and responsibilities should be designated for receiving and returning all loaned items. This may include a reprocessing area or site of patient use (e.g. operating room), where applicable.
• Instrumentation packaging should include a transport/loan list that identifies the items being delivered, which may include:

○ Identification of the device/set

○ Number and types of instruments/implants (especially to include pictures of the set with devices identified)

○ Signature of the individual delivering the items

○ Signature of the individual receiving the items

○ Signed verification that the devices/device set have been previously reprocessed

○ A copy of the device manufacturer's written handling and processing instructions

• If delivered ready for patient use, devices should be inspected prior to use in accordance with the facility's policies (Chapter 7).

• If the device/set requires reprocessing, normal facility protocols for cleaning, disinfection and/or sterilization, and distribution should be followed. Loaned devices may require specific procedures, including disassembly, cleaning, sterilization and transport to a site of use. This is often due their size, weight and device/set complexity. For example, device sets may need to be completely disassembled prior to cleaning/rinsing/disinfection and reassembled in preparation for sterilization. The weight of metal in larger sets is often too great to be sterilized as one tray, resulting in inadequate sterilization and wet packs (Chapter 11, in the section on troubleshooting steam sterilization problem). Lifting and transporting of such trays can also pose a safety risk to staff.

• Procedures should be in place to allow the devices to be tracked within a facility.

In conclusion, due to the increase in technology and use of loaned device sets, such items are becoming more frequently used in healthcare facilities. The use and reprocessing of loaned devices/sets should be managed effectively. It is therefore important to identify and understand the complete process and all potential problems that may arise. A set management program requires close collaboration between the lender and the facility using the set, to include all staff that may be required to handle these devices during their use/re-use. To ensure accountability, a written agreement between the facility and the device/set supplier should be in place to cover the entire process from receipt of the loaned items to their return.

A surgical implant is defined as a critical device that may be used to support, enhance, replace or repair a missing, abnormal or damaged structure within the body. They can be further defined as:

• Having a minimum use in the patient of three months

• Penetrating living tissue

• Having a physiologic interaction

• Being retrievable

This definition excludes short-term implantable devices such as most catheters (defined as a thin flexible tube that is inserted into a part of the body to inject or drain away fluid or to keep a passage open). They are also considered separate to a transplant (or bio-implant), which is the introduction of foreign tissue. An implant is generally man-made, to include metal, plastic, ceramic or other materials and in some cases can include skin, bone or other body tissues. Bio-implants made from skin, bone or other body tissues, are commonly used in maxillo-facial orthopedics, reconstructive prosthetics, cardiac prosthetics (artificial heart valves), skin and cornea. In some cases implants contain electronics, for example artificial pacemakers and cochlear implants, these are called "active" implants and are generally powered using batteries or other energy sources. Implants can be designed to deliver medications, monitor body functions, or provide support to organs and tissues. They can be permanent (e.g. hip replacements/dental implants/stents) or they can be temporary, being removed once they are no longer needed (such as chemotherapy ports or pins/plates to repair broken bones).

Implant surgery is not always 100% successful due to a number of associated risks. These include difficulty in surgical placement or removal, infection, rejection (a reaction to the materials used in implants) and implant failure. Infections are common and are due mainly to skin contamination at the time of surgery, but may also be due to an otherwise contaminated implant device (e.g. due to inappropriate handling or reprocessing). Due to the nature of orthopedic surgery (Chapter 3) this is probably the area in which the largest number of implants are used; it is also an area where implants may not always be adequately reprocessed, due to the wide variety of pins, screws, small plates and other small orthopedic implants that are needed. These implants are often repeatedly reprocessed in loaned device racks or trays (Figure 15.7).

Orthopedic implants are devices that are placed over or within bones to hold a fracture or a prosthesis that would replace a piece or whole part of a joint or bone. There are many types of orthopedic implants available, including specific procedures involving the hip, knee, shoulder, elbow and other bones. Some examples are interlocking nails, screws, wires and pins; mini, small and large fragment implants; cannulated screws; angled blade plates; hip/knee/shoulder prosthesis; etc. Concerns have been raised that many of these smaller implants are continually reprocessed (e.g. pins, plates,

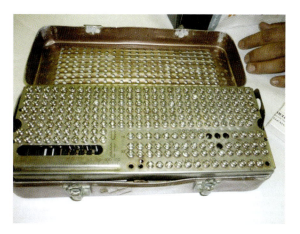

Figure 15.7 A set of loaned orthopedic screw implants.

implant failure depend on the critical nature of the implant, and its position in the body. Thus, heart valve failure is likely to threaten the life of the individual, while breast implant or hip joint failure is less likely to be life-threatening.

Overall, facilities should ask device manufacturers for the recommended number of re-use or reprocessing cycles, or lifespan of implantable screws, wires and plates (i.e. the number of times the item can be cleaned and re-sterilized without compromising functionality). Care should also be taken to carefully follow device manufacturers' instructions regarding the safe reprocessing of such sets, including their inspection following cleaning. Overall, it is optimal for facilities to consider the use of individually reprocessed and presented sterile screws.

screws), but are not individually tracked or adequately decontaminated, and as a result may not be safe for patient use. Many of these devices are classified as "single use", which means they must not be re-used following contact with a patient (see the section on single use devices, earlier in this chapter). This also means that they should only be reprocessed once, prior to first being handled/used, which is not the case in most theaters. Because the surgeon does not know what size plate or screws he will need at the time of a patient procedure, a large assortment is provided for each surgery. Often a surgeon may measure or start using a particular plate or screw that is then replaced in the set and a larger or smaller size used for the procedure. Due to costs, these pins/plates/screws are merely rinsed (if practical) and returned to the set holder, in theatre. When the holder is returned to a reprocessing area, it is typical for only the missing screws to be replaced and the whole set reprocessed for the next patient use. As a result many of these sets can circulate for many years with the same screws, having being reprocessed many times. As mentioned previously, residues that could build up on reprocessed implants over time can potentially contribute to implant failures and other problems, such as through infection or inflammation/toxic reactions in the patient.

There is also a concern that in repeated reprocessing implants can become corroded and weakened. This has clear implications for increasing implant failures over time. In many cases such implants may be better described as being for "limited re-use" (see the section on single-use devices, earlier in this chapter). The consequences of

Surgical and medical laundry

Laundering of surgical/medical linens and textiles should follow the same chain of events as the reprocessing of any other surgical/medical devices. These have been previously outlined in Chapter 8 (in the section on textiles and laundry) and Chapter 9 (in the section on laundry) to include (Figure 15.8):
• Post-procedure sorting and separation of waste from materials to be reprocessed (Chapter 7, in the section on post-procedure sorting)
• Safe transport to a reprocessing site (Chapter 7, in section on transportation post-procedure)
• Cleaning (Chapter 8, in the section on textiles and laundry)
• Disinfection and drying (Chapter 9, in the section on laundry)
• Inspection (Chapter 8, in the section on textiles and laundry) and packaging (if applicable)
• Sterilization (Chapter 11) if required (e.g. if used directly or contacting critical devices used directly for patient procedures)
• Safe transport to storage and/or site of patient use
Textiles and linens can be designed for single use or re-use. Re-usable surgical textiles are generally made from various grades and weaves of cotton with or without special waterproofing treatments. Re-usable items can be become heavily soiled during medical/surgical use and should be safely handled, cleaned, disinfected or even sterilized prior to their use with another patient. It is therefore important to ensure that an in-house or external laundry is used that is capable of handling such

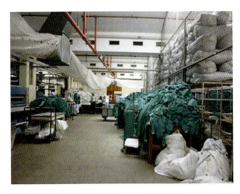
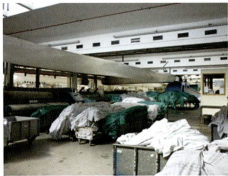

Contaminated surgical laundry is sorted and weighed.

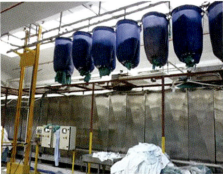
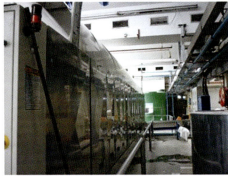

The weighed laundry is transported to the washer-disinfector.

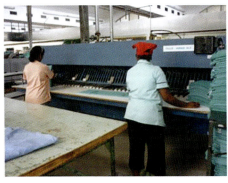
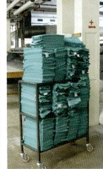

After inspection laundry is ironed, folded and ready for use or for further sterilization.

Figure 15.8 Various stages of a laundry process.

materials and ensuring an efficient cleaning and decontamination process is applied. The healthcare facility should have a medical/surgical textile re-use policy in place, as well as a tracking and monitoring system that will monitor the number of times that the item passes through the laundering process. The number of decontamination cycles to which these materials can be subjected varies, but can generally be assumed to be between 55 and 300 cycles.

The healthcare facility, and any external laundering facility, has a health and safety obligation to prevent the risk of infection to staff handling contaminated textiles. Only authorized personnel should be allowed in storage, dispatch or laundering areas. As with instruments, all textiles that have been exposed to patient use, whether they may appear to be used or not, are assumed to be soiled, and therefore contaminated. When used/contaminated surgical laundry is handled, it is important that the worker is well protected and wearing the correct protective equipment (PPE), as they are often at a higher risk of being exposed to contaminants than those dealing with contaminated instruments. All staff working in the receiving/sorting area must wear the appropriate PPE, for example waterproof aprons and gloves, and should be fully trained in operating any associated laundry equipment. There is also the very real risk of potential harm to laundry staff and damage to surgical textiles by a failure of the end user to separate "sharps" from dirty surgical laundry before it is placed in laundry bags. Sharps and waste segregation procedures must be in place, as well as adequate PPE to protect staff dealing with used textiles from these risks (Chapter 13).

The laundry area should follow the same design recommendations as a device reprocessing facility (Chapter 1, in the section on the design of a decontamination area). For example, the receiving/sorting area should be functionally separated from the area handling cleaned/disinfected textiles. Functional separation can often be achieved by using pass through washer-disinfectors (often referred to as washer-extractors or continuous tunnel washers). It is also recommended that contaminated surgical laundry (such as drapes, gowns and towels) are laundered and kept functionally separated from general hospital laundry.

The laundering process has many of the same essential processes as medical/surgical devices, with the addition of separate drying, ironing and folding stages. On receipt of contaminated laundry items should be sorted, weighed and placed into the dedicated washers or washer-disinfectors. Heavily contaminated soiled textiles are often recommended to be pre-washed (sluiced), to remove as much organic material as possible prior to loading into the washer; this practice may often be recommended to be more safely performed as a pre-treatment step in the washer-disinfector. This will assist in stain removal. Staining is a concern not only due to difficulty in cleaning and disinfection/sterilization, but also in that visually stained textiles are not acceptable to patients/staff. If stains cannot be removed the items must be discarded according to the healthcare facility policy. Loading the correct weight of material into a washer is important to ensure adequate cleaning/disinfection. The way the washers are loaded is a critical step; if they are not loaded according to manufacturer guidelines (e.g. too heavy or too light) the laundry process will not be efficient. The washing process is generally followed by a thermal and/or chemical disinfection cycle. A typical heat disinfection process includes holding the load for a minimum of ten minutes at 65°C (150°F) or three minutes at 71°C (160°F). The cleaning and disinfection cycle will depend on the equipment design, validation and can even vary depending on the load (as defined by the equipment manufacturer). For chemical disinfection, the entire process (including washing, dilution and disinfection) is often recommended to be capable of reducing the viable count of microorganisms by 5 $\log_{10}$. Laundry washer-disinfectors will require routine testing and maintenance to ensure their safe operation (Chapter 8 and 9).

Drying is an important step in the laundry decontamination process. The most widely used method is by using heat and extractor based drying, with or without tumble dryers, as this process can also be efficient in further reducing microorganisms. In the absence of a mechanical dryer, air drying in full sunlight is also an option. Wet textiles should be dried as soon as possible following decontamination, to prevent the growth of microorganisms. Once dried, textiles should be protected from cross-contamination during ironing, folding, transport and storage. Working surfaces in the clean area (e.g. table tops, trolleys and ironing equipment) should be kept clean of visible soil, dust and lint. Before or during ironing and folding, textiles should be visually inspected for staining and damage. Any stained textiles should be rejected and discarded for aesthetic reasons according to the healthcare facility policy. Any damaged or torn items should also be removed from service and/or sent for mending according to laundry protocol. Damage is usually repaired using heat patches; tears must not be sewn as this only serves to increase the number of holes. Following inspection, textiles are ironed and folded. When ironing, care should be taken not to contaminate items on the floor or other surfaces.

When transporting unwrapped textiles, following the decontamination process, they should be placed into dedicated clean surgical laundry carts or hampers and covered, the textiles should remain covered at all times during transport. If carts do not have a solid bottom or sides, they should be lined with an impervious plastic/paper or cover. It is recommended that decontaminated textiles are stored in a clean storage area on slatted shelving 1–2 inches (2.5–5 cm) from the walls, 6–8 inches (15–20 cm) from the floor and 12–18 inches (30–45 cm) from the ceiling to allow for circulation of air and periodic cleaning. Textiles for use in higher risk patient procedures (such as in the operating room within or adjacent to the sterile core; Chapter 3, Principles of aseptic (or "sterile") technique) are recommended to be packaged and sterilized by an appropriate sterilization process (Chapter 11). Laundry sterilization processes include the use of steam and dry heat.

Devices known or suspected to be contaminated with prion material

Prions are unusual infectious agents (Chapter 5, in the section on prion and other infectious proteins). They are considered infectious proteins, and are strongly implicated in causing a group of rare diseases known as transmissible spongiform encephalopathies (TSEs), with the most common example being Creutzfeldt-Jakob disease (CJD). Other disease examples include Gerstmann–Sträussler–Scheinker syndrome (GSS), fatal familial insomnia (FFI) and variant Creutzfeldt-Jakob disease (vCJD). Variant Creutzfeldt-Jakob disease is a similar yet distinct disease in humans, which is particularly notable as it is strongly suggested to have been transferred to humans from eating meat from animals with another prion disease, bovine spongiform encephalopathy (BSE or more commonly known as "mad cow disease"). Overall, these diseases are considered very rare, with a typical risk in a population being 1–3 cases in a million people.

Transmissible spongiform encephalopathies are known to be transferred through contaminated tissues (particularly brain and other nervous tissues/organs) on items such as re-usable devices, and are considered to have a higher resistance to decontamination methods. For these reasons, in most countries in the world (including older recommendations by the World Health Organization, WHO published in 1999[1]), additional precautions and handling procedures are recommended in known or suspected cases of prion disease. These are briefly considered in this section, with cross-references to other sections of the book that consider this subject.

Prion diseases are transmissible through re-usable devices; this has been confirmed clinically and experimentally in the laboratory. Due to the long incubation times associated with the development of prion diseases and their difficulty in diagnosis, it is currently unknown what the true risks of device-associated prion transmission are. Although the research into these diseases and their implications to patient safety are ongoing, such patient safety risks can be significantly reduced by routine decontamination practices. To date, particular

care is taken to estimate such risks, based on the knowledge that a particular patient is known to be or suspected of developing a prion disease. Special decontamination procedures are recommended when re-usable devices are used in such cases, although in some countries the recommendation exists that any such devices be removed from use (or destroyed). In general, most national and international recommendations include:

- Develop, document and implement a policy regarding the handling of devices and materials used on patients with known or suspected prion disease.
- As part of the policy, any potential risk groups (such as patients with a family history or with clinical signs suspected to indicate a prion disease) should be identified with clinical staff and these patients should be specially tracked during their time at the facility.
- Devices used on a person known or suspected to have a prion disease risk may require special handling. This is particularly the case when devices are used for any high-risk surgical procedures. A high-risk procedure is considered to be any procedure that contacts tissues that are known to contain potentially high doses of the prion agent. These include the brain, spinal cord and certain major nerve tissues (such as the optic nerve associated with the eye). It is recommended in such cases that:
  - Disposable devices are used and, if not available, that a facility should strongly consider safe disposal (incineration) of any devices used.
  - Re-usable devices should be decontaminated using specific procedures. These include rigorous cleaning (Chapter 8, in the section on devices known or suspected to be contaminated with prion material), chemical decontamination (e.g. with 1–2 N NaOH for one hour; Chapter 9, in the section on environmental disinfection) and/or elongated steam sterilization (e.g. 134°C for 18 minutes; Chapter 11, in the section on prion sterilization). Some of these methods are, however, considered damaging to devices, in particular high concentrations of NaOH.
- Procedures and devices that are considered to have a lower risk, such as those used for other surgical procedures (e.g. with blood contact and/or contacting other tissues) are sometimes recommended to be similarly discarded or reprocessed, and in other cases to be decontaminated according to normal facility practices. Non-critical devices are not considered to present a patient risk and are also recommended to be routinely decontaminated.

---

[1] WHO infection control guidelines for transmissible spongiform encephalopathies (2000). Report of a WHO consultation, Geneva, Switzerland, 23–26 March 1999. WHO/CDS/CSR/APH/2000/3. http://www.who.int/csr/resources/publications/bse/WHO_CDS_CSR_APH_2000_3/en/

It is practical for such a specific prion policy to be developed and applied within a facility. Consideration should be given to any country-specific guidelines or recommendations in the policy implementation. There is, however, much debate regarding the safety and efficacy of these general recommendations. The reasons for this debate include:

• Known (diagnosed) or suspected cases of prion diseases are only considered part of the at risk population. For example, 80% of CJD cases alone are known to be sporadic (or not associated with any known risk factors) and the incubation time of the disease before clinical signs can be a very long period. Therefore many more patients may be incubating these diseases but will not be identified for some time.

• Recent research with sensitive methods to be able to detect the prion agent may be present in various other patient tissues, depending on the stage of the disease. The levels of detection are low, depending on the stage of the disease, but can include blood, lymph nodes and muscle. Although the levels of prion contamination are dramatically lower than those observed in brain tissue, the significance of such low-level contamination is uncertain.

• Some of the methods recommended (in particular immersion in NaOH, a strong alkali or elongated steam sterilization) are not recommended by device manufacturers. Such treatment may damage devices and lead to other patient complications. Although such methods have been tested under laboratory conditions their safety/efficacy may not be tested for clinical use.

• Prions are now known to be very difficult to clean from surfaces. It is a fact that the use of some chemistries in specific cleaning processes can significantly reduce prion contamination levels, but in other cases they appear to render the material *more difficult* to decontaminate. The reasons for this are currently unknown.

• Cleaning (with some chemistries) followed by steam sterilization (e.g. at 134°C for 4 minutes or 18 minutes) can be a very effective method of prion decontamination. But, as already highlighted above, this will depend on the cleaning process used.

In consideration of various guidelines and published data at the time of writing the following recommendations can be made:

• A facility policy should be in place that describes the handling and potential reprocessing of devices used on patients with or suspected to have a prion disease. The facility should be periodically reviewed and, if necessary, updated to ensure it is current with country-specific guidelines and research.

• Facilities should consider the implementation of routine decontamination procedures that provide standard precautions to reduce any risks of prion decontamination. This can include specific cleaning, disinfection and sterilization products/processes that have been shown to reduce the risks of prion contamination. Care should be taken to carefully inspect any such efficacy claims to include their associated application (temperatures, contact conditions/times, etc.).

• Prions are regarded as being infectious proteins; however, methods that are known to inactivate or degrade proteins, such as specific enzymes (proteases) and heat may NOT be effective against prions. Any data claims against prions should be carefully inspected to ensure it substantiates efficacy against these agents.

• Special handling and decontamination procedures may be considered with devices used on known or suspected cases of prion disease. These should be particularly considered when used in high-risk surgical procedures associated with the brain, spinal cord or posterior eye. Consider the use of disposable devices/items where possible. Difficult to clean items should be discarded. Re-usable items may be cleaned with a cleaning process (with a specific chemistry) shown to be effective against prions, followed by a high or low temperature sterilization process shown to be effective (e.g. 134°C for 18 minutes).

• Do not allow devices to dry prior to decontamination. It has been shown that drying of prion contaminated soil can render the device harder to decontaminate.

• Cleaning recommendations have been considered in detail in Chapter 8, in the section on devices known or suspected to be contaminated with prion material. Cleaning chemistries and processes used should be supported with data that shows that such products have been shown to reduce the risks of prion contamination. Ensure that devices are correctly rinsed and prepared for subsequent disinfection/sterilization.

• Disinfection recommendations have been considered in detail in Chapter 9, in the section on environmental disinfection. High concentrations of chemicals such as NaOH and NaOCl have been shown to be effective as disinfection agents against prions, but can lead to device damage; they are not recommended for use. Moist heat disinfection has been shown to have little benefit in prion decontamination. Any disinfection method that could lead to protein fixation, such as dry heat, aldehydes and alcohols should not be used. Any alternative disinfection methods and/or chemicals should be supported by research data.

• Steam sterilization is considered as an effective method and is considered in more detail in Chapter 12, in the section on prion sterilization. Steam cycles that are considered to be effective include pre-vacuum cycles at 134°C/274°F for 18 minutes, gravity displacement cycles at 121°C/250°F for one hour and pre-vacuum cycles at 134°C/274°F for four minutes (when shown to be effective in combination with an effective cleaning process). Dry heat sterilization should be avoided.

• Some low temperature sterilization processes have been shown to reduce the risk. These include liquid chemical peracetic acid (depending on the formulation and even then only to reduce the risk; Chapter 11, in the section on liquid chemical peracetic acid) and hydrogen peroxide gas processes (Chapter 11, in the section on hydrogen peroxide gas). As highlighted earlier, any low temperature sterilization process claiming to be effective should be supported by research data. Also, any chemical used that could lead to protein fixation, such as formaldehyde and ethylene oxide should not be used.

It is anticipated that in the coming years the understanding of prion diseases and their successful decontamination will be better understood. This will allow for the development of more practical guidelines and standards to control the risks of prion decontamination and the introduction of standard precautions to reduce their risks in parallel with other infectious agents.

Index

A Practical Guide to Decontamination in Healthcare, First Edition. Gerald McDonnell and Denise Sheard.
© 2012 Gerald McDonnell and Denise Sheard. Published 2012 by Blackwell Publishing Ltd.

Keep up with critical fields

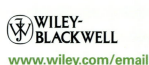
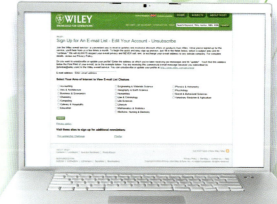

17841